acute surgical management

acute surgical management

editors

Hwang Nian Chih
Singapore General Hospital

London Lucien Ooi
National Cancer Centre, Singapore

World Scientific

SGH PGMI
SGH Postgraduate Medical Institute

Published by

World Scientific Publishing Co. Pte. Ltd.
5 Toh Tuck Link, Singapore 596224
USA office: Suite 202, 1060 Main Street, River Edge, NJ 07661
UK office: 57 Shelton Street, Covent Garden, London WC2H 9HE

British Library Cataloguing-in-Publication Data
A catalogue record for this book is available from the British Library.

Library of Congress Cataloging-in-Publication Data
Acute surgical management / editors, Nian Chih Hwang, London Ooi.
p. ; cm.
Includes bibliographical references and index.
ISBN 981-238-681-5 (alk. paper)
1. Medical emergencies. 2. Surgery, Operative. 3. Wounds and injuries--Surgery.
4. Therapeutics, Surgical. I. Hwang, N. C. (Nian Chih), 1960– II. Ooi, London.
[DNLM: 1. Emergencies. 2. Surgical Procedures, Operative. 3. Wounds and Injuries--surgery. WO 700 A1897 2004]
RC87.A346 2004
616.0215--dc22

2003063108

Printed by FuIsland Offset Printing (S) Pte Ltd, Singapore

Contents

Foreword

One of the most important functions of the Singapore General Hospital (SGH) is Teaching & Training. In fact, SGH prides itself in being responsible for the biggest share in postgraduate medical training in Singapore. It is well known that SGH is the first hospital responsible for both Undergraduate and Postgraduate Medical teaching in Singapore. With the publication of this book, we confirm our strong commitment to this long tradition in Medical Education.

In the choice of topics for the book, we took into consideration what is current and relevant in surgical practice in a very busy tertiary acute General Hospital (where half of the admissions comes through the portal of the Emergency Department and where the other half is electively admitted). The final content depended, to a great extent, on the choice of Surgeon Authors who were authorities in the topics they wrote. These were busy clinicians and teachers and under the dedicated supervision of our editor who are an anaesthesiologist and a surgeon, we hope this book will be treasured by all who train in surgery at SGH.

The prime purpose of this book is to educate. The reason why we need to educate is to produce the next and subsequent generations of surgeons who will be required to look after patients, not only in Singapore but also, to a smaller extent, the surrounding region. The other important reason in producing this book is to document the current practice of surgery for posterity, so that those who come after can build on the processes and structure that have been put into place. Finally, the strongest of reasons for this book is for the care of our patients. It is because of them and for them that this is published, so that we can always strive to improve their care.

Boon-Keng Tay

Preface

Singapore General Hospital (SGH) is the largest public sector hospital in Singapore. Established in 1821, SGH serves as the nation's main tertiary care and acute care hospital. Within the grounds of SGH are 21 specialty departments with close links to the four national centres (National Cancer Centre Singapore, National Heart Centre, Singapore National Eye Centre and the National Dental Centre) within the same compound. With a strong tradition of clinical excellence, SGH has been intimately involved in the training and teaching of both undergraduate medical students from the National University of Singapore and post-graduate students in the various specialties and sub-specialties of medicine since the days when the Medical Faculty was located at the Sepoy Lines (the current location of the Ministry of Health). SGH also prides itself on having extended training opportunities to clinical fellows and students from all over the world.

The chapters in this book are written by surgeons, radiologists and anaesthesiologists from this hospital. Together with basic surgical principles, the unique local experiences and perspectives are presented. There are two parts to this book. Part I of the book deals with the principles of management of acute surgical emergencies. These emergencies include craniofacial, otorhinolaryngological, cardiovascular and thoracic, gastrointestinal, gynaecological, urological, perianal, orthopaedic and hand, as well as those involving the soft tissue and skin. The importance of computed tomography imaging in blunt abdominal trauma and the role of interventional radiology in acute haemorrhage; as well as peri-operative anaesthetic care of the patient requiring acute surgical management are described in Part II of the book.

London Lucien Ooi
Nian-Chih Hwang

PART I
ACUTE SURGICAL MANAGEMENT

Section I

Craniofacial Emergencies

1

The Acute Management of Head Injuries

Alvin Hong

Cerebral Perfusion

The brain weighs 1500 g (2% body weight) and receives 15% of the cardiac output. It also uses 20% of the body's total oxygen consumption. Unlike other organs, there are minimal stores of oxygen and high energy phosphates, and these must be provided to the brain via the bloodstream. Hence, cerebral blood flow must be maintained. It can be described as a general equation of flow:

$$\text{Cerebral blood flow (CBF)} = \frac{\text{cerebral perfusion pressure (CPP)}}{\text{cerebrovascular resistance}}$$

The cerebral blood vessels are able to autoregulate, such that changes in CPP are matched by changes in cerebrovascular resistance, resulting in a constant cerebral blood flow. This occurs at the level of the arterioles. If CPP drops, these vessels dilate so that CVR drops proportionally, and CBF remains constant.

Cerebral perfusion can be affected if the arterial pressure is low and/or the intracranial pressure is high.

Cerebral perfusion pressure
$$= \text{mean arterial pressure} - \text{intracranial pressure}$$

Mean arterial pressure
$$= 1/3(\text{systolic pressure} - \text{diastolic pressure}) + \text{diastolic pressure}$$

Autoregulation maintains CPP over a range of mean arterial pressure levels between 60 and 150 mmHg.

The autonomic nervous system affects the range of CPP over which autoregulation works. Patients with chronic hypertension have the range set upwards, so care must be taken when lowering the blood pressure of a patient with chronic hypertension.

The maintenance of cerebral perfusion underlies the acute management of head injuries. Primary damage (i.e. damage occurring at the scene of the accident) has already occurred, and cannot be influenced by the clinician. The prevention of secondary damage, from hypoxia, hypotension and raised intracranial pressure, gives the patient the best chance of recovery.

Raised ICP

Raised intracranial pressure can occur from an expanding haematoma (extradural, subdural, intracerebral) or from brain swelling.

The skull can be considered as a "box" containing the intracranial contents. These include the meninges, the neurones, the glial cells, the blood vessels, the extracellular fluid (ECF) and the cerebrospinal fluid (CSF). The Monro-Kellie doctrine says that if a space-occupying lesion (such as a haematoma) is added to this "box", the pressure will rise unless an equivalent volume is removed. However, this "box" opens into the spinal canal via the foramen magnum, and the initial displacement of an equivalent volume of CSF from the cranial cavity to the spinal canal allows compensation to occur. The intracranial pressure (ICP) remains normal until no more CSF can be displaced. Decompensation then occurs; the ICP rises rapidly, then cerebral blood flow decreases, and the patient loses consciousness.

Unfortunately, there is no easy method of determining when a patient is about to decompensate. Hence clinicians must be acutely aware of the possibility of the rapid deterioration of an alert patient with a space-occupying lesion.

Brain Herniation

Raised ICP can affect the brain by affecting cerebral blood flow or by causing brain herniation.

Brain tissue will herniate across an opening if there is a pressure gradient across this opening. This can occur in four situations:

(1) *Cingulate or subfalcine herniation*

The cingulate gyrus is part of the limbic system, and clinical effects cannot be seen easily. But the distal part of the anterior cerebral artery can be compressed. This supplies the part of the motor cortex that controls the leg, and hence the patient develops contralateral leg weakness.

(2) *Unilateral transtentorial or uncal herniation*

The most medial part of the temporal lobe, the uncus, can herniate across the tentorial hiatus. Compression of the parasympathetic fibres that lie on the surface of the oculomotor nerve, results in an ipsilateral fixed dilated pupil. Compression of the midbrain leads to loss of consciousness. The posterior cerebral artery runs through the tentorial hiatus, and kinking of this vessel results in an occipital lobe infarct. The patient later notices a contralateral homonymous hemianopia that is usually macular sparing. The cerebral peduncle of the same side can be compressed, leading to a contralateral hemiplegia. However, the cerebral peduncle of the opposite side can also be compressed by the free edge of the tentorium, producing an ipsilateral hemiplegia. Post-mortem studies can show the groove on the peduncle, known as Kernohan's notch. This means that the side of the paralysis is less useful to localise the side of the problem. The side of the blown pupil is better.

(3) *Central transtentorial herniation*

This occurs when the cerebral hemispheres are so swollen that both temporal lobes herniate into the posterior fossa. In addition to bilateral fixed dilated pupils, coma, no limb movement and occipital lobe infarction, the perforators coming off the top of the basilar artery are stretched. These supply the hypothalamus, which consequently becomes ischaemic. Diabetes insipidus results, and this is often seen in the terminal stages of a severe head injury.

(4) *Tonsillar herniation*

If the posterior fossa pressure is high, the cerebellar tonsils can herniate through the foramen magnum, compressing the medulla. In addition to loss of consciousness, the cardiovascular and respiratory centres are affected, leading to a labile blood pressure and irregular breathing.

Cushing Reflex

When the hypothalamus is ischaemic due to poor brain perfusion, the sympathetic centre becomes more active, acting on the heart to increase cardiac output, and on the arterioles to increase peripheral resistance. Blood pressure rises as a protective reflex to increase cerebral perfusion. This rise in blood pressure activates the stretch receptors in the carotid sinuses, causing the normal reflex activation of the parasympathetic nervous system, with a bradycardia. Hence the Cushing reflex results in a rising blood pressure associated with a bradycardia. This is seen in the terminal stages of an acute head injury.

The Immediate Management of a Head Injured Patient

To prevent secondary damage from hypoxia and hypotension, resuscitate patient first, according to generally accepted principles, i.e.

- Airway
- Breathing
- Circulation

Thereafter a rapid neurological assessment is made, including:

- Glasgow coma score, which is an assessment of conscious level (see Fig. 1).
- Pupillary response.
- Pattern of limb movements (posturing, asymmetry).
- Brainstem reflexes (corneal, oculocephalic, gag).

The cervical spine is also assessed for possible injuries (see Figs. 2 and 3), because trauma that is sufficient to produce a severe head injury may also cause a spinal injury.

EYE OPENING

4 spontaneous
3 to speech
2 to pain
1 none

SPEECH

5 oriented
4 confused
3 inappropriate
2 incomprehensible
1 none

BEST MOTOR RESPONSE

6 obeys commands
5 localises to pain
4 withdrawal to pain
3 abnormal flexion (decorticate)
2 extension (decerebrate)
1 no movement

Total: 3 to 15

Fig. 1 Glasgow coma scale.

- Antero-posterior and lateral views.
- Open mouth view if C1 and C2 cannot be seen on a-p view.
- In multisystem trauma, lateral view as an initial screening investigation (but needs review after resuscitation and stabilisation as it does not exclude a cervical spine injury).[4]

- GCS 15 if:
  - neck pain or tenderness
  - neurological deficit not due to an intracranial or peripheral problem
  - mechanism of injury suggests a spinal injury

- GCS 14 or less if:
  - normal X-rays, but significant neck pain, lateral flexion and extension views done by the patient[3,4]
  - normal X-rays but neurological deficit that might be caused by the cervical spine, X-ray entire spinal column (a-p and lateral views of thoracic and lumbosacral spine) and refer to specialist for admission[3,4]

Fig. 2 Indications for cervical spine X-rays.[2–4]

- C7/T1 if not seen on plain X-rays (despite optimisation of shoulder position).
- C1 and C2 if GCS 8 or less, or if cannot be seen on a-p or open mouth view, to be done at time of CT head scan (need to specify on CT request form).

Fig. 3 Indications for CT scan of the cervical spine.[2,3]

Any further investigations, including skull X-rays and CT brain scans, are ordered if there is a clinical suspicion of an intracranial injury, to confirm an intracranial haematoma(s) or brain swelling that may require specific medical and/or surgical treatment, in order to preserve cerebral perfusion. The indications for these tests depend on the likelihood of finding significant abnormalities.

Indications for Investigations and Admission

The following questions are most commonly asked:

(1) When to do skull X-rays?
(2) When to order a CT head scan?
(3) When to order a CT head scan for epileptics or drunks?

(4) When to allow home?
(5) When to admit to the Observation Ward (if available)?
(6) When to admit to the General Ward?
(7) When to admit to the High Dependency Unit?
(8) When to admit to the Intensive Care Unit?
(9) When to intubate?
(10) When to give mannitol?
(11) When to hyperventilate?
(12) When to give phenytoin?

When should skull X-rays be done?[2,5]

A skull fracture increases the chance of an intracranial haematoma by 400 times, and historically, this has led to hospital admission to observe all patients with skull fractures. But the significance of a skull fracture, without looking at the clinical picture, is less useful because there will be subgroups where the clinical picture will make the chance of an intracranial injury low or high. Guidelines for skull X-rays taking into account the clinical presentation exist[5] but with the widespread availability of CT scanners, these have been superceded by newer recommendations for CT brain scans.

Skull X-rays should include antero-posterior and lateral views, with the Towne's view for occipital trauma, and an oblique view for a suspected depressed fracture. It should be done for all patients with GCS 13 and 14, and those with GCS 15 if the following are present:

(1) Mechanism of injury suggests a severe blow.
(2) Full thickness scalp laceration or boggy haematoma.
(3) Loss of consciousness (any period of time).
(4) Loss of memory.
(5) Vomiting.
(6) Inadequate history.
(7) Difficulty in clinical assessment, for example, alcohol intoxication, epilepsy, uncommunicative children.
(8) Depressed fracture or foreign body suspected.

When should CT head scans be done?[2,6,7]

CT scans have revolutionised the management of head injuries by identifying collections of blood that cannot be seen on plain X-rays and cerebral angiograms. The indications include:

(1) All skull fractures.
(2) Signs of skull base fracture.[a]
(3) Deteriorating conscious level.
(4) Neurological signs.
(5) Seizure.
(6) Patients with GCS 15 with a persistent severe headache, persistent vomiting, and/or neurological signs.
(7) Patients with GCS 13 to 14 and who fail to improve after four hours of observation.
(8) Patients with GCS 13 to 14 who need a general anaesthetic for another reason, e.g. orthopaedic injury.
(9) All patients with GCS 12 or lower.

CT head scans in an intoxicated or post-seizure patient[2]

This is a difficult group of patients to manage, as they would already be drowsy. They should be scanned if they have a GCS 13 to 14, and fail to improve after four hours of observation, of if any of the above indications are found.

Criteria for discharge from Emergency Department

All patients with GCS 15 with no indications for observation or admission, and all patients with GCS 15 with no neurological symptoms, can be allowed home. They should be told to return if they develop a severe headache, drowsiness, vomiting, seizure or a neurological

---

[a]Signs of a skull base fracture include periorbital bruising, subconjunctival haemorrhage, epistaxis or CSF rhinorrhoea, mastoid bruising (Battle's sign), bloody or CSF otorrhoea.

deficit. Ideally, an "advice sheet" is given to a responsible second person, to watch for these warning signs.

Indications for admission to emergency observation ward or general ward

Patients are observed in order to detect evolving intracranial events, such as an expanding haematoma, that may require treatment. Such patients include those with:

(1) Headache.
(2) Non-specific dizziness.
(3) Scalp haematoma, laceration, contusion, abrasion.
(4) Loss of consciousness.
(5) Soft tissue facial injury.
(6) Vomiting.
(7) Alcohol or drug intoxication.
(8) Unreliable or inadequate history.
(9) Age less than 3 (unless injury is very trivial).
(10) Patients with bleeding tendencies e.g. anticoagulation, thrombocytopenia.

In the observation ward, the management should include:

(1) Monitoring the GCS half hourly for two hours, then every hour thereafter.
(2) Review at four hours (extra care of patients with bleeding tendencies).
(3) Nil by mouth.
(4) Intravenous hydration (if clinically indicated).

Indications for admission to general ward

Head injured patients with any of the following should be admitted for observation in the general ward:

(1) Fracture on skull X-ray.
(2) High speed injury.
(3) Signs of skull base fracture.
(4) Possible skull penetration or depressed skull fracture.
(5) Suspected child abuse.
(6) Patients on emergency observation ward who have been assessed by the senior doctor as requiring admission.

A CT brain scan should be ordered if indicated.
On the ward, the patient should be managed as follows:

(1) Blood samples are taken for full blood count, and analysis of serum urea and electrolyte concentrations, prothrombin time and partial thromboplastin time.
(2) Blood is taken for "Group and Save".
(3) The GCS is assessed half hourly for two hours, then every hour thereafter.
(4) Hourly blood pressure (BP) and pulse rate.
(5) Nil by mouth.
(6) Intravenous infusion (if clinically indicated).

Indications for admission to high dependency area

Head injured patients with any of the following should be admitted to the High Dependency Unit (HDU) where closer monitoring is present:

(1) Depressed (GCS 12 or less) or decreasing conscious level.
(2) Multiple fractures.
(3) Serious facial injury.
(4) Post-traumatic seizure.
(5) Severe co-morbidities.
(6) CT brain scan findings of intracranial pathology with significant mass effect and/or signs of brain swelling (loss of grey/white differentiation, loss of perimesencephalic cisterns, loss of cortical sulci).

The management in the High Dependency Unit should include:

(1) Obtaining blood samples for full blood count and the analysis of serum urea and electrolyte concentrations, prothrombin time and partial thromboplastin time.
(2) Obtaining blood for "Group and Save".
(3) Obtaining a chest X-ray and a 12-lead electrocardiograph (ECG).
(4) Monitoring the GCS half hourly for two hours, then every hour thereafter.
(5) Hourly measurements of fluid input and urine output.
(6) Continuous ECG, BP, pulse, arterial oxygen saturation monitoring.
(7) Nil by mouth.

Indications for admission to intensive care unit

Head injured patients who require mechanical ventilatory support or who have cardiovascular instability requiring support, should be admitted to the intensive care unit (ICU).

The management in the ICU should include:

(1) Obtaining blood samples for full blood count and analysis of serum urea and electrolyte concentrations, prothrombin time and partial thromboplastin time.
(2) Obtaining blood for "Group and Save".
(3) Obtaining a chest X-ray and a 12-lead electrocardiograph (ECG).
(4) Monitoring the GCS half hourly for two hours, then every hour thereafter.
(5) Hourly measurements of fluid input.
(6) Inserting a urinary catheter for hourly measurements of urine output.
(7) Continuous monitoring of the ECG, arterial oxygen, and capnography.

(8) Invasive monitoring of BP and pulse via an arterial line.
(9) Nil by mouth.
(10) Naso-gastric tube (oro-gastric if a skull base fracture is suspected).
(11) Monitoring of peripheral temperature.
(12) Insertion of central venous catheter and monitoring of central venous pressures (CVP).
(13) Fluid replacement with normal saline (avoid 5% glucose).
(14) Monitoring of blood glucose concentration every six hours.

The management of these patients should be adjusted judiciously to achieve the following:

(1) Arterial oxygen partial pressure (PaO_2) greater than 60 mmHg[1].
(2) Arterial carbon dioxide partial pressure ($PaCO_2$) at chosen range but not less than 30 mmHg[1].
(3) Systolic BP greater than 90 mmHg[1].
(4) Intracranial pressures (if measured) less than 20 mmHg[1].
(5) Cerebral perfusion pressures more than 60 mmHg (if ICP is measured).
(6) Blood glucose levels of 4 to 10 mmol/l.
(7) Maintaining core temperature between 36 and 37°C.
(8) No seizures.

Indications for intubation[4]

Head injured patients with any of the following should be intubated:

(1) Severe facial fractures.
(2) A GCS between 3 and 8.
(3) Arterial oxygen partial pressures less than 60 mmHg.
(4) Systolic blood pressure less than 90 mmHg.
(5) Signs of transtentorial herniation (see below).
(6) Suspicion of neurological deterioration not due to extra-cranial explanations.

Indications for mannitol[1]

Mannitol is a high-molecular-weight sugar that can be administered to lower the ICP. By exerting an osmotic effect, extracellular fluid is removed from the brain.

Mannitol is indicated if there is evidence of transtentorial herniation or progressive neurological deterioration. The signs of transtentorial herniation include unilateral or bilateral pupillary dilatation, asymmetric pupillary reactivity, and abnormal motor posturing (decorticate, decerebrate or no movement).

If intracranial pathology with significant mass effect, and/or signs of brain swelling (loss of grey/white differentiation, loss of perimesencephalic cisterns, loss of cortical sulci) have been identified after a CT scan of the brain, mannitol therapy should also be instituted.

Mannitol should not be routinely administered for extradural haematomas (as the volume of haemotoma may enlarge) unless signs of herniation are detected and the conscious level has deteriorated and the patient requires airway maintenance and ventilatory support, prior to surgical evacuation of the haematoma.

Mannitol is available as a 20% (20 g per 100 ml or 5 ml per g) solution and is administered at 0.5 g per kg per dose. A 70 kg patient would require 35 g (175 ml) of mannitol. As mannitol therapy will result in an osmotic diuresis, a urinary catheter should be inserted prior to starting mannitol.

Mannitol should be administered over 30 minutes. The onset of action is approximately 15 to 30 minutes, with maximal effect seen at 90 minutes. As the effect of each dose lasts for up to four hours, the administration of mannitol can be repeated every four hourly.

As mannitol therapy can result in a hyperosmolar state leading to renal hypoperfusion and renal dysfunction, fluid input and output should be monitored and balanced with the use of normal saline solution to avoid hypovolaemia. Daily serum urea and electrolytes concentrations should be monitored, and the serum osmolarity kept below 320 mOsm. The serum osmolarity should be routinely monitored after two days of therapy, and sooner if renal impairment is suspected.

Mannitol is contraindicated if there is congestive cardiac failure or pulmonary oedema.

Indications for hyperventilation ($PaCO_2$ 30 to 35 mmHg)[1]

The cerebral blood vessels constrict when the arterial CO_2 is lowered, leading to decreased cerebral blood volume in the cranium, lowering ICP.

After intubation, ventilate with tidal volume of 8 ml per kg, 10 breaths per minute, 100% oxygen. Arterial blood gases should be measured after 15 minutes of initiating mechanical ventilation, and the $PaCO_2$ should be maintained between 35 to 40 mmHg.

With transtentorial herniation or progressive neurological deterioration, the minute ventilation should be adjusted to maintain $PaCO_2$ at between 30 to 35 mmHg. Hyperventilation should also be done if the ICP is higher than 20 mmHg, despite mannitol therapy (and surgical decompression or a repeat CT scan of the brain should be considered if this is unsuccessful).

Indications for phenytoin[1]

Phenytoin therapy is indicated in head injured patients with increased risk of developing early (within first week) post-traumatic seizures. These patients may have any of the following:

(1) Seizure within 24 hours of injury.
(2) A GCS of less than 10.
(3) Penetrating head wound.
(4) Depressed skull fracture.
(5) Extradural haematoma.
(6) Acute subdural haematoma.
(7) Cerebral contusion.

The adult loading dose is 15 mg/kg (1050 mg for a 70 kg patient). The physician should administer the initial intravenous dose of 500 mg at a rate of not more than 50 mg per minute with ECG and BP monitoring. The dose is repeated after 12 hours. The side effects to expect include cardiovascular and central nervous system depression, with arrhythmias, hypotension, cardiovascular collapse and respiratory arrest.

The adult maintenance dose thereafter is at 4 mg/kg/day (280 mg for a 70 kg patient). Monitor the serum phenytoin concentrations after two days. If the dose is 300 mg or more per day, increase at 30 mg intervals. The therapeutic serum level is between 10 and 20 μg/ml, and at this level, a small dosage change can result in a large level change so that any increments should be small.

Neurosurgical Treatment

Medical treatment options include:

(1) Mannitol therapy (see above).
(2) Hyperventilation (see above).
(3) Hypertensive therapy to maintain cerebral perfusion pressure above 60 mmHg if other measures to lower ICP are unsuccessful.
(4) Barbiturate therapy to suppress cerebral metabolism. However, there are potential problems with hypotension, and its efficacy is not clearly established.

Surgical options include:

(1) The insertion of an ICP monitor (to allow measurement of cerebral perfusion pressure).
(2) The insertion of an external ventricular drain (to allow drainage of CSF to lower ICP).
(3) Surgical evacuation of haematomas (extradural, acute subdural, intracerebral contusions).
(4) Decompressive craniectomy.

This is best left to the neurosurgeons to manage, and is outside the scope of this book.

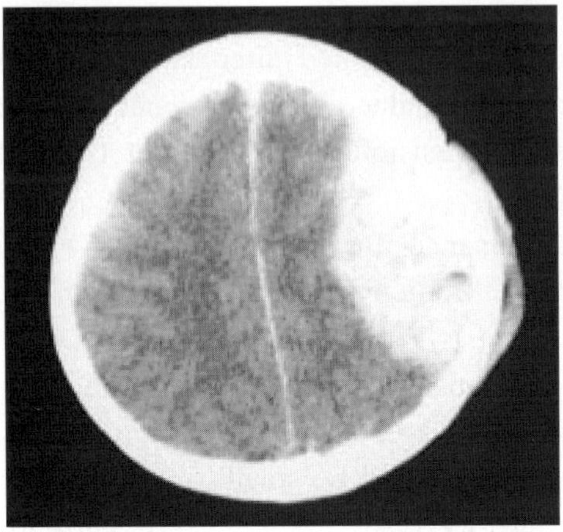

CT scan of an extradural haematoma.

Specific Traumatic Intracranial Haemorrhages

Extradural haematomas

This is usually associated with a skull fracture. Bleeding occurs into the potential space between the dura and the skull. This may take time to occur, and a lucid interval may be found, before clinical deterioration occurs. Because the pathology is essentially outside the brain, the prognosis is good provided the haematoma is evacuated soon enough.

Acute subdural haematomas

Bleeding occurs into the subdural space, lying between the dura and the arachnoid. This can occur in two circumstances:

(1) Bleeding from a torn bridging vein, especially in the elderly. This can sometimes occur slowly so that there is a lucid interval. Prognosis can be good if the clot is evacuated early.

(2) Bleeding from underlying damaged brain matter. The prognosis depends on the underlying brain damage, as well as any delay in evacuating the clot.

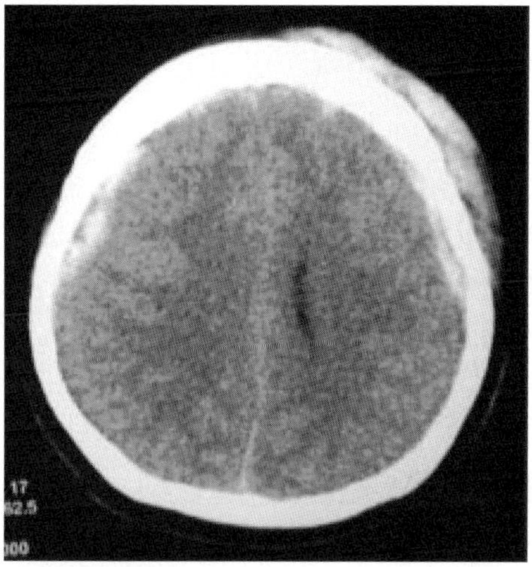

CT scan of bilateral acute subdural haematomas.

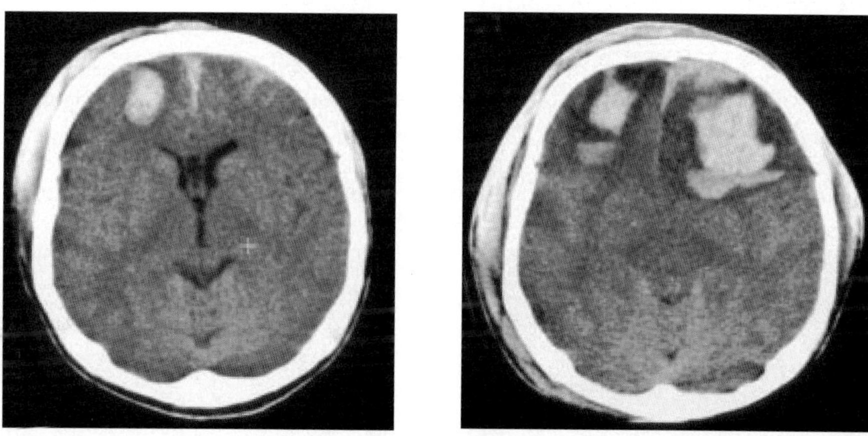

CT scan of a brain contusion: on first day, and after 24 hours.

Intracerebral contusions

These typically occur in the frontal and temporal lobes, probably due to the bony prominences in the floor of the anterior and middle cranial fossae. They begin as small haemorrhages which coalesce into larger ones with mass effect. Together with the surrounding oedema that develops after 24 hours, delayed clinical deterioration can occur. The prognosis depends on the severity as well as the location of the haemorrhages.

Diffuse axonal injury

This refers to diffuse injury to the brain, with resultant generalised brain swelling without any large haemorrhages. The prognosis is variable as the damage to the brain cannot be localised. Long-term cognitive problems are common.

Chronic subdural haematomas

A subset of acute subdural haematomas begin to enlarge. A membrane surrounds these acute subdural clots, and recurrent bleeding from this membrane is the cause of the enlargement. It is postulated that the breakdown products of clot lysis inhibits platelet aggregation. Enlargement of the haematoma due to osmotic absorption of fluid may also contribute. Prognosis is usually good provided the haematoma is evacuated soon enough, usually via some burr holes.

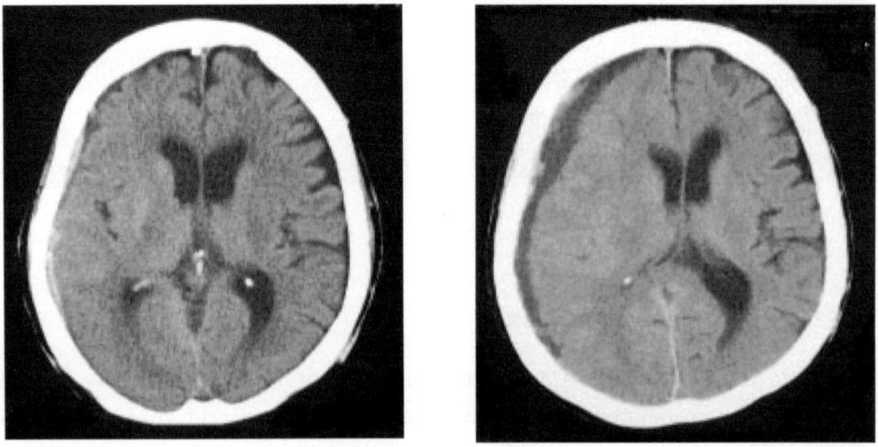

CT scan of a small asymptomatic right acute subdural haematoma that became a symptomatic chronic subdural haematoma after 6 weeks.

References

1. Brain Trauma Foundation, American Association of Neurological Surgeons, Joint Section on Neurotrauma and Critical Care (1996). Guidelines for the management of severe head injury. *J Neurotrauma* **13**, 641–734.
2. Scottish Intercollegiate Guidelines Network (2000). Early management of patients with a head injury. SIGN secretariat, Royal College of Physicians, 9 Queen Street, Edinburgh EH2 1JQ (*www.sign.ac.uk*).
3. Eastern Association for the Surgery of Trauma, USA (1998). Practice management guidelines for identifying cervical spine injuries following trauma (*www.east.org*).
4. American College of Surgeons (1997). *Advanced Trauma Life Support Student Manual*, 6th Ed. USA: American College of Surgeons.
5. Masters *et al.* (1987). Skull X-ray examinations after head trauma. Recommendations by a multi-disciplinary panel and validation study. *New Engl J Med* **316**(2), 84–91.
6. Stiell *et al.* (2001). The Canadian CT Head Rule for patients with minor head injury. *Lancet* **357**, 1391–1396.
7. Newcombe *et al.* (1999). The management of acute neurotrauma in rural and remote locations. *J Clin Neurosci* **6**(1), 85–93.

2

Intra-cerebral Haemorrhage in Adults

John Thomas

Introduction

Intracerebral haemorrhages (ICH) are catastrophic events that often present as the sudden onset of neurologic deficit in previously well patients. The overall incidence is about 12–15 cases per 100,000/year. Under the age of 45, ICH is rare — less than 2 per 100,000/year. The

Table 1 Causes of Intracerebral Haematomas

I. Traumatic
  Non-iatrogenic
  Iatrogenic (e.g. peri-operative)

II. Spontaneous (non-traumatic)
  Hypertension
  Vascular anomaly — cerebral aneurysm, AVM, cavernous malformation
  Haemorrhagic conversion of cerebral infarction
  Cerebral amyloid angiopathy
  Coagulopathy — constitutional, drug related
  Tumour — primary or metastatic or leukaemia
  Drug abuse

incidence of ICH increases significantly after age 55 years, and doubles with each decade of age until age of more than 80 where the incidence is 25 times that for the total population (350 per 100,000/ year). The incidence of ICH is higher among the Japanese, Chinese and African Americans. There is conflicting evidence of a sexual bias, with some studies suggesting a higher incidence in women. This chapter will discuss spontaneous, non-traumatic haemorrhages (Table 1)[1] within the brain parenchyma (ICH proper).

Initial Clinical Approach to the Patient

The common situation is when the patient is brought to the emergency department for symptoms suggestive of stroke that is, with sudden neurologic deficit. Patients with ICH may also present with headaches, seizures, confusion or drowsiness. Apart from the common ABC's of resuscitation, the first clinical assessment should include the following parameters:

(1) Glasgow Coma Score (GCS).
(2) Pupillary size, reaction to light and any pupillary asymmetry
(3) Blood pressure, pulse rate.
(4) A rating of the power in each of the four limbs according to the MRC 6 point (0 to 5) rating scale.

These are the parameters that are commonly charted in the "Head Chart." The main parameter that will determine the course of action is the GCS. Any patient with significantly impaired consciousness (a GCS of less than 13) will need more careful evaluation. This is the first clinical clue that the diagnosis may be a cerebral haemorrhage rather than the much more common ichaemic stroke. A history of deterioration of the GCS over a short time (for example, previously talking but now obtunded) is very suspicious of ICH. In such patients and in comatose patients (a GCS of less than or equal to 8), one will have to determine the appropriateness of securing the patient's airway via endotracheal intubation.

The patient's age, history of serious pre-existing illness (e.g. malignancy, serious organ failure) and presenting neurologic status should be considered prior to endotracheal intubation. In general, the age limit of 70 years is an initial guide. Most patients older than this who present in coma due to stroke or ICH are unlikely to do well despite aggressive treatment. In these patients the decision to intubate may be deferred until the information from the CT brain scan is available.

The need to intubate the patient also carries the possibility that urgent surgical intervention may be necessary. It is therefore important that baseline blood studies be done when intravenous access is made. These would include Full Blood Count, serum Urea/Electrolytes, Prothrombin Time/Partial Thromboplastin Time, Blood Group and Crossmatch.

The next important assessment that should be made in the intubated patient is whether the comatose state is due to raised intracranial pressure. Brainstem infarcts and haemorrhages can result in coma without raising intra-cranial pressure (ICP) due to disruption of the reticular activating system (RAS). The finding of asymmetry in the pupils or limb movements or response especially in the presence of a raised blood pressure (systolic pressure greater than 180 mmHg) is very suggestive of a mass lesion (for example, dilated left pupil with right hemiplegia). A single bolus dose of 100 ml of intravenous 20% mannitol is a useful measure to control high ICP in this setting. Urinary catheterisation is absolutely necessary before administration of mannitol. Mannitol is contraindicated in heart failure and endstage renal failure because fluid overload may result. Mild hyperventilation (to achieve a Pco_2 of 30–35 mmHg) will also help to reduce raised ICP as will head elevation of 15° to 30°.

After these initial measures, a CT brain scan should be performed as soon as possible to determine the appropriate management for the patient.

In the majority of cases, endotracheal intubation is not necessary and the clinical picture will be that of an uncomplicated stroke. The diagnosis of intra-cerebral haemorrhage in these patients is unlikely to be made prior to the results of the CT brain scan. It is good to keep in mind that 80% of strokes are due to ischaemic events, and thus the CT will show a haemorrhage in about one-fifth of patients.

Prior to the CT scan the history may be of some use in suggesting that a haemorrhage is present. In general the neurologic deficit with ICH is characterised by a smooth progressive onset over minutes to hours (as the haematoma enlarges and reaches stable size) whereas with embolic or ischaemic events, the deficit is maximal at onset (when the blood flow is occluded). Severe headache, vomiting and alteration of consciousness are more common in ICH.

The other major clinical clue in the history is the presence of a clotting disorder. This may be due to an underlying haematologic disease or the therapeutic use of anticoagulant medication (warfarin or low molecular weight heparin). Aspirin and the other anti-platelet agents do not usually predispose the patient towards cerebral haemorrhage, although they can potentially allow a larger haemorrhage to form once the bleeding starts.

The use or abuse of drugs, especially sympathomimetic, agents should also be kept in mind especially if the patient is young (Table 2).

Table 2 Causes of Intracerebral Haemorrhage by Age (in Descending Order of Frequency)

I.	Young adults (< 45 years)
	Vascular malformation
	Cerebral aneurysm
	Drug abuse (cocaine, amphetamines, alcohol)
II.	Middle-aged adults
	Vascular malformation
	Tumour
	Aneurysm
III.	Elderly (> 65 years)
	Hypertension
	Tumours
	Amyloid angiopathy
	Coagulopathy
	Aneurysm or arteriovascular malformation (AVM)

These drugs can predispose them to both ischaemic or haemorrhagic events.

Imaging

A CT brain scan is the best tool to ascertain the presence of ICH. MRI is not the ideal initial investigation to evaluate cerebral haemorrhage. ICH is seen as a high density area within the brain substance. The high density on CT is due to the high haematocrit of formed haematoma (60–90%) and the consequent high iron concentration. It is possible for the haematoma to be less distinct if severe anaemia is present or if the blood has not clotted.

Haematoma volume carries prognostic significance. Most haematomas smaller than 25 ml in volume are associated with much less parenchymal damage and a higher likelihood of good neurologic recovery with conservative management. Haematomas greater than 60–70 ml are usually associated with coma and poorer outcome despite aggressive treatment. Haematoma volume is usually approximated by a modified ellipsoid volume equation:

$$\text{Modified ellipsoid volume} \approx \tfrac{1}{2}\,(A \times B \times C)$$

where A, B and C are the maximum length, breadth and height of the clot measured off the CT scan.

The CT scan also allows a useful classification of ICH into lobar and deep haemorrhages. Lobar haemorrhage (Fig. 1) is seen in the cortex and subcortical white matter of the cerebral or cerebellar hemispheres. In contrast, deep haemorrhages (Fig. 2) are seen in the basal ganglia (caudate nucleus and putamen), thalamus, brainstem and deep nuclei of the cerebellum. Lobar haemorrhages are more likely to be associated with structural abnormalities than deep haemorrhages. With large haemorrhages it may be difficult to make the distinction between lobar/deep ICH. The distribution of ICH is summarised in Table 3.

With reference to Table 3, the main difference in the distribution of haematomas in the general population as compared to hypertensive patients is the higher incidence of deep haematomas (putamen,

Table 3 Common Sites for Intracerebral Haemorrhage

Location	Hypertensive Patients (%)	General Population (%)
Lobar	18	20–50
Putamen	61	40–50
Thalamus	12	5–20
Cerebellum	8	5–10
Brainstem	1	1–5

thalamus and brainstem) in hypertensive patients. The lobar location is more associated with other causes, such as amyloid angiopathy, AVM, neoplasm and drug abuse rather than with hypertension.

Damage to the internal capsule on CT scan is of prognostic importance. Haemorrhages extending through the internal capsule are likely to produce permanent neurologic deficit. Haematomas which merely compress the internal capsule are more likely to be associated with neurologic improvement.

Haemorrhage in the cerebellum (Fig. 3) has to be evaluated very carefully. There is the risk that a patient who is relatively well may suddenly develop cerebral herniation and succumb because the posterior cranial fossa is a small compartment and is very intolerant even of small volume changes. A haematoma of 30 ml can lead to death if it is in the posterior cranial fossa.

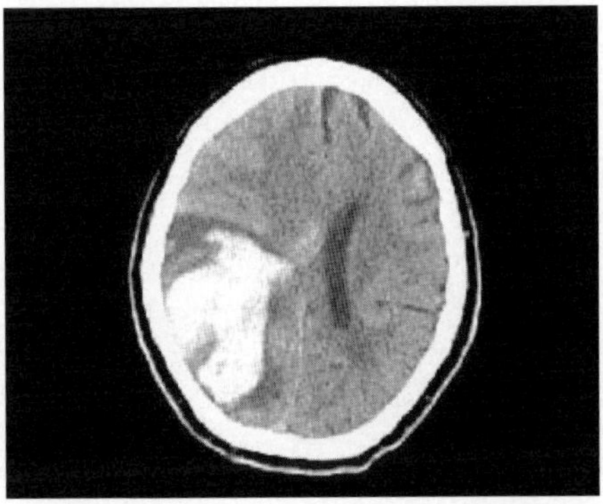

Fig. 1 Right parietal ICH (lobar).

The CT scan will also show if the ICH has led to CSF pathway obstruction and hydrocephalus.

General Pathophysiology

The initial clinical effects of an intracerebral haematoma are due to the direct destruction and displacement of the surrounding brain tissue. The haematoma volume and location therefore have a direct correlation with the degree and type of initial tissue destruction.

The mechanisms of secondary tissue injury include rebleeding, cerebral oedema and hydrocephalus. These may lead to cerebral

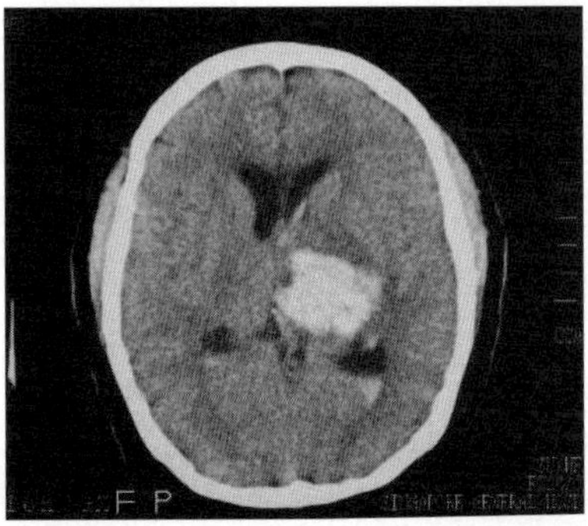

Fig. 2 Left thalamic ICH (deep).

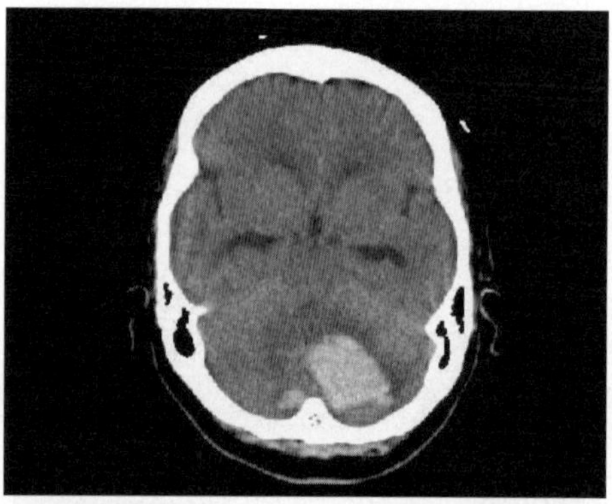

Fig. 3 Left cerebellar ICH (greater than 3 cm diameter).

herniation (coning). On the cellular level experimental studies have shown decreased local cerebral blood flow, hyperaemia, dysautoregulation, and blood-brain barrier disruption in the brain surrounding haematomas. These events are thought to initiate a cascade of biochemical processes that precipitate cellular metabolic disruption and eventual cell death.

The biochemical cascades are thought to be similar to what happens in cerebral ischaemia. Current management therefore seeks to optimise the related physiologic parameters (such as blood pressure, cardiac output, temperature, cerebral blood flow, blood glucose) that may reduce this biochemical secondary tissue injury.

A number of experimental animal models[2] have led to the idea that removing even small haematomas can reduce the peri-haematoma ischaemic changes that lead to further brain loss. The randomised clinical surgical trials thus far performed, however, have not shown benefit over medical management for small (less than 25 ml) and large (more than 60–70 ml) haematomas (but the trials have been criticised for small sample sizes and methodological problems).

The pathogenesis of ICH in hypertensive patients is thought to be related either to the formation and rupture of microaneurysms (0.2–1.0 mm size, Charcot-Bouchard aneurysms) or hypertension-induced medial degeneration (lipohyalinosis or fibrohyalinosis). Both pathologies are found in the perforating arteries supplying the basal ganglia, thalamus, pons and cerebellum. These perforating arteries are direct-end-arteries coming off the main cerebral vessels, and are exposed to higher pressures than the distal) end-arteries supplying the cerebral cortex.

Cerebral amyloid angiopathy is a unique form of cerebro-vascular disease where there is abnormal amyloid deposition in cerebral vessels, but is not associated with systemic amyloidosis. It primarily affects the elderly. The weakened affected vessels are prone to spontaneous rupture. The haemorrhages typically have a lobar distribution with the basal ganglia and thalamus spared.

ICH is well known to be related to drug abuse (cocaine, amphetamines). The bleeding with these agents usually occurs minutes to hours after drug use, and is typically subcortical (lobar). The mechanism is related to transient severe increases in sympathetic output and blood pressure. Cerebral vasculitis is another cause of ICH, usually related to amphetamine misuse. Mycotic aneurysms are another potential cause especially in intravenous drug users.

Bleeding into cerebral tumours is relatively uncommon, occurring in less than 1% of all lesions. Benign tumours rarely haemorrhage. Most lesions that bleed are malignant primary (glioblatoma multiforme) or metastatic tumours. Metastases from bronchogenic carcinoma, choriocarcinoma and renal cell carcinoma have a higher propensity to bleed.

Management Paradigms for Intracerebral Haemorrhage

Acute medical management

This involves stabilising the cardiorespiratory system (intubation if necessary), controlling elevated intra-cranial pressure (head elevation, mild to moderate hyperventilation, intravenous mannitol), preventing and treating seizures (for lobar haemorrhages only) and controlling significantly raised blood pressure. Coagulopathies will have to be acutely corrected to prevent the risk of haematoma expansion.

Blood pressure is considered to be the most important factor in determining the risk of rapid expansion of a cerebral haematoma or rehaemorrhage. The aim of treatment is to achieve systolic blood pressures of or less than 160 to 180 mmHg and diastolic blood pressures of or less than 95 to 100 mmHg initially and allow slow correction thereafter, over several days, to the ideal long term levels for the patient. The common agents used in the acute situation include sublingual nifedipine, intravenous labetolol and, in refractory cases, intravenous trinitroglycerin (GTN). Most chronic hypertensive patients have impaired cerebral autoregulation and require a higher blood pressure than normal for optimum brain perfusion. Therefore, acute overtreatment of high blood pressure can result in relative cerebral hypoperfusion and ischaemia with deleterious consequences.

There is no evidence that corticosteroids are efficacious for patients with ICH and in general are not used.

Urgent surgical intervention

Urgent intervention is considered for stuporous or comatose patients who are not moribund (GCS 12 to 6), with good pre-morbid history and who are at high risk of further deterioration. The aims of surgery are the preservation of life and the prevention of further deterioration of neurologic function. Surgical candidates are usually younger patients in whom the CT brain scan does not show severe brain damage, and have a good prognosis. Surgery, though, usually does not restore severe neurologic deficit. Involvement of the dominant cerebral hemisphere (usually the left), age > 75, GCS ≤ 5, deep (thalamic and brainstem) haemorrhages and large clots greater than 60 ml in size are poor prognostic indicators. Such patients may not be offered surgery after discussion with their families. In surgical candidates, depending on the problems defined on the CT brain scan, the intervention may be haematoma evacuation (via craniotomy, burr hole or stereotactic aspiration), drainage of hydrocephalus, decompression via bone flap removal, or a combination of some or all of the above.

Cerebellar haematomas are treated more urgently than comparable lobar ICH both because these are more likely to worsen without surgery and because these is a much better outcome. Most surgeons would intervene for clots greater than 3 cm in diameter, especially if the GCS is less than 14.

Delayed surgical intervention

This involves patients who are clinically well (GCS ≥ 13) upon presentation to hospital, managed conservatively initially, but who later deteriorate either in terms of poorer conscious level or worsening neurologic dysfunction. Intervention is considered if the GCS should worsen by 2 points or more. The deterioration may be due to haematoma enlargement, brain swelling or hydrocephalus. CT brain scan is required to evaluate the cause of deterioration and determine the correct course of intervention.

The role of haematoma evacuation to restore neurologic deficit or improve neurologic recovery (in the absence of deterioration in GCS) is controversial but is under investigation.

Initial conservative management with further investigation

The investigations are cerebral angiography and MRI brain scan. These are reserved for patients with atypical clinical or radiological features. The atypical features may suggest the possibility of recurrent haemorrhage or an underlying lesion or tumour.

The common clinical feature that deserves investigation is a haemorrhage (in any location) in a young patient (under 45 years). In these patients the possibility that a brain vascular malformation may underlie the haemorrhage needs to be excluded by cerebral angiography. This is performed electively unless urgent surgical intervention is planned, in which case the angiogram should be done urgently as well. Other atypical radiological features that merit angiography include lobar haemorrhage, calcification in the region of the haematoma and multiple haemorrhages. If the index of suspicion is high, an initial negative cerebral angiogram will be repeated after six weeks or so. The delayed study allows re-evaluation after most of the clot has been lysed and removed.

MRI brain scan is usually best deferred till six to eight weeks after the haemorrhage to allow for haematoma resorption and better discrimination. Ideally it should follow all atypical cases with negative cerebral angiograms to rule out tumours (primary or metastatic) and cavernous angiomas (which are usually not seen on angiograms).

Once discovered, vascular malformations may be treated by surgical excision, endovascular embolisation, stereotactic radiosurgery or by a combination of these modalities. Tumours are usually treated with surgical excision or biopsy followed by radiotherapy and chemotherapy where appropriate.

Risk factor control and rehabilitation

This is by far the most common treatment paradigm used for patients in our practice. The presence of hypertension, diabetes mellitus and hyperlipidemia needs to be evaluated in all patients as modifiable risk factors for ICH due to degenerative cerebrovascular disease. Smoking is another important modifiable risk factor.

Conclusion

Intracerebral haematomas continue to challenge clinicians. In the last decade, much has been done to elucidate the biochemical cascades that lead to secondary brain injury after an ICH but this has not yet been translated into efficacious new treatment. Minimally invasive surgery combined with computerised image-guided surgical navigation techniques have significantly reduced the morbidity of surgical treatment of ICH. Combined clinical management teams involving neurologists, neurosurgeons, rehabilitation physicians, nurses, speech, occupational and physiotherapists and social workers have provided holistic management approaches for these patients. One of the main hopes for improved outcomes remains new techniques of augmenting brain repair mechanisms.

References

1. Hamilton MG, Zabramski JM (1995). Intracerebral haematomas. In *Neurovascular Surgery*. Carter LP, Spetzler RF (eds.) McGraw-Hill Inc., pp. 477–496.
2. Nehls DG, Mendelow AD, Graham DI, Teasdale GM (1990). Experimental intracerebral haemorrhage: early removal of spontaneous mass lesion improves late outcome. *Neurosurgery* **27**, 674.

3

Paediatric Neurosurgical Emergencies: A Problem-Based Approach

Keith YC Goh

Introduction

The doctor who practises in a large general hospital does not frequently encounter neurosurgical emergencies in children. In most countries, these cases are usually diverted to the nearest children's hospital, where trained paediatric doctors are available to deal with the special problems which this patient group presents. However, there will be occasional situations when the critically ill child presents to the adult doctor and first-line treatment must be quickly instituted. It is therefore necessary for frontline medical staff to be equipped with the basic knowledge of common paediatric neurosurgical emergency conditions so that life-saving treatment can be initiated without delay.

The purpose of this chapter is to discuss these conditions from a problem-based perspective, to provide guidance in formulating logical management plans when faced with such clinical situations, and to describe the treatment options, which can be initiated by the general surgeon, prior to referral to the neurosurgeon.

The neurosurgical conditions in this chapter will mainly be confined to disorders of the brain, in which emergencies inevitably present with impaired consciousness. Acute paediatric spinal cord conditions rarely present as emergencies except in the setting of trauma or vascular events, and in these, the principles of management are the same as for adults.

Approach to the Drowsy Child

One of the most commonly encountered scenarios is that of the drowsy child. As in all clinical situations, it is important to go through the steps of taking a good history, and performing a complete physical examination, according to well-established clinical priorities. Airway, breathing and circulation must be assessed first, and immediate treatment instituted if necessary. Hypoxia and hypotension are significant secondary insults to the brain, and all efforts must be made to minimise these.[1,2]

The neurologic examination is performed in two stages. First, the degree of impaired consciousness is determined by referencing the Glasgow Coma Scale (GCS), which is the universally accepted clinical scoring system for coma assessment.[3] Three components are assessed, i.e. eye, verbal and motor responses (Table 1). A GCS score of 3 indicates that the patient is in deep coma, while a fully conscious and

Table 1 The Glasgow Coma Scale (GCS)

Points	Best Eye Opening	Best Verbal Response*	Best Motor Response
6	–	–	Obeys
5	–	Oriented	Localises pain
4	Spontaneous	Confused	Flexion withdrawal
3	To speech	Inappropriate words	Abnormal flexion (decorticate)
2	To pain	Incomprehensible sounds	Extension (decerebrate)
1	None	None	None

*Children younger than two years should receive full verbal scoring if they cry after stimulation.

alert patient has a score of 15. In children who are younger than two years of age, verbal skills are not well developed, and the GCS has been adapted to take this into consideration.[4] A full score in the verbal response category is therefore given if the child cries after stimulation. It should be noted that the GCS is an indicator of global conscious level, and cannot be used to follow a focal neurologic deficit, and that the scores are related to "best" responses. This is important for purposes of decision-making and eventually, prognosis.

If the GCS is 8 or below, it is preferable to intubate and ventilate the patient because airway protection is impaired. Pupillary size and

Table 2 Aetiology of Coma

Neurosurgical Causes	Non-neurosurgical Causes
Head trauma Intracranial haematomas Cerebral oedema	*Epilepsy*
Hydrocephalus Obstructive Communicating	*Metabolic/Electrolyte disorders* Drug overdosage Endocrine disorders Organ failure
Neoplasia Supratentorial tumours Infratentorial tumours	*Neoplasia* Disseminated carcinomatosis Haematologic malignancies
Vascular disorders Haemorrhagic conditions, e.g. Arteriovenous malformations, aneurysms Ischaemic conditions, e.g. Infarcts, Moya-moya disease	*Vascular disorders* Thrombo-embolism Vasculitis Infarct
Infection Brain abscess Subdural empyema Ventriculitis	*Infection* Meningitis Encephalitis Septicaemia
	Pseudo-coma Psychiatric causes Neuromuscular disease

responses are then examined, followed by checking for the presence or absence of neurologic deficits.

Based on the patient history and physical examination, it will be possible to make a few differential diagnoses as to the probable aetiology of the impaired consciousness (Annex 1) (Table 2). At this point, radiologic investigations are needed to confirm the diagnosis and cause of the coma.

Annex 1 Management Algorithm for the Drowsy Child

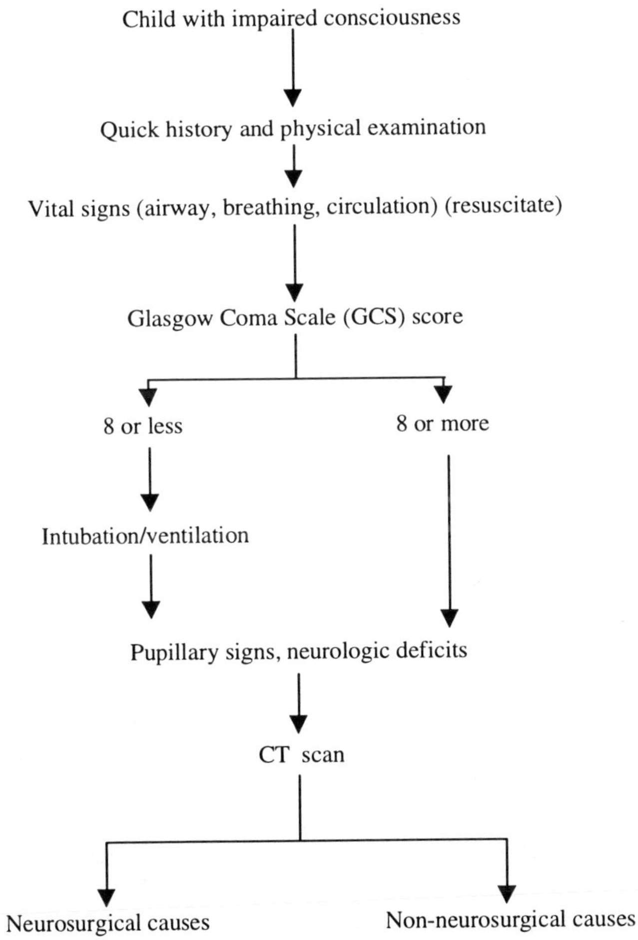

Radiologic Investigations

In the emergency setting, the most important investigation is a computer-tomographic (CT) scan of the brain.[5] Plain X-rays have been shown to be of minimal value in detecting a mass lesion in the brain, and time should not be wasted in organising this at the expense of a CT scan.[6] Modern CT machines are able to perform a scan within one to two minutes, and this provides valuable information to the neurosurgeon as to whether surgical intervention is immediately required.[7] Magnetic resonance imaging (MRI) scans also have no place in the emergency setting, as these take too much time and effort to organise for a ventilated patient.[8]

It is important to exclude neurosurgically-related causes because rapid neurosurgical intervention may be required, and because unnecessary delays which lead to poorer outcomes, can be reduced.

Temporising Measures

While waiting for the neurosurgeon to arrive, or for the transfer to a neurosurgical unit, several important measures can be initiated to protect the brain and improve the patient. The overwhelming need is to reduce intracranial pressure (ICP) until definitive treatment can be provided. This can be done by hyperventilating the patient, administering osmotherapy (mannitol), elevating the head of the patient, and in certain situations, administering steroids. The role of prophylactic anticonvulsants is somewhat controversial. However, when there has been a clearly witnessed convulsion, there is no doubt that medication should be started. Similarly, in cases where there is the likelihood of seizures (such as compound depressed fractures or temporal lobe tumours), or where neurosurgical intervention is imminent, anticonvulsants should also be started.

Head Trauma

Paediatric head trauma accounts for a large number of emergency room attendances and hospital admissions. Fortunately the majority of these patients have minor head injuries, and almost all recover fully. Since the various types of head trauma and intracranial haematomas and their treatment have already been described in the chapter on head injuries, this section will focus on the approach to the head-injured child; identify subtypes unique to children; and emphasise some of the differences from adults.

In assessing the head-injured child, the first important step is to try to determine the risk of intracranial haemorrhage. A good history and physical examination are mandatory. Studies have shown that in the small percentage of children who sustain significant intracranial injury, the most common mechanism is a fall from a height greater than the patient's height; with the clinical presentation of impaired or reduced consciousness.[5] A post-traumatic seizure is not predictive of intracranial haemorrhage, although conventional teaching has mandated CT scans in this situation.[9–11]

Once a risk category is assigned, i.e. low-risk, medium-risk or high-risk (Table 3), then the management algorithm becomes logical (Annex 2). Low-risk patients are treated conservatively and can be

Table 3 Risk of Intracranial Haemorrhage or Injury*

Low Risk	Medium Risk	High Risk
GCS 15	GCS 13-14	GCS 12 or less
Mild or no headache	Progressive headache	Drowsiness
Vomiting (less than 3 times)	Vomiting (more than 3 times)	Focal neurologic signs
Transient loss of consciousness (seconds)	Loss of consciousness (minutes)	Multiple trauma
Mild scalp injury	Possible depressed fracture	Penetrating injury
	Signs of skull base fracture	
	Associated facial fracture	
	Neonate or child younger than 2 years	

*Adapted from the Ministry of Health, Singapore, Clinical Practice Guidelines 2001 on "Head Injury in Children".

Annex 2 Management Algorithm for Paediatric Head Injury Based on Risk Assessment*

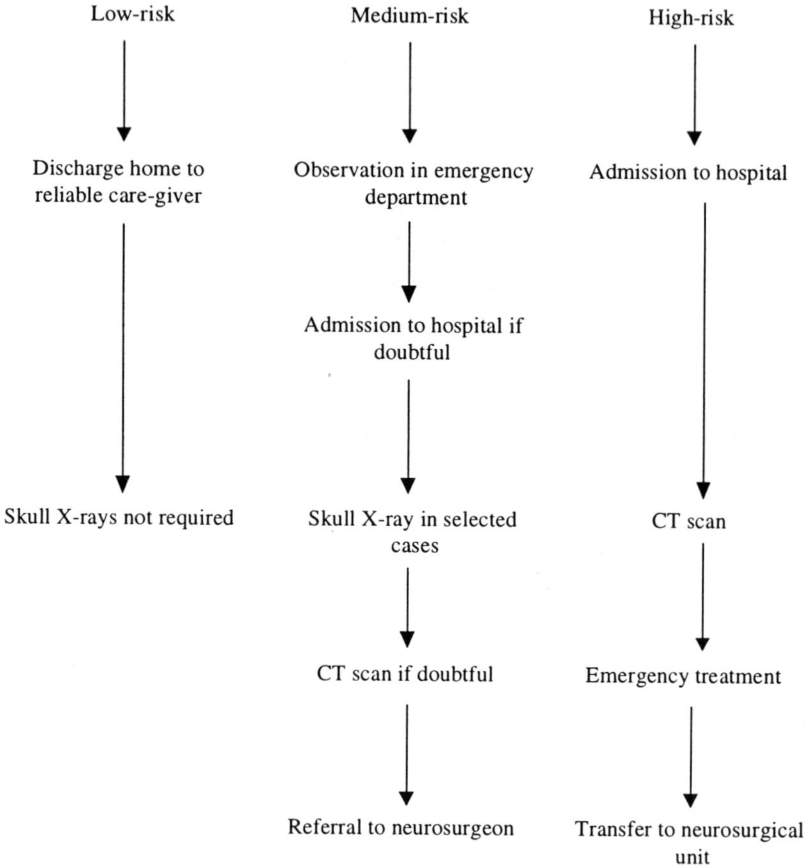

*Adapted from the Ministry of Health, Singapore, Clinical Practice Guidelines 2001 on "Head Injury in Children".

discharged. Some medium-risk patients are observed in hospital and will undergo CT scans if there are concerns of possible intracranial injuries. High-risk patients will need intensive management and are best transferred to a paediatric neurosurgical intensive care unit for definitive treatment.

It is appropriate at this point to describe certain age-specific syndromes which are unique to the paediatric population. Of note are the "shaken baby" syndrome and "ping-pong" fractures in infants;

"growing" fractures in young children; and "paediatric concussion" syndrome in the older child.

"Shaken baby" syndrome refers to the clinical features found in an infant who has been abused or inflicted with injuries from violent shaking.[12] There is often a doubtful history of minor trauma or no trauma; seizures; apnoea; evidence of blunt impact to the head; skeletal or soft tissue injuries; and retinal haemorrhage. In the acute stage, CT scan findings typically show subarachnoid haemorrhage or acute subdural haematomas (Fig. 1). In cases where there has been repeated injury, the CT scan can show chronic subdural collections and cerebral atrophy (Fig. 2). These children sometimes present in extremis, with deep coma or status epilepticus. Resuscitation is required, followed by urgent neurosurgical intervention. Despite this, the outcome is usually poor, with high mortality rates.

In infants and toddlers (age less than two years), linear fractures and cephalohaematomas are common, even with seemingly minor trauma. "Ping-pong" fractures are depressed fractures which occur because of the relatively thin cranial vault. The surgeon can easily elevate them by making a small adjacent burr-hole, then levering the depressed segment of bone upwards. This springs back into place in a similar manner to a ping-pong ball. In this age group, "growing"

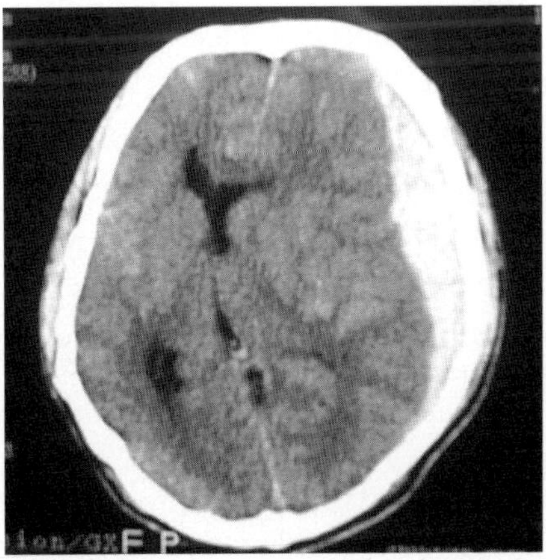

Fig. 1 CT scan of the brain showing a left acute subdural haematoma.

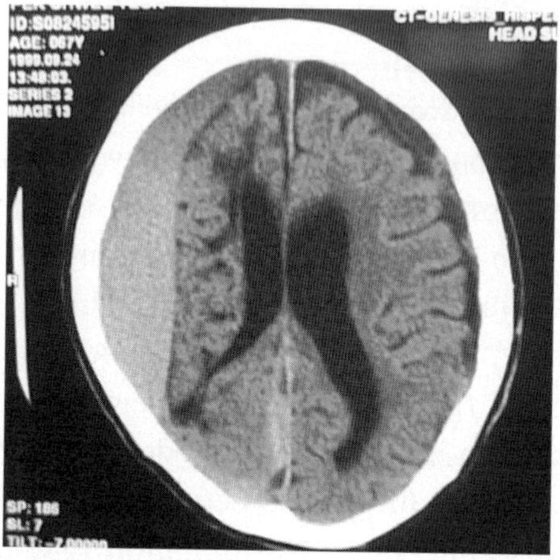

Fig. 2 CT scan showing a chronic subdural haematoma with accompanying cerebral atrophy.

fractures are sometimes also encountered. Most linear skull fractures heal without sequelae. However in cases where the injury has been relatively severe, and there is an underlying dural laceration, the force of the growing brain or an associated underlying cyst, causes the bony defect to enlarge or "grow". If left untreated, large areas of bone loss and herniated brain can develop.

Finally, in older children (between three and eight years), a syndrome of impaired consciousness has been described after a head injury, but with normal CT scan findings. The clinical hallmark of a concussion is a brief loss of a consciousness, followed by the return to essentially normal mentation.[13] However in this group of children, they appear to worsen after the concussion, with symptoms of lethargy, irritability, nausea and vomiting. CT scans are essentially normal, and these children gradually improve over a few days.

Hydrocephalus

Hydrocephalus is most easily understood as the abnormal accumulation of cerebrospinal fluid (CSF) from either a structural obstruction to

Table 4 Aetiology of Hydrocephalus

Obstructive Hydrocephalus	Communicating Hydrocephalus
Congenital	*Infection*
Aqueduct stenosis	Meningitis
Myelomeningocoele	Ventriculitis
Dandy-walker malformation	
Tumours	*Haemorrhage*
Intraventricular tumours	Intraventricular haemorrhage
Posterior fossa tumours	Subarachnoid haemorrhage
Brainstem tumours	
Post-surgical removal	
	Idiopathic
	Congenital

CSF flow, or a failure of absorption at the level of the arachnoid granulations in the dural venous sinuses, where most of the absorption takes place (Table 4). In most paediatric cases, the onset of hydrocephalus is gradual, with the children presenting with a noticeably larger-than-average head size, and the paediatrician noting a head circumference greater than the 97th percentile. Clinical features are usually subtle, and have been ignored or missed for some time. There may be developmental delays such as slowness to talk or walk. However in children with significantly raised intracranial pressure, the fontanelle will be palpably tense, and there will be papilloedema (although the absence of papilloedema does not exclude raised intracranial pressures or ICP) with "sunset" eyes (Fig. 3).

The emergency presentation of hydrocephalus with altered consciousness commonly occurs in the following situations:

(1) *Posterior fossa tumours*

This will be discussed further in the section on brain tumours. Hydrocephalus occurs because the tumour obstructs the flow of CSF, usually at the aqueduct or fourth ventricle.

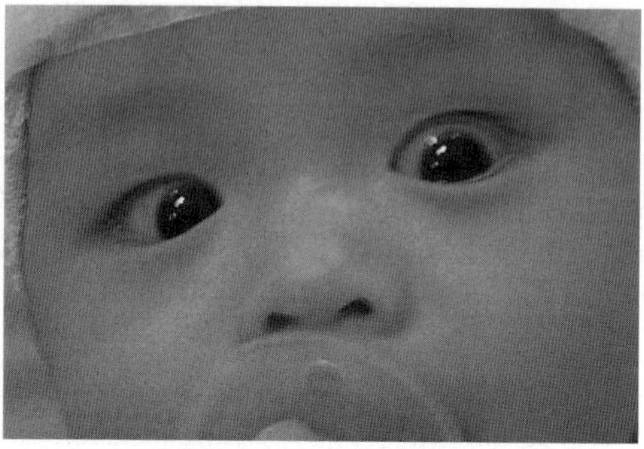

Fig. 3 "Sunset" eyes.

(2) *Infection — meningitis, ventriculitis*

Bacteria alter the CSF absorption abilities of the arachnoid granulations, leading to communicating hydrocephalus.

(3) *Intraventricular haemorrhage*

Blood products affect the arachnoid granulations in a similar manner as bacteria.

(4) *Previous CSF shunt which has malfunctioned*

The child who is used to normal ICP's from being shunted, tends to become rapidly obtunded when the shunt malfunctions. This has been postulated as due to changes in the pressure-volume compliance of the shunted brain, but is generally not well understood.

Congenital hydrocephalus seldom requires emergency surgical intervention because the fontanelle is still open and the skull sutures have not closed yet.

Based on the patient history, clinical examination and CT scan, diagnosis is usually easily made. CT scan appearances of large ventricles are characteristic (Figs. 4 and 5). The definitive treatment is to re-establish or divert the CSF flow, and there are several methods of achieving this. The time-tested conventional method is to insert a

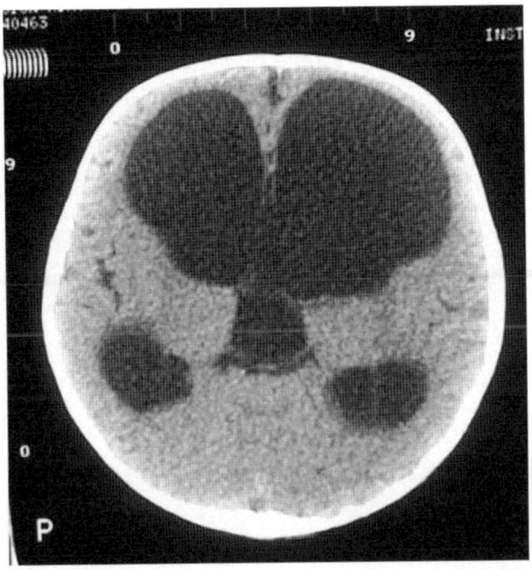

Fig. 4 Axial CT scan of the brain showing large lateral ventricles.

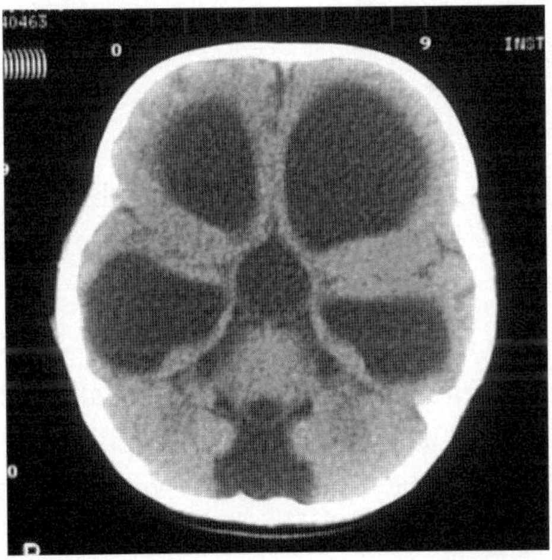

Fig. 5 Axial CT scan of the brain showing a large rounded third ventricle in addition to large frontal and temporal horns of the lateral ventricles.

shunt, with the safest being the ventriculo-peritoneal (VP) shunt. In this operation, a small-calibre silicon tubing is inserted into the ventricle, connected to a flow- or pressure-regulated valve, and then subcutaneously tunnelled to the abdomen where it is inserted into the peritoneal

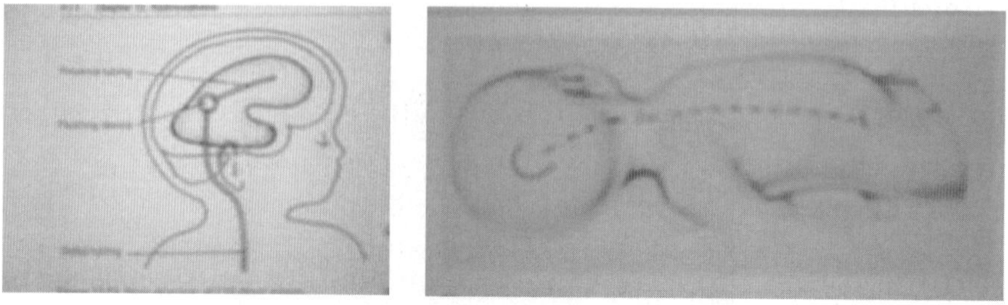

Fig. 6 Diagramatic representation of VP shunt.

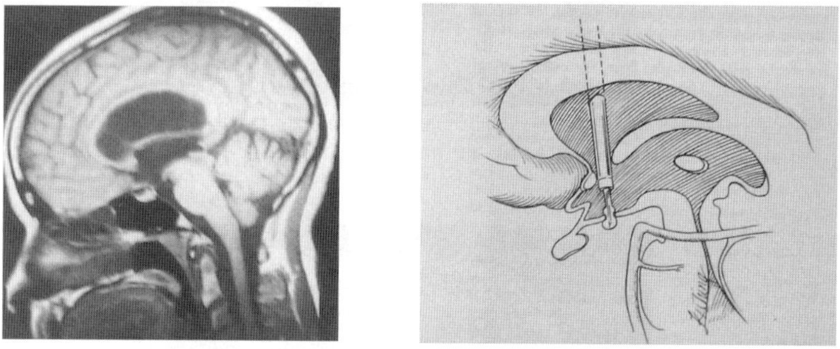

Fig. 7 Endoscopic third ventriculostomy.

cavity (Fig. 6). In cases where the peritoneal cavity is unsuitable, a ventriculo-atrial (VA) shunt is inserted.

In certain cases of obstructive hydrocephalus where the level of obstruction is at the aqueduct, another option is to fenestrate an opening in the floor of the anterior third ventricle, thus allowing CSF flow to be diverted to the front of the brainstem. This procedure is performed with a neuro-endoscope, and is called an endoscopic third ventriculostomy (Fig. 7). If successfully performed, a shunt does not have to be inserted.

All these surgical procedures require the expertise of a neurosurgeon, and it is therefore prudent in these situations to quickly refer the child to the neurosurgical unit. Temporising measures to reduce ICP are intubation with hyperventilation, osmotherapy with mannitol, and lumbar puncture (for communicating hydrocephalus).

Tumours

Paediatric brain tumours are the second most common form of cancer in children after leukaemias (incidence 20%), with about 60% occurring in the posterior fossa.[14] Most cases usually escape diagnosis until they grow to a large size because of the elasticity of the infant skull, adaptability of the developing nervous system to compensate for neurologic deficits, and difficulty in examining a child who is usually uncooperative. As such, these patients present more insidiously with vague headaches, subtle neurologic deficits, failure to thrive, large heads or developmental regression.

The tumours which present suddenly or in a catastrophic manner are usually tumours of the posterior fossa which cause obstructive hydrocephalus (Fig. 8), or tumours which have spontaneously haemorrhaged. The most common tumours are medulloblastoma, brainstem glioma, cerebellar astrocytoma and ependymoma (Fig. 9). Although radiologic appearances may suggest the tumour type, the definitive test is histologic examination of the surgically resected specimen.

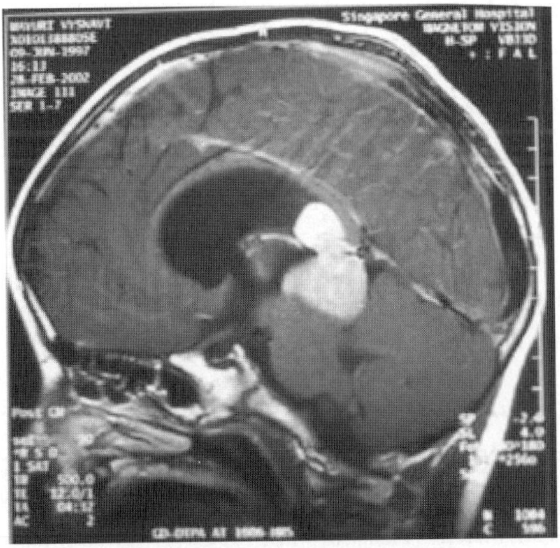

Fig. 8 Posterior fossa tumour causing hydrocephalus.

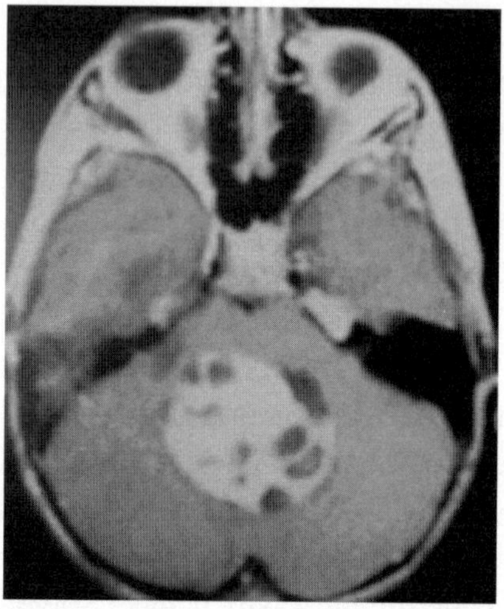

Fig. 9 MRI scan of the brain showing an ependymoma of the fourth ventricle.

Priorities in management are as follows:

(1) *Resuscitation of the patient*

Airway protection, ventilation and circulatory support, depending on the GCS and haemodynamics.

(2) *Stabilisation of the blood-brain barrier*

As a temporising measure, high-dose steroids (dexamethasone) should be given according to body weight.

(3) *Reduction of ICP*

Osmotherapy with mannitol is a reasonable temporising measure, but not very effective.

(4) *CSF diversion*

This requires transfer to a paediatric neurosurgical unit for definitive treatment. The CSF diversion procedure can be an endoscopic third ventriculostomy, external ventricular drain or VP shunt.

(5) *Tumour resection*

The definitive treatment is then scheduled for the next available date.

Infection

Infections of the central nervous system (CNS) can occur in children because of the immature blood-brain barrier and weaker immune system as compared to adults. Meningitis, which is the most common type of CNS infection, is usually treated with antibiotics, in doses sufficient to cross the blood-brain barrier and specific to the causative pathogen. These cases become neurosurgical emergencies only if hydrocephalus or ventriculitis develops as previously mentioned, and a CSF diversion procedure has to be performed.

Brain abscesses and subdural empyemas (Figs. 10 and 11) arise in three ways:

(1) *Haematogenous Spread*

Children with cyanotic heart disease and cardiac shunts are predisposed to abscess proliferation because of the hypoxic environment and the loss of the filtering effects of the lungs.

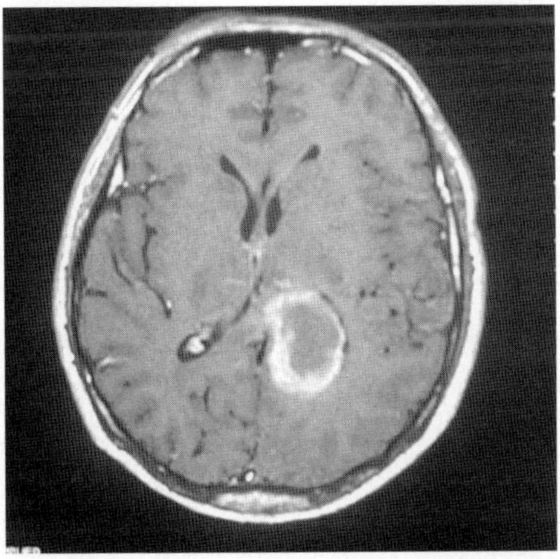

Fig. 10 MRI showing a brain abscess.

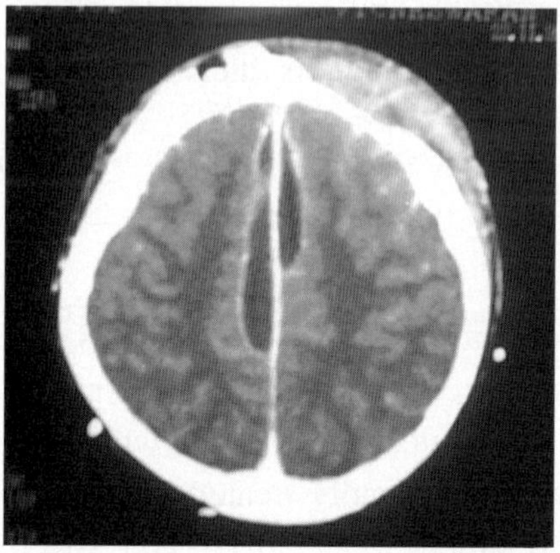

Fig. 11 CT scan showing the parafalcine collections typical of subdural empyema.

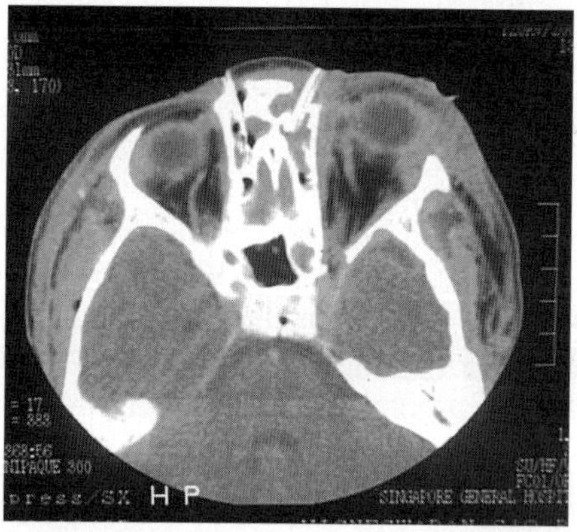

Fig. 12 CT scan showing paranasal sinusitis requiring drainage.

(2) *Contiguous Spread*

Paranasal sinusitis, otitis media or mastoiditis can spread by local osteomyelitis or phlebitis of emissary veins into the brain[15] (Fig. 12).

(3) *Following Head Trauma or Neurosurgery*

Open fracture, fractures or surgery traversing air sinuses and any form of penetrating trauma can result in intracranial infection. This is especially so if there is a CSF leak.

As in all neurosurgical conditions, the indications for surgery are raised ICP from mass effect, causing deteriorating conscious level. However the surgical techniques of brain abscess aspiration and drainage of subdural empyemas are beyond the scope of the general surgeon and require transfer to a neurosurgical unit.[16] Temporising measures are as stated in previous sections, and it is preferable that antibiotics are not started until proper specimens are obtained for cultures. In all these cases, it is important to treat the underlying aetiology, such as sinusitis or mastoiditis.

Vascular Events

These occur rarely in children and can be either haemorrhagic or ischaemic in aetiology. The common surgical causes are arteriovenous malformations, aneurysms, angiomas and Moya-moya disease. The same principles of managing these cases applies, as previously described, paying attention to airway protection, reducing ICP by various methods, starting anticonvulsants, and then transferring the patient to a neurosurgical unit.

In neonates, particularly premature babies, intracranial haemorrhage can occur because of the highly vascular germinal matrix tissue of the developing brain. Surgical intervention is not usually required unless there is a significant intraventricular component causing hydrocephalus, or a posterior fossa component causing brainstem compression. If there is communicating hydrocephalus without a haematoma in the brain, serial lumbar punctures can be sufficient to tide the baby over this episode.

Congenital Disorders

A large number of congenital malformations can be present and discovered at birth. However the only conditions which require urgent neurosurgical intervention are open neural tube defects or myelomeningocoele and open encephalocoeles. Again, these are beyond the scope of the general surgeon, and require paediatric neurosurgical expertise. The most important principle of treatment in this situation is in the protection of the neural elements and soft tissue by carefully applied, non-traumatic and non-adhesive dressings, prophylactic antibiotics, and rapid transfer for definitive treatment.

Conclusions

While it is true that paediatric neurosurgical conditions require highly specialised care, a good outcome for patients who present in the emergency room is dependent on competent medical care, based on sound fundamental knowledge. Some of the important principles of management have been outlined in this chapter, and are well within the realm of every frontline doctor.

References

1. Miller JD, Sweet RC, Narayan R, Becker DP (1978). Early insults to the injured brain. *JAMA* **240**, 439–442.
2. Manley G, Knudsen MM, Morabito D, Damron S, Erickson V, Pitts L (2001). Hypotension, hypoxia and head injury. *Arch Surg* **136**, 1118–1123.
3. Teasdale G, Jennett B (1974). Assessment of coma and impaired consciousness: a practical scale. *Lancet* **2**, 81–84.
4. Reilly PL, Simpson DA, Sprod R (1988). Assessing the conscious level in infants and young children: a paediatric version of the Glasgow Coma Scale. *Child's Nerv Syst* **4**, 30–33.
5. Read HS, Johnstone AJ, Scobie WG (1995). Skull fractures in children: altered conscious level is the main indication for urgent CT scanning. *Injury* **25**(5), 333–334.
6. Lloyd DA, Carty H, Patterson M, Butcher CK, Roe D (1997). Predictive value of skull radiography for intracranial injury in children with blunt head injury. *Lancet* **349**, 821–824.
7. Feuerman T, Wackym PA, Gade GF (1998). Value of skull radiography, head computed tomography, and admission for observation in cases of minor head injury. *Neurosurgery* **22**, 449–453.

8. Raimondi AJ (1998). Trauma. In *Pediatric Neurosurgery*, 2nd Ed. Raimondi AJ (ed.) Berlin: Springer-Verlag, Chap. 13, pp. 415–459.
9. Greenes DS, Schutzman SA (1999). Clinical indicators of intracranial injury in head-injured infants. *Pediatrics* **104**, 861–867.
10. Borczuk P (1995). Predictors of intracranial injury in patients with mild head trauma. *Ann Emerg Med* **25**, 731.
11. Teasdale GM, Murray G, Anderson E, Mendclow AD, MacMillan R, Jennett B, Brookes M (1990). Risks of acute intracranial haematoma in children and adults: implications for managing head injuries. *Br Med J* **300**, 363–367.
12. Duhaime AC, Gennarelli TG, Thibault LE, Bruce DA, Margulies SS, Wiser R (1987). The shaken baby syndrome. A clinical, pathological, and biomechanical study. *J Neurosurg* **66**, 409–415.
13. Duhaime AC (1999). Closed head injury without fractures. In *Principles and Practice of Pediatric Neurosurgery*. Albright AL, Pollack IF, Adelson PD (eds.) New York: Thieme Publishers, pp. 799–802.
14. Allen JC (1985). Childhood brain tumours: current status of clinical trials in newly diagnosed and recurrent disease. *Ped Clin N Am* **32**, 633–651.
15. Giannoni C, Sulek M, Friedman EM (1998). Intracranial complications of sinusitis: a pediatric series. *Am J Rhinol* **12**, 173–178.
16. Nathoo N, Nadvi SS, van Dellen JR, Gouws E (1999). Intracranial subdural empyemas in the era of computed tomography: a review of 699 cases. *Neurosurgery* **44**, 529–536.

4

Acute Management of Craniofacial Trauma

Vincent KL Yeow
Andrew Tay

Introduction

The management of complex craniofacial trauma has rapidly evolved over the past two decades, with several factors contributing to improved outcomes and early restoration of pre-trauma appearance and function. Advances in diagnostic imaging have facilitated accurate preoperative diagnosis and surgical planning. Technological advances in fixation devices and alloplastic implants have resulted in a broad range of treatment options. The emphasis in surgical treatment has shifted from a conservative approach with delayed operative repair, to an early, aggressive, single-stage approach. The modern principles of management of facial trauma, adopted from established craniofacial methods of exposure and bone manipulation, include early one-stage repair, complete exposure of all fracture fragments, precise anatomic fixation, immediate bone grafting, and definitive soft tissue management.

Aetiology and Associated Injuries

The aetiology of facial injuries include falls, motor vehicle accidents, industrial accidents, interpersonal violence and athletic injuries. Facial injuries are frequently associated with trauma to other systems.[1,2] In particular, the incidence of concomitant closed head injury has been reported as 55%,[3] while skull base fractures were reported in 21% to 33% of patients with facial fractures.[4] Cervical spine injury is less frequent, occurring in 1.3% to 5.5% of patients with facial fractures.[5] The incidence of ocular injury associated with facial fractures ranges from 25% to 29%.[6,7]

Initial Evaluation

Trauma victims are evaluated and treated according to the protocol of Advanced Trauma Life Support® (ATLS®). All life-threatening conditions are identified in the initial evaluation and treated immediately.

Head and neck trauma victims are considered to have a cervical spine injury until a lateral cervical spine (C-spine) film proves otherwise. Therefore, neck stabilisation with a cervical collar is mandatory until C-spine injury is ruled out or documented. There are three life-threatening facial emergencies (Fig. 1):

(1) Respiratory obstruction
(2) Haemorrhage
(3) Pulmonary aspiration

Airway management

The most common cause of airway obstruction is tongue retropositioning in an unconscious patient. Other situations which may result in airway obstruction include unstable mandibular and maxillary fractures, massive trauma with severe swelling, and haemorrhage into the airway.

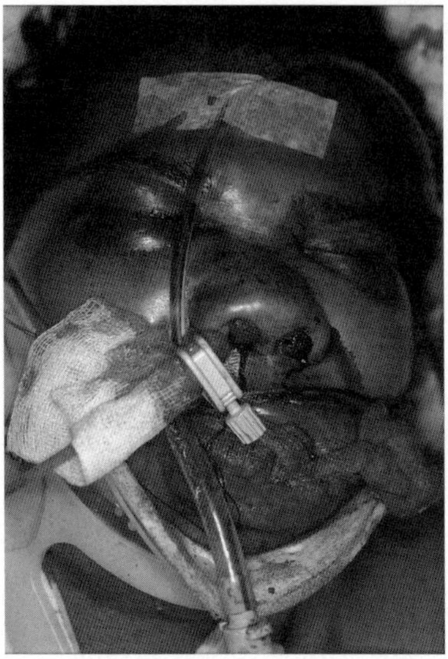

Fig. 1 Multiple facial fractures following motor vehicle accident. Severe facial swelling, haemorrhage and unstable mandibular fractures have necessitated orotracheal intubation. Nasal packs and Foley catheter in the posterior nasal space were necessary to control haemorrhage.

Conscious patients that are able to give appropriate verbal responses demonstrate clinically that their airway is patent, ventilatory status is adequate and that there is adequate blood supply to the brain.

Intubation or other manoeuvres to secure the airway must be accomplished without hyper-extension of the neck, to avoid injury to the C-spine. Emergency surgical access to the airway may be achieved by means of a cricothyroidectomy, while tracheostomy is generally performed under controlled conditions in an operating room once other life-threatening conditions have been stabilised.

Haemorrhage

During initial evaluation, haemorrhage that is contributing to significant blood loss or is compromising the airway can usually be controlled effectively with direct pressure. Surgical clamps should not be blindly placed into areas of bleeding as this can result in damage to other vital structures, such as the facial nerve.

Nasopharyngeal bleeding can often compromise the airway, and the source is usually difficult to identify. Various techniques of creating a tamponade effect to control nasopharyngeal bleeding have been employed, and the materials used can range from gauze packing strips to Foley's catheter. The Foley's catheter can be passed through the nasal cavity and into the nasopharynx. Once correctly positioned, the balloon is inflated and the catheter is withdrawn, allowing the inflated balloon to come into apposition with the posterior nasal choanae, thus causing the tamponade effect.

In maxillary (LeFort) fractures, manual reduction and placement of intermaxillary fixation may control profuse nasopharyngeal bleeding.

If the above methods are unsuccessful, angiographic demonstration and embolisation of bleeding points may control haemorrhage. If this fails, surgical exploration and haemostasis may be necessary. Failure to identify specific points of haemorrhage in the maxillofacial region may necessitate ligation of the external carotid artery or superficial temporal artery.

Pulmonary aspiration

In craniofacial trauma, the collection of blood in the pharynx from upper airway haemorrhage, and regurgitated gastric contents, or displaced structures (most commonly teeth) may be aspirated. Urgent gastric decompression after securing the airway is often necessary. In addition, where there is hard tissue avulsion, most notably in the dentoalveolar region, a chest film is imperative to rule out aspiration of teeth and bone.

Assessment of Craniofacial Trauma

The anatomic assessment of the extent of craniofacial trauma is undertaken only after the patient has undergone initial evaluation, resuscitation and stabilisation. This more thorough physical examination is completed before the patient is sent for diagnostic imaging.

In cases of isolated craniofacial trauma, this is generally quite straightforward but in cases of multiple trauma, aspects of this secondary examination and diagnostic imaging may need to be delayed, sometimes for days. The goal of this comprehensive assessment is to identify all the pathology present, and obtain a complete diagnosis upon which a definitive treatment plan can be formulated.

The clinical examination should begin with an evaluation for symmetry and deformity. Facial injuries should be considered in three categories:

(1) Soft tissue injuries
(2) Soft tissue injuries associated with bony fractures
(3) Facial fractures alone

Soft tissue injuries range from minor superficial wounds or abrasions to severe soft tissue injuries as a result of shotgun wounds. All lacerations must be examined no matter how small or insignificant. Such facial lacerations may be the only sign of penetrating injuries to the eye, nose, ear or cranial cavity. Evaluation of structures in the line of lacerations is important. The facial nerve and parotid duct are examined in lateral lacerations, and the lacrimal duct system are examined in medial periorbital trauma.

Ecchymosis in specific locations is suggestive for particular fractures. Post-auricular bruising or Battle's sign is associated with base-of-skull fractures of the middle cranial fossa. Sublingual bruising is usually pathognomonic for mandibular fractures. Subconjunctival haemorrhage and a palpebral haematoma in conjunction with or without underlying crepitus suggest a fracture of the nose, zygoma, orbit, nasoethmoid or frontal region.

Palpation of all the bony surfaces should be performed in an orderly manner from the top down. Palpable steps, crepitus, tenderness and mobility are all indicative of an underlying fracture.

Ocular assessment should include evaluation of globe position, enophthalmos, eye movements and diplopia. Unequal globe levels and diplopia usually indicate either an orbito-zygomatic fracture or an orbital blowout fracture. Eye movements should be assessed to determine if any entrapment of the extraocular muscles has occurred. There may also be restriction of eye movements and visual loss when the orbital apex is involved.

Fractures of the facial bones can also be diagnosed on the basis of malocclusion of the teeth or an open bite deformity. This is due to a displaced fracture of the maxilla or the mandible. In addition, mandibular fractures are associated with pain, deviation with movement, trismus and an inability to occlude properly. Any missing teeth also suggests dentoalveolar fractures and the risk of displaced teeth, which may have migrated to the upper airway, posing a significant risk of pulmonary aspiration. Condylar mobility can be assessed by placing a finger in the ear canal. Mobility of the middle third of the face in relation to the skull is indicative of a fracture of the LeFort type.

A quick evaluation of the sensory and motor nerve functions of the face will often highlight fractures of the midface, orbit and base of skull. In addition, fundoscopic examination and a complete examination of the globe is necessary to identify penetrating globe injuries and traumatic orbital neuropathy that will require an urgent ophthalmic consult. Finally tympanoscopy will identify any blood in the middle ear which is indicative of a base of skull fracture. This may be associated with cerebrospinal fluid (CSF) rhinorrhoea or otorrhoea.

Diagnostic Imaging

Imaging studies are indispensable in the evaluation of the patient with craniofacial trauma. Even though the clinical evaluation may demonstrate obvious fractures and suggest a standard type of management, a thorough radiological examination should be performed. In view of the high incidence of litigation arising from such injuries, it is of prime importance to have a thorough documentation of all bone injuries even if treatment is not required.

Emergency room radiographic examination of these patients consists of a routine series of skull films. These include the following views: posteroanterior, lateral, Water's, submental vertex view, reverse Towne's view and oblique mandibular views. Lastly, if possible, a panoramic view of the mandible (orthopantomogram (OPG) or Panorex®) is helpful in mandibular fracture evaluation.

Routine computed tomography (CT) scanning provides data in the axial plane only. With the advent of spiral CT scanners, it is now possible to obtain three-dimensional CT films that are reformatted to allow evaluation of facial fractures in the axial, coronal as well as sagittal planes. This augments evaluation and improves definition of the bony anatomy to allow more accurate fracture diagnosis, treatment planning and finally, outcome analysis.

Classification and Features of Facial Fractures

Facial fractures can broadly be grouped according to their anatomic location. The face can be divided into the upper, middle and lower thirds. The bony components of the upper face include the frontal sinuses medially, and the lateral frontal-temporal supraorbital segments. The middle face consists of the naso-ethmoid orbital region, maxilla and maxillary alveolus centrally, and the orbito-zygomatic complexes laterally. The lower face includes the mandible and its alveolar process. The features of the above groups of fractures will be briefly characterised.

Frontal sinus fractures

These injuries are usually the result of high velocity impacts, such as from motor vehicle accidents. They are commonly associated with other injuries, in particular, to the brain and cervical spine. Clinical signs suggestive of frontal sinus fractures include forehead and supraorbital ridge lacerations, which should be probed in a sterile fashion, and palpable bony deformities. In severe injuries where posterior table fractures are associated with dural tears, cerebrospinal fluid rhinorrhea may be observed. Plain radiographs, in particular the lateral and Caldwell views, may show fracture lines or air-fluid levels. High-definition CT scans will allow definitive diagnosis to be made, as the extent of injury to the anterior and posterior walls of the frontal sinus and the fronto-nasal ducts can clearly be identified (Fig. 2).

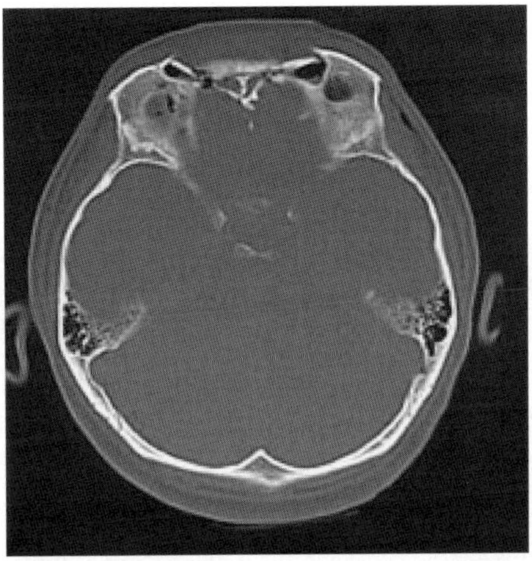

Fig. 2 Frontal sinus fracture. CT scan in axial plane demonstrates fractures of both anterior and posterior walls, with involvement of the fronto-nasal ducts.

Naso-orbito-ethmoid fractures

This fracture pattern should be suspected in cases of central midface trauma. Physical findings include localised ecchymoses, lacerations and oedema in the nasal and periorbital regions, loss of nasal projection and height, and traumatic telecanthus. Palpation may reveal crepitus and bone movement at the nasal bridge and directly over the canthal ligaments. Bimanual palpation, using a blunt-tipped instrument (for example, an artery forceps) placed intranasally against the intranasal portion of the medial orbital rim and with the palpating index finger placed over the medial canthal insertion, may provide useful information about the stability of the central fragment. If naso-orbito-ethmoid fractures are suspected, CT scans are essential.

Orbito-zygomatic fractures

In low-velocity injuries such as a fall or punch to the face, these injuries are usually isolated, whereas in high velocity injuries, associated injuries to other components of the facial skeleton, and to other systems, should be suspected. Clinical examination may reveal facial asymmetry, in particular flattening of the malar eminences (Fig. 3), a palpable bony step along the zygomatic arch or orbital rim, and numbness of the cheek and upper lip. Ocular assessment may reveal

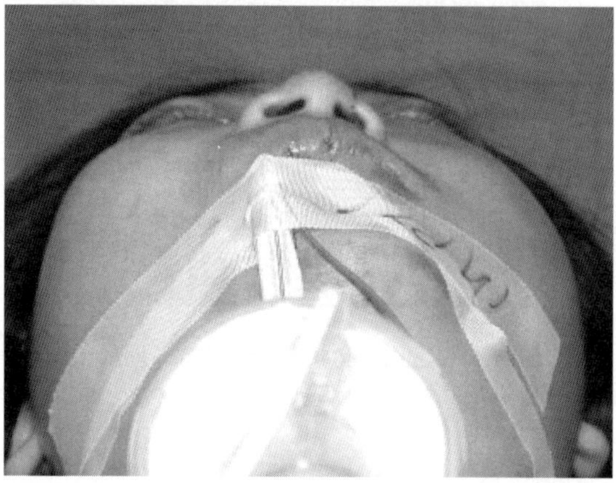

Fig. 3 Left orbito-zygomatic fracture. Depression of the left malar eminence is visible.

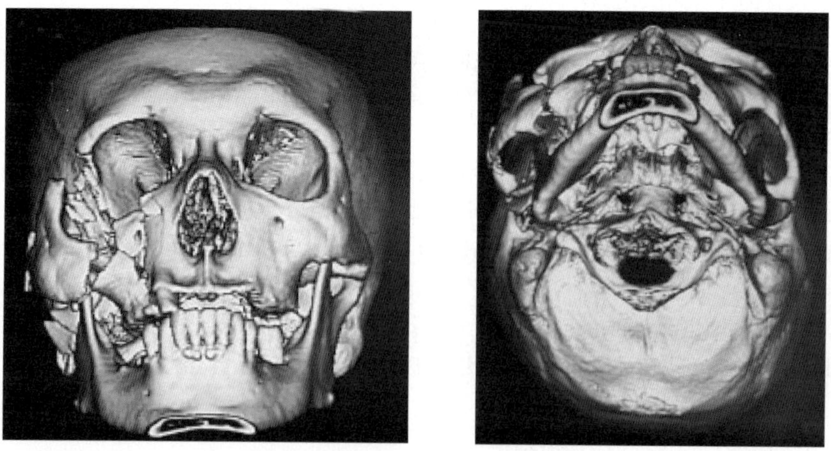

(A) (B)

Figs. 4(A) and (B) Right orbito-zygomatic fracture 3-D reformatted CT scan shows a comminuted, displaced injury with fractures at the 5 articulations of the zygoma with the adjacent craniofacial skeleton, namely the zygomatico-maxillary buttress, inferior orbital rim, zygomaticofrontal suture, sphenozygomatic suture and zygomatic arch.

enophthalmos, diplopia and limitation of extraocular movements. Jaw movement should be assessed to exclude malocclusion, suggesting associated maxillary or mandibular fractures; and trismus, in cases of coronoid process impingement caused by a displaced zygomatic arch.

Plain X-rays providing useful information are the occipito-mental (OM) views, and the submental-vertex (SMV) views. The OM view assesses displacement at the inferior orbital rim and zygomatico-maxillary buttress, while the SMV view allows visualisation of the zygomatic arch. Computed tomography scans (Fig. 4) should be performed for patients in whom clinical evaluation suggests injury to the internal orbit (floor and walls); with comminuted fractures or who had high-velocity injuries, and who are suspected to have injury to other facial bones.

Maxillary fractures

Maxillary fractures are commonly the result of high-velocity injuries, such as motor vehicle accidents. Clinical findings include periorbital haematoma, nasopharyngeal bleeding, intra-oral lacerations and malocclusion, and in particular, an anterior open bite. Mobility of the maxillary dental arch is diagnostic of a maxillary fracture, and may occur at

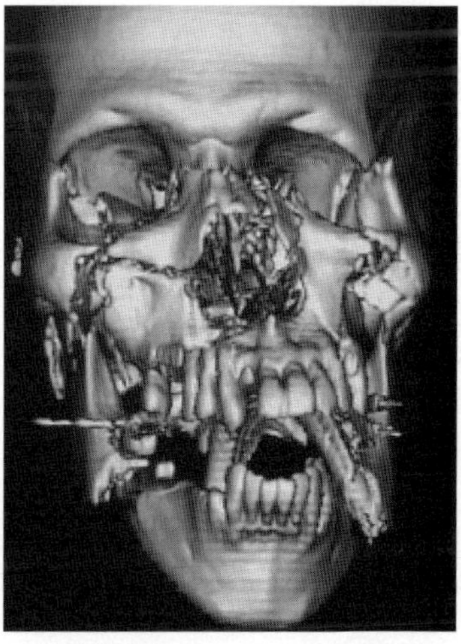

Fig. 5 Severe facial fractures following a motor vehicle accident, with complete disruption of the facial architecture. Complex midface fractures including bilateral LeFort I, II and III fractures.

different levels. In the LeFort I fracture, a tranverse fracture separates the maxillary alveolus at the lower margin of the pyriform aperture. The LeFort II fracture separates a pyramid-shaped central fragment containing the maxillary dentition from the remainder of the orbits and upper craniofacial skeleton. The LeFort III fracture, or craniofacial dysjunction, separates the maxilla at the level of the floor of the orbits and nasoethmoid region. A split palate may be accompanied by a palatal laceration, and excess or differential movement of the maxillary alveolus.

Cerebrospinal fluid rhinorrhea may be observed in LeFort II and III fractures. Computed tomography scans are essential for accurate diagnosis and surgical planning (Fig. 5).

Mandibular fractures

Due to its prominence the mandible is particularly susceptible to trauma and is one of the most commonly fractured facial bones. Common causes include motor vehicle accidents and assaults, and there is a high likelihood of fracture at more than one anatomic site of the mandible.[8] Unlike fractures of the middle and upper face, fractures of the mandible are frequently associated with contamination from oral

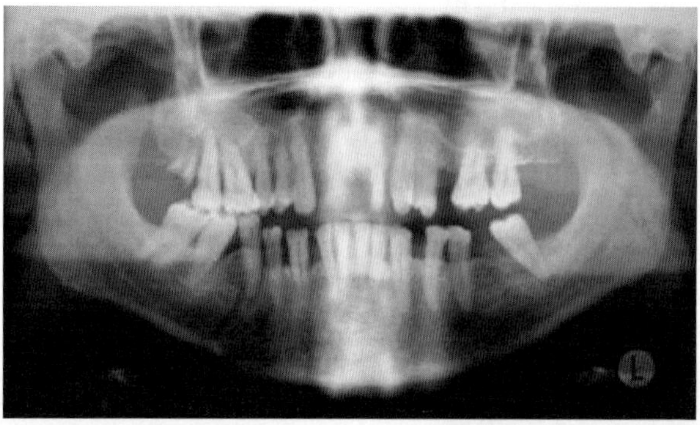

Fig. 6 An orthopantomogram (OPG) demonstrates the entire mandible from condyle to condyle. In this case there is a fracture of the right horizontal ramus (body) and left ascending ramus, following an assault.

secretions. Clinical symptoms and signs suggestive of mandible fractures include pain, swelling, tenderness, external or intraoral lacerations, malocclusion, fractured or missing teeth, gaps, level discrepancies in dentition, and mobility. Plain X-rays that should be obtained include the antero-posterior view and oblique views to visualise the condylar areas. The OPG is the single most useful X-ray (Fig. 6), but requires special dental facilities and patient cooperation. Due to the high likelihood of contamination by intraoral bacteria, antibiotics should routinely be prescribed.

Treatment of Soft Tissue Injuries

With the exception of uncontrolled haemorrhage, most types of soft tissue injuries are not life threatening. Many facial wounds are complex and are compounded by the nature of the anatomy that is disrupted. All facial wounds are potentially contaminated even in the cleanest of environments, and the administration of tetanus toxoid vaccination or as a booster is necessary.

Under adequate anaesthesia (either local or general) adequate toilet of the wound is achieved. The mechanism of injury determines the extent of tissue damage suffered by the wound edges. The management of the facial wound is determined by the quality of the blood supply, the uniqueness of the tissues, the degree of contamination and the timing from injury to repair.

General principles of facial wound repair are:

(1) Sharp debridement of devitalised tissue and of any ragged edges to convert the traumatic wound as much as possible into a fresh surgical wound.
(2) Removal of all dirt and embedded foreign material.
(3) Evacuation of all haematomas and securing of haemostasis.
(4) Careful closure of the wound in layers.
(5) Repair of any injured ducts and or nerves.
(6) Restoration and alignment of normal anatomic landmarks such as lip margins, eyelids, eyebrows, and nostrils.

(7) Even distribution of tension and avoidance of closure under tension.
(8) Eversion of wound edges.
(9) Careful apposition of all skin edges.

The tissues of the face are very unique and are fortunately endowed with good vascularity. As such, marginally perfused wound edges can be preserved to maximise the available tissue for wound closure and reconstruction. Therefore, conservation of these tissues by judicious debridement is imperative. This allows for an ultimately better aesthetic result in the long term.

Loss of tissue, or avulsion injuries, may prevent primary wound closure without distortion of the local anatomy. In these cases, if the defect is small, mobilisation of adjacent tissue, or the use of local flaps, may help achieve primary closure. In cases of moderate to severe tissue loss, the use of skin grafts or regional flaps and or free tissue transfer is a surgical option that is usually performed secondarily.

Any injury to the facial nerve should be identified prior to surgery. The wound should then be explored, the cut ends identified and freshened before primary repair performed under an operating microscope. If there is any nerve gap that cannot be bridged by mobilisation of the nerve ends, primary nerve grafting should be performed.

The parotid duct runs alongside the buccal branch of the facial nerve. Therefore, buccal branch paralysis should highlight the possibility of associated parotid duct injury. All lacerations of the parotid duct must also be identified in the wound, the duct stented and primarily repaired under the operating microscope. The stent is then removed per-orally after two to three weeks.

Lacerations near the medial canthus may also sever the lacrimal system. The duct ends can be identified by irrigating the wound with saline. This causes the cut end of the duct to dilate and become identifiable. The cut ends of the duct are intubated with fine silastic tubing with one free end extruding into the nasal cavity. Repair of the duct is performed over the tubing. The stent is then removed after two to three weeks.

Management of Craniofacial Fractures

The goal in the management of the patient with facial fractures is to re-establish the projection, height, and width of the facial structures.[9] Surgical treatment is usually performed at the earliest possible time, once the patient is stabilised and radiographic examination is complete. In cases where surgery is to be delayed for medical reasons, soft tissue lacerations are repaired first in order to minimise facial scarring.

Facial photographs, preferably with the patient smiling, will allow the surgeon to appreciate the facial symmetry and skeletal proportions prior to surgical reduction. In addition, the photographs enable the identification of the premorbid occlusal relationship, and the existence of any pre-existing telecanthus, or other facial anomalies of the patient.

Surgical planning includes the placement of incisions for access and exposure of the underlying facial fracture. Co-existing facial lacerations are often useful for fracture exposure. The common surgical approaches include transconjunctival or subciliary, coronal, maxillary and or mandibular buccal sulcus. In addition, a variety of submandibular or retromandibular incisions may be used. From a combination of these incisions, the entire facial skeleton can be exposed and any facial fracture anatomically reduced under direct vision for rigid fixation (Fig. 7).

Several basic dentoskeletal relationships must be established to restore aesthetic and functional facial balance and harmony. These are (1) the anteroposterior (AP) relationship between the midface and the base of skull; (2) the occlusal relationship between the teeth of the maxilla and the mandible; and (3) the vertical distance (midface height) between the maxillary dentoalveolar arch and the inferior orbital rims.

Different sequences of reduction and stabilisation of multiple facial fractures have been proposed. The central zone concept advocates that

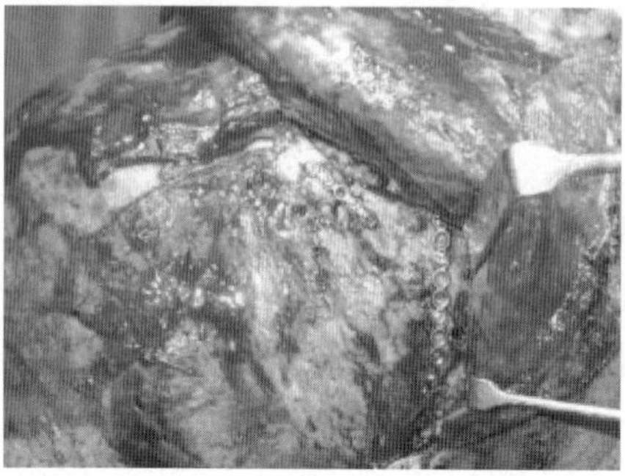

(A)

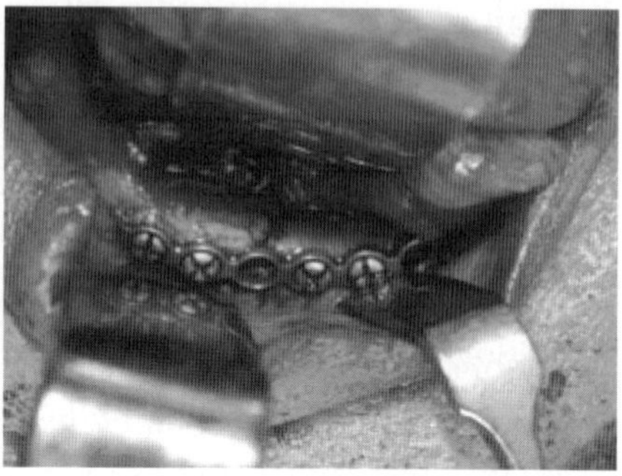

(B)

Figs. 7(A) and (B) Surgical exposure of the craniofacial skeleton for fracture reduction and fixation. **(A)** The coronal approach allows exposure of the upper and middle facial skeleton, including the frontal and supraorbital regions, the orbit and zygomatic arch. In this case, fractures of the zygomatic arch and frontozygomatic process are exposed and fixed. **(B)** The subciliary approach exposes the inferior, medial and lateral orbital rims and the orbital floor. Here, a fracture of the inferior orbital rim has been exposed and fixed.

stabilisation of fractures is initiated centrally, with regards to the naso-ethmoid region, the maxillary and mandibular alveolus, and the horizontal portion of the mandible.[10–12] Central facial width is established with accurate reduction of the naso-ethmoid area, followed by correct positioning and stabilisation of the zygomas. In the lower face, occlusion is established, followed by reconstruction of the vertical (ramus and condylar) and horizontal units of the mandible. The lower and upper facial units are united at the LeFort I level by plating of the anterior maxillary buttresses.

In contrast, Gruss and colleagues[13–15] have proposed that reconstruction is initiated with reduction and stabilisation of the outer facial frame, using the zygomatic arches as the basic reference point. Accurate reduction of the zygomatic arches results in correct positioning of the zygomatic complexes and re-establishment of the correct facial width and antero-posterior projection. The upper inner facial frame is repaired within this outer frame. Correct midfacial width and projection is established with reduction of the anterior maxillary buttresses.

Occlusion is then restored, followed by reduction and fixation of the horizontal and vertical components of the mandible.

Inter-maxillary fixation with careful attention to the occlusal relationship will restore the pretraumatic occlusal relationship. While reduction and rigid fixation of mandibular fractures is essential for the re-establishment of the dental occlusion, the correction of maxillary dentoalveolar fractures is not dependent on the synchronous reduction and fixation of the accompanying maxillary fractures.

Reconstruction of the naso-maxillary and the zygomatico-maxillary buttresses with rigid fixation and bone grafting, where indicated, will finally restore the pretraumatic midfacial height.[16,17] This is essential especially in cases of bilateral subcondylar fractures that are to be treated conservatively. The reconstitution of the midfacial height coupled with intermaxillary fixation effectively permits the restoration of adequate mandibular height that has been lost due to the subcondylar fractures. Multiple complex craniofacial fractures often are complicated by bony defects in regions where the bone is thin and brittle. The force of the trauma often causes the bone in these regions such as the orbit, anterior maxillary wall, nasal and naso-ethmoid to shatter and thereby lose its strength and continuity. This manifests in herniation of orbital contents or cheek soft tissue into the maxillary antrum with resultant enophthalmos or soft tissue deformities. Primary

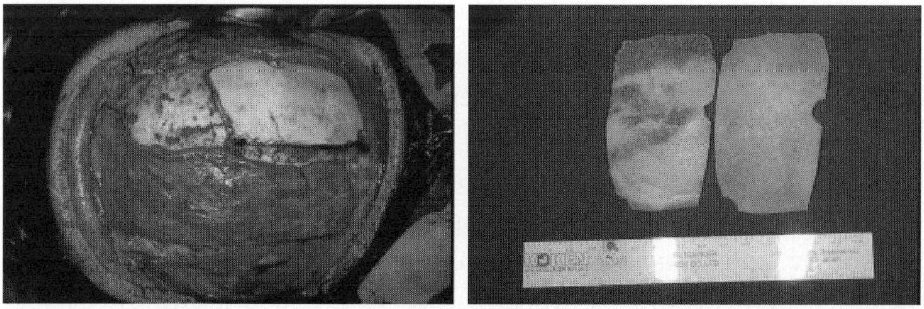

(A) (B)

Figs. 8(A) and (B) Large quantities of split-thickness, monocortical bone can be harvested from the calvarium, with minimal donor site morbidity, for use in primary reconstruction of traumatic defects of the orbits, upper and midface.

bone grafting with split calvarial bone grafts (Fig. 8) can be used to reconstruct such defects immediately.[16] Other surgical options include the use of titanium meshes, resorbable sheets and other alloplasts for reconstruction.

References

1. Haug RH, Prather J, Indresano AT (1990). An epidemiologic survey of facial fractures and concomitant injuries. *J Oral Maxillofac Surg* **48**(9), 926–932.
2. Lim LH, Lam LK, Moore MH, Trott JA, David DJ (1993). Associated injuries in facial fractures: review of 839 patients. *Br J Plast Surg* **46**(8), 635–638.
3. Davidoff G, Jakubowski M, Thomas D, Alpert M (1988). The spectrum of closed-head injuries in facial trauma victims: incidence and impact. *Ann Emerg Med* **17**(1), 6–9.
4. Slupchynskyj OS, Berkower AS, Byrne DW, Cayten CG (1992). Association of skull base and facial fractures. *Laryngoscope* **102**(11), 1247–1250.
5. Davidson JS, Birdsell DC (1989). Cervical spine injury in patients with facial skeletal trauma. *J Trauma* **29**(9), 1276–1278.
6. Jabaley ME, Lerman M, Sanders HJ (1975). Ocular injuries in orbital fractures. A review of 119 cases. *Plast Reconstr Surg* **56**(4), 410–418.
7. Gossman MD, Roberts DM, Barr CC (1992). Ophthalmic aspects of orbital injury. A comprehensive diagnostic and management approach. *Clin Plast Surg* **19**(1), 71–85.
8. Tay AG, Yeow VK, Tan BK, Sng K, Huang MH, Foo CL (1999). A review of mandibular fractures in a craniomaxillofacial trauma centre. *Ann Acad Med Singapore* **28**(5), 630–633.
9. Manson PN, Clark N, Robertson B, Slezak S, Wheatly M, Vander Kolk C, Iliff N (1999). Subunit principles in midface fractures: the importance of sagittal buttresses, soft-tissue reductions, and sequencing treatment of segmental fractures. *Plast Reconstr Surg* **103**(4), 1287–1306.

10. Markowitz BL, Manson PN (1989). Panfacial fractures: organisation of treatment. *Clin Plast Surg* **16**(1), 105–114.
11. Kelly KJ, Manson PN, Vander Kolk CA, Markowitz BL, Dunham CM, Rumley TO, Crawley WA (1990). Sequencing LeFort fracture treatment (Organisation of treatment for a panfacial fracture). *J Craniofac Surg* **1**(4), 168–178.
12. Manson PN, Clark N, Robertson B, Crawley WA (1995). Comprehensive management of pan-facial fractures. *J Craniomaxillofac Trauma* **1**(1), 43–56.
13. Gruss JS, Phillips JH (1989). Complex facial trauma: the evolving role of rigid fixation and immediate bone graft reconstruction. *Clin Plast Surg* **16**(1), 93–104.
14. Gruss JS, Van Wyck L, Phillips JH, Antonyshyn O (1990). The importance of the zygomatic arch in complex midfacial fracture repair and correction of posttraumatic orbitozygomatic deformities. *Plast Reconstr Surg* **85**(6), 878–890.
15. Gruss JS, Bubak PJ, Egbert MA (1992). Craniofacial fractures. An algorithm to optimise results. *Clin Plast Surg* **19**(1), 195–206.
16. Gruss JS, Mackinnon SE, Kassel EE, Cooper PW (1985). The role of primary bone grafting in complex craniomaxillofacial trauma. *Plast Reconstr Surg* **75**(1), 17–24.
17. Gruss JS, Mackinnon SE (1986). Complex maxillary fractures: role of buttress reconstruction and immediate bone grafts. *Plast Reconstr Surg* **78**(1), 9–22.

5

Emergencies in Oral and Maxillofacial Surgery

Asher Lim
Luan-Yook Teh

Introduction

It is common for the Emergency Department to handle problems related to the face and oral cavity. The patients may present in the Emergency Room with oro-facial pain, swelling or injuries due to trauma or infection. The oro-facial problem or condition may be the sole complaint or part of a multisystem involvement, as in trauma or systemic disease conditions.

Triage of Patients

Triage of these patients must be based on the chief complaint, regardless of whether there is profuse haemorrhage and whether the airway and circulation are compromised. During triage, the patient may be categorised as emergency, urgent or non-emergency cases.

Emergency cases

This group of patients presents with complaints, vital signs, illness or injury consistent with an acute, potentially life or limb-threatening condition that requires immediate evaluation or treatment to prevent mortality or increased morbidity. For example, patients with maxillofacial fractures may present with airway obstruction or severe haemorrhage. Patients with Ludwig's angina associated with an odontogenic cause may present with respiratory distress.

Urgent category

Patients of this category present with complaints, vital signs, illness, or injury consistent with an acute, potentially life or limb-threatening condition requiring evaluation or treatment within a few hours to prevent mortality or increased morbidity. For example, patients with oro-facial infections and deep fascial space infection in the head and neck region may progress to develop respiratory distress if not treated early.

Non-emergency category

Patients present with complaints, vital signs, illness, or injury consistent with a subacute or chronic and not life or limb-threatening condition that does not require evaluation or management within 24 hours to prevent increased morbidity.

Oral and Maxillofacial Trauma

Oro-facial trauma may be categorised into:

(1) Fractures of the mandible and the mid-face skeleton.
(2) Dento-alveolar injuries.
(3) Oro-facial soft tissue injuries. (Only the management of hard tissue injuries will be described in this chapter.)

Fractures of the Mandible and the Mid-face Skeleton

The management of trauma involving the maxillofacial region is always challenging and demanding. The ABCs of resuscitation must be strictly adhered to in the preliminary assessment and management of a patient with maxillofacial trauma.

Patients who have sustained mandibular fractures may develop associated airway obstruction because of the presence of blood and debris, or the loss of tongue support resulting from the mandibular fractures. In an unconscious patient, the tongue may have fallen back, obstructing the oropharynx. The backward displacement of the tongue may be associated with unfavourable bilateral fractures of the body or symphysis of the mandible; or with comminuted fractures of the mandible.

If an unstable neck injury has not been excluded, lifting the mandible forward using the chin-lift or jaw thrust manoeuvers, together with the insertion of an oral airway, may relieve the airway obstruction. Patency of the airway may also be restored by placement of a mattress suture or a towel clip through the tongue, and applying gentle forward traction; or by pulling the fractured jaw segments forward. Wiring of the badly displaced fracture fragments may be done to temporarily immobilise the fracture fragments.

In patients with maxillary LeFort I, II or III fractures, the fractured maxilla may be displaced downward and posteriorly, causing impingement of the soft palate against the pharyngeal wall. This can compromise the airway. Airway obstruction can be relieved by using fingers to reach behind the hard palate and pulling the fractured maxilla forward and upward. This action may also be achieved by tying wires around the teeth to allow the maxilla to be pulled forward and upward.

The presence of foreign bodies, debris, tooth fragments and blood in the oral cavity can compromise the airway and should be removed by applying gentle sweeping movements with a finger or by suction. Broken dentures, avulsed or fractured teeth should be kept, as subsequent reconstitution of a whole denture or tooth may rule out the possibility of inhaled fragments. If missing teeth or an oral prosthesis is not accounted for, a chest radiograph is imperative to exclude pulmonary aspiration.

Blood may accumulate rapidly at the pharynx, due to bleeding from the fractured oro-facial bone or soft tissue lacerations. Suction is used to help locate any bleeding point that may be amenable to pressure packing or ligation of the bleeding vessel. Temporary wiring of badly displaced fracture fragments may help to control haemorrhage at the fracture site. In cases where haemorrhage persists, and the airway is threatened, endotracheal intubation should be attempted by a competent operator.

After the patient's airway is secured and bleeding controlled and cervical spinal cord injuries have been excluded, the maxillofacial region is then evaluated for injuries. Whenever possible, the events relating to the injury should be elicited as they provide clues to the type of injuries. Clinical evaluation should be sequential and organised, from "top-down and inside-out". The maxillofacial examination must include the following components: skeletal and soft tissue, and the dentition.

Mid-facial trauma involving the orbital region requires thorough examination as early management to avoid visual impairment is crucial in some cases. A thorough ocular examination should be performed. Any abnormal or equivocal findings should prompt an ophthalmological consultation. Injuries that cause "bleeding behind the eye", such as intraconal bleeding can cause anterior ischaemic optic neuropathy and retrobulbar haemorrhage can result in blindness. Patients with retrobulbar haemorrhage may present with proptosis, a tense globe, marked chemosis, ophthalmoplegia, dilated pupil, loss of direct pupil reflex, retention of consensual light reflex, pain in the eye, and deteriorating vision or blindness. Surgical decompression is mandatory. Lateral canthotomy, a simple and quick maneuver can help to relieve some of the intraocular pressure. Local anaesthetic solution is injected into the region of the lateral canthal tendon. Using a pair of small sharp scissors, dissect towards the lateral orbital rim and the lateral canthal tendon is then snipped.

Fractures of the malar complex and orbital bone that do not threaten blindness do not need immediate treatment even though these are usually associated with severe periorbital oedema, chemosis, and sub-cojunctival haemorrhage.

Early definitive treatment of maxillofacial fractures is required in the following situations to reduce morbidity: (i) when there is uncontrolled bleeding from the fracture site (Fig. 1), (ii) when the displaced

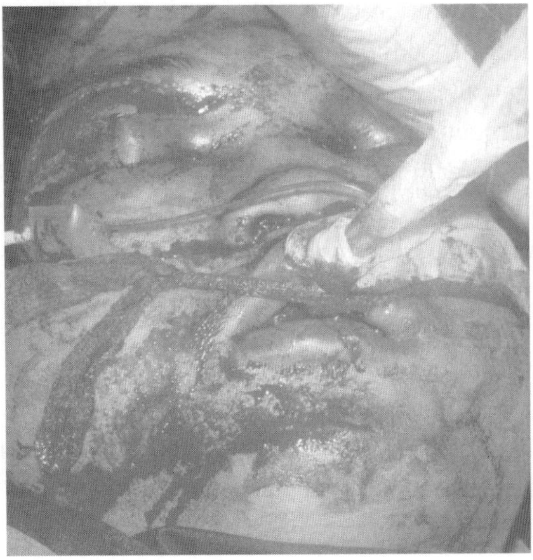

Fig. 1 Uncontrolled haemorrhage associated with maxillo-mandibular fractures.

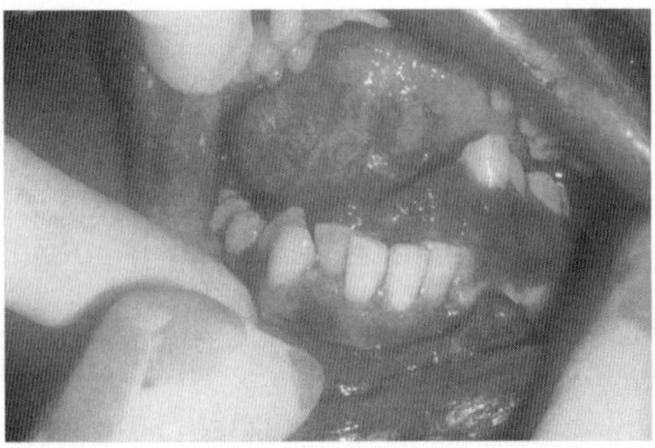

Fig. 2 Compound mandibular fracture with severely displaced segments interfering with occlusion.

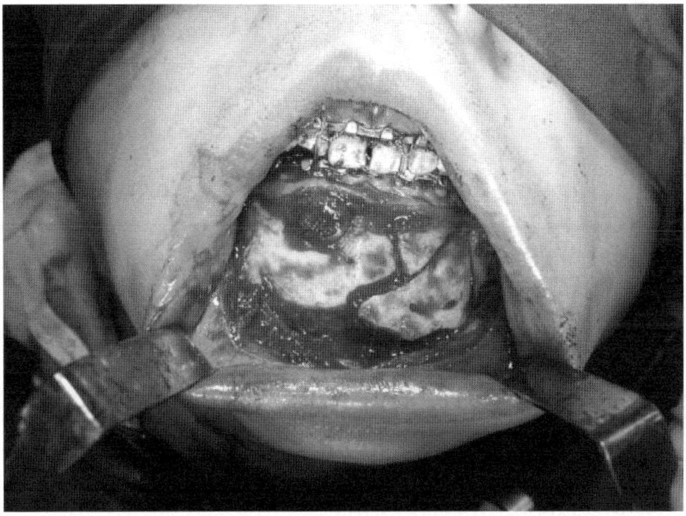

Fig. 3 Compound and comminuted fractures of the mandibular requiring early treatment.

fractured jaw segments interfere with the airway or occlusion (Fig. 2), (iii) when the fracture sustained is compound (Figs. 2 and 3), and (iv) when there is severe paraesthesia resulting from nerve injury associated with the fractures. Treatment of maxillofacial fractures is by reduction, immobilisation and fixation of the fractures.

Dento-alveolar injuries

Dento-alveolar injuries are injuries involving the alveolar bone (the teeth-supporting bone) or the teeth. Dento-alveolar fractures require urgent treatment as delayed management will increase morbidity, due to loss of the alveolar bone and teeth. Dento-alveolar fractures may be isolated or part of a jaw fracture. Derangement in occlusion, displaced teeth and laceration of the overlying mucosa are some of the signs of dento-alveolar fracture. Palpation of the alveolus is done to elicit the presence of bony step deformity or crepitus. Radiographic examination including the orthopantomogram (OPG) and occlusal radiographs provides valuable information.

Types of dento-alveolar injuries

This classification of dento-alveolar injuries was first developed by the World Health Organization (WHO) in 1978 and modified by Andreason.[1]

(1) Fractured teeth

Crown fractures: Uncomplicated — involving only enamel or enamel and dentine.
Complicated — involving enamel, dentine and pulp.

Crown/root fractures: Uncomplicated — not involving pulp.
Complicated — involving pulp.

(2) Non-displacement injuries of teeth

Concussion injuries: The tooth is not displaced from its normal position, is not mobile, and is very sensitive on percussion.

Subluxation injuries: Evidence of abnormal tooth mobility but there is no evidence of displacement.

(3) Displacement injuries of teeth

Displaced or dislocated teeth from their socket can be classified as follows:

Extrusive luxation or partial avulsion
Intrusive luxation
Lateral luxation
Complete luxation

(4) Alveolar bone fracture

Comminuted fractures of the alveolar bone.

Fractures of the buccal or lingual plates of the alveolar process.

Fractures of the alveolar process, resulting in mobility of an entire segment of teeth and bone.

Dento-alveolar bone fracture associated with fractures of the maxillary and/or mandibular bone.

Table 1 Time to Treat to Reduce Morbidity

Type of Injury	Time to Treat Within
Complicated crown fractures	3 hours
Uncomplicated crown fractures with exposed dentine	48 hours
Complete luxation (avulsion)	1 hour
Alveolar bone fracture	1 hour

Management of dento-alveolar injuries

The prognosis of the injured dento-alveolar components depends on the amount of time that has elapsed from the injury to the time of definitive treatment. Dento-alveolar injuries involving tooth crown fractures with pulp exposed, complete luxation (avulsion) of teeth and alveolar bone fracture, all require urgent treatment. Table 1 shows the "time to treat" to reduce morbidity.

(1) Management of fractured teeth

Complicated crown fractures may be evident when there is bleeding from the pulp chamber of the teeth. Bacterial contamination of the pulp can result in part or all of the pulp becoming necrotic. It has been found that when dental treatment is instituted within the first three hours of the pulp exposure, the extent of pathologic pulpal changes can be limited to the first 2 mm of the pulp, thereby possibly sparing the patient from the necessity of root canal therapy.[2]

Root fractures of teeth are best detected by clinical examination and confirmed with dental radiographs. The crown of the tooth may be mobile when the fracture is near the coronal third of the root. However, when the root fracture is in the middle third or apical third, there may be no increase in mobility. Percussion or pressure applied on these teeth may elicit severe pain. Bleeding from the gingivae may be suggestive of a root fracture.

Extraction of teeth is recommended when the root fracture involves the coronal or middle third of the root. Apical third root fracture is managed by splinting of the fractured tooth/teeth to the adjacent non-fractured teeth after repositioning the tooth to its normal position. A rigid splint using only composite or wires with composite is placed for a period of two to three months. Between 20% to 44% of the teeth with root fractures require endodontic treatment and between 22% to 60% undergo root resorption.[3]

In primary teeth, no treatment is recommended for apical third root fracture because the coronal two thirds are usually stable. For coronal third root fracture in primary teeth, extraction of the crown with the coronal third root is recommended and the apical portion of the root is left to resorb.

(2) Management of displaced teeth

Extrusive and lateral luxation of permanent teeth will require re-positioning of the teeth to their normal position before a non-rigid splint is placed. The splint is left *in situ* for about two to three weeks. Extruded or laterally displaced primary teeth that are mobile or interfere with occlusion are extracted to avoid damage to the permanent dentition.

The management of intruded teeth depends on the degree of root formation and the severity of intrusion. Intruded teeth usually do not increase in mobility. If the root formation is incomplete, no treatment is required. Generally, the teeth will re-erupt in 1 to 2 months' time. Intruded teeth with closed apices that are firm do not require immediate treatment.

For intruded teeth associated with dento-alveolar fracture, re-positioning with splinting of teeth/alveolar bone is done. In cases of severely intruded teeth associated with comminuted dento-alveolar fracture, extraction of the involved teeth is recommended.

The prognosis of a completely luxated tooth is highly dependent on the time that had elapsed prior to the tooth receiving definitive treatment. When a patient presents with a traumatic tooth avulsion in the Emergency Department, a dental surgeon is to be called at the earliest possible moment. Every effort should be made to re-implant the tooth within the first 15 to 20 minutes from the time of avulsion to maximise successful re-implantation[3] (Figs. 4A and B). While waiting for the tooth to be re-implanted, the tooth should be stored in

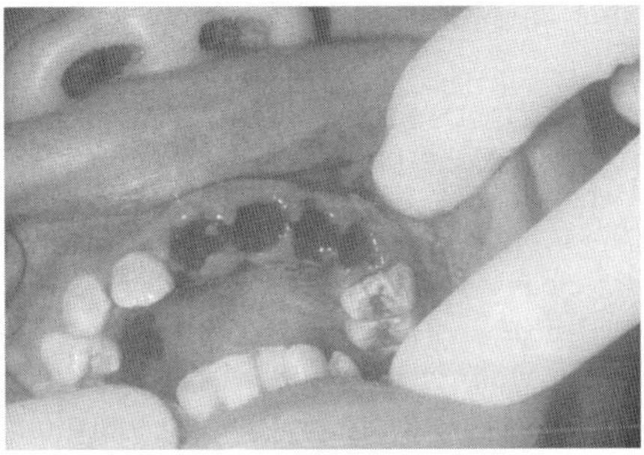

Fig. 4A Avulsion of teeth due to trauma.

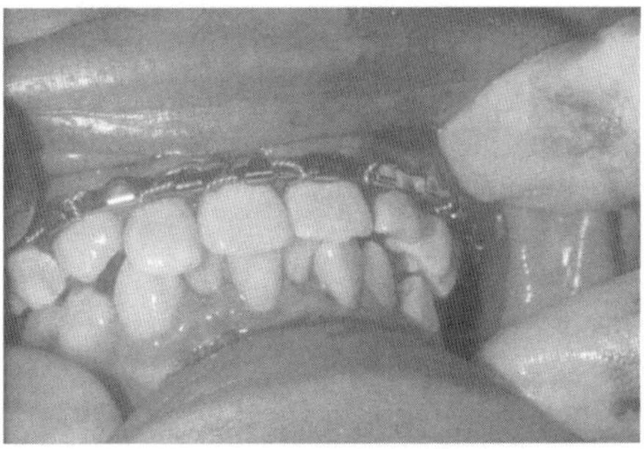

Fig. 4B Early re-implantation and splinting of avulsed teeth.

an appropriate medium. Suggested media in order of preference are fresh milk, saliva (either in the vestibule of the mouth or in a container into which the patient spits), physiologic saline or water. Hank's Balanced Salt Solution (HBSS), a cell culture medium in special transport containers, has shown superior ability to maintain the viability of the periodontal ligament on the avulsed tooth for an extended period.[4] However, the Hank's solution is generally not available at the site of the accident/injury. Table 2 provides a summary of the management of avulsed teeth.

(3) Management of alveolar bone fracture

Alveolar bone fracture can be divided into the following categories:

Table 2 Management of an Avulsed Tooth

Time Lapse from Injury to Treatment	Tooth with Closed Root Apex	Tooth with Open Root Apex
Less than 60 minutes	The tooth socket and root surface are cleansed with saline. If there is a displaced fracture of the socket wall, reposition it with a suitable instrument. Tooth is re-implanted followed by semi-rigid splinting for 7 to 10 days.	Cleanse the tooth and the socket with saline. Soak the tooth in doxycycline for 5 minutes. Examine the tooth socket. If there is a displaced fracture of the socket wall, reposition it with a suitable instrument. The tooth is re-implanted gently followed by semi-rigid splinting for 7 to 10 days.
More than 60 minutes	Remove the periodontal ligament. Cleanse the socket with saline. If there is fracture of socket wall, reposition it with a suitable instrument. Immerse the tooth in 2.4% sodium fluoride solution acidulated to a pH 5.5 for 5 minutes. If possible, perform root canal treatment before re-implantation. Semi-rigid splint is placed for 7 to 10 days.	Re-implantation is not recommended.

- Comminuted fractures of the alveolar bone
- Fractures of the buccal or lingual plate of the alveolar process
- Fractures of the alveolar process, resulting in mobility of an entire segment of teeth and bone
- Dento-alveolar bone fractures associated with fractures of the maxilla and/or mandible

Dento-alveolar fractures usually present with associated gingival injuries. The fracture is reduced by manually repositioning the involved teeth and alveolar bone segment to the proper arch alignment and applying a rigid splint for about six to eight weeks to allow bone healing. Surgical reduction is necessary when segments cannot be properly re-aligned manually. This can be done under local or general anaesthesia.

In comminuted alveolar bone fracture, removal of the crushed alveolar bone and re-contouring of the intact alveolar bone, together with the extraction of the associated teeth may be necessary. Complications associated with alveolar bone fractures include development of pulp necrosis of the involved teeth (75%), development of root resorption of the involved teeth (11%), and loss of marginal bone support of involved teeth (13%). Studies have shown that complications are more likely to develop when fracture reduction and splinting are delayed beyond one hour from time of injury.[1] Thus treatment of dento-alveolar fracture must be provided at the earliest possible time to reduce patient suffering, pain, loss of teeth and its associated morbidity and expense.

Odontogenic Infections

Odontogenic infection is defined as infection originating from the tooth. It is one of the most common causes of infection involving the deep fascial planes of the head and neck.[5]

Odontogenic infections may arise from a carious tooth, a periodontally involved tooth, a dental cyst, an odontogenic tumour, or following an oral-surgical procedure. Infection from the tooth may spread beyond the root apex and its supporting tissue, the gingivae and periodontal ligament, into the alveolar process of the maxilla or mandible. The bacteria and inflammation can propagate and spread through the medullary spaces until the cortical plate of the jaw bone is reached and eventually perforated. The spread of infection is along the path of least resistance, following the anatomical fascial planes. Odontogenic infection can track deeply into the head and neck fascial spaces. The pathways for the spread of infection into surrounding deep fascial spaces are illustrated in Fig. 5.

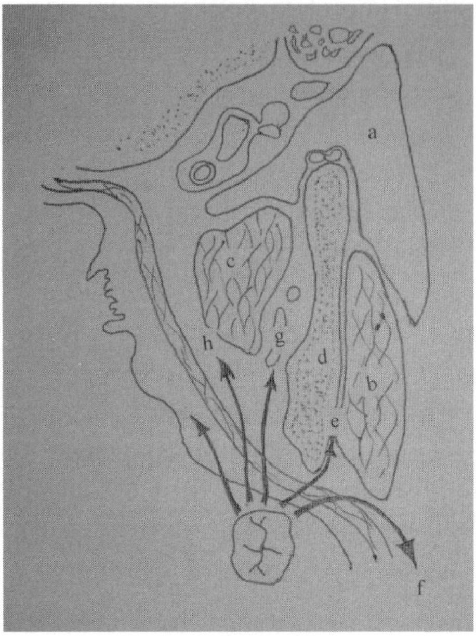

Fig. 5 Pathways of spread of odontogenic infections to deep fascial spaces in the head and neck region: (a) parotid gland, (b) masseteric muscle, (c) medial pterygoid muscle, (d) ramus of mandible, (e) submasseteric space, (f) to buccal space, (g) to pterygomandibular space, and (h) to pharyngeal space.

When a patient presents with a painful swelling of the face and neck, the emergency physician must have a high index of suspicion for an odontogenic infection. Deep fascial space infections of the head and neck can quickly progress to threaten and obstruct the airway. Thus, timely consultation with a dental surgeon or an oral and maxillo-facial surgeon can be life-saving.

A careful examination of the head and neck is done to locate the cause of swelling and to see if there is any difficulty in breathing. Infection in the pharyngeal, pterygo-mandibular, sublingual or submandibular spaces may threaten the airway. Breathing difficulty that worsens by the hour indicates the need for emergency intervention. It is also important to ask if there is any dysphagia. A history of dysphagia is suggestive of swelling/oedema around the oro-pharyngeal region.

The examiner should inspect for swelling in the mouth and investigate the cause of the infection — a carious or broken tooth, root stumps, or periodontal disease. Pericoronitis (inflammation of the soft

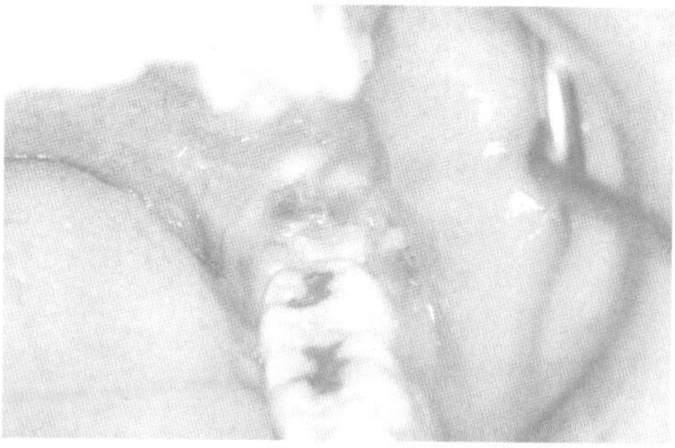

Fig. 6 Pericoronitis associated with the lower left wisdom tooth.

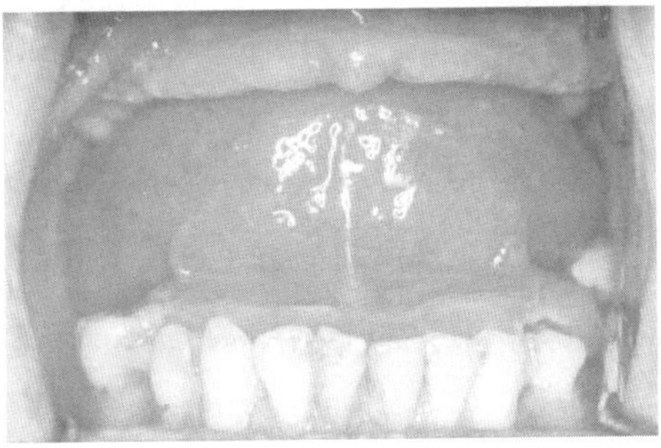

Fig, 7 Sublingual space infection causing the floor of mouth and tongue to be raised.

tissue covering the crown of a partially erupted tooth) is one of the most common causes of odontogenic infection. It is common to have pus exuding from the pocket between the soft tissue and the tooth. The lower third molar is the tooth most commonly involved (Fig. 6). The presence of trismus may hinder intra-oral examination.

In sublingual-space infections, the floor of mouth and tongue may be raised (Fig. 7). In pterygomandibular space or lateral pharyngeal space infection, the uvula can deviate to the contralateral side, and the anterior tonsillar pillar on the affected side is swollen, tender and red.

Computer tomography (CT) provides accurate evaluation of head and neck fascial space infection (Fig. 8). Contrast-enhanced CT has

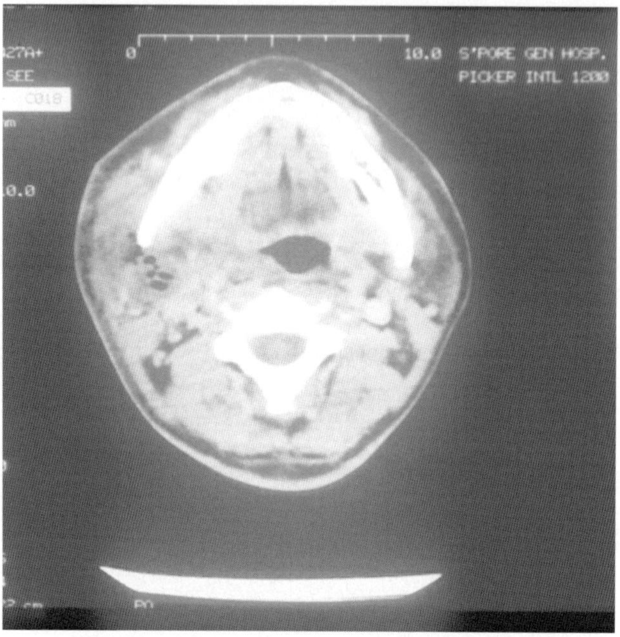

Fig. 8 Computer tomography showing pus collections in the submasseteric and submandibular spaces.

become the imaging modality of choice for head and neck deep fascial space infection because CT scans can precisely localise the site of pus collection. If CT is not available, plain X-ray films are the next best option. Postero-anterior and lateral soft tissue radiographs of the neck may reveal significant swelling or oedema in the oro-pharyngeal region, suggestive of airway obstruction. The soft tissue thickness of the retropharyngeal tissue over the second cervical vertebra and the sixth cervical vertebra on a lateral soft tissue radiograph of the neck should be 6 mm or less and 20 mm or less respectively.[6] An increase of the soft tissue thickness indicates presence of retropharyngeal swelling and a potential threat to the airway. An orthopantomogram is a highly valuable X-ray of the jaws as it can help to rapidly identify the underlying pathology associated with the infection (Fig. 9).

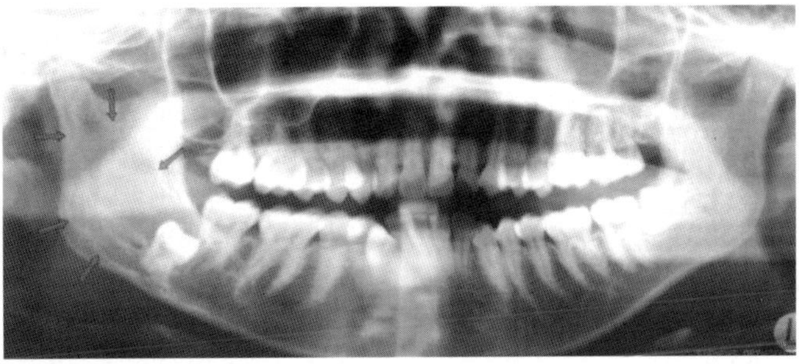

Fig. 9 Orthopantomogram of a patient who presented with buccal and submasseteric space infections associated with a keratocyst of her right angle and ramus of mandible.

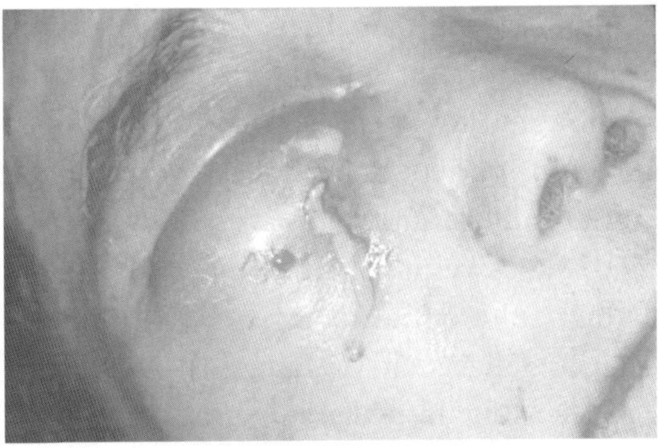

Fig. 10 Periorbital abscess of odontogenic origin — incision and drainage of pus done.

Management of odontogenic infection

The treatment of odontogenic infection includes incision and drainage of pus (Fig. 10), removal of the causative agent, and supportive measures such as antimicrobial therapy, pain relief and fluid replacement if necessary.

Odontogenic infections causing severe swelling involving the pharyngeal wall, the sublingual and submandibular spaces can compromise the airway. Early treatment is important to prevent airway obstruction. In patients who are likely to have complete airway obstruction, endotracheal intubation with or without the aid of fibre-optic scope, cricothyroidotomy or tracheostomy may be required. Factors to be taken into consideration in the management of the airway are:

- The presence of trismus that may limit transoral intubation
- The need to maintain the protective airway reflexes during intubation
- The possibility that the passage of an endotracheal tube could cause a distended abscess to rupture into the airway
- The need to quickly establish an effective seal against potential aspiration of infected material

Incision and drainage of the abscess can be done under local or general anaesthesia, preferably general anaesthesia when deep spaces are involved. Incision and drainage is done at the point where swelling is most fluctuant and gravity-dependent. Two specimens should be taken for a bacterial culture and sensitivity test. A broad area of skin over the portion of the swelling that is most likely to produce pus is prepared with iodine solution. After one to two minutes, the iodine is removed using sterile gauze. An 18-gauge or larger bore needle is then advanced through the skin into the infection site, and pus or cellular fluid is aspirated. The aspirate is sent for aerobic and anaerobic culture. The deep infected space may be reached using a pair of sinus forceps to establish drainage following incision. Saline irrigation of the infected space is done to remove necrotic tissue and to reduce the bacteria count. Drains may be inserted and secured with suture.

Brooke *et al.*[7] found that 50% of odontogenic deep fascial space infections yielded only anaerobic bacteria, whereas 44% yielded a mixed aerobic and anaerobic flora.[7] Only 6% of their cases yielded a pure culture of aerobic bacteria. Sakamoto *et al.*[8] showed that odontogenic infections usually result from a synergistic interaction among several bacterial species, usually consisting of streptococcus and anaerobic gram-negative rods.[8]

The antimicrobials of choice for the treatment of odontogenic infections are intravenous penicillin and metronidazole or oral amoxycillin

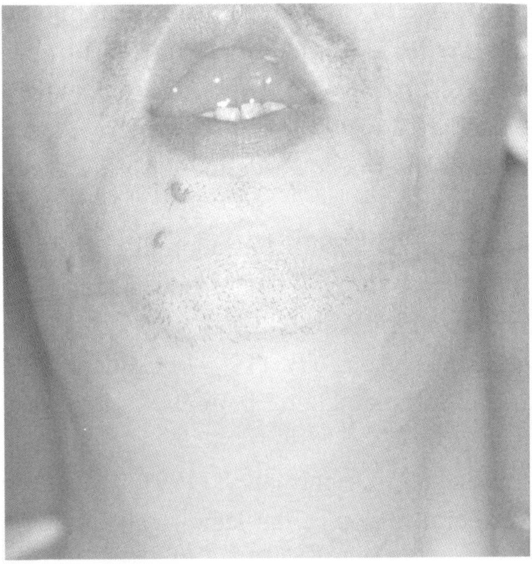

Fig. 11 Ludwig's angina involving the submandibular, sublingual and submental spaces (bilateral).

and metronidazole. These should be given while awaiting the bacteriological report.

There have been reported cases of complications and mortality associated with odontogenic infection. Ludwig's angina (Fig. 11) and descending necrotising mediastinitis may be life-threatening. Cavernous sinus thrombosis, brain abscess and orbital abscess may arise from infection from the oro-maxillary region, resulting in severe morbidity. It is thus important to treat severe odontogenic infections as an emergency or urgent case.

References

1. Andreason JO, Andreason FM (1994). Classification, etiology and epidemiology. In *Textbook and Color Atlas of Traumatic Injuries to the Teeth*, 3rd Ed. Andreason JO, Andreason FM (eds.) Copenhagen: Munksgaard.

2. Cvek M (1978). A clinical report on partial pulpotomy and capping with calcium hydroxide in permanent incisors with complicated crown fracture. *J Endod* **4**, 232.
3. Barrett EJ, Kenny DJ (1997). Avulsed permanent teeth: a review of the literature and treatment guidelines. *Endod Dent Traumatol* **13**, 153–163.
4. Trope M, Friedman S (1992). Periodontal healing of replanted dog teeth stored in Viaspan; milk and Hank's Balanced Salt Solution. *Endod Dent Traumatol* **8**, 183–188.
5. Biederman GR, Dodson TB (1994). Epidemiological review of facial infections in hospitalized patients. *J Oral Maxillofacial Surg* **52**, 1042.
6. Hang RH, Wible RT, Lieberman J (1991). Measurement standards for the prevertebral region in the lateral soft tissue radiograph of the neck. *J Oral Maxillofac Surg* **49**, 1149.
7. Brooke I, Frazier EH, Gher ME (1991). Aerobic and anaerobic microbiology of periapical abscess. *Oral Microbial Immunol* **6**, 123.
8. Sakamoto H, Kato H, Sato T (1998). Semiquantitative bacteriology of closed odontogenic abscesses. *Bull Tokyo Dent Coll* **39**, 103.

Section II

Otorhinolaryngological Emergencies

6

Management of Epistaxis

Dharambir S Sethi
Jern-Lin Leong

Introduction

Epistaxis is one of the common presenting complaints in otorhinolaryngology practice. The incidence of epistaxis in the general population may be difficult to determine, as the majority of episodes go unreported, resolving with conservative self-management. Most patients seeking medical assistance are treated as outpatients and discharged. A smaller subset of patients may present with a single severe episode that will not stop, or with several persistent recurrences. Others may present with a potentially life-threatening haemorrhage. These patients may require immediate evaluation, identification of the aetiology, and emergent initiation of treatment to avoid hypotension, hypoxia, anaemia, aspiration or death.

Commonly, epistaxis may occur from the vascular plexus on the anterior part of the nasal septum. In geographical regions with low humidity or in air-conditioned environments, dryness and crusting of the nasal mucosa may cause epistaxis. In the majority of these patients bleeding can be controlled with simple measures such as application of manual pressure by pinching the nostrils together.

Epistaxis originating from the posterior portion of the nasal cavity, or patients in whom the bleeding site cannot be identified, may be difficult to manage owing to the site of bleeding, the quantity of blood loss, and often-serious underlying illnesses. This chapter will focus on the management of epistaxis from a pragmatic point of view. Evaluation of the patient with epistaxis, and consideration of appropriate differential diagnosis, as well as underlying aetiologies, will be discussed. Emphasis will be on the emergent management of a patient presenting with exsanguinating epistaxis. Methods of traditional as well as more recent innovative techniques will be reviewed. Detailed specific management of systemic causes of epistaxis, hereditary haemorrhagic telangiectiasia, and foreign bodies in the nasal cavity, have been excluded from this chapter.

Anatomy

An understanding of nasal vascular anatomy is essential to effectively and safely utilise newer technologies. Open surgical procedures, endoscopic evaluation with treatment, and angiographic techniques, all demand an accurate knowledge of endonasal and maxillary anatomy as well as the anatomy of multiple arterial systems supplying the nasal lining and structures.

The nasal cavity is a rich vascular bed, with blood supply originating from the internal and external carotid arteries (Fig. 1). The external carotid serves as the major contributor, and provides blood to the nose primarily through the maxillary artery, and secondarily via the facial artery. The external carotid artery divides and terminates as the superficial temporal artery and the internal maxillary artery. The internal maxillary artery passes deep to the neck of the mandible, through the infratemporal fossa, deep or superficial to the lateral pterygoid muscle. The artery then enters the pterygopalatine fossa inferolaterally via the pterygomaxillary fissure (Fig. 2). Within the pterygopalatine fossa the maxillary artery courses in a serpentine manner within a pad of fat. The maxillary artery and its branches are generally more anterioinferior within the pterygopalatine fossa than the

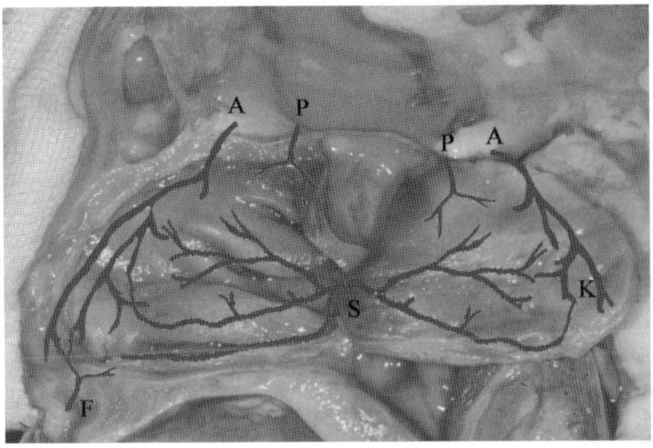

Fig. 1 Blood supply of the lateral nasal nose and nasal septum. A = anterior ethmoid artery, P = posterior ethmoid artery, S = sphenopalatine artery, F = facial artery, and K = Keisselbach's plexus on the nasal septum.

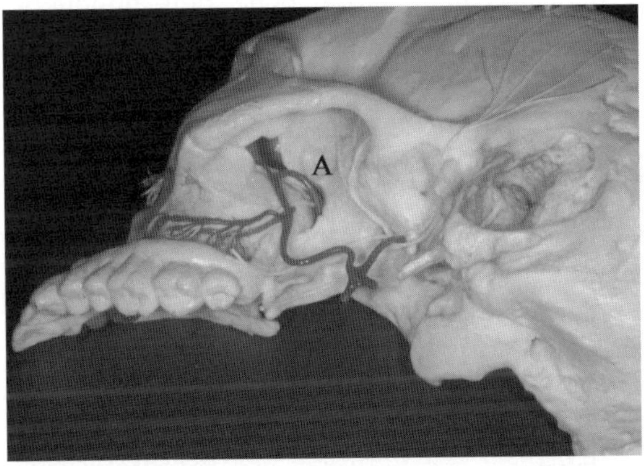

Fig. 2 Internal maxillary artery as it enters the pterygopalatine fossa (A).

maxillary, and vidian nerves form an anatomic point that facilitates maxillary artery ligation for epistaxis. The internal maxillary artery terminates into five branches within the pterygopalatine fossa. These are: posterior-superior alveolar, descending or greater palatine, infraorbital, pharyngeal, and pterygoid canal arteries. The descending palatine artery may have two or three branches, the largest serving as the greater palatine artery of the greater palatine canal. The lesser palatine artery passes through the lesser palatine foramen and supplies blood to the soft palate. The greater palatine artery takes a circuitous course to the nose by first passing inferiorly through the greater palatine canal and foramen, and then travelling within the lateral hard palatal mucosa. The bilateral paired arteries meet anteriorly in the midline, and pass superiorly through the single midline incisive foramen to supply the nasal septum and floor of the nose.

At or distal to the sphenopalatine foramen, the maxillary artery bifurcates into the sphenopalatine and posterior nasal arteries (Fig. 3). The sphenopalatine foramen is oval-shaped with a longer vertical diameter of 6.5 mm (range, 5 to 8 mm) and the shorter horizontal diameter of 4.5 mm (range, 3.0 to 7.0 mm). It is located at the posterior end of the superior meatus (85%) or middle meatus (5%), or bridged by the basilar lamina of the middle turbinate (10%). As the perpendicular plate of the palatine bone runs obliquely from behind forward, the plane of the foramen forms an angle with the sagittal plane ranging from 0° to 30°.

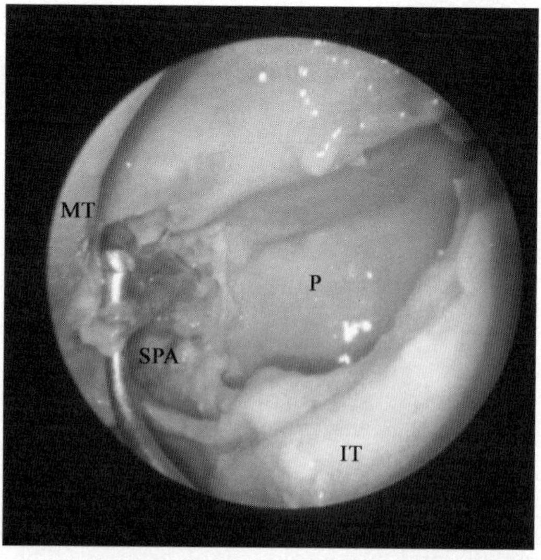

Fig. 3 Endoscopic view of the left sphenopalatine artery as it exits the sphenopalatine foramen in a cadaver specimen. P = posterior wall of the maxillary sinus, IT = inferior turbinate, MT = middle turbinate, and SPA = sphenopalatine artery.

The sphenopalatine artery supplies the septal mucosa and in the region of the anteriorinferior septum anastomoses with the greater palatine artery, the anterior ethmoid artery, and the nasal branch of the facial, thus forming Kiesselbach's plexus or Littles's area. The posterior nasal artery supplies the lateral nasal wall and the turbinates. Superiorly it anastomoses with the ethmoid arteries. Inferiorly it anastomoses with the pharyngeal arteries branches of the maxillary artery, thus forming Woodruff's naso-nasopharyngeal plexus.

The internal carotid artery contributes to the blood supply of the internal nose via the ophthalmic artery. The ophthalmic artery is the first major intracranial branch of the internal carotid artery. It arises just posterior to the optic canal, and enters the optic canal inferior to the optic nerve but within its dural sheath. It exits the dura at the anterior end of the optic canal to enter the bony orbit. Within the orbit, it divides into a number of branches including the anterior and posterior arteries, supplying the superior nasal septum and lateral nasal wall. Both arteries pass through the periorbital fascia through the

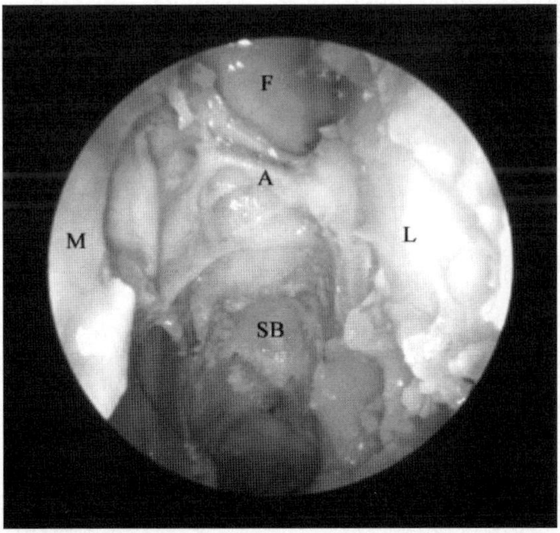

Fig. 4 Endoscopic view of the left anterior ethmoid artery in a cadaver specimen. F = fovea ethmoidalis, L = lamina papyrecea, M = middle turbinate, SB = skull base, and A = anterior ethmoid artery.

shared wall of the medial orbital and the lateral fovea ethmoidalis bone along the frontoethmoidal suture line, at the level coinciding with the cribriform plate (Fig. 4). The posterior ethmoid artery enters the posterior ethmoid foramen. The distance from the optic canal to the posterior ethmoid foramen varies from 2 to 9 mm as noted by Harrison.[1] It is 4 to 7 mm 80% of the time. The anterior ethmoid artery enters the anterior ethmoid foramen 14 to 22 mm posterior to the maxillolacrimal suture more than 80% of the time.[2] The distance of the anterior ethmoid foramen from the optic canal varies from 14 to 35 mm.[3] The distance between the anterior and posterior ethmoidal foramina is also variable. The anterior ethmoid artery is absent 7% to 14% of the time.[2] The posterior ethmoid artery is absent 31% of the time.[2] The anterior and posterior ethmoid vessels pass through ethmoid air cells and give rise to medial and lateral branches. The medial branches of the ethmoid arteries supply the superior septum and Little's area. The lateral branches of the ethmoid arteries supply the superior and middle turbinates.

In summary, nasal cavity vascular anatomy is complex and variable with numerous arterial anatomotic systems, thus explaining in part why treatment failures and late recurrences are common. A greater understanding of vascular anatomy and possible variants will expedite successful treatment in light of increasing endoscopic evaluation and treatment by practising otolaryngologists.

Epidemiology

No local epidemiological data is available. Review of the literature, however, reveals some interesting epidemiological characteristics. A U.S. health examination survey from 1972 of 6672 adults revealed a 7% to 14% incidence of epistaxis.[4] A Scandinivian survey from 1974 of 410 people found a 60% incidence of at least one episode of epistaxis during one's lifetime, a 6% incidence requiring medical attention, and an annual incidence of 15% for men and 9% for women.[5] A Finnish study from 1974 of 1724 patients with epistaxis revealed a higher male incidence of 58% versus 42% for women; overall, 71% of the patients were over 50 years of age.[6]

Aetiology

Epistaxis occurs within the anterior nasal region 90% to 95% of the time.[7] The majority of cases are secondary to manipulation, relatively cold temperatures with low humidity, and/or chronic use of nasal decongestion spray. A single and minor episode of epistaxis with an otherwise normal history and physical examination, does not warrant an extensive evaluation. In contrast, a severe episode or recurring epistaxis should prompt further investigation to rule out some of the aetiologies. The aetiologies may be divided into two broad categories: local and systemic factors.

Local factors

Mechanical or traumatic causes

Trauma is one of the most common causes of epistaxis. Children or adults with habitual digital manipulation have a higher incidence of epistaxis of the anterior cartilaginous nasal septum. Continuous mucosal trauma devitalises the perichondrium with resultant cartilage exposure and perforation. Septal perforation induces turbulence, impairs laminar airflow, and results in drying, scab formation, and subsequent bleeding. Isolated trauma to the nose or in adjacent regions such as the sinuses, orbit, and middle ear may manifest as nasal haemorrhage. Severe life-threatening midface and base-of-skull fractures may result in exsanguinating arterial haemorrhage. Massive epistaxis in a patient presenting with a classic triad of prior monocular blindness, ipsilateral orbital fractures, and delayed epistaxis with a recent or distant history of head trauma, should alert the clinician to probable post traumatic pseudoaneurysm of the internal carotid artery. Bleeding after septorhinoplasty, endoscopic sinus operations, or turbinate resection can result from mucosal surfaces or from a major vessel. Both decongestants and steroid sprays can address acute dryness and bleeding.

Septal deformity

Septal deflections and spurs also may produce nasal dryness, crusting, and subsequent epistaxis. Padgam[8] analysed the position of bleeding points in relation to septal anatomy in patients with a septal deflection, and found that the bleeding site was anterior to the septal deflection in 83%. He also noted that posterior bleeding occurred only in patients with normal or widely patent nasal airways.

Inflammatory disease

Local inflammatory reactions due to acute respiratory infections, chronic sinusitis, allergic rhinitis, and environment irritants such as tobacco smoke, may alter the normal mucus protective blanket and underlying mucosa, allowing for dryness, crusting, exposure, and haemorrhage. Bleeding of inflammatory origin is generally a blood-streaked mucus, but it may become an active epistaxis depending on the degree of inflammation.

Tumours

Benign and malignant neoplasms of the nose, sinuses and nasopharynx may present with epistaxis. Nasopharyngeal carcinoma deserves a special mention for its high incidence among the Chinese population. In Singapore, the incidence among the Cantonese is 18.2 per 100,000 in males and 7.5 per 100,000 in females.[9] The symptom of epistaxis in these patients should prompt an endoscopic evaluation for nasopharyngeal cancer (Fig. 5). Epistaxis is a frequent presenting sign of an angiofibroma, which is a benign, locally invasive, highly vascular tumour (Fig. 6). Manipulation and biopsy of this tumour should be avoided because of the potential for haemorrhage. Contrast computed tomography (CT) and magnetic resonance imaging (MRI) should be used for diagnosis and treatment planning.

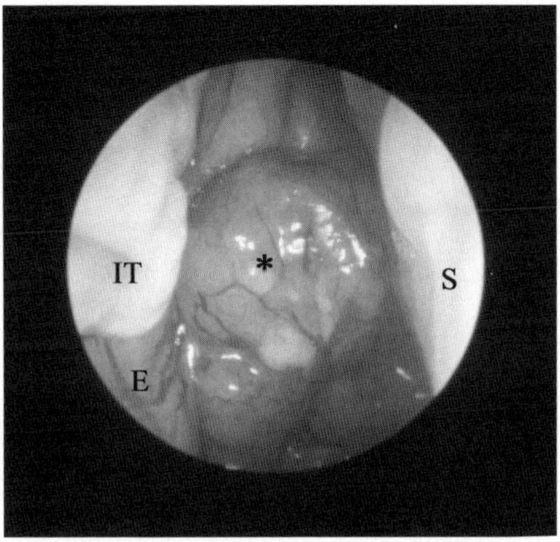

Fig. 5 Endoscopic examination revealed a nasopharyngeal carcinoma in a patient who presented with epistaxis. IT = inferior turbinate, E = eustachian tube, S = posterior part of the nasal septum, and * = exophytic nasopharyngeal carcinoma.

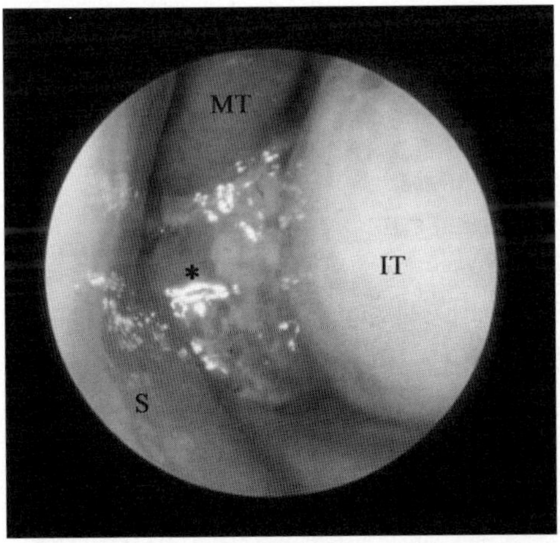

Fig. 6 An angiofibroma noted in the left nasal cavity of a patient who presented with persistent epistaxis. IT = inferior turbinate, S = nasal septum, MT = middle turbinate, and * = indicated the angiofibroma.

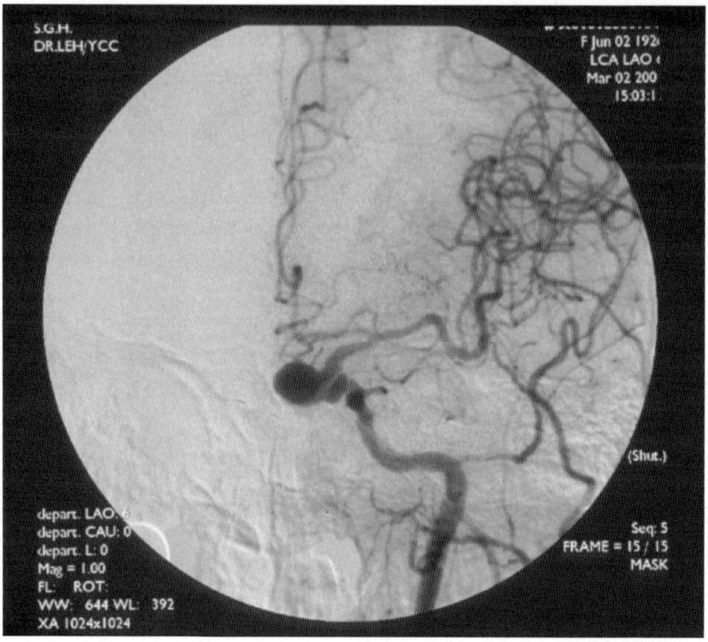

Fig. 7 An aneurysm of the internal carotid artery in a patient presenting with epistaxis. The patient gave history of a head injury about ten years earlier.

Aneurysms

Intracavernous aneurysms of the internal carotid artery may be post-traumatic or non-traumatic in origin.

Epistaxis in patients with non-traumatic aneurysm is rare, but large aneurysms may be mistaken for a tumour and result in fatal haemorrhage with biopsy. Post-traumatic aneurysms more commonly cause epistaxis, often delayed (Fig. 7).

Systemic causes

Coagulation deficits

Congenital or acquired coagulopathies may cause epistaxis that is difficult to manage until the underlying clotting disorder is corrected. Congenital coagulopathy should be suspected in the presence of a positive family history, easy bruisability, and a history of prolonged bleeding from lacerations, dental extractions, or minor trauma.

von Willebrand disease

The most common hereditary bleeding disorder associated with epistaxis is von Willebrand's disease (vWD). This disease is inherited in an autosomal dominant pattern, and manifests clinically with mucocutaneous haemorrhage, excessive bleeding after trauma or surgery, and epistaxis. Epistaxis is the most common symptom of vWD, affecting approximately 60% of those with the disorder. Other symptoms may be easy bruising (40%), menorrhagia (35%), gingival bleeding (20%). Under normal conditions, the von Willebrand factor (vWF) induces platelet aggregation when the subendothelium is exposed as in a vessel injury. The increased bleeding time seen in vWD is due to vWF being functionally aberrant or quantitatively deficient. Although bleeding tests are useful as screening tests, laboratory diagnosis is most commonly made with qualitative immunoelectrophoresis or an enzyme-linked immunoassay. Management depends on the severity of the disease and the clinical setting. Replacement therapy with cryoprecipitate and possibly platelets, sufficient to normalise the Duke bleeding time and factor VIII coagulant activity, is recommended for seven to 10 days after major surgical procedures, and four to six days after minor procedures.[10]

Acquired coagulopathies may be drug- or disease-mediated. Numerous medications affect coagulation as their intended therapeutic effect or as a side effect. Drug or disease-mediated thrombocytopenia tends to produce spontaneous bleeding when platelet counts are between 10,000 to 20,000/mm^3. Counts below 10,000/mm^3 are associated with severe bleeding.

Vitamin K is essential for the synthesis of prothrombin and factors VII, IX and X. Vitamin K deficiency as a result of diet, disease or medications may produce severe or fatal bleeding. Liver disease is a common cause of impaired coagulation, with reduced levels of all coagulation factors except factor VIII. In the absence of liver disease, alcohol may be a factor in those with epistaxis. An association between high alcohol use and epistaxis has been confirmed by McGarry.[11]

Hereditary haemorrhagic telangiectiasia

Hereditary haemorrhagic telangiectiasia (Osler-Weber-Rendu disease) is an autosomal dominant disease manifested by diffuse mucocutansous telangiectiasia and arteriovenous malformation. Incidence is about 1 or 2 per 100,000. The angiodysplasia of hereditary haemorrhagic telangiectiasia affects vessels from capillaries to large arteries, producing telangiectiasia, arteriovenous malformations, and aneurysms. Localised areas in capillaries are lined by a single endothelial layer and lack elastic tissue, resulting in vessel fragility and impaired vasoconstriction. Telangiectiasias occur throughout the body on mucous membranes and skin. Hereditary haemorrhagic telangiectiasia also demonstrates arteriovenous fistulae and aneurysms, with locations in the lung, central nervous system, liver, and bowel often being clinically significant. Recurrent epistaxis is the most common manifestation, and an early sign of hereditary haemorrhagic telangiectiasia.[12]

Arteriosclerotic vascular disease

The higher incidence of epistaxis noted in the higher age group may be due to arteriosclerotic disease seen in these patients. Hypertension is often thought to be an contributing factor but an actual increase in frequency or severity of epistaxis in hypertensive groups has not been shown.[4,8,13]

Management of Epistaxis

The vascular anatomy of the nose, and clinical observation, has led to the division of epistaxis into anterior and posterior locations. Anterior epistaxis has a bleeding site visible on anterior rhinoscopy and almost always originates from Kiesselbach's area on the anterior septum. The majority of bleeding sites (82%) in all age groups are anterior and accessible to local treatment. Bleeding sites not visible on anterior rhinoscopy traditionally have been assumed to originate posteriorly from the posterior nasal septum or vicinity of the sphenopalatine foramen. The use of fiberoptic endoscopes is invaluable in identifying the precise anatomical locations of these bleeding sites.

The degree, site and aetiology of the epistaxis, as well as the clinical state of the patient, dictate thc expediency and aggressiveness of the initial treatment.

General measures

An accurate patient history is essential. Specific history about location, severity, duration and frequency of bleeding should be obtained. The history should also include questions regarding underlying medical conditions, family history, medications, tobacco and alcohol use to discover factors that may be causing epistaxis, or that may affect management. A general physical examination and thorough head and neck evaluation is then performed. Anterior rhinoscopy should be done both before and after topical anaesthesia and vasoconstriction. Flexible or rigid endoscopy examination is then performed to visualise the bleeding site. Laboratory evaluation for assessment of blood loss, fluid status, coagulopathy, or underlying systemic disease should be initiated. Imaging studies including CT or MRI scanning may be needed to evaluate for neoplasms and for assessment of anatomy for possible surgical access.

Management of exsanguinating epistaxis

Exsanguinating epistaxis may be life threatening. It may result following severe midfacial trauma with laceration of the maxillary artery. The injury is often associated with multiple system trauma. The patient requires immediate evaluation, aggressive resuscitation, control of airway, followed by control of bleeding and concurrent fluid or crystalloid replacement. Anterior and posterior nasal packing may be necessary to stop the bleeding. Often, unstable midfacial fractures may confound the surgeon's ability to tightly pack these areas, resulting in continued exsanguination. In such situations, ligation of the external carotid artery under local anaesthesia may have to be considered.

Persistent bleeding in spite of aggressive packing may represent disseminated intravascular coagulation, which requires early recognition and treatment. In certain cases, emergent angiography with embolisation may be necessary and can be considered. In patients with recurrent or massive epistaxis, particularly if there is a past history of head injury or sphenoid surgery, a pseudoaneurysm of the intracavernous carotid artery has to be excluded. The latent period from initial trauma to haemorrhage may vary from days to years with 87% bleeding within six months. A mortality rate of 30% in this group of patients is associated with inadequate and delayed diagnosis and improper treatment. The diagnosis can be established with emergent angiography and lifesaving embolisation. The majority of patients presenting to the otolaryngologist are haemodynamically stable. The anatomical site of the bleeding may be anteriorly or posteriorly located in the nose. Anterior bleeding occurs primarily in the Little's area and is more often venous in origin. Posterior epistaxis occurs primarily in the region of the posterior septum, followed in frequency by the posterior lateral nasal wall, and is more often arterial in origin. Specifically, the site of the posterior epistaxis is more frequently (60% to 65%) on the posterior septum compared to the lateral wall.

Determination of the bleeding site is most readily performed with both the patient and physician being relatively comfortable and with protective clothing and eye protection. The patient should be in a sitting position and the examiner equipped with an adequate light source; suction, anaesthetic solution, packing material and cautery should be available. The patient's nose is examined both before and after vasoconstriction. Topical anaesthetic and vasoconstrictor agents are applied via cotton pledgets or neurosurgical cottonoids. Topical cocaine 4%, is excellent for this purpose. If cocaine is not available, a 1:1 mixture of oxymetazoline and xylocaine 4% may be used.

Identification of most anterior bleeding sites can be accomplished with illumination and exposure from a head light, a nasal speculum, bayonet forceps, a Frasier's suction for the nasal cavity, and a Yankauer suction for the oral cavity blood clots. Posterior bleeding sites may be more difficult to visualise and a 30° endoscope will enhance visualisation and identification. Identification of the specific bleeding site, provides the opportunity for localised therapy such as localised cautery and mini-packing, which is less painful for the patient, has a lower failure rate, and allows for out patient management or a shorter hospitalisation.

Cautery

Silver nitrate cauterisation

After adequate anaesthesia and vasoconstriction are achieved, chemical cautery may be used. Once the bleeding site has been identified, lidocaine on a small piece of cotton is applied over the bleeding site to obviate the burning sensation before cauterisation. Silver nitrate on an applicator stick is then applied to the vessels leading to the bleeding site, over a circumferential area of 2 to 3 mm, and then onto the site itself. To prevent further burning of normal tissue, the silver nitrate can be neutralised with the application of sodium chloride, thereby converting silver nitrate to silver chloride. Finally, a thin layer of one of the absorbable materials like Surgicel® or Gelfoam® is placed over the cautery site to act as a temporary scab, and prevent desiccation of the cauterised mucosa. This method of chemical cautery is highly successful with Kremp and Noorily, noting a 65% success rate with administration of oxymetazoline alone, and an additional 18% success rate with use of silver nitrate and oxymetazoline in emergency room patients.[14]

Electric cauterisation

Electrocautery is an alternative method of managing anterior epistaxis, noted to be equally as effective as silver nitrate.[15] Electrocautery

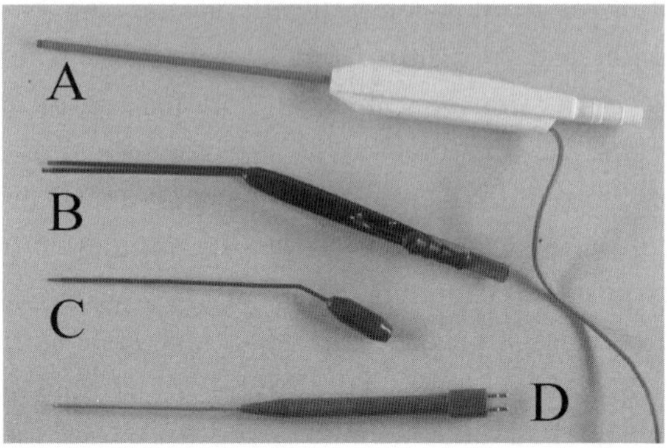

Fig. 8 Cautery units. A = disposable monopolar with suction, B = bipolar forceps with suction, C = monopolar probe, and D = co-axial bipolar probe.

usually requires local rather than topical anaesthesia as it induces a deeper penetration and more tissue destruction than silver nitrate. Monopolar electrocautery units are malleable and designed with suction, allowing for continuous clearing of blood from the field. A bipolar bayonet forceps cautery in the anterior nose may allow for a more controlled cauterisation with less depth of tissue injury compared to monopolar cautery. The drawback with the bipolar bayonet forceps cautery compared to monopolar suction cautery is the limited access to the posterior nasal region because of the width of the bipolar forceps handle/tip. Coaxial bipolar cautery units have become available and allow for posterior nasal cavity access but lack suction. (Fig. 8) For all types of cautery, repetitive cauterisation increases the likelihood of septal perforation. Therefore, a precise identification of the bleeding site is imperative. Light petroleum gauze packing, impregnated with antibiotic ointment or absorbable packing like Surgicel®, is useful to cover the area, decrease infection risk, and maintain local moisture.

Laser photocoagulation

Laser photocoagulation is also useful in the treatment of anterior septal bleeding, but it may not be available for emergent use in the office, clinic or emergency room. Its use has been reported for patients with hereditary haemorrhagic telangiectiasia.

Nasal packing — Anterior

When cautery is unsuccessful in controlling acute anterior epistaxis, packing may be necessary. Anterior nasal packing can constitute a traditional ribbon gauze pack, prefabricated expandable packs or intra-nasal balloons applied to an identified or unidentified bleeding site. Alternatively, an identified bleeding site may be managed with a "mini" pack applied directly to the bleeding site, thereby decreasing patient discomfort. If a bleeding site cannot be identified, then a traditional anterior nasal pack may provide haemostasis. The traditional anterior pack is available as petroleum gauze (0.5 × 72 inches) coated with an antibacterial ointment. After adequate vasoconstriction and anaesthesia, the gauze strip is accordion-layered beginning on the floor of the nose, with each layer placed far enough posteriorly and tightly enough to prevent loss into the nasopahrynx. Both ends of the packing should be retained anteriorly (Fig. 9). Telfa packing can also be coated

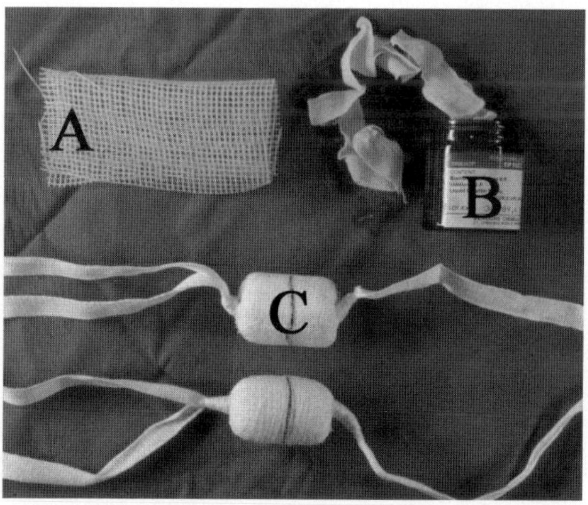

Fig. 9 Nonabsobrable packing materials. A = Tulla-Gras packing, B = bismuth iodine ribbon gauge, and C = posterior nasal bolster.

with antibacterial ointment, rolled, and placed into the nasal cavity. Placing a single layer of absorbable material such as Surgicel® or Gelfoam® over the known bleeding site, followed by packing material, may prevent rebleeding after pack removal two to four days later (Fig. 10).

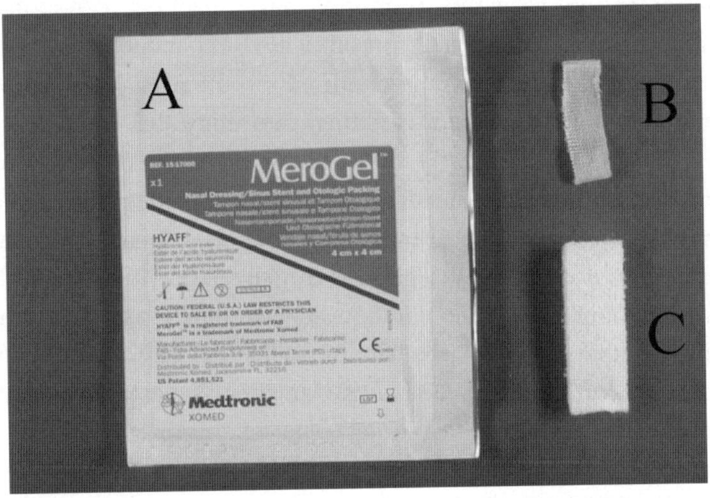

Fig. 10 Absorbable materials used alone or in conjunction with packing or cautery. A = Merogel®, B = Surgicel®, and C = Gelfoam®.

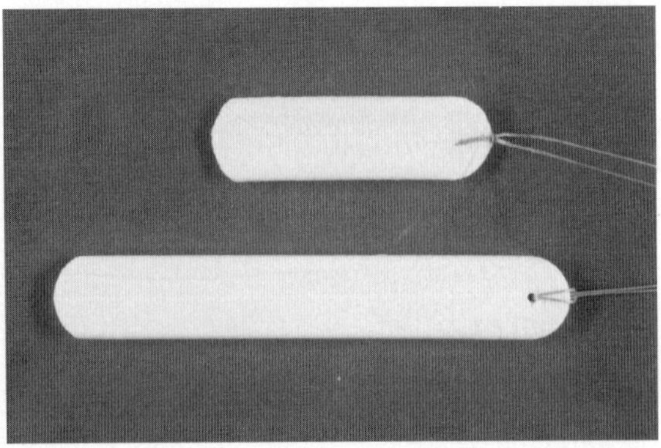

Fig. 11 Nonabsorbable hydrophilic and expanding nasal packs (Merocel®).

Newer nasal packing materials have become available that expand several times in volume with hydration, providing tamponade. These hydrophilic and compressed sponges are generally made of hydroxylated polyvinyl actal (Merocel®; Fig. 11) and polyvinyl alcohol (Expandcell®). Although these can be placed more quickly, these may not be adequate pressure in the appropriate areas. Use of oxymetazoline to hydrate it, and periodically thereafter may be helpful. Administration of oral antibiotics to prevent sinusitis should be considered. Gauze packing usually is removed in two to five days. Merocel® is usually removed in two days. All packs should be rehydrated prior to removal. Multiple sizes are available. Some nasal packs come with attached drawstrings and integrated airways to facilitate nasal respiration with the packing in place. Corbridge *et al.*[16] conducted a prospective randomised trial comparing Merocel® nasal packing with ribbon gauze impregnated with bismuth subnitrate and iodoform paste for the control of epistaxis. These demonstrated no difference in insertion or removal discomfort, haemostasis, or complication in a study of 49 patients.

Patients with chronic mucosal pathology from hereditary haemorrhagic telangiectiasia, coagulation disorders, or leukaemia should be managed conservatively. It may be preferred to avoid the trauma of cautery and nasal packing, particularly if the coagulopathy cannot be treated. In these patients, a vasoconstrictor alone may be helpful. Microfibrillar bovine topocollagen (Avitene®) or oxidised cellulose (Surgicel®) may be placed directly on the bleeding site and left in place. Avitene® is available in a 5 mm syringe applicator to facilitate placement more posteriorly in the nose in conjunction with the use of an endoscope.

Treatment of posterior epistaxis

Posterior epistaxis treatment traditionally has been a step-wise approach of non-surgical treatment with anterior and posterior packing, followed by arterial ligation in those with packing failures. In recent years, with the advent of endoscopes and availability of interventional radiological techniques, the management of epistaxis has changed, providing minimally invasive alternatives. Familiarity with rigid endoscopes has promoted better definition of bleeding sites and popularised the use of posterior endoscopic cauterisation. The availability of interventional radiologists has increased the use of vessel embolisation.

Nasal packing — Posterior

Posterior nasal packing is indicated for patients failing anterior nasal packs, or who, upon evaluation, have previously known posterior bleeding. As the procedure may cause considerable discomfort and airway manipulation, the patient's co-operation is essential. Careful instructions must be given to the patient. Intravenous access and mild sedation are recommended unless medically contraindicated. Some patients may need to be taken to the operation room for placement of a proper pack.

A posterior nasal pack (Fig. 9) may be a traditional gauze pack or an inflatable balloon pack. The traditional posterior nasal pack is composed of rolled gauze. The pack should be of adequate size to occlude the posterior choana but not interfere with swallowing. The posterior nasal pack is generally used in conjunction with an anterior pack to stabilise it. The nose and the pharynx of the patient are anaesthetised, and the patient may be sedated with a short-acting sedating agent. A posterior nasal pack is prepared by rolling a medium tonsillar sponge into a bolster of adequate size to fill in the nasopharynx. Three strings are sutured to it. Two small rubber catheters are passed through the nasal cavity on each side, and pulled out through the mouth. The two strings of the posterior nasal pack are tied or sutured to the catheters on each side, and the pack is then pulled into the posterior nasopharynx by traction on the nasal end of the catheter. The pack is guided into the posterior choana by a finger or a long curved clamp. The trailing string is left dangling out of the mouth and is taped to the cheek. Anterior packing is placed, and the nasal ties tied over a dental roll or placed over a columellar bolster. The packing is left in place for three to four days and is removed via the oropharynx.

All patients with a posterior pack should be admitted and monitored in an appropriate hospital setting. Nasal packing has been shown to increase nocturnal episodes of hypoxia and may induce or exacerbate obstructive sleep apnoea. Pulse oximetry is recommended to monitor oxygen saturation. Maintaining of body fluids is important as most patients may experience difficulty in swallowing. Most patients are treated with antibiotics to prevent infection. Adequate pain control is essential.

To remove the pack, the anterior strings of the posterior nasal pack are untied or cut. A tongue blade is used to depress the tongue and the oropharyngeal string is pulled out of the mouth removing the pack. If patients fail packing, they may be candidates for further intervention described subsequently, or the physician may undertake a different initial procedure based on the clinical presentation.

Balloon packs

Several inflatable balloon packs have become available (Fig. 12). These have the advantage of being easier to place, and are therefore preferred by the novice. The concept is the same as traditional nasal

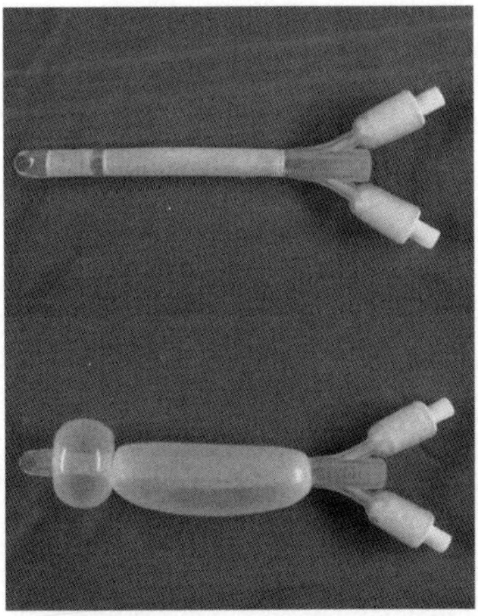

Fig. 12 Balloons used for epistaxis.

packing; by placement of air or saline into the balloon, pressure is applied to the lateral nasal wall and septum. Newer types of nasal balloon packs include double balloons — balloons that allow continued respiration through an integral hollow center. A potential drawback of the balloon pack is the inability to place pressure against the actual site of bleeding.

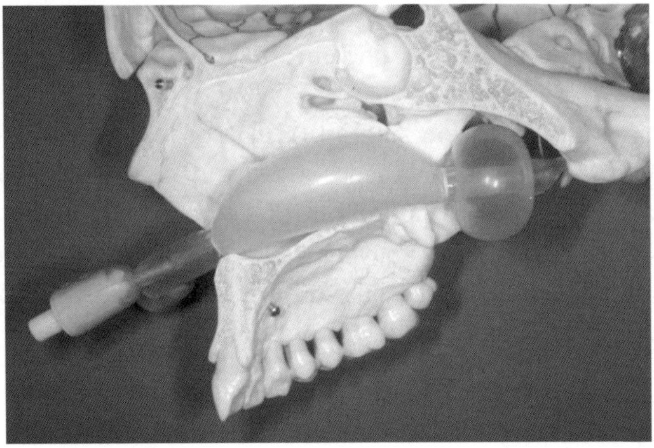

Fig. 13 Inflated balloon of the Foley's catheter placed in the nasopharynx.

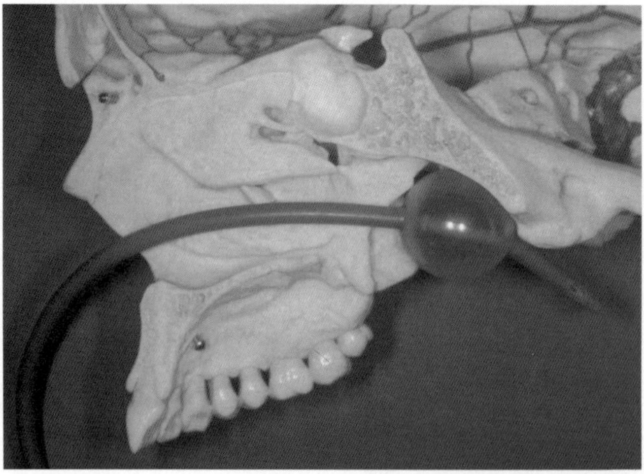

Fig. 14 Position of the inflated balloon in the nasal cavity and nasopharynx. This is a double balloon with an integral hollow center that allows continued respiration.

Foley's catheter as a balloon pack

A Foley's catheter may be used as an alternative to other epistaxis balloons (Fig. 14). A size 12 French or 14 French Foley catheter with a 30 ml balloon is suitable for posterior nasal packing. The catheter is placed through the bleeding nostril into the nasopharynx. The balloon is inflated with 8 to 15 ml of water, and anterior traction is applied. It is better to use water for balloon inflation because deflation will occur with time if air is used. Overinflation of the balloon should be avoided because it will displace the palate downward, interfere with patient swallowing and comfort, and prevent proper balloon placement in the posterior choanae. An anterior pack is then placed. With continued anterior traction on the catheter a C-clamp is placed against the anterior pack and tightened to maintain tension. Complications of posterior nasal packing and balloon tamponade include alar and columellar necrosis if the packing is placed too tightly or the strings are tied too tightly against the alar and columella. Appropriate measures should be taken to prevent these complications.

Endoscopic management

The excellent illumination and visualisation provided with fibreoptic endoscopes have introduced a new era of epistaxis management. Rigid and flexible endoscopes enable visualisation of regions in the nasal cavity that were not readily seen with a head light or nasal speculum. The use of endoscopes has facilitated a more precise definition of bleeding sites. Flexible fibreoptic nasopharyngoscope use for visualising posterior epistaxis and cauterising with silver nitrate or trichloroacetic acid was first reported in 1987[17] and since then there have been several reports on the use of endoscopes for managing epistaxis. The flexible scope allows excellent visualisation of the posterior nasal cavity but instrumentation when cauterising the bleeding site can be cumbersome. The author prefers to use rigid endoscopes as instrumentation is easier. A 4.0 mm 30° telescope is used to identify the bleeding site. Topical vasoconstriction and anaesthesia are induced after the bleeding site has been localised. If the bleeding site is located posteriorly, a 22-gauge spinal needle is used to inject lidocaine and epinephrine locally. An insulated suction cautery unit is then used to electrocoagulate the bleeding site. With this technique, the senior author has managed several bleeding sites on the posterior nasal septum, middle meatus, inferior meatus, nasal floor, and face of the sphenoid. The success rate of posterior endoscopic cauterisation is reported in the 80% to 90% range. Endoscopic management of epistaxis requires expertise compared to that for nasal packing. Proper instrumentation may not be optimal in emergency departments, where most of these patients are encountered. It may not be suitable in emergent situations, where epistaxis is profuse and occludes visualisation.

Arterial ligation

Ligation of the arterial blood supply is an effective method of epistaxis control. Ligation traditionally has been a management choice when packing has failed. The choice of a specific vessel to ligate is usually dictated by the observed site, or the most likely site of bleeding, based on history taking.

External carotid artery ligation

Ligation of the external branch of the carotid artery is a relatively straightforward approach to decreasing blood flow to the more distal maxillary artery, compared to sphenopalatine artery ligation. It can be performed under local anaesthesia and done without specialised equipment. The procedure may be considered in patients who are poor anaesthetic risks, and patients with exsanguinating epistaxis. The disadvantage is the lack of control of potential collateral circulation, which will maintain high maxillary blood pressure. A high rate of rebleeding with external carotid artery ligation (45%) was noted on long-term follow-up by Stafford and Durham.[18]

The external carotid artery is approached via a horizontal incision between the hyoid and upper border of thyroid cartilage. Superior and inferior subplatysmal flaps are elevated, and the sternocleidomastoid muscle is retracted posteriorly. The internal jugular vein is retracted, exposing the carotid bifurcation. Exposure of the internal carotid artery for several centimetres and dissection of the external carotid, identifying its branches, ascending pharyngeal, superior thyroid and lingual arteries before ligation, prevents ligation of the internal carotid artery by mistake. Suture ligation of the external carotid artery is performed with heavy silk. To reduce the failure rate of the procedure, external carotid artery ligation can be combined with anterior ethmoid artery ligation. In a ten-year follow-up of patients who had external artery ligation, 45% of the patients failed treatment.[18] However, another study reported a nine-year follow-up with a 7% failure rate in patients who had external carotid artery and anterior ethmoid artery ligation without any significant complications.[19]

Internal maxillary artery ligation

Internal maxillary artery ligation has been the most popular method of arterial ligation over the past several decades. Ligation of this branch of the external carotid artery causes a decrease in the intravascular pressure gradient, resulting in homeostasis of the posterior nasal cavity unless anatomosis exists, with continued high pressures. The internal maxillary artery is usually approached transantrally. A transoral approach also has been described.[20] Preoperative radiographic assessment of antral size is necessary because a hypoplastic antrum is a contraindication to this approach.

The antrum is entered via a Caldwell-Luc approach. A large bony opening should be made and a self-retaining retractor is placed using an operating microscope. The posterior maxillary sinus wall is identified, and a laterally based U-shaped mucosal incision outlined with a long guarded needle tip cautery, and elevated off the posterior antral wall. The posterior sinus wall is opened with a drill or mallet and chisel, and widened with Kerrison's rongeurs. The posterior maxillary wall is then removed. The posterior periosteum is carefully opened. The vessels of the pterygopalatine fossa are dissected and elevated with blunt hooks, and two haemoclips placed on each vessel. The internal maxillary, sphenopalatine, and descending palatine arteries should be double clipped and not divided.[21] It may be necessary to remove the orbital process of the palatine bone to gain exposure of the sphenopalatine foramen and the arterial vessels.

Gelfoam® is placed over the posterior wall, and the mucosal incision is closed. An antral window or middle meatal antrostomy may be considered, for drainage of the sinus. All nasal packing placed before the procedure is then removed to ascertain the success of the procedure. Reported success rates of transantral maxillary artery ligation range from 75% to 100%.[22–24] Possible reasons for failure of this procedure include variability of arterial branching within the pterygopalatine fossa, and failure to identify all branches. Combining anterior ethmoid artery ligation with maxillary artery ligation has been recommended.[21,22] However, McDonald and Pearson evaluated their patients long term and found no additional benefit with anterior ethmoid artery ligation.[25]

Sphenopalatine artery ligation

In 1982, Simpson *et al.* described an approach to ligate the sphenopalatine artery without entering the pterygopalatine fossa.[26] The medial posterior inferior maxillary wall and the orbital process of the palatine bone is removed. The sphenopalatine artery and vidian nerve are exposed. The vidian nerve is dissected free and the vessel ligated. An endoscopic modification of Simpson's technique of isolation and ligation of the sphenopalatine artery has also been reported.[27] An endoscopic uncinectomy and middle meatal antrostomy facilitate exposure. Mucosa is then elevated from the posterior part of the middle meatal antrostomy between the middle and the inferior turbinates. The posterior margin of the sphenopalatine foramen, formed by the orbital process of the palatine bone is identified. Careful dissection will identify the sphenopalatine artery as it exits the sphenopalatine foramen. The orbital process of the palatine bone and the part of the medial part of the posterior wall of the maxillary sinus may be removed with rongeurs for better exposure. The artery is then clipped or coagulated for control of bleeding.

Ethmoid artery ligation

When the bleeding site is superior to the middle turbinate, the anterior and posterior ethmoid arteries may have to be ligated to decrease blood flow to the upper nasal vault from the internal carotid artery system. It is generally performed in conjunction with ligation of the maxillary artery or the external carotid artery. Kirchner *et al.* first described anterior and posterior ethmoid artery anatomy and ligation in 1961.[2] A circumlinear incision is normally made between the inner canthus and midline of the nose (Lynch incision). The periosteum is incised and elevated, retracting the orbital periosteum laterally. The frontoethmoid suture line is followed in the posterior direction about 14 to 22 mm to the anterior ethmoid artery and its foramen. The artery can be managed by bipolar cautery or neurosurgical clips before division. The usually smaller posterior ethmoid artery is located further posteriorly located at an average of 33 mm from the anterior lacrimal crest, although the distance may be highly variable (range: 26 to 39 mm).

The optic nerve lies 4 to 7 mm more posterior to the posterior ethmoid foramen. Alternatively, these vessels may be accessed intranasally using an endoscope. A complete ethmoidectomy has to be performed exposing the ethmoid roof. The anterior and the posterior ethmoid vessels are identified and coagulated with bipolar cautery (Figs. 13 and 14). Interventional radiological techniques, such as angiography and embolisation, are unable to access these branches of the ophthalmic artery. Surgical access remains an important procedure in patients requiring ethmoid artery ligation.

Arterial embolisation

In 1974, Sokoloff *et al.* reported percutaneous angiography and selective embolisation of the maxillary artery for localising and controlling

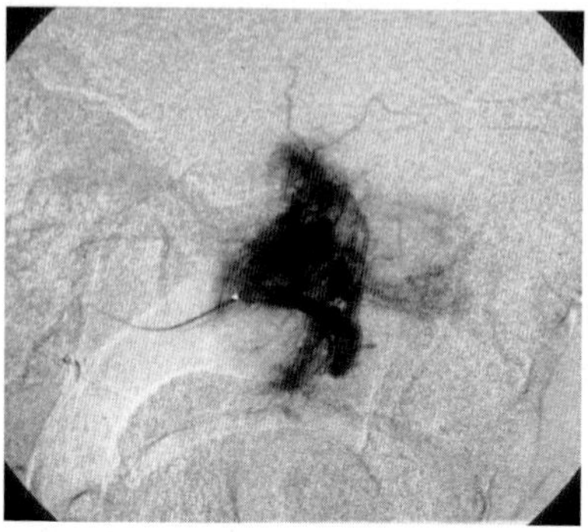

Fig. 15 Pre-embolisation angiogram in a patient with persistent epistaxis.

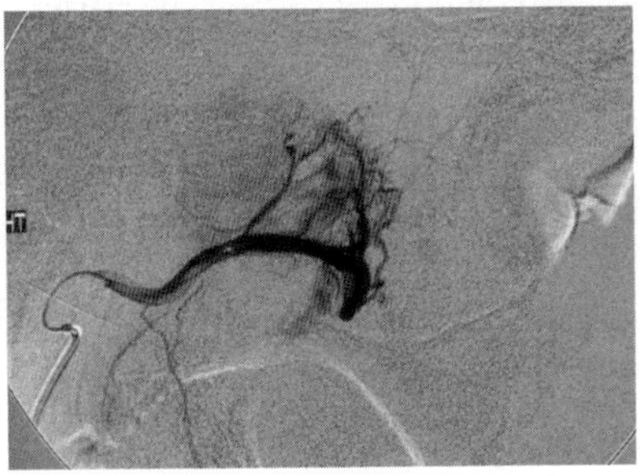

Fig. 16 Post-embolisation angiogram in the same patient.

recalcitrant epistaxis.[28] Since then, the increasing availability of interventional radiologists has made arterial embolisation (Figs. 15 and 16) an option for primary treatment of epistaxis and for surgical failures.

In 1991, Vitek reported a success rate of 87%, with isolated distal branch maxillary artery embolisation.[29] Additional embolisation of the facial artery resulted in 97% control.[29] Similar results have been reported by others.[30–32] The advantages of angiography and embolisation include: shorter hospitalisation; application of local versus general anaesthesia, ability to treat surgically inaccessible vessels, ability to manage surgical failures due to development of arterioarterial anastomotic collaterals; and the relatively high success rates. However, the technique is not as useful in cases of ethmoid artery bleeding, vascular anomalies, or severe atherosclerosis and the facility may not be available at all centres.

Short-term failures may be attributed to dominant anterior, and/or, posterior ethmoid arteries, dominant ipsilateral facial arteries, or, contralateral collateral maxillary artery branches. Dominant anterior, and/ or, posterior ethmoid arteries, may require external surgical ligation or endoscopic coagulation. Additional embolisation of the ipsilateral facial artery has been shown to reduce the short-term failure rate of this interventional procedure.[29] Numerous embolisation materials are used, including polyvinyl alcohol, Gelfoam® particles and coiled springs. Potential but rare complications include skin necrosis, blindness ophthalmoplegia, facial pain/oedema, paresthesia or paralysis, and cerebral embolisation with hemiplegia. Groin haemotoma is the most common complication. Two of the series reported a single case of a cerebrovascular accident[30,32] and one case of retinal artery occlusion.[30]

A comparison of transantral maxillary artery ligation with embolisation reviewing multiple factors showed a success rate of 94% and no major complications for 16 patients who underwent embolisation, and 87% success rate and no major complications for five patients undergoing ligation.[24]

Conclusion

Patient education will help prevent many episodes of epistaxis. Discussion of the importance of humidity in dry climates, restraint from the practice of digital manipulation, avoidance of airborne irritants and control of allergies may avert many episodes of epistaxis. Locally placed petrolatum or antibiotic ointment may help those with dry intranasal mucosa. Measures such as tapering the usage of topical steroid nasal sprays, too obtain maximum therapeutic benefit but decrease risk of nasal mucosal dryness and epistaxis. In patients with epistaxis, the use of nasal mucosal vasoconstriction alone may suffice. Anteriorly located bleeding sites can be managed with chemical or electrocautery. Nasal tamponade may be required in patients with recalcitrant epistaxis or a posteriorly located bleeding site. Surgical management including ligation of the internal maxillary or the sphenopalatine artery may be necessary in some cases. This may be combined with ligation or cauterisation of the ethmoid arteries where there is presumed ethmoid artery bleeding that could not be treated with embolisation, or where the presence of severe atherosclerosis limits angiocatheter access. Endoscopic management of epistaxis allows us to identify the bleeding site and institute specific treatment in some cases. Endoscopic ligation of the sphenopalatine combined with ethmoid artery ligation offers a minimally invasive alternative. Percutaneous angiography and selective embolisation may be used in patients who are poor anaesthetic risks.

Sentinel epistaxis in a patient with recent history of head trauma, especially with unilateral blindness and orbital fracture, should alert the physician of the potential for internal carotid artery pseudoaneurysm.

References

1. Harrison DFN (1981). Surgical approach to the medial orbital wall. *Ann Otol Rhinol Laryngol* **90**, 415–419.
2. Kirchner JA, Yanagisawa E, Crelin ES. (1961) Surgical anatomy of thc cthmoidal artcries. *Arch Otolaryngol* **74**, 382–386.
3. McQueen CT *et al.* (1995). Orbital osteology: a study of the surgical landmarks. *Laryngoscope* **105**, 783–788.
4. Weiss NS (1971). Relation of high blood pressure to headaches, epistaxis and selected other symptoms. *N Engl J Med* **287**, 631–633.
5. Petruson B (1974). Epistaxis: a clinical study with special reference to fibrinolysis. *Acta Otolaryngol* **317**(Suppl. 3), 1–73.
6. Juselius H (1974). Epistaxis. *J Laryngol Otol* **88**, 317–327.
7. Viducich RA, Blanda MP, Gerson LW (1995). Posterior epistaxis: clinical features and acute complications. *Ann Emerg Med* **25**(5), 592–596.
8. Padgam N (1990). Epistaxis: anatomical and clinical correlates. *J Laryngol Otol* **104**, 308–311.
9. Lee HP, Day NE, Shanmugaratnam K (1988). Trends in cancer incidence in Singapore 1968–1982. *IARC Scientific Publication, Lyon, IARC*, No. 91.

10. Williams WJ *et al.* (1990). *Hemotology*, 4th Ed., New York: McGraw-Hill.
11. McGarry GW, Gatehouse S, Vernham G (1995). Idiopathic epistaxis, haemostasis and alcohol. *Clin Otolaryngol* **20**(2), 174–177.
12. Peery WH (1987). Clinical spectrum of hereditary haemorrhagic telangiectiasia (Osler-weber-Rendu disease). *Am J Med* **82**, 989–997
13. Loftus BC, Blitzer A, Cozine K (1994). Epistaxis, medical history and the nasopulmonary reflex: what is clinically relevant? *Otolaryngol Head Neck Surg* **110**, 363–369.
14. Krempi GA, Noorily AD (1995). Use of oxymetazoline in the management of epistaxis. *Ann Otol Rhinol Laryngol* **104**, 704–706.
15. Toner JG, Walby AP (1990). Comparison of electro and chemical cautery in treatment of epistaxis. *J Laryngol Otol* **104**, 617–618.
16. Corbridge RJ, Djazaeri B, Hellier WPL, Hadley J (1995). A prospective randomized controlled trial comparing the use of merocel nasal tampons and BIPP in the control of acute epistaxis. *Clin Otolaryngol* **20**, 305–307.
17. Borgstein JA (1987). Epistaxis and the flexible nasopharygoscope. *Clin Otolaryngol* **12**, 49–51.
18. Stafford P, Durham JS (1992). Epistaxis and efficacy of arterial ligation and long term outcome. *J Otolaryngol* **21**(4), 252–256.
19. Waldron J, Stafford N (1992). Ligation of the external carotid artery for severe epistaxis. *J Otolaryngol* **21**(4), 249–251.
20. Maceri DR, Makielski KH (1984). Intraoral ligation of the maxillary artery for posterior epistaxis. *Laryngoscope* **94**, 737–741.
21. Pearson BW, Mackenzie RG, Goodman WS (!969). The anatomical basis of transantral ligation of maxillary artery in severe epistaxis. *Laryngoscope* **79**, 969–984.
22. Metson R, Lane R (!988). Internal maxillary artery ligation for epistaxis: an anlysis of failures. *Laryngoscope* **98**, 760–764.
23. Shaw CB, Wax MK, Westmore SJ (1993). Epistaxis: a comparison of treatment. *Otolaryngol Head Neck Surg* **109**, 60–65.

24. Strong EB, Bell DA, Johnson LP, Jacobs JM (1995). Intractable epistaxis: transantral ligation versus embolisation: efficacy review and cost analysis. *Otolaryngol Head Neck Surg* **113**, 674–678.
25. McDonald TJ, Pearson BW (1980). Follow-up on maxillary artery ligation for epistaxis. *Arch Otolaryngol* **106**, 635–638.
26. Simpson GT, Janfaza P, Becker GD (1982). Transantral sphenopalatine artery ligation. *Laryngoscope* **92**(1), 001–1005.
27. White PS (1996). Endoscopic ligation of the sphenopalatine artery (ELSA): a preliminary description. *J Laryngol Otol* **110**(1), 27–30.
28. Sokoloff J, Wickbom I, McDonald D, Brahme F, Georgen TG, Goldberger LE (1974). Therapeutic percutaneous embolisation in intractable epistaxis. *Radiology* **111**, 285–287.
29. Vitek J (1991). Idiopathic intractable epistaxis: endovascular therapy. *Radiology* **181**(1), 113–116.
30. Elden L, Montanera W, Terbrugge K, Willinsky R, Lasjaunias P, Charles D (1994). Angiographic embolisation for treatment of epistaxis: a review of 108 cases. *Otolaryngol Head Neck Surg* **111**(1), 44–50.
31. Elahi MM, Parncs LS, Fox AJ, Pelz DM, Lee DH (1995). *Arch Otolaryngol Head Neck Surg* **121**(1), 65–69.
32. Tseng EY, Narducci CA, Willing SJ, Sillers MJ (1995). Angiographic embolisation for epistaxis: a review of 114 cases. *Laryngoscope* **108**, 615–619.

7

Managing the Difficult Airway in an Emergency Setting

Ruban Poopalalingam
Nian-Chih Hwang
Eugene Chin

Introduction

Adept airway management is an essential skill for any doctor to acquire, particularly for those who are involved with resuscitation and emergencies. In this chapter, it is assumed that the reader has adequate basic airway management skills such as the triple manoeuvre (head tilt, jaw thrust, and chin lift) to maintain the upper airway, manual ventilation via a facemask with or without the use of oral or nasal airway, and endotracheal intubation under direct laryngoscopy. Therefore these will not be described. Instead, this chapter will focus on the recognition of the patient with a potentially difficult laryngoscopy, and the various techniques of securing the difficult airway in the emergency setting.

Indications for Tracheal Intubation

Other than to facilitate muscle paralysis and mechanical ventilation during general anaesthesia, indications for tracheal intubation can be broadly classified into the following categories.

Airway maintenance and protection

(1) Airway maintenance — Patients who are unable to maintain a patent airway and are therefore at a risk of hypoxia and hypercapnia. This would include patients with inhalational burns who may potentially develop airway compromise.
(2) Airway protection — If the patient is unconscious, the risk of regurgitation and pulmonary aspiration exist.[1] Patients who are at risk of pulmonary aspiration of oral or gastric contents, such as those with Glasgow Coma Scale of 8 or less, require either a cuffed endotracheal tube or tracheostomy to protect the airway.

Ventilation mechanics and gas exchange

(3) For ventilatory insufficiency — The criteria for ventilatory support are as follows:
    - Respiratory rate > 35 per minute
    - Tidal volume < 5 ml per kg
    - Vital capacity < 15 ml per kg
    - Maximum inspiratory force < −25 cm H_2O
    - $P_aO_2 < 60$ mmHg with FiO_2 0.6
    - $P_aCO_2 > 60$ mmHg
    - Dead space > 0.6
(4) For patients who require positive airway pressure to assist in oxygenation and ventilation, such as patients with pulmonary oedema.
(5) For tracheo-bronchial toilet. Tracheal access is required to assist in clearing secretions from the airways of patients with impaired cough mechanism.

Part of management strategy

(6) For generation of hypocapnia. Neurosurgical patients may require transient hyperventilation to reduce intracranial pressure while definitive neurosurgical measures are taken.

Recognising a Potentially Difficult Direct Laryngoscopy

Tracheal intubation becomes less straightforward if the glottis is not easily seen during direct laryngoscopy. For the glottis to be seen during direct laryngoscopy using a conventional curved blade laryngoscope, the following manoeuvres are necessary:

- Forward flexion of the neck.
- Extension of the atlanto-occipital joint.
- Maximal mouth opening without resistance.
- Leftward and submandibular displacement of the tongue.
- Elevation of hyoid bone.
- Elevation of epiglottis.

The interplay of the various manoeuvres allows the oro-laryngeal axes to be aligned, and thus provides optimum condition for direct laryngoscopy and tracheal intubation. It is important to be able to identify the patient with a potentially difficult tracheal intubation if conventional direct laryngoscopy is to proceed. If difficult tracheal intubation can be predicted early, then preparation can be made to increase the chance of successful tracheal intubation. Table 1 shows the anatomical features which may allow the reader to predict difficult tracheal intubation. From experience, a combination of retrognathia, small mouth opening, protruding incisors, reduced atlanto-occipital extension, will invariably result in a grade IIb or worse laryngoscopic view.

The presence of supraglottic pathologies such as epiglottitis and submandibular abcess (Ludwig's angina) can also result in difficult tracheal intubation. For patients with such conditions, a team approach

Table 1 Suboptimal Conditions for Direct Laryngoscopy

Anatomical Features	Significance
Protruding upper incisors with over-riding of maxillary teeth anterior to mandibular teeth, worse if loose	Laryngoscope blade has to be introduced into the mouth in a cephalad direction
Limited anterior excursion of mandible	Restricted temporo-mandibular joint movement: inability to subluxate the jaw anteriorly during laryngoscopy
Limited mouth opening with inter-incisor distance less than 3 cm or 2 ordinary-sized fingerbreadth in the adult patient (inter-canine distance should be measured if incisors are absent): evidence of trismus, temporo-mandibular joint disease, previous trauma, or radiotherapy of the region)	Restricted temporo-mandibular joint movement: difficult to insert the 2 cm flange of laryngoscope blade between teeth
Mallampati Class III or IV oropharyngeal class (Fig. 1)*: tongue is large in relation to size of oropharyngeal cavity	Decreases oropharyngeal volume and room for both blade and endotracheal tube
Palate appears very narrow: the highly arched palate is narrow	Decreases oropharyngeal volume and room for both blade and endotracheal tube
Thyromental distance less than 6 cm or 3 ordinary-sized fingerbreadth in the adult patient: evidence of retrognathia	Reduction of submandibular space: tongue cannot be fully displaced into this space during laryngoscopy
Poor compliance of submandibular space: evidence of fibrosis (radiation, scar formation), submandibular swelling (abscess, tumour)	The tongue cannot be displaced into this space during laryngoscopy
Short, thick neck	Decreases the ability to align the axes of the upper airway

Table 1 (*Continued*)

Anatomical Features	Significance
Limited range of movement of head and neck, and inability to assume the "sniff" position: anterior neck flexion less than 35°, extension at atlanto-occipital joint less than 80°: spondylosis	Decreases the ability to align the axes of the upper airway
Possible cervical instability: evidence of severe rheumatoid arthritis affecting the stability of C_1–C_2 cervical vertebrae, or cervical spine trauma	Decreases the ability to align the axes of the upper airway

*The original Mallampati score has three classes; the scoring was later modified by Samsoon and Young into four classes (Fig. 1).[7,8]

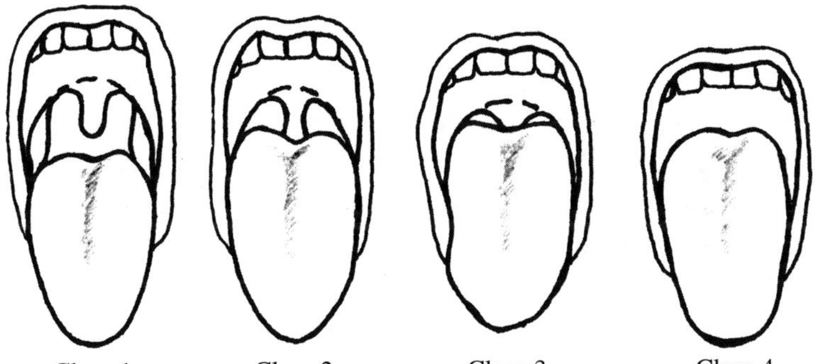

Fig. 1 Modified Mallampati's classification of pharyngeal appearance.

Class 1: The tonsils, palatopharyngeal arches, uvula, soft and hard palates are seen.
Class 2: The palatopharyngeal arches, uvula, soft and hard palates are seen.
Class 3: The soft and hard palates are seen.
Class 4: Only the hard palate is seen.

with the otorhinolaryngologist (ENT surgeon) is *mandatory* to provide optimum outcome.

Many anaesthesiologists still make use of the laryngeal grading obtained during direct laryngoscopy first described by Cormack and

Table 2 Cormack and Lehane Classification of Laryngoscopic Views

Grade I	The epiglottis can be lifted up during direct laryngoscopy and the vocal cords including the anterior commissure, and the arytenoids can be seen.
Grade II*	The epiglottis can be lifted up during direct laryngoscopy but the anterior commissure cannot be seen, only the posterior portion of the vocal cords and the arytenoids can be seen.
Grade III	The epiglottis cannot be lifted up during direct laryngoscopy and the vocal cords and the arytenoids cannot be seen.
Grade IV	The epiglottis cannot be seen, only the retropharyngeal wall can be seen.

*Some investigators have further divided Grade II into a and b. In Grade IIa, only part of the glottis is seen, and in Grade IIb, only the arytenoids or the very posterior origin of the cords are visible.

Lehane (Table 2), although other methods of scoring the laryngeal views have been described in recent years.[2–5] If the patient has had anaesthesia and surgery before, the previous anaesthesiologists may have documented any difficulty in direct laryngoscopy or tracheal intubation. In most centres, the laryngeal grading is documented preoperatively. Hence, if medical records (anaesthetic charts and case notes) are available, they should be reviewed. Alternatively, the patient could be asked if he or she had been told by the previous anaesthesiologist about difficulty in managing his or her airway.

The incidence of difficult airway is eight to 10 times higher in obstetric patients, possibly due to decreased range of head and neck movement, increased size of tongue, and laryngeal oedema. The sub-optimal laryngoscopy condition is made worse by the presence of full dentition, large breasts, and the fervent one-handed application of the Sellick's manoeuvre (or commonly known as cricoid pressure).[16]

Ideally, the Sellick's manoeuvre should be applied via a bimanual approach, that is, with the palm of one hand supporting the back of the neck while cricoid pressure is applied with the fingers of the other hand. A commonly observed practice is to have the anaesthetic assistant apply cricoid pressure in a single-handed downward approach using the head-rest or pillow, or worse, the operating table, as a counter-pressure. With an over-enthusiastic single-handed application of Sellick's manoeuvre, extension at the atlanto-occipital joint becomes restricted; and what would have been easy direct laryngoscopy can be converted to difficult laryngoscopy.

Considerations in Securing the Airway in an Emergency Setting

For the physician who is inexperienced in emergency airway management, help from an anaesthesiologist is recommended for these patients.

Awake, sedated or anaesthetised?

The decision to secure the airway with the patient awake or anaesthetised should be made in relation to the indication for tracheal intubation.

The upper airway is better maintained in the awake patient. If the management of the airway is expected to be difficult when the patient is rendered unconscious, and if insufficient skilled assistants are available, then the airway should be secured with the patient awake. Although endotracheal intubation in the awake patient is more time-consuming and generally more uncomfortable for the patient, it is the safest approach.

If management of the airway is not expected to be difficult when the patient is rendered unconscious, sedative (diazepam or mida-zolam) or anaesthetic agent (thiopentone, propofol or etomidate) may be administered prior to tracheal intubation to reduce patient's anxiety. However, the physician should be familiar with the pharmacology of the drugs that are administered. For example, the hypotensive effect due to the administration of these agents in the hypovolaemic patient must be expected and fluid therapy should be instituted to minimise the hypotensive effect. Sedation of the patient brings with it other problems. One common problem encountered in the deeply sedated patient is that breathing becomes shallow and apnoea may even occur. Arterial oxygen saturation decreases as a result of atelectasis of the lungs, shunting of venous blood, and venous admixture. In the lightly sedated patient, any airway manipulation may result in laryngospasm and breath holding.

In the event that the use of muscle relaxant is contemplated, as a safeguard against the "cannot intubate and cannot ventilate" scenario from developing, it is always prudent to assess that mask ventilation is possible before paralysing the patient. Knowing that manual ventilation via the facemask is possible will reassure the physician that he or she can continue to ventilate and oxygenate the patient in the event that tracheal intubation is unsuccessful. The management of the "cannot intubate and cannot ventilate" scenario will be discussed under the "Unpredicted difficult direct laryngoscopy" section.

In the event of lack of expertise, *Do Not Sedate or Paralyse the Patient.*

Gastric regurgitation and pulmonary aspiration

Unless certain about the fasting period prior to airway management, it is safer to assume that the patient has not been adequately fasted and has a full stomach.

If a nasogastric tube has been inserted as part of the overall management plan of the patient, it is better to aspirate as much gastric contents as possible before airway management. It should then be removed so that when cricoid pressure is applied during intubation of the unconscious patient, occlusion of the upper oesophagus will be more effective. If awake intubation is intended, then the nasogastric tube need not be removed.

Techniques of securing the airway

The options available for emergency airway management depend on whether the patient is to be intubated awake or unconscious; on the expertise of the attending physician; and on the available facilities, equipment and assistance. The technique of tracheal intubation should be one that the doctor is most comfortable with.

For the awake patient, besides intubation under direct laryngoscopy (with or without external laryngeal manipulation and the aid of the stylet or the gum elastic bougie), tracheal intubation can be guided by either flexible fibreoptic laryngoscopy, or via a guide-wire in the retrograde technique of intubation, or the breath sounds in blind nasal intubation technique. Both the fibreoptic guided tracheal intubation and the retrograde technique of tracheal intubation are suitable for patients whose head and neck have to be maintained in the neutral position. If direct laryngoscopy is difficult, and the other options are not possible, tracheostomy can be performed under local anaesthesia.

If sedation of the patient before tracheal intubation is feasible, then more options are available to secure the airway. Other than those techniques already listed for intubation in the awake patient, tracheal intubation can be guided by rigid fibreoscopy; or the intubating laryngeal mask airway; or the transillumination of the Trachlight®.

When it is recognised that death from asphyxia as a result of upper airway obstruction is imminent, a cricothyroid puncture with a 14-gauge needle and plastic cannula assembly, followed by insufflation of air or oxygen through the cannula, may be life-saving. As soon as possible, a tracheostomy should be performed so that the airway is protected and ventilation and gas exchange can be optimised. More details are provided about transtracheal jet ventilation under the "Unpredicted difficult direct laryngoscopy" section. For information on tracheostomy please refer to Chapter 8.

Psychological preparation of the patient

Adequate psychological preparation is important to obtain maximal patient cooperation and to allay anxiety. The patient should be informed about the events leading up to tracheal intubation and the inability to vocalise once the endotracheal tube is in place. The decision to sedate the patient after tracheal intubation will depend on the overall management plan.

Care and monitoring of the patient

Oxygen supplementation should be provided while the airway is being secured but without interfering with the process of securing the airway. Oxygen can be delivered to the patient's nose and mouth via any oxygen delivery system (nasal prongs or anaesthetic breathing circuit), or via the suction channel of the fibrescope, if one is used. An intravenous access is mandatory.

Monitoring of the patient should consist of arterial oxygen saturation (with pulse oximetry), blood pressure, heart rate, and electrocardiography.

Predicted Difficult Direct Laryngoscopy

Tracheal intubation with a flexible fibreoptic laryngoscope

Flexible fibreoptic guided tracheal can be performed via either the nasal or oral route and in the awake or sedated patient. For safety reasons, the airway should preferably be secured with the patient awake and for comfort reasons, via the nasal route. The preparation of the patient and the choice of the endotracheal tube are discussed below.

Preparation of the upper airway

Cotton pledgets soaked with lignocaine 10% with phenylephrine or cocaine 4% applied along the hard palate in the nasal passage can provide both topical anaesthesia and vasoconstriction of the inferior turbinate and nasal mucosa. In order to avoid exceeding toxic limits of lignocaine application, only the nasal passage intended for airway manipulation need be prepared.[9] Vasoconstriction of the nasal mucosa and inferior turbinate of the intended nasal passage prevents epistaxis. Vasoconstriction of the inferior turbinate will also provide more space for the passage of both the fibrescope and the endotracheal tube.

Topical lignocaine 10% can be sprayed onto both oral and pharyngeal surfaces to anaesthetise the region.

Bilateral superior laryngeal nerve blocks can be performed, by injecting one to two millilitres of lignocaine 1% at each superior cornu of the hyoid bone, to anaesthetise the larynx. Another two to three millilitres of lignocaine 2% can be injected through the cricothyroid membrane into the trachea during inspiration, taking advantage of the deep inhalation and coughing immediately following the injection to distribute the anaesthetic solution throughout the trachea. Although briefly described here, these two steps are not necessary for the success of fibreoptic guided tracheal intubation. Besides, with nerve blocks, the protective airway, cough and swallowing reflexes will be impaired. Usually, this region can be topically anaesthetised with the "inject-as-you-go" technique.

In the inject-as-you-go technique, a 5 ml syringe of lignocaine 2% is attached to the biopsy channel of the fibrescope. The lignocaine solution is intermittently injected through the fibrescope as the tip of the fibrescope approaches the laryngopharynx and the glottis.

The administration of an antisialogogue agent such as hyoscine hydrobromide or glycopyrrolate to dry the oral mucosa, can improve the duration of topical anaesthesia. The maximum dose of lignocaine *without* the addition of epinephrine is 3 mg/kg and should not be exceeded.

Preparation of the equipment

The external diameter of the insertion tube of the fibreoptic laryngoscope or bronchoscope determines the size of the endotracheal tube that can be used. Generally, the bronchoscope has a larger diameter insertion tube. The function of various parts of the fibrescope, such as the angulation control, the optics, and the light guide, should be checked before use.

The usual Magill endotracheal tube, anatomical preformed endotracheal tube and armoured endotracheal tube can be used for fibreoptic guided tracheal intubation. Although it is generally easier to guide a non-bevelled armoured endotracheal tube over the fibrescope and through the glottis, the technique of rotating the endotracheal tube 90° anticlockwise axially before railroading the endotracheal tube into the glottis will avoid the tip of the bevelled-endotracheal tube coming into contact with the vocal cords and the arytenoids during intubation.

As the endotracheal tube connector is the narrowest portion of the endotracheal tube, the size of the endotracheal tube prepared for intubation should be at least half to one millimetre larger than the diameter of the insertion tube of the fibrescope. Lubricating the insertion tube before passing it through the endotracheal tube will make removal of the fibrescope easy after tracheal intubation. The endotracheal tube should also be lubricated before tracheal intubation.

Fibreoscopy

Although expertise at fibrcoscopy is acquired through practice, some useful advice is given here. The anatomical structures should be identified as soon as fibreoscopy has started, to avoid "getting lost". As light is projected forwards through the fibrescope, near objects will be lighted up, and far objects will appear darker, keep the intended airway passage in the centre of the view. Any blood and secretions should preferably be suctioned through a separate large bore suctioning tube and not through the suction channel of the flexible fibrescope. After passing the fibrescope into the trachea, the patient may cough if the trachea has not been topically anaesthetised. Do wait until the patient has stopped coughing before passing the endotracheal through the glottis. While coughing, the glottis alternates between closing and opening. Trauma to the larynx may occur if the endotracheal tube is forcefully pushed into the tracheal while the patient is coughing or breath-holding. As mentioned before, rotating the endotracheal tube 90° anti-clockwise axially before railroading the endotracheal tube into the glottis, will avoid the tip of the bevelled-endotracheal tube coming into contact with the vocal cords and the arytenoids during intubation. After intubation, use the fibrescope to check the position of the tip of the endotracheal tube to exclude endo-bronchial intubation. While withdrawing the fibrescope, do not touch the angulation control, to avoid accidentally damaging the distal segment of the fibrescope.

Tracheal intubation with a rigid fibreoptic laryngoscope

These laryngoscopes are suitable for tracheal intubation via both the oral and nasal routes. With a rigid anatomical design, and incorporation of fibreoptics to view the glottis, the rigid fibreoptic laryngoscope gives better control of the soft tissues. In order to reduce the gag reflex and stress to the patient, the patient should be sedated for this technique of intubation. Examples of these laryngoscopes include the WuScope®, Glidescope®, Upsherscope® and the Bullard® laryngoscope.[10] Both these laryngoscopes have ports for suctioning, oxygen insufflation and instillation of local anaesthetic solution. While the use of the Bullard laryngoscope results in less head extension and cervical spine, extension than conventional laryngoscopes, the WuScope allows tracheal intubation without movement of the cervical spine, and is advantageous in patients with cervical spine injuries.[11,12] As with the flexible fibreoptic laryngoscope, blood and secretion can obscure the view via the fibreoptics.

The retrograde tracheal intubation technique

This technique is especially useful in the patient with limited neck mobility, who requires an emergency airway, and where visualisation of the vocal cords is prevented by blood secretions or anatomical anomaly.[13]

The upper airway of the patient is prepared as for flexible fibreoscopy.

The cricothyroid or the cricotracheal membrane is pierced with a 16-gauge needle at a cephalad angle and a suitable-size guide wire is advanced cephalad until it exits from the nose or the mouth. The endotracheal tube is then advanced over the wire, guided via the nose or mouth into the trachea while the distal end of the wire is clamped outside the neck. A common problem encountered is that the acute angulation assumed by the guide-wire causes the endotracheal tube to be obstructed by the arytenoids as it slides over the guide-wire. This can be overcome by rotating the endotracheal tube 90° anti-clockwise as it passes the vocal cords; the same technique is applied as for passing the endotracheal tube over the bougie or fibrescope.

Alternatively, the guide-wire can be threaded through the working channel of a flexible fibreoptic laryngoscope which has already been loaded with an endotracheal tube. The flexible fibrescope can then be advanced over the guide-wire into the trachea. After confirming the correct location of the fibrescope, the endotracheal tube can then be passed over the fibreoptic laryngoscope and into the trachea. With this technique, the correct location of the endotracheal tube can be confirmed visually before the removal of the guide-wire.

The obvious relative contraindications include pretracheal infection, coagulopathy, laryngo-tracheal disease, poor anatomical landmarks and pretracheal mass.

Blind nasal intubation

This technique has to be carried out in the spontaneously breathing patient. The upper airway is prepared as for flexible fibreoscopy and general lubrication of the endotracheal tube is highly recommended for a successful intubation.

The patient's head should be placed in the sniffing position. Air movement through the endotracheal tube should be continuously felt, heard or monitored by capnography. The endotracheal tube is slowly advanced during inspiration. If no airflow is detected through the endotracheal tube, it should be withdrawn until air flow is detected again. Manoeuvres such as external laryngeal pressure, extension at the atlanto-occipital joint, inflating the cuff of the endotracheal tube in the laryngopharynx, using a flexible tip endotracheal tube or the use of a stylet, may help guide the endotracheal tube more anteriorly into the glottis.

Tracheal intubation through an intubating laryngeal mask

The intubating laryngeal mask airway was created as an airway system with better intubation characteristics than the conventional laryngeal mask airway. Like the conventional laryngeal mask airway, it has an elliptical cuff that will form a low pressure seal in the laryngopharynx around the laryngeal inlet.[14] When placed accurately, the laryngeal mask airway supersedes the combination of facemask and an oral airway by providing the airway and freeing the hand. One advantage that the intubating laryngeal mask airway has over the conventional laryngeal mask airway is that the use of the intubating model eliminates the need for head and neck manipulation during placement.

The principal features of the intubating laryngeal mask airway system are an anatomically curved, rigid airway tube with an integral guiding handle, an epiglottic elevating bar replacing the mask bars, a guiding ramp built into the floor of the mask aperture, and a modified silicone tracheal tube developed for use with the device.[15]

The patient has to be anaesthetised for the placement of the intubating laryngeal mask airway. In a local study involving anaesthetised patients, blind tracheal intubation with the modified silicone endotracheal tube through the intubating laryngeal mask airway was successful in 97% of patients — 50% on the first attempt, 42% on the second and 5% on the third. Success was improved by pulling the metal handle of the intubating laryngeal mask airway towards the intubator in an "extension" manoeuvre, if intubation was not possible on the first attempt.[16]

Tracheal intubation with a Trachlight®

This device comprises three parts: a reusable handle, a flexible wand, and a stiff retractable stylet. The wand is a flexible plastic shaft with a bright light bulb at the distal end. This bulb provides transillumination of the soft tissue of the neck. Tracheal intubation can be accomplished in ambient light in most cases. As the illuminating light enters the trachea, it remains bright and circumscribed. If the tip enters the oesophagus, the light becomes diffused. The retractable stylet allows the device to be shaped into a hockey stick, which directs bright light against the anterior wall of the larynx and the trachea. It also permits manoeuvrability when railroading the endotracheal tube in the trachea.

Several factors impair its usefulness; these include obesity, neck tumours, blood and secretions and anterior cervical scars from previous neck operations. The Trachlight® does have some limitations. As it is a light-guided technique in which there is no direct visualisation of the upper airway structures, it should be avoided in patients with known anatomical abnormalities of the upper airway, and used with caution in patients in whom transillumination of the anterior neck may not be achieved adequately. As with any intubating technique, successful intubation using the Trachlight® relies on the preparation of the patient and the operator's skill and experience.[17] It is obvious that this technique is difficult to carry out in the awake patient.

Unpredicted Difficult Direct Laryngoscopy

In the event that the initial tracheal intubation under direct laryngoscopy fails, and the patient had been anaesthetised and paralysed, the facemask should be reapplied and the patient should receive oxygen and ventilation to maintain gas exchange. The degree of difficulty of laryngoscopy should be assessed and one optimal or best attempt at laryngoscopy (described below) should be made. The amount of bleeding and laryngeal oedema increases after every attempt at intubation. Therefore it is prudent to stop attempting to intubate the trachea after a few failed attempts while ventilation can still be maintained. Otherwise, persistent and prolonged attempts at intubation may result in the inability to ventilate the patient via facemask as well — that is the "cannot intubate and cannot ventilate" scenario. *Patients do not die from failure to intubate, but rather, from a failure to stop trying to intubate.*

Optimal or best attempt at laryngoscopy

The laryngoscopy should be performed by an experienced laryngoscopist. If possible, the patient should be placed in an optimal "sniff"

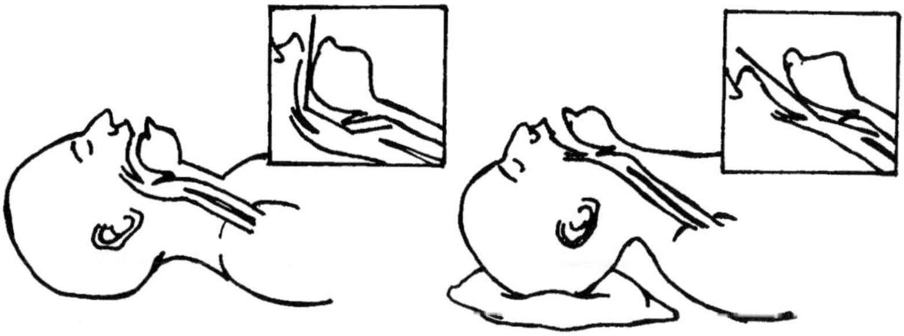

(a) (b)

Fig. 2 The alignment of the oral, pharyngeal and laryngeal axes. (a) Head and neck in neutral position. The oral, pharyngeal and laryngeal axes are not aligned. (b) "Sniff position". With a pillow under the head, and the neck flexed and atlanto-occipital joint extended, the oral and pharyngeal axes are in alignment. With displacement of the tongue towards the left and the submental space during direct laryngoscopy, one should then be able to visualise the glottis.

position, which should allow alignment of the oral, pharyngeal and laryngeal axes into a straight line during direct laryngoscopy (Fig. 2). It may involve placing a pillow, or blanket, or folded towels under the patient's shoulders, scapula, nape of the neck and head maximising flexion of the neck and extension of the atlanto-occipital joint. Optimal external laryngeal manipulation often improves the view of the glottis in difficult laryngoscopy.

Depending on the preference of the individual physician, either a malleable stylet or a gum elastic bougie can be used to guide the endotracheal tube into the trachea. The malleable stylet can be inserted into the endotracheal tube to increase the curvature of the tube. Care should be taken not to allow the distal end of the stylet to protrude past the endotracheal tube as it could traumatise and lacerate the trachea during tracheal intubation. The distal tip of the gum elastic bougie is already angulated to facilitate intubation of the "anterior" larynx. This angulation should not be corrected as a broken bougie is useless. Sometimes during railroading of the endotracheal tube over the bougie, the tube may impinge on the vocal cords and resist passing into the trachea. This can be resolved by rotating the endotracheal tube 90° anti-clockwise before passing the tube through the glottis.

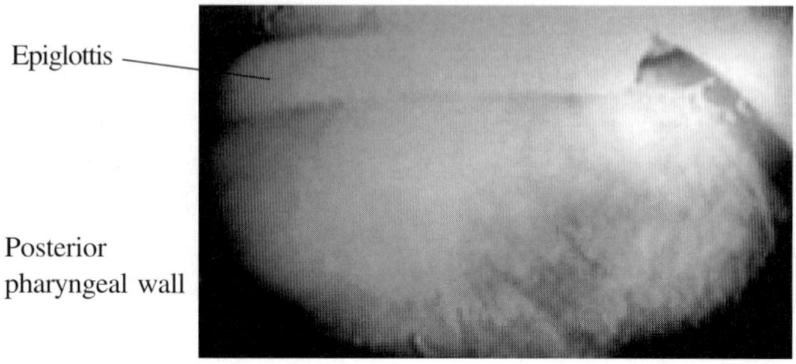

Fig. 3 Grade III laryngeal view. The epiglottis cannot be lifted during direct laryngoscopy and is seen as apposing against the retropharyngeal wall.

The curved Macintosh laryngoscope blade should be long enough to put tension on the hyo-epiglottic ligament, while the straight Miller blade must be long enough to trap the epiglottis against the tongue. A Macintosh blade is better when there is little upper airway room, and the Miller blade is useful when the incisors are large, mandibular space is limited and the epiglottis is floppy. A one-time change of the type of blade can be made if necessary. For a Grade III laryngeal view (Fig. 3), the tip of the curved Macintosh blade can be pushed into the oesophagus and then slowly pulled back until part of the glottis is seen. Without altering the laryngoscope position, a gum elastic bougie is introduced into the trachea to guide the endotracheal tube into the trachea. If only the arytenoids are seen with this manoeuvre, the tactile sensation, arising from the tip of the bougie coming into contact with the tracheal cartilage as the bougie is passed into the trachea, may help to confirm the correct placement of the bougie.

Cannot intubate and cannot ventilate scenario

"Cannot ventilate by mask" refers to the scenario when a reasonably experienced practitioner cannot maintain a life sustaining amount of gas exchange in the patient. "Cannot intubate" means that the same practitioner cannot intubate the trachea of the patient within a life-sustaining amount of time. The incidence is 0.01 to 2 per 10,000. This is a true life threatening emergency and gas exchange must be restored immediately. The options to manage the "cannot intubate and cannot ventilate" situation involve the use of the laryngeal mask airway, transtracheal jet ventilation, surgical airway or the Combitube®.

Laryngeal mask airway

The laryngeal mask airway has worked well as a ventilatory device in the "cannot intubate and cannot ventilate" scenario, and has been included in the American Society of Anesthesiologists' Management of Difficult Airway Algorithm.[18] However, the laryngeal mask airway remains a supraglottic device, which means that it cannot relieve glottic or subglottic airway obstructions, and cannot guarantee a seal against pulmonary aspiration of gastric contents. Its placement should then become a conduit for the fibrescope and subsequent guided tracheal intubation. If the intubating laryngeal mask airway (LMA Fastrach®) is used, the trachea can be intubated with the modified silicone endotracheal tube guided through the airway device.

Some complications that have been associated with its use include failed insertion, gastric insufflation, airway trauma, laryngospasm, bronchospasm, regurgitation and pulmonary aspiration. Malposition of the laryngeal mask airway can increase the risk of aspiration. The incidence of aspiration associated with the use of this device is two in 10,000.[19] The incidence of failed placement of the laryngeal mask airway is one to five percent, but this decreases with increased experience.

Laryngeal mask airway Proseal® is the most recent variation designed with a posterior modified cuff. This modification incorporates a channel which can be used for gastric tube placement or as an escape conduit for regurgitant fluid. Theoretically, it should minimise the risk of pulmonary aspiration. Furthermore, the modified posterior cuff improves the laryngeal seal and allows positive pressure ventilation with higher airway pressures than the conventional laryngeal mask airway.

Transtracheal jet ventilation

This method provides a temporary method of ventilation of the lungs while a more definite airway is established. The basic equipment includes over-the-needle catheter, a Luer® lock adaptor, a non-compressible oxygen tubing and a pressurised oxygen source. The complications include barotraumas, breath-stacking due to inadequate exhalation, tissue emphysema, pneumothorax and carbon dioxide retention.

Surgical airway

After exhausting one's personal repertoire of techniques, simply repeating the failed methods will lead to progressive laryngeal and pharyngeal oedema and potential airway obstruction with little chance of success. The remaining options would include surgical airways, such as percutaneous or surgical tracheostomy and surgical cricothyroidotomy. These would be described in Chapter 8.

Oesophageal-tracheal Combitube®

Several guidelines including that of the European Resuscitation Council, American Heart Association and American Society of Anesthesiologists have included the Combitube® as a primary rescue device in "cannot intubate and cannot ventilate" situations.[20] The oesophageal-tracheal Combitube® is a well established device in emergency medicine, providing adequate ventilation and oxygenation without the need for direct laryngoscopy with a low risk/benefit ratio.[21] The Combitube may be a suitable alternative to the laryngeal mask for use in resuscitation by unskilled staff.[22] The main advantage of the Combitube® is that it protects the airway and facilitates high airway pressure ventilation when placed correctly.[23] However, its use is associated with a higher incidence of postoperative dysphagia, sore throat, haematoma and mucosal lacerations compared to the laryngeal mask airway and indeed tracheal intubation.[24] This has been attributed to the pressure exerted on the anterior pharyngeal wall by the 85 ml pharyngeal cuff of the Combitube®. In patients whose necks are immobilised in rigid cervical collars, the success rate of placement is low.[25] The paediatric size Combitube® is currently not commercially available.

Confirmation of Correct Endotracheal Tube Placement

Visualisation of the endotracheal tube entering the glottis, detection of sustained exhaled carbon dioxide with capnography, in conjunction with auscultation of the axillae and epigastrium, can quickly confirm successful tracheal intubation. If the fibrescope had been used to guide tracheal intubation, visualisation of the tracheal cartilage, carina and the tip of the endotracheal tube through the fibrescope confirms correct endotracheal tube placement.

Documentation

The doctors involved in the management of the difficult airway must communicate this experience to future doctors so that complications from an airway incident can be averted in future. The airway difficulty must be carefully explained to the patient and relatives, impressing upon them to communicate this to future doctors. In addition, a detailed note explaining the difficulty or a medic alert card or bracelet for difficulty airway may be given to the patient. There should also be proper and prominent documentation of the difficult airway in the casenotes.

Patients who have had an intubation via direct laryngoscopy should have their laryngoscopic view grading documented in the casenotes or the anaesthetic charts. This grading has been shown in a local study to provide a reliable guide for future airway management in these patients.[26]

Conclusion

Recognition of the difficult airway, though not always possible, is crucial to prevent an airway catastrophe. The routine use and practice of more specialised airway devices will improve performance and reduce complications. Each device has its unique properties that are advantageous in some situations and limiting in others.

References

1. Mendelson CL (1946). The aspiration of stomach contents into the lungs during obstetric anesthesia. *Am J Obstet Gynecol* **52**, 191.
2. Cormack RS, Lehane J (1984). Difficult tracheal intubation in obstetrics. *Anaesthesia* **39**(11), 1105–1111.
3. Yentis SM, Lee DJ (1998). Evaluation of an improved scoring system for the grading of direct laryngoscopy. *Anaesthesia* **53**(11), 1041–1044.
4. Ochroch EA, Hollander JE, Kush S, Shofer FS, Levitan RM (1999). Assessment of laryngeal view: percentage of glottic opening score versus Cormack and Lehane grading. *Can J Anaesth* **46**(10), 987–990.
5. Cook TM (2000). A new practical classification of laryngeal view. *Anaesthesia* **55**(3), 274–279.
6. Sellick BA (1961). Cricoid pressure to control regurgitation of stomach contents during induction of anaesthesia. *Lancet* **2**, 404.
7. Mallampati SR (1983). A clinical sign to predict difficult tracheal intubation. *Can J Anesth* **30**, 316–317.
8. Samsoon GLT, Young JRB (1987). Difficult tracheal intubation: a retrospective study. *Anaesthesia* **42**, 487–490.
9. Hwang NC. *Fiberoptic Guided Tracheal Intubation — A Practical Approach* (1995). Singapore: McGraw-Hill Book Company (ISBN 0-07-113379-8).
10. Gorback MS (1991). Management of the challenging airway with the Bullard laryngoscope. *J Clin Anesth* **3**, 473–477.
11. Hastings RH, Vigil AC, Hanna R, Yang B-Y, Sartoris DJ (1995). Cervical spine movement during laryngoscopy with the Bullard, Macintosh, and Miller laryngoscopes. *Anesthesiology* **82**, 859–869.

12. Wu T, Chou H (1994). A new laryngoscope: the combination intubating device. *Anesthesiology* **82**, 1085.
13. Gupta B, McDonald JS, Brooks JH, Mendenhall J (1989). Oral fiberoptic intubation over a retrograde guidewire. *Anesth Analg* **68**(4), 517–519.
14. Braude N, Clements EA, Hodges UM, Andrews BP (1989). The pressor response and laryngeal mask insertion. A comparison with tracheal intubation. *Anaesthesia* **44**(7), 551–554.
15. Brain AI, Verghese C, Addy EV, Kapila A (1997). The intubating laryngeal mask. I: development of a new device for intubation of the trachea. *Br J Anaesth* **79**(6), 699–703.
16. Chan YW, Kong CF, Kong CS, Hwang NC, Ip-Yam PC (1998). The intubating laryngeal mask airway (ILMA): initial experience in Singapore. *Br J Anaesth* **81**(4), 610–611.
17. Hung OR, Stewart RD (1995). Lightwand intubation: I — a new lightwand device. *Can J Anaesth* **42**(9), 820–825.
18. Benumof JL (1996). Laryngeal mask airway and the ASA difficult airway algorithm. *Anesthesiology* **84**, 686–699.
19. Brimacombe JR, Bery A (1995). The incidence of aspiration associated with the laryngeal mask airway: a meta-analysis of published literature. *J Clin Anesth* **7**(4), 297–305.
20. Agro F, Frass M, Benumof J, Krafft P, Urtubia R, Gaitini L, Guiliano I (2001). The esophageal tracheal combitube as a noninvasive alternative to endotracheal intubation. A review. *Minerva Anesthesiol* **67**(12), 863–874.
21. Frass M, Frenzer R, Zdrahal F, Hoflehner G, Porges P, Lackner F (1987). The esophageal tracheal combitube: preliminary results with a new airway for CPR. *Ann Emerg Med* **16**, 768–772.
22. Yardy N, Hancox D, Strang T (1999). A comparison of two airway aids for emergency use by unskilled personnel. The Combitube® and laryngeal mask. *Anaesthesia* **54**, 181–183.
23. Pepe PE, Zachariah BS, Chandra NC (1993). Invasive airway techniques in resuscitation. *Ann Emerg Med* **22**, 393–403.
24. Oczenski W, Krenn H, Dahaba AA, Binder M, El-Schahawi-Kienzl, Kohout S, Scharz S, Fitzgerald RD (1999). Complications

following the use of the Combitube®, tracheal tube and laryngeal mask airway. *Anaesthesia* **54**, 1161–1165.

25. Mercer MH, Gabbott DA (1998). Insertion of the Combitube®s airway with the cervical spine immobilised in a rigid cervical collar. *Anaesthesia* **53**(10), 971–974.
26. Koh DLK, Ip-Yam CP, Kong CF, Chew STH (2000). Evaluation of a modified grading system for direct laryngoscopy: our preliminary experience in Singapore. *SGH Proceedings* **9**, 79–82.

8

Tracheostomy

Abhilash Balakrishnan

Introduction

Although descriptions of incisions into the windpipe have been made between 2000 and 1000 B.C. in Hindu and Egyptian Sacred texts,[1] the first tracheostomy is attributed to Asclepiades of Persia in 100 B.C. It was reserved as an emergency procedure with limited success, and the operation became known as the "scandal of surgery" until its definitive description and technique was refined by Chevalier Jackson in 1909 A.D.[2]

The term tracheotomy simply means an opening in the trachea whilst a tracheostomy implies communication with the overlying skin. The words are often used interchangeably, and in a practical sense there is no difference between the two.

Indications

The main indications for a tracheostomy are:

(1) Upper Airway Obstruction
(2) Airway Support
(3) Tracheobronchial Tree Protection and/or Toilet

Details of these are found in Tables 1 and 2. In this institution, the majority of tracheostomies are done for patients with prolonged intubation in the Surgical or Medical Intensive Care Units (SICU and MICU), imminent obstruction from a carcinoma of the larynx, and as a prophlylatic measure in severe deep neck infections with possibility of airway compromise.

It is well documented that mucosal damage can take place within 72 hours of endotracheal intubation.[3] The recommended period for conversion to a tracheostomy is about a week and in our department it is usually done within the first week. This has resulted in less morbidity after extubation. Medical patients who have chronic obstructive airway disease, may have a poor cough reflex and are unable to deal

Table 1 Causes of Upper Airway Obstruction

I. Congenital
- Subglottic stenosis
- Tracheal hypoplasia
- Vocal cord paralysis

II. Acquired

Traumatic
- Blunt trauma to neck and larynx
- Severe facial trauma
- Foreign bodies
- Burns/corrosive injury to face, upper aerodigestive tract

Infective
- Epiglottitis
- Deep neck infections
- Ludwig's angina
- Diptheria

Neoplastic
- Tumours of pharynx, tongue, larynx
- Haemangioma
- Respiratory papillomatosis
- Tracheal tumour

Miscellaneous
- Angioneurotic oedema

Table 2 Indication for Assisted Ventilation/Pulmonary Toilet

Congenital
- Cardiac anomalies
- Hypoplastic lungs

Traumatic
- Head injury
- Crushed chest
- Shocked lungs

Infective
- Tetanus
- Poliomyelitis
- Pneumonia

Neoplastic
- Brain tumour
- Spinal cord tumour

Miscellaneous
- Adult respiratory distress syndrome
- Cardiac failure
- Pulmonary failure
- Guillain-Barre syndrome

with their secretions. A tracheostomy decreases the dead space and thus decreases the respiratory effort required and allows nursing staff or family members to clear the bronchial secretions adequately. Quality of life and personal hygiene are also thus improved.

Types of Tracheostomy

Elective

Most tracheostomies done in this hospital are elective as a planned procedure done in the operating theatre. Many of the patients are already intubated, especially those from the MICU. There is *almost* no place for bedside tracheostomies (except in the situations mentioned below) with all its attendant risks and morbidity in current day surgical practice. Bedside tracheostomies are to be condemned, as problems can arise even in experienced hands, and should always be done in optimal surroundings for the patients' benefit and well being.

Urgent

This situation arises in the Singapore General Hospital when patients with a confirmed diagnosis of laryngeal carcinoma, having refused all treatment, are admitted from A&E with increasing stridor and obvious respiratory distress. They are often difficult to intubate due to an obstructing large tumour and an "awake" tracheostomy under local anaesthesia has to be done, sometimes in a semi-sitting position.

Emergency

Also known as a "slash tracheostomy" in the US, this should only be performed in the rare situation where a patient collapses in the ward, intubation has been attempted and failed, and a cricothyrotomy set is unavailable. No physician without prior experience should attempt a tracheostomy, as it is a dangerous procedure in untrained hands.

Whilst most tracheostomies are of a temporary nature, some may be permanent, for example patients with bilateral vocal cord palsies or severe Obstructive Sleep Apnea who do not want any definitive surgical procedures.

Surgical Anatomy

It is important to appreciate the relevant anatomy before a tracheostomy is contemplated. Regardless of whether a horizontal or vertical skin incision is used, the eventual dissection is in the midline. The various layers of the neck that are traversed are listed in Table 3.

In a patient with a thin neck, each of these layers can be well delineated. The following anatomical points must be borne in mind during the surgery to avoid mishaps.

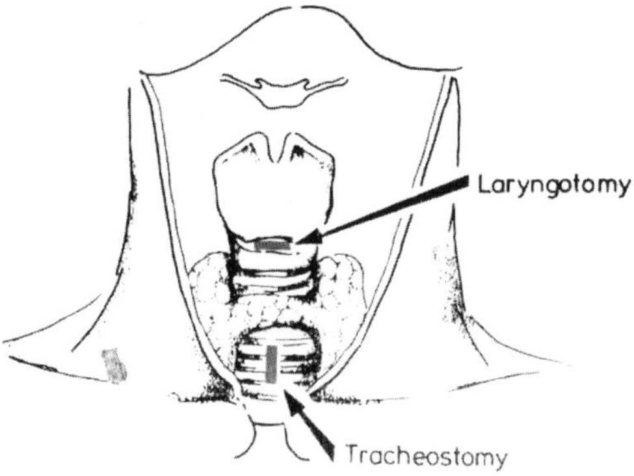

Fig. 1 Surgical anatomy and incision sites.

Table 3 Traversal of Various Layers of the Neck

Skin
Subcutaneous fat
Superficial layer of superficial cervical fascia
Platysma
Superficial layer of the deep cervical fascia
Strap muscles
Pretracheal fascia
Isthmus of thyroid
Pretracheal fascia
Trachea

(1) The isthmus of the thyroid overlies the second, third and fourth tracheal rings. This may have to be divided and suture ligated as it is very vascular.
(2) A pair of anterior jugular veins lies under cover of the platysma. These may need to be ligated.
(3) Paratracheal structures at risk include the carotid vessels, the internal jugular vein, and recurrent larygeal nerves, especially if the surgeon does not keep strictly to the midline.
(4) The cupola of the pleura is drawn up into the neck when it is extended in positioning the patient. Damage to this can cause a tension pneumothorax.

(5) The brachiocephalic trunk or innominate artery crosses left to right anterior to the trachea at the thoracic inlet, and may also expand into the neck during extension.
(6) The larynx consists of three large cartilages, of which the thyroid and cricoid are the most important during tracheostomy.

Surgical Procedure

Preoperative

A full blood count and a coagulation profile may be useful in certain patients, especially those with bleeding disorders. A haematological consultation is mandatory to correct these, and a platelet count of at least 60×10^9/L is necessary before an intubated patient is converted to a tracheostomy.

In the anaesthetised patient, the neck should be extended with a shoulder roll placed in the interscapular area. This allows for at least 6–10 rings of the trachea to be brought up into the neck. Surface markings are the cricoid cartilage superiorly and the suprasternal notch inferiorly (Fig. 2).

The surgeon should personally choose the appropriate size tracheostomy tube, test it and ensure that the cuff is patent before starting the

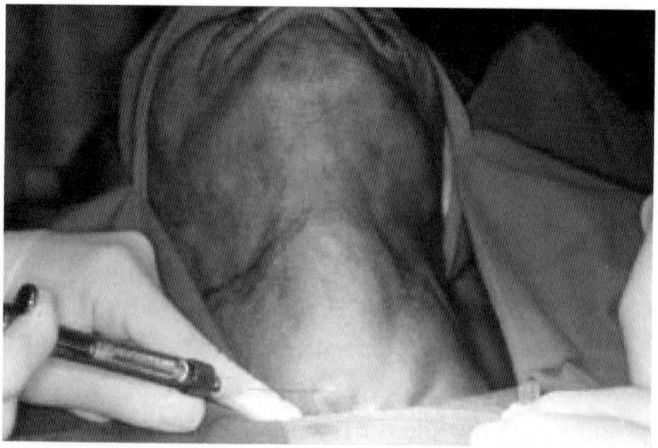

Fig. 2 Surface marking and local anaesthesia.

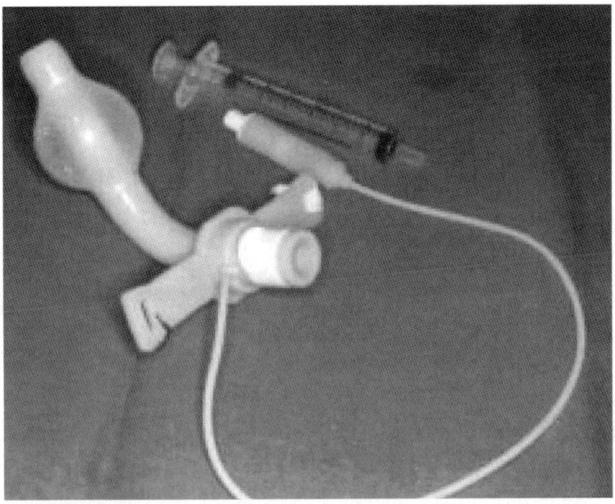

Fig. 3 Cuffed tube being tested.

procedure (Fig. 3). In a fresh tracheostomy, it is safer to use a cuffed tube, as the patient may continue to need post-op ventilation and also to prevent aspiration of secretions and blood.

Intraoperative

If the operation is done under local anaesthesia, it would be prudent to have an anaesthetist monitoring the patient and providing sedation as necessary. If the operation is done under general anaesthesia, the surgeon should co-ordinate with the anaesthetist when he is ready to have the tube removed for insertion of the tracheostomy tube. Tracheostomy is not an operation to be done by a single operator; an assistant is absolutely necessary.

The patient is cleaned and draped in such a way that the anaesthetist can have easy access to the airway without sacrificing sterility in the surgical field. A transvenous skin incision is made between the cricoid cartilage and suprasternal notch. Bleeding can be decreased if the incisional site is injected subcutaneously with a solution consisting of lignocaine® 1% with 1:80,000 Adrenaline using a dental syringe. In patients with chronically progressive airway obstruction, for example carcinoma of the larynx, there is a good deal of venous congestion, and troublesome bleeding may be encountered. The incision is extended through subcutaneous tissue and platysma until the superficial layer of the deep cervical fascia is reached (Fig. 4). If the pair of anterior jugular veins are in the way, these are clamped, divided and ligated. From here on the incision continues in the vertical plane, using electrocautery or retractors to separate the strap muscles along their median raphe until the thyroid gland is reached (Fig. 5). Here,

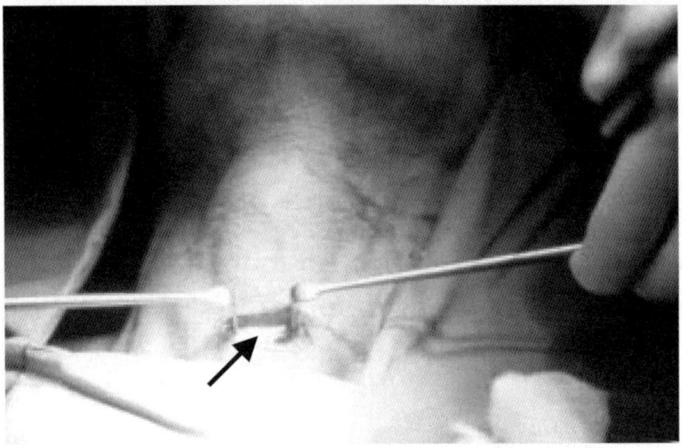

Fig. 4 Transverse skin incision exposing the superficial layer of deep cervical fascia.

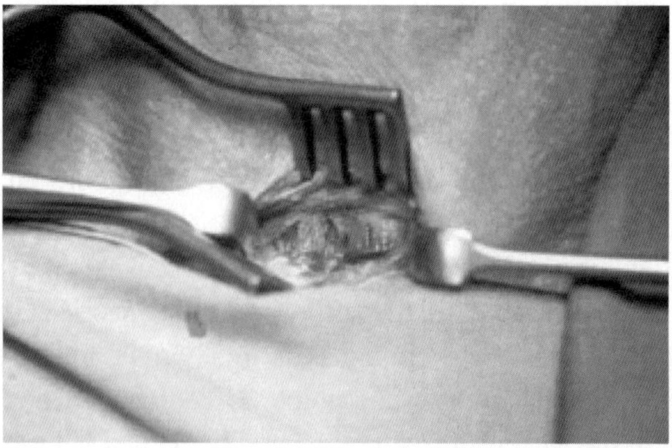

Fig. 5 Strap muscles being separated in the vertical place.

a few options are available. If the thyroid gland overlies mainly the thyroid cartilage, the isthmus can be retracted superiorly using a cricoid hook, but if it overlies the cricoid cartilage and upper tracheal rings, it is better to suture ligate the isthmus to expose the trachea (Fig. 6).

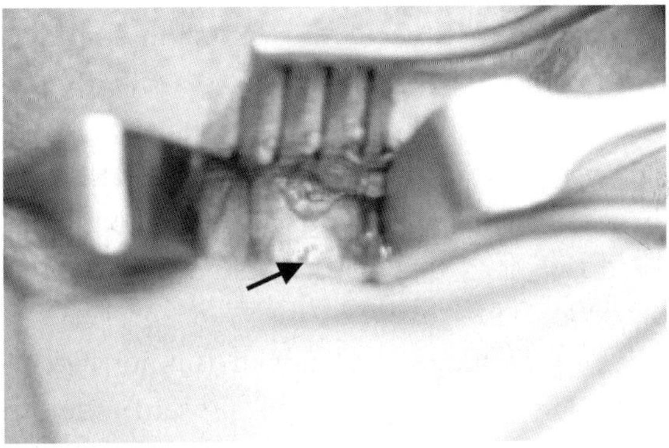

Fig. 6 Exposure of the isthmus of the thyroid gland.

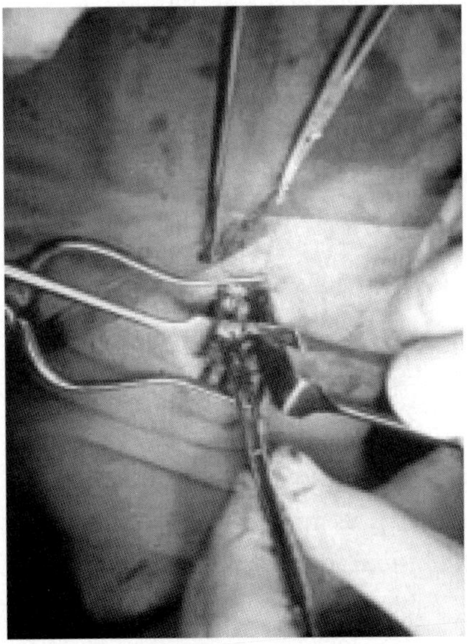

Fig. 7 Removing a circular piece of tracheal cartilage.

Once the trachea is reached, the cricoid cartilage is identified, and the anaesthetist is alerted that the trachea is about to be entered. Remove a circular ring of cartilage between the 2nd and 3rd rings or the 3rd and 4th rings, just enough to admit the previously tested tracheostomy tube (Fig. 7). There is no danger of tracheal stenosis as minimal tracheal tissue is removed. Variations of this opening include an inferior based (Björk) flap. The merits of these will not be discussed here, but excellent reviews are found in literature.[4,5] Once the trachea is entered, blood and secretions are sucked out as the suction catheter is withdrawn. This should be done sparingly as one does not want to deplete the oxygen in the lungs. A patient with tracheostomy done under local anaesthesia may undergo an apnoeic phase as the trachea is entered due to a loss of the respiratory drive from a sudden decrease in carbon dioxide levels of inspired air.

Once the ring of cartilage is removed (taking care not to cut into the underlying endotracheal tube when present), the tracheal dilator is used to guide the previously chosen tracheostomy tube into the trachea. Most tubes also have an obturator in the inner lumen and this helps to slip the tube into the trachea. The cuff of the tracheostomy tube is inflated and the appropriate connector is handed to the anaesthetist to continue ventilation of the patient. The tube is then secured firmly by tapes with the neck flexed and the shoulder roll removed. The flanges of the tracheostomy tube are stitched down to prevent accidental decannulation. The incision is *not* closed, so as to minimise the risk of subcutaneous emphysema and pneumomediastinum. A soft gauze is placed on either side beneath the flange to soak secretions and blood.

Choice of tube

An age-appropriate tube should be used. Both the Portex® and Shiley® cuffed tubes are suitable. These have low pressure, high volume cuffs to minimise tracheal damage. The technical data of these tubes for adolescents and adults are given in Table 4. It is important not to choose too large or too long a tube as these can erode the anterior

Table 4

Portex® Tracheostomy Tubes, Blue Line, Siliconised PVC, Profile Cuff, 15 mm Connectors*

Sizes I.D. (mm)	O.D. (mm)
6.0	8.3
7.0	9.7
7.5	10.4
8.0	11.0
9.0	12.4
10.0	13.7

Shiley®, Low Pressure Cuffed Tracheostomy Cannulae with Disposable Inner Cannula, Sterile*

Size	I.D. (mm)	O.D. (mm)
4	5.0	9.4
6	6.4	10.8
8	7.6	12.2
10	8.9	13.8

*Technical data information from Portex® and Shiley® catalogues.

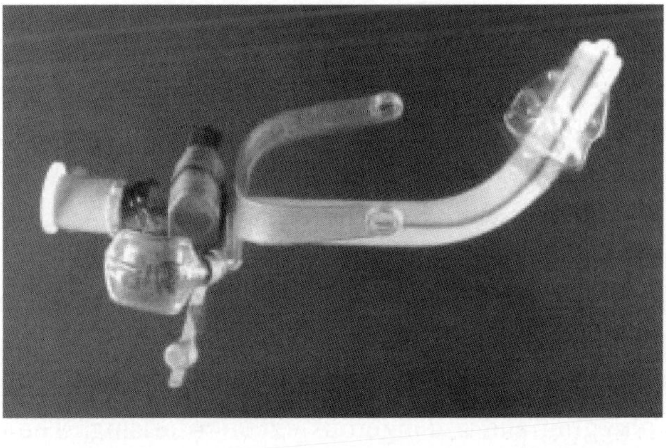

Fig. 8 Adjustable flange tracheostomy tube.

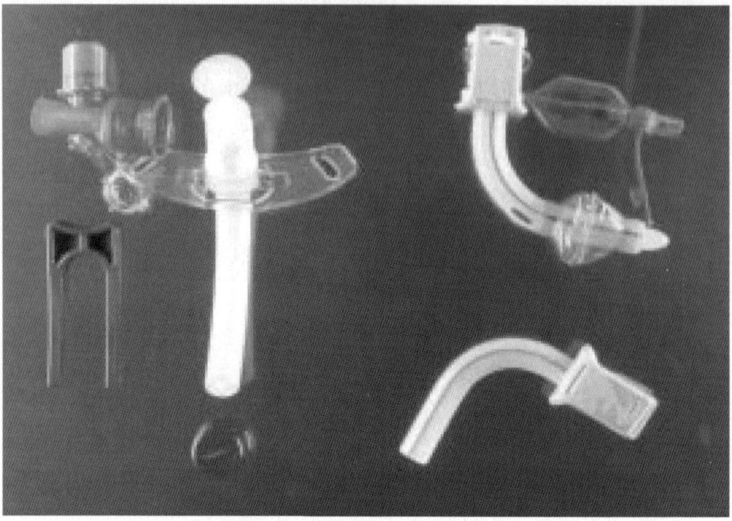

Fig. 9 Various tracheostomy tubes and connectors.

tracheal wall with dire consequences. However in certain instances a longer length may be necessary, for example, in patients with a very fat neck, an adjustable flange Portex® tracheostomy tube is available (Fig. 8). Some of the different tubes, both cuffed and non-cuffed are shown below with the various adaptors and connectors (Fig. 9).

Postoperative care

If in spite of a tracheostomy, ventilation is difficult and the patient continues to have airway obstruction, then either a pneumothorax must be suspected, or there is distal airway obstruction below the tracheostomy site. As a tracheostomy tube is a foreign body, copious secretions are produced in the first few hours to days. Frequent suction is necessary to prevent secretions from blocking off the tube, but this should be done with care, and only along the length of the tube. Humidified air, saline or mucolytic drops may decrease the possibility of mucous plugging and a dangerous situation arising. The cuff which is usually inflated for about 24 hours, should be deflated for about

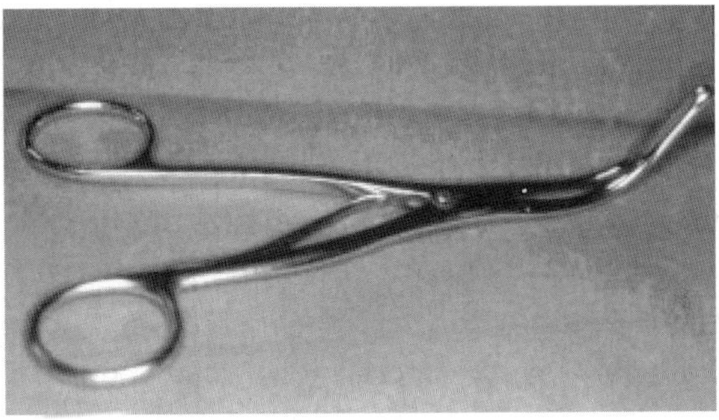

Fig. 10 Tracheal dilator.

5 minutes hourly to reduce the risk of tracheitis and pressure necrosis by the tracheostomy tube. Otherwise there may be trauma to the tracheal wall and risk of tracheal stenosis. A chest X-ray should be done in the immediate post-operative period to exclude a pneumothorax. The patient is to be observed for 24 hours in the high dependency area before transferring out into the general wards. Those needing ventilatory support will remain in the intensive care unit.

Every patient with a fresh tracheostomy should have a tracheal dilator and spare tube by the bedside (Fig. 10) Both of these can be life-saving in the situation of a dislodged or blocked tracheostomy tube.

The tracheostomy tract is fairly well formed by about 4–7 days. A first tube change is made, and if the patient is not on a ventilator, to a non-cuffed tube. It is preferable to use one with an inner tubc, as these can easily be removed if blocked, still leaving a patent airway. The inner tube should be cleaned at least once a day or ideally every eight hours. Non-cuffed tubes without an inner tube should be changed daily. The flanges need not be stitched down, and can be taped down with velcro tracheostomy tapes which are very stable.

As soon as the cuff is deflated or the patient is weaned off the ventilator, he can be trained to phonate by putting his fingers to occlude the tube as long as there is no significant laryngeal oedema. Patients who need long term tracheostomy can be evaluated by the speech therapist to have a Passy-Muir valve fitted, provided they do not have subglottic stenosis. This is a one-way valve that close automatically during exhalation for speech and open on inspiration. The patient must also be advised that there will be initial difficulty with swallowing as coordination is decreased by difficulty in laryngeal elevation after a tracheostomy.

If the patient needs a long term tracheostomy he and his family members are taught routine tracheostomy care and arrangements are made for them to either purchase or rent a suction machine and catheters.

Complications

In modern surgical practice, the mortality rate for tracheostomy in adult patients has remained below 5% and total complication rate is between 14–66%.[6] Higher morbidity and mortality rates seem to arise in tracheostomies done in the emergent state in the ICU situation and in children.

Immediate

Troublesome bleeding during surgery, apnoea due to loss of hypoxic respiratory drive and pneumothorax have all been mentioned previously.

Intermediate

(1) Primary or secondary haemorrhage is possible from a slipped ligature or increased blood pressure post-operatively. This may require a return to the operating theatre for haemostasis.
(2) Mucus plugging of the tube due to copious secretions can be a threat in the early days especially before changing to a tube with an inner cannula.
(3) Accidental decannulation is always a serious problem even if the tube is well secured. Should this happen, attempt to keep the

tracheostome open and reintroduce a spare tracheostomy tube. It is dangerous to continue if several attempts have failed because the possibility of creating a false passage into the anterior mediastinum is a reality. If this fails, a nasogastric tube or a small tube can be passed. Attempts can also be made with a flexible fibreoptic nasopharyngoscope with a tracheostomy tube as a sheath to be passed under direct vision — if all else fails, manually ventilate the patient with 100% oxygen, reintubate and rush to the operating theatre to re-establish the tracheostomy site.

(4) Subcutaneous emphysema is usually around the tracheostomy site below the hyoid bone and above the suprasternal notch. This is the main reason why no suturing of the incision should be done. If this happens, remove all sutures and tight packings immediately. Unnecessary dissection beyond the midline during surgery will also increase the risk of the emphysema spreading into multiple fascial and tissue planes.

Late complications

(1) *Haemorrhagic*

Sudden bleeding after an established tracheostomy is an ominous sign. This is often a "sentinel" bleed indicating the possibility of a tracheo-innominate artery fistula resulting from erosion of the anterior tracheal wall. Occasionally bleeding may be from granulation tissue secondary to infection around the stoma site. Appropriate emergency measures include group and cross matching the patient's blood, inspection with a flexible nasopharyngoscope and alerting the operating theatre and the thoracic surgeon.

(2) *Difficult decannulation*

This may be a result of tracheal stenosis, an obstructing granuloma, tracheomalacia or bilateral vocal cord paralysis. Evaluation of the larynx and trachea under anaesthesia may be necessary to determine the cause so that appropriate therapy can be instituted.

(3) *Laryngeal/tracheal stenosis*

During tracheostomy, no incision is made over the cricoid and 1st tracheal ring. Injury to these structures may lead to development of subglottic stenosis. Tracheal stenosis can result from overzealous removal of tracheal tissue, the use of inappropriate sized tracheostomy tubes or the prolonged use of cuffed tubes.

(4) *Tracheocutaneous fistula*

This is rare in most patients when the tracheostomy is temporary in nature. Occasionally a formal excision of the fistulous tract may be necessary. It would however be prudent to do an endoscopic evaluation of the larynx and trachea prior to closure of the fistula to ensure that there is no proximal or residual obstruction.

(5) *Tracheostomy scar*

It is often said that a transverse incision leaves a better "cosmetic" scar. As cosmesis is the least important consideration when a tracheostomy is indicated, it is useful to know that both the vertical or transverse incision leaves a small but visible scar and this is usually due to the tracheostome rather than the type of skin incision made.

Decannulation

This is considered when the need for a tracheostomy ceases to exist, and is usually decided by the surgeon. The protocol is to first downsize to a smaller tube for the first 24 hours. If this is tolerated then the tube is spigoted for 12 hours at first and then throughout the day including during sleep. If the patient tolerates this, then the tube is removed and the incision site is covered with a light gauze (Fig. 11). The whole process of decannulation takes about 3–4 days and the wound site usually heals within a week. Wherever there is uncertainty or decannulation fails, then an endoscopic assessment of the upper and lower airways may be necessary.

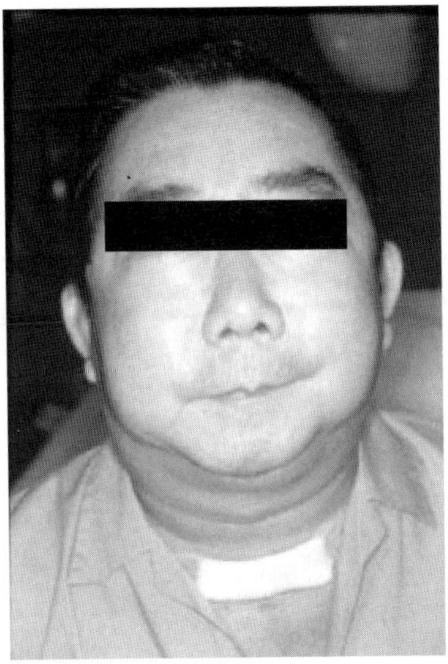

Fig. 11 A decannulated patient.

Paediatric Tracheostomy

Although the basic surgical principles remains the same, because of the absolute and relative differences in anatomy, there are subtle differences. Children have short necks, their larynx is high up in the neck and when the neck is in the extended position, the pleura, the brachiocephatic trunk and the thymus are all drawn up into the neck. Only a vertical incision is made to create an opening into the trachea. Prolene® stay sutures are placed on either side of the incision laterally to enable quick replacement if the tracheostomy tube becomes displaced. No tracheal tissue is ever removed as this will lead to tracheal stenosis. In mild to moderate cases of subglottic stenosis, alternatives to paediatric tracheostomy exist.[7]

Alteration to Tracheostomy

Cricothyroidotomy

Cricothyroidotomy (laryngotomy), or sometimes called minitracheostomy, is often touted as an easier alternative to a formal tracheostomy

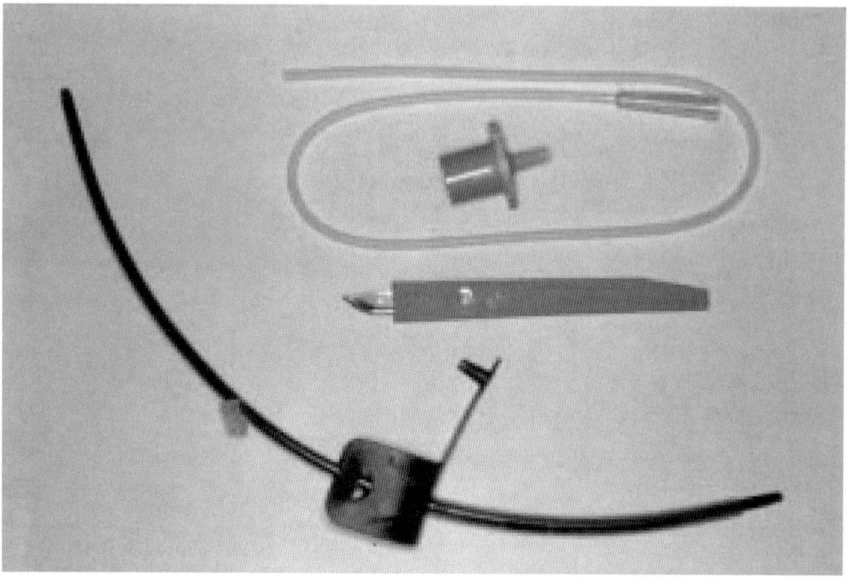

Fig. 12 Cricothyroidotomy set.

in the emergent situation. Nothing can be further from the truth. In a course conducted by the author on cadavers, even experienced otolaryngologists who had never done this procedure, took some time to successfully cannulate the trachea. So while the apparent simplicity of the procedure accounts for the perceived popularity, the higher risk of complication, like tracheal stenosis, makes it less attractive except in the truly emergency situation. A cricothyroidotomy set is usually available in the Accident and Emergency and the Ear, Nose and Throat wards (Fig. 12). A cricothyroidotomy should be converted to a formal tracheostomy as soon as possible.

Percutaneous Tracheostomy

Several variations of this technique exist: Percutaneous Dilatation Tracheostomy,[8] Rapitrach,[9] and Guide Wire Dilating Forceps Techniques.[10] All are based on the Seldinger guide wire technique using various dilators to form the tracheostome. It gained popularity in the ICU where intensivists perform it on critically ill patients who may need prolonged ventilation. There is, however, a similar learning curve as in any airway access surgery, and thus this procedure is contraindicated in the following situations:

(1) Emergency access in acute airway distress
(2) Uncorrectable bleeding disorders
   - Platelet count less than 60×10^9/L
   - Bleeding time more than 10 minutes
(3) Abnormally distorted neck anatomy
   - Previous surgical scar
   - Tumours
   - Gross thyroid enlargement
(4) Suspected tracheomalacia
(5) Obese and fat neck obscuring landmarks
(6) Paediatric age group patients

The "open" tracheostomy remains the gold standard for airway access in all situations.

Tubeless tracheostomy

Essentially this is the tracheal opening stitched to the overlying skin flaps, resulting in a permanent stoma. This is usually done in patients with severe obstructing sleep apnoea who do not want any surgical intervention, and is a reversible procedure.

Acknowledgements

I would like to express my deepest gratitude to Ms. Rajakumari N, Secretary to Surgical Specialities, KK Women's and Children's Hospital for her invaluable assistance in typing this manuscript.

References

1. Frost EAM (1976). Tracing the tracheostomy. *Ann Otol Rhinol Laryngol* **85**, 618.
2. Jackson C (1909). Tracheostomy. *Laryngoscope* **19**, 285–290.
3. Whited RE (1984). A prospective study of laryngotracheal sequelae in long-term intubation. *Laryngoscope* **94**, 367.
4. Lulenski GC, Batsakis JG (1975). Tracheal incision as a contributing factor to tracheal stenosis: an experimental study. *Am J Otol* **84**, 781–786.
5. Lulenski GC, Batsakis JG (1979). Management of flap tracheostomy: an experimental study. *Arch Otolaryngol* **105**, 260–263.
6. Stauffer JL, Olson DE, Petty TL (1981). Complications and consequences of endotracheal intubation and tracheotomy: a prospective study of 150 critically ill adult patients. *Am J Med* **70**, 65–76.
7. A Balakrishnan. Cricoid split: an alternative to paediatric tracheostomy. *Ann Acad Med* 1992.
8. Ciaglia P, Firsching R, Syniec C. (1985) Elective percutaneous dilatational tracheostomy. A new simple bedside procedure; preliminary report. *Chest* **87**(6), 715–719.
9. Schachner A, Ovil Y, Sidi J (1989). Percutaneous tracheostomy — a new method. *Crit Care Med* **17**(10), 1052–1056.
10. Griggs WM, Worthley LI, Gilligan JE (1990). A simple percutaneous tracheostomy technique. *Surg Gynecol Obstet* **170**(6), 543–545.

9

Management of Ingested Foreign Bodies

Wong-Kein Low
Hin-Ngan Tay

Introduction

Foreign body (FB) ingestion represents the largest number of urgent otolaryngology referrals in Singapore. The majority of these patients are managed as outpatients in the Emergency Department. Most ingested FBs transit through the gastro-intestinal tract uneventfully, and get passed out without the need for medical intervention. The others get impacted in the process, usually in the upper aero-digestive tract or oesophagus; and have to be removed by the otolaryngologist. Fish bones form the commonest type of FB ingested in Singapore. There is a tendency for fish bones to be lodged in the pharynx, where they can easily be removed in the Emergency Department. In the event of more distal impaction in the oesophagus, endoscopic removal under general anaesthesia may be required. Ingested FBs if unrecognised or inappropriately managed, can result in potentially life-threatening complications.

Epidemiology

In Singapore, 600 to 1200 cases of FB ingestion per year are seen in the Emergency Departments of hospitals. In a local study, fish bones constituted more than 80% of ingested FBs.[1] Ingested fish bones are commonly lodged in the tonsils (31.8–39.7%), base of the tongue (18.2–40.2%) and the cervical oesophagus (7.1–13.9%). The high incidence of fish bone ingestion is attributed to the common local practice of eating fish unfilleted. Locally, fish bone ingestion in children is common because they are frequently fed porridge cooked with fish. Fish porridge is often considered nutritious for the growing child by parents; but the fish bones may inadvertently be fed to the child. In the West, ingestion of coins and toy parts has been reported to be more common.[2] Other frequently ingested FBs in Singapore include chicken/duck bones (5.0%), pork/beef/mutton bones (1.8%) and prawn/crab shells (1.8%).

Presentation

Odynophagia and throat discomfort are the most frequent presenting symptoms in adults. In young patients who are unable to express themselves, refusal to eat or drink may be the presenting complaint. Dysphagia as a solitary symptom is uncommon.

The onset of pain is usually immediate following ingestion of the FB. The site of pain gives a good indication of the side and level of impaction. Patients with pain in the oral region or the upper part of the neck are more likely to have FBs impacted in the tonsils or tongue base. More than two-thirds of patients with FBs in the posterior pharyngeal wall, piriform fossae or cervical oesophagus experience pain in the lower part of the neck.[3] FBs in the thoracic oesophagus tend to produce retro-sternal symptoms.

Patients sometimes present with the complications that result from FB ingestion. These include para- or retro-pharyngeal abscesses, mediastinitis and complications associated with migration of the FB such as injury to major blood vessels.[4] In Singapore, major complication rates have been reported to be 2.5–7%, with at least one mortality encountered every one to two years.[5] An ingested fish bone may occasionally be seen emerging from the skin in the neck, weeks after its ingestion.[6]

It is emphasised that it is not uncommon for patients presenting with complications of FB ingestion, not to volunteer a history of its ingestion. Some would have forgotten about the FB, which may have been ingested some time ago. Others may not think the FB is relevant to the presenting complaint. It is therefore important that the attending physician be vigilant of this condition and a history of FB ingestion should actively be sought, should an index of suspicion exists.

Management in the Emergency Department

A good history and physical examination are essential in the initial assessment of the patient. Relevant information includes the type of foreign body, time of its ingestion, the presence of dysphagia or odynophagia and localisation of pain. With the oral cavity and pharynx well anaesthetised (e.g. with topical cocaine 4% spray), most patients can be adequately examined. FBs lodged in the tonsils can be seen on tongue depression and easily removed with a pair of forceps. The base of tongue and hypopharynx can usually be well inspected by indirect laryngoscopy, using the laryngeal mirror in the oropharynx. If in doubt, examination is supplemented by transnasal flexible pharyngolaryngoscope. An FB identified can usually be removed by a specially designed FB forceps, such as the Nagashima forceps. Sometimes, FBs can only be seen and removed by direct laryngoscopy under local anaesthesia. It is only in the occasional patient that general anaesthesia in the operating theatre is required to remove FB lodged at this level.

For FBs impacted more distally in the piriform fossae or cervical oesophagus, laryngeal rock and water drinking test are two useful clinical tests, which have a sensitivity of more than 72–82% in detecting a FB impacted at that level. A lateral neck x-ray would confirm the diagnosis in most cases, as most fish bones are radio-opaque (Fig. 1). To detect radiolucent bones and in cases where extensive

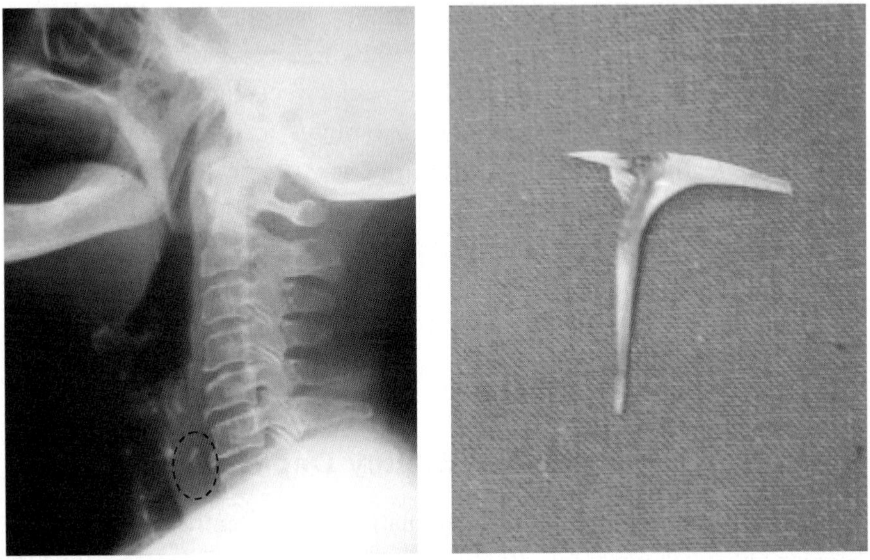

Fig. 1 Fishbone impacted in cervical oesophagus. Seen on plain lateral neck x-ray (circled). Fishbone removed intact and corresponds with x-ray image.

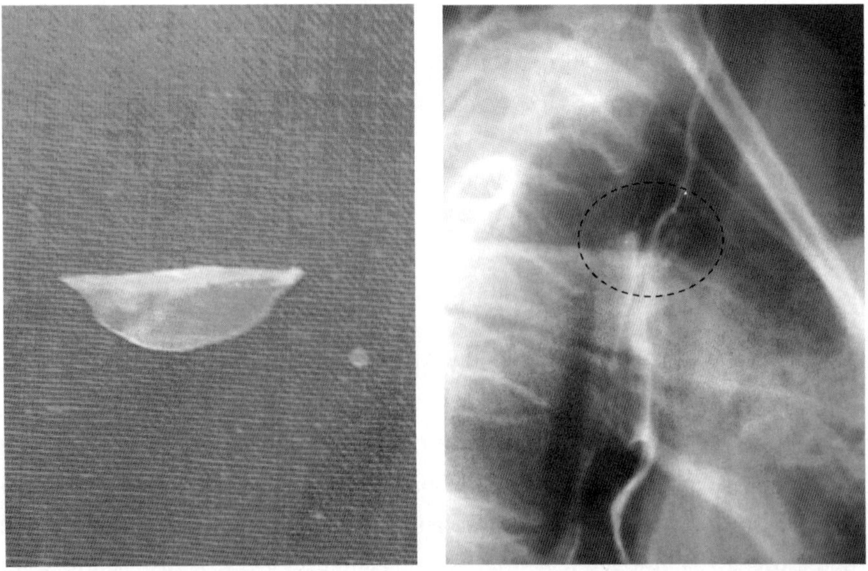

Fig. 2 Fishbone seen on barium swallow. The fishbone shown on the left was impacted in the thoracic oesophagus as illustrated on the barium swallow (circled).

laryngeal calcification makes interpretation of an impacted FB difficult, barium swallow may be indicated (Fig. 2). Even barium swallow has its limitations, with high false positive and negative rates of 6.5% and 16%, respectively. Thus if the patient is very symptomatic and the above examinations are negative, a CT scan which is highly sensitive and specific in detecting ingested FBs, is indicated.[7,8]

FBs impacted further distally in the thoracic oesophagus are usually difficult to detect on plain chest x-rays. When there is an index of suspicion of FB impacted at this level, a barium swallow or CT scan is mandatory.

Management in the Operating Theatre

Fortunately, most patients with ingested FBs do not require surgical intervention in the operating theatre. There are three main categories of surgical intervention by the otolaryngologist for ingested foreign bodies:

(1) rigid endoscopy for removal of FBs impacted in the oesophagus;
(2) migrated FBs requiring surgical exploration of the neck; and
(3) drainage of associated deep neck abscesses.

Rigid oesophagoscopy

The rigid endoscope has traditionally been used for removal of FBs impacted in the oesophagus. It is an excellent tool for locating and removing FBs, particularly in the cricopharynx, where manipulation of the scope can very effectively expose FBs which are hidden in mucosal folds or are partially embedded. In addition, removing FBs within the lumen of the rigid scope protects the oesophagus, as the process of simply pulling an unprotected sharp-edged FB out of the oesophagus can cause further injury to the oesophagus mucosa. Although the flexible oesophagoscope has been used in the removal of FBs in the oesophagus, the rigid scope is still superior in locating and removing FBs, particularly in the upper oesophagus. Flexible oesophagoscopy although uncomfortable, has the advantage of not requiring general anaesthesia and is superior in negotiating curves. Protective sheaths have been specifically designed to protect the oesophageal mucosa from sharp-edged FBs, during their removal by flexible oesophagoscopy.

We still routinely use rigid endoscopy for the removal of FBs impacted in the oesophagus. Indications for flexible endoscopy include patients who are unfit for general anaesthesia and distal oesophageal impaction, especially in patients with spinal abnormalities which render rigid endoscopy difficult.

Pre-operative preparation

It is important that the surgeon carefully assesses the patient prior to the operation. In particular, the following should be noted:

(1) Assess the cervical spine: This includes a good history and examination, to exclude cervical spinal disorders. Atlanto-axial instability or subluxation, as in rheumatoid arthritis, may result in serious complication with neck extension during intubation and endoscopy. Prominent anterior osteophytes may obstruct the advancement of the endoscope, increasing the risk of iatrogenic perforation.

(2) Assess the teeth: Loose teeth may be dislodged during endoscopy. Dental crowns especially of the upper incisors may be dislodged. Prominent upper incisors can make the procedure more difficult.

(3) Assess the chest: A chest x-ray is indicated in FBs impacted in the thoracic oesophagus. A widened mediastinum will alert the surgeon to the possibility of mediastinitis, especially if it is accompanied by gas shadows.

(4) Assess the FB: The neck x-ray is reviewed to ensure that the FB is centrally located in the lumen of the oesophagus and not outside. Localisation of the pain with respect to the side and

level is important in helping the surgeon locate the FB during endoscopy. In fact, just before induction of anaesthesia, the persistence of pain should be re-confirmed, as it is possible that the FB could have been dislodged while the patient is waiting for the procedure. A history of haematemesis may give a clue that the FB has penetrated a major blood vessel.

Informed consent includes explaining the risk of general anaesthesia, damage to dentition and the possibility of infection and abscess formation even after removal of the FB. Iatrogenic oesophageal perforation with reported rates of 0.15–0.5% and mortality rates of 0.1%, is potentially a serious complication.[9,10] Patients with FB impaction due to oesophageal strictures are especially at risk and a history suggestive of oesophageal strictures must be actively sought.

Intra-operative procedure

The patient is in a supine position with a shoulder roll and the neck slightly extended. If a "South" — pointing anatomical preformed endotracheal tube is not available, the endotracheal tube should be turned caudally to minimise interference with the procedure (Fig. 3). An armoured tube may be used to prevent compression of the tube during oesophagoscopy. Sufficient depth of anaesthesia and paralysis are important to allow easy maneouvering of the oesophagoscope and also to prevent complications like bronchospasm or iatrogenic perforation.

The oesophagoscope should be lubricated and inserted in the midline with the uvula as a good point of reference. Leverage should be on the surgeon's thumb, which is placed in the midline and never on the patient's teeth. After negotiating the oesophageal inlet, further advancement should be slow and the lumen kept central. Foreign bodies are most commonly found at the three anatomical narrowings in the oesophagus: the cricopharyngeus (16 cm), the aortic arch (23 cm) and the left bronchus (27 cm). Once the foreign body is encountered, the appropriate forceps is used for extraction. If the foreign body can pass

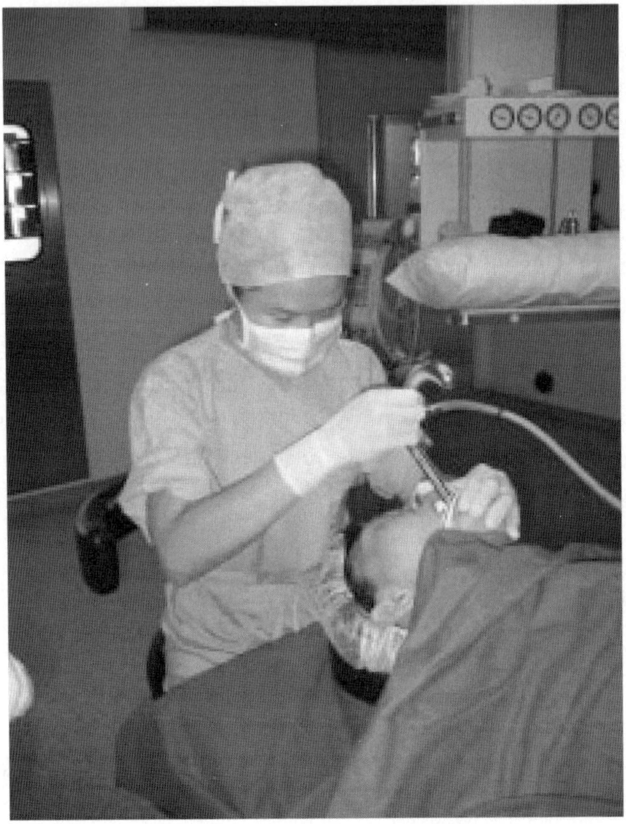

Fig. 3 Rigid oesophagoscopy in progress.

through the lumen of the oesophagoscope, it can be removed with the scope in place. Otherwise, it should be retracted as much as possible into the scope, with any sharp points sheathed and forceps, scope and foreign body removed as a unit. Large FB such as dentures may have to be cut into smaller pieces before they can be safely removed. Excessive force applied on stubbornly impacted foreign bodies could cause a perforation, especially in patients with strictures. After removal of the FB, it should be inspected to ensure that it is intact. Comparison of its dimensions with x-rays and CT scans is mandatory. Care is also taken to ensure that multiple FBs have been removed.

A situation for concern is when the FB is seen perforating the oesophageal wall, particularly if it is at the level of the aortic arch. If it is associated with significant bleeding and pulsation, the opinion of a cardiothoracic surgeon's must be sought immediately. He may decide on a formal exploration using an external approach as a major vessel is likely to have been punctured. Failure to address the vascular injury when endoscopically removing the FB, may lead to torrential bleeding and exsanguination.

In the event of a negative scope even after two passes, no further attempt should be made, to avoid further trauma to the oesophagus. The FB could have been dislodged or migrated outside the oesophageal lumen. In patients with FBs seen on x-rays to be lodged at the level of the cricopharynx, it is important to ensure that the FB is not impacted in the piriform fossa. If the FB is still not found, the patient is reversed and further evaluated radiologically in the ward.

Should there be significant mucosal trauma or suspicion of oesophageal perforation, a naso-gastric should be inserted before discontinuing anaesthesia. Dentition should also be checked after the procedure to ensure that none has been dislodged.

Post-operative care

After successful removal of the FB, the patient is observed in the general ward for sub-cutaneous emphysema and evidence of sepsis. Feeding can soon commence if there has been minimal trauma to the oesophagus, either by the foreign body or secondary to the oesophagoscopy. Should there be significant trauma, the patient is fed through the previously inserted naso-gastric tube for a few days. Before commencing feeding orally, the absence of oesophageal leakage should be confirmed with barium swallow (Fig. 4).

In the event of a failure to locate the FB endoscopically, the relevant x-rays must be repeated to confirm that the FB has indeed been dislodged. Dislodgement of the FB is not unusual, secondary to a combination of relaxation of oesophageal musculature during general anaesthesia and manipulation. If the foreign body is still present in the

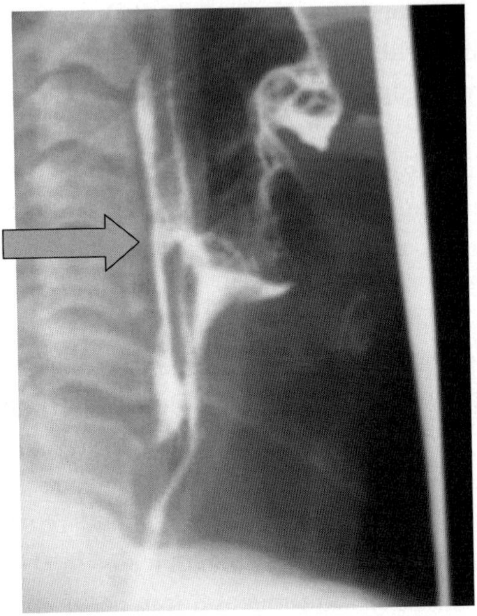

Fig. 4 Oesophageal perforation following removal of impacted fishbone via rigid oesophagoscopy. This complication, which can be caused by fishbone perforation of the oesophageal wall or traumatic extraction, is demonstrated here by the leakage of barium into the retropharyngeal space on barium swallow.

same location, extraluminal migration is likely and the patient is managed as for a migrated FB.

Surgery for migrated foreign bodies in the neck

An FB is suspected to have migrated out of the lumen of the oesophagus if:[11]

(1) It is not centrally located in the oesophagus as seen on lateral neck x-ray;
(2) The patient experiences improvement or resolution of the initial pain, and yet an FB is seen radiologically;
(3) A negative endoscopy but the FB is still present radiologically; and

(4) The FB is a needle-like fish-bone which is thin and has a sharp, pointed leading end.

Pre-operative preparation

A CT scan (preferably fine cuts of at least 3 mm with soft tissue windows) not only shows the size, orientation and position of the FB, it also demonstrates the location of the FB in relation to surrounding structures. Useful landmarks include carotid sheath, thyroid gland, thyroid and cricoid cartilages and the hyoid bone.

Pre-operative counselling for a neck exploration includes the possibility of failure in locating the foreign body, and complications of the operation such as injury to the recurrent laryngeal nerve and sympathetic chain.

Rigid endoscopy is usually performed as well and the relevant pre-operative preparation as described previously for rigid endoscopy, applies.

Intra-operative procedure

A rigid endoscopy is performed as described previously. Endoscopy before exploring the neck is useful for two reasons:

(1) It confirms that FB has completely migrated out of the lumen of the oesophagus. By appropriately manipulating the end of the rigid endoscope, it is sometimes possible to reveal the tip of the FB. It can then be removed by a pair of forceps endoscopically, without the need to proceed to a neck exploration.
(2) It identifies the site of luminal exit by the FB, for example, a puncture mark or an area of granulation may be present. The tip of the rigid endoscope can later be placed at this site where it can be palpated from the neck during exploration. This gives an indication of the exact location of the FB.

A nasogastric tube is inserted before commencing the exploration. The level of the incision is determined by the location of the foreign body as indicated on the CT scan. Exploration should be systematic and follow the anatomical neck spaces the foreign body is suspected to be in. Locating the foreign body has been described as "searching for a needle in a haystack", but this may be aided by taking reference from the surrounding structures and comparing with the x-rays and CT scans as well as from endoscopic guidance. Intra-operative clues include induration and oedema surrounding the foreign body or even a small pocket of suppuration containing the foreign body. An oesophagotomy may be required if the FB is lodged submucosally. Because of mucosal oedema, it is often difficult to be able to palpate a FB embedded beneath the mucosa. A useful technique to locate such a FB is to grip and lift the mucosa with a pair of forceps, in the area where the FB is suspected to be. If the FB is embedded beneath, mucosal tenting by the whole FB will be observed.

After the FB has been retrieved, if an oesophagotomy was performed, it can be closed with absorbable sutures in a watertight fashion. We usually use 3/0 Vicryl in a continuous closure. Any tear in the oesophagus due to foreign body perforation may be repaired in a similar way. Meticulous haemostasis and lavage must be performed to decrease the risk of haematoma or abscess formation. The decision whether to insert drains is dependent on the extent of contamination, and the amount of intra-operative bleeding. The nasogastric tube is left *in situ*, so that the patient can be fed through it post-operatively.

Post-operative care

Our patients are usually nursed and monitored in the high dependency ward after neck exploration. Intravenous antibiotics should be continued for a week.

If indicated, radiological investigations are repeated to confirm that the foreign body has been completely removed and to exclude any space occupying lesion, e.g. haematoma or seroma compressing the trachea.

Feeding is through the nasogastric tube until the surgeon is satisfied that it is safe to feed orally. In the case where the oesophagus has been breached, a barium swallow to exclude leakage is done seven to ten days after the operation, before feeding the patient per-orally. Resumption of feeding should proceed gradually, the patient being fit for discharge once normal oral feeding is tolerated without problems.

Drainage of deep neck abscesses

In a local series, 27% of neck abscesses were found to be secondary to FBs[12] (Fig. 5). Thus when patients present with a history of foreign body ingestion associated with systemic symptoms of fever, or signs like trismus, oedema and swelling intra-orally or externally, the index of suspicion for the presence of a deep neck space infection should

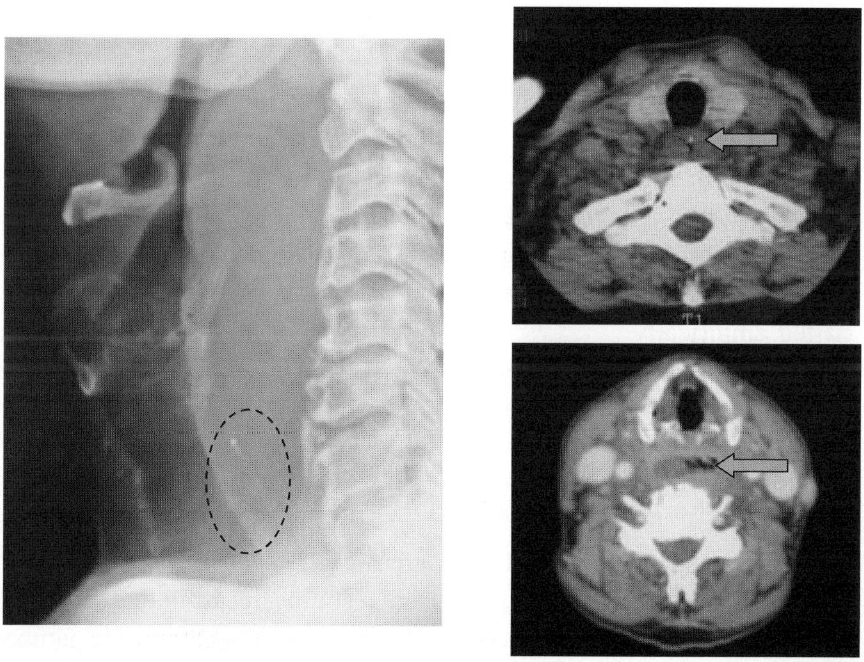

Fig. 5 Fishbone impacted in cervical oesophagus with retropharyngeal abscess formation. Fishbone (circled) seen in plain lateral neck x-ray with widening of retropharyngeal space. Fishbone (arrow) seen in top CT scan. Retropharyngeal abscess with pockets of air (arrow) seen in lower CT scan.

be very high. Similarly, when a patient presents with a deep neck abscess, a history of FB ingestion must be actively sought. These patients require not only urgent surgical drainage of the abscess but also removal of the causative FB.

Pre-operative preparation

Airway compromise is a major consideration in patients who develop deep neck abscesses. The abscess can potentially block the upper airway, and infection can also spread to the supra-glottis and glottis. The airway must be monitored and if necessary secured by intubation or tracheostomy. Even if tracheostomy is not indicated on admission, consent for it should be obtained in case airway is compromised later. Another major consideration is the development of septicaemic shock. The vital signs must be carefully monitored and the patient resuscitated if necessary.

Upon admission, aerobic and anaerobic blood cultures should be taken and intravenous antibiotics started immediately. A study in Singapore revealed both Gram-negative and -positive organisms causing deep neck abscesses: *Klebsiella* (32%), *Pseudomonas aeruginosa* (14%), *Staphylococcus aureus* (9%) and *alpha-Streptococcus* (5%). An antibiotic which is broad-spectrum, should therefore be started empirically.

CT scans of the neck provides essential information for the surgeon in planning and draining the abscess (Fig. 5).

Intra-operative procedure

Patients should be intubated with great care, to ensure that intra-oral rupture of the abscess does not occur, resulting in aspiration of infectious material. An experienced anaesthetist should perform the intubation as swelling and distortion of pharyngeal and laryngeal anatomy could make intubation difficult. A traumatic attempt at endotracheal intubation may aggravate the oedema and increase airway compromise. If intubation is impossible, a tracheostomy may be performed. A nasogastric tube should also be inserted prior to commencement of surgery.

Guided by CT scan and clinical findings, the appropriate skin incision is made. The abscess is approached by blunt dissection along tissue planes. In the case of para-pharyngeal abscesses, per-oral drainage has been described. However, a per-oral approach provides limited access and difficulty in locating a deeply located FB. In all cases, purulent material should be sent for cultures to tailor subsequent antimicrobial therapy. An effort should be made to locate the FB causing the infection. Usually, the FB is found within the abscess or impacted and perforating the oesophageal wall leading to the abscess. Rigid oesophagoscopy may be required to remove a foreign body impacted in the oesophagus.

If the abscess has tracked downwards into the mediastinum via the danger space, the cardiothoracic surgeon should be consulted regarding the most appropriate modality of drainage. A thoracotomy might be required in such cases.

Drains should be inserted and the skin either loosely sutured together or packed open. The principle behind this is to maintain adequate drainage of the cavity to allow healing and prevent reaccumulation of the abscess. The nasogastric tube should be left *in situ*.

Post-operative care

After drainage of neck abscesses, all patients are monitored closely in our high dependency ward. The emphasis is again on monitoring of airway and vital signs. Broad-spectrum antibiotics should be continued until cultures are ready, when the therapy can be targeted towards the organisms isolated.

If a Penrose drain was inserted, it should be withdrawn by 1 cm daily. For neck wounds that are packed, daily wash and packing with chlorhexidine gauze should be done. Absorptive dressings such as Kaltostat and other alginates may be used for heavily exuding wounds. They are also believed to improve the micro-environment of the wound to aid healing. Wounds with remnant necrotic tissue or slough may be dressed with hydrophilic gels like Duoderm or Intrasite to facilitate debridement or autolysis. Once the drains are out, the wound is clean, and the infection cleared, secondary suture can be performed.

For tracheostomised patients, the tracheostomy should be maintained until the infection has been cleared. The cuffed portex tube can be exchanged to a Shiley's double lumen tube for improved patient comfort and ease of care. Weaning should be gradual and started only after the surgeon is confident that the risk to the airway has passed, after inspecting the upper airway.

Conclusion

Fish bone ingestion is common in Singapore, where fish is a staple and eaten unfilleted. If lodged in the aero-digestive tract, the majority are in the tonsils or the base of the tongue, where they can easily be removed in the Emergency Department. Fish bones impacted in the oesophagus are especially dangerous, as they can potentially cause infection and abscess formation as well as fistula formation into vital structures like the great vessels, possibly resulting in mortality. Recognition of these patients is facilitated by a high index of suspicion and a complete workup, both clinical and radiological. Timely removal based on sound surgical principles is essential, to avoid dire consequences.

References

1. Lim CT, Quah RF, Loh LE (1994). A prospective study of ingested foreign bodies in Singapore. *Arch Otolaryngol Head Neck Surg* **120**(1), 96–101.
2. A Arana, B Hauser, S Hachimi-Idrissi, Y Vandenplas (2001). Management of ingested foreign bodies in childhood and review of the literature. *Eur J Pediatr* **160**, 468–472.
3. Ciriza C, Garcia L, Suarez P *et al.* (2000). What predictive parameters best indicate the need for emergent gastrointestinal

endoscopy after foreign body ingestion? *J Clin Gastroenterol* **31**(1), 23–28.

4. Nandi P, Ong GB (1978). Foreign bodies in the oesophagus: review of 2394 cases. *Br J Surg* **65**, 5–9.
5. Loh KS, Tan LKS, Smith JD, Yeoh KH, Fang D (2000). Complications of foreign bodies in the oesophagus. *Otolaryngol Head Neck Surg* **123**, 613–616.
6. Low WK (1999). Clinical diagnosis of an unusual cause of a cutaneous neck mass. *ORL* **61**, 364–366.
7. Watanabe KI, Kikuchi T, Katori Y *et al.* (1998). The usefulness of computed tomography in the diagnosis of impacted fish bones in the oesophagus. *J Laryngol Otol* **112**, 360–364.
8. Eliashar R, Dano I, Dangoor E, Braverman I, Sichel J-Y (1999). Computed tomography diagnosis of esophageal bone impaction: a prospective study. *Ann Otol Rhinol Laryngol* **108**, 708–710.
9. Hsu WC, Sheen TS, Lin CD, Tan CT, Yeh TH, Lee SY (2000). Clinical experiences of removing foreign bodies in the airway and oesophagus with a rigid endoscope: a series of 3217 cases from 1970 to 1996. *Otolaryngol Head Neck Surg* **122**, 450–454.
10. Berggreen PJ, Harrison ME, Sanowski RA, Ingebo K, Noland B, Zierer S (1993). Techniques and complications of esophageal foreign body extraction in children and adults. *Gastrointest Endosc* **39**, 626–630.
11. Chee LWJ, Sethi DS (1999). Diagnostic and therapeutic approach to migrating foreign bodies. *Ann Otol Rhinol Laryngol* **108**, 177–180.
12. Sethi DS, Stanley RE (1994). Deep neck abscesses — changing trends. *J Laryngol Otol* **108**, 138–143.

Section III

Cardiovascular and Thoracic Emergencies

10

Blunt Cardiac Injury

Yeong-Phang Lim
Richard Lupinski
Yeow-Leng Chua

Introduction

Blunt cardiac injury forms the majority (80%) of cardiac trauma that comes through the Accident and Emergency Department (Table 1). Most of these are sustained through high-speed road traffic accidents or falls from significant heights. These patients usually have concomitant multiple injuries. Another cause of cardiac contusion is from closed chest cardiopulmonary resuscitation. With more efficient and improved pre-hospital trauma systems, more severely-injured patients are surviving to a hospital facility, and so patients with severe life threatening cardiac injuries that are potentially salvageable may present in extremis. Most series report 15% to 75% incidence of myocardial injury in patients with blunt chest trauma.[1]

There were 31 cases of blunt cardiac injuries presenting in Singapore General Hospital over a four-year period from 1998 to 2001, of which 21 died and 14 survived.[2] Review of autopsy reports on patients that died revealed eight cases of cardiac rupture and 13 cases of significant myocardial contusion. Pathologies found on

Table 1 The Spectrum of Blunt Cardiac Injury is Summarised in the Table Below

Site of Injury	Acute Presentation	Delayed Presentation
Myocardium		
	Contusion (partial/full thickness)	Aneurysm
	Cardiac rupture	Pseudoaneurysm
	Atrial/ventricular septal rupture	
Conduction tissue		
	Atrial tachyarrhythmia	
	Bundle branch block	
	Complete heart block	
	Ventricular arrhythmias	
Coronary vessels		
	Acute thrombosis/occlusion	Coronary artery aneurysm/ pseudoaneurysm
	Coronary artery fistula	
Valve tissue		
	Valvular leaflet tear	
	Chordae tendinae rupture	
	Mitral valve papillary muscle dysfunction	
Pericardium		
	Laceration	Pericarditis
	Haemopericardium	
	Reactive effusion	Constrictive pericarditis

autopsy included rupture of the inter-atrial septum, tricuspid valve laceration and aortic valve transection. Two survivors were operated upon for right ventricular rupture, and the rest of the survivors had clinically diagnosed cardiac contusion.

Pathology

Blunt cardiac injury causes a whole range of pathologic patterns that may vary considerably in extent and location. The lesions may be subepicardial, subendocardial or transmural with or without cardiac rupture. Microscopically there is myocyte fragmentation with haemorrhage into the interstitium. Small arteries or arterioles may be disrupted. There may be myocardial necrosis that is usually patchy. Acute myocardial contusion is often considered similar to acute myocardial infarction but with important differences. There is subsequent coagulative necrosis and patchy scarring, which gives a better prognosis than myocardial infarction. Damage to the coronary intima or even the intima of vein grafts in patients with previous bypass grafting, may also occur, giving rise to coronary thrombosis and myocardial infarction.

The mechanisms of injury may be multi-factorial:

(1) Compression of the heart between sternum and vertebral column, causing direct pressure to the heart.
(2) Sudden acceleration or deceleration, causing tears at the junction of fixed and mobile parts of the heart, for example, at the atrio caval junction.
(3) Sudden increased hydraulic pressure transmitted from a force in the extremity or abdominal veins, causing rupture of the right atrium.
(4) Sudden increase in intra thoracic pressures, causing subendocardial injury.
(5) Sudden increase in intra abdominal pressure, causing cardiac contusion/rupture.
(6) Myocardial contusion, necrosis and rupture.
(7) Penetration from fractured ribs or sternal fragments.

Diagnosis

Symptoms

The diagnosis of severe blunt cardiac injury is often difficult to make, as patients are admitted to the hospital with many concomitant injuries — especially chest wall injuries, lung contusion and/ or pneumothoraces which may cause severe chest pain and dypsnoea. The patient may present in low output state, though in the setting of a trauma patient, hypovolaemia is the most common cause of low cardiac output. There is a significant decrease in cardiac output in patients with significant myocardial contusion.[3] Patients with significant regurgitation from torn valves or shunts from septal defects may also present in pulmonary oedema. There may also be cardiac arrhythmias or conduction disorders depending on the location of contusion. A high index of clinical suspicion is required to make the diagnosis. A diagnosis of cardiac contusion must be ruled out in the presence of other significant acceleration/deceleration injuries such as aortic transection, tracheobronchial tears, a lacerated diaphragm or ruptured spleen.

Signs

There may be tell-tale bruising on the anterior chest wall or petechial haemorrhages over the chest/neck, suggestive of significant crush injury. Distended neck veins in the presence of significant blood loss prior to resuscitation, is suspicious of tamponade. The typical Beck's triad of elevated jugular venous pressure, hypotension and muffled heart sounds and pulsus paradoxicus is often not seen. A new systolic murmur in the presence of cardiac failure or pulmonary oedema may be indicative of acute valvular regurgitation or an acute septal defect which requires urgent echocardiography.

Investigations

The electrocardiogram is the most common modality of diagnosis. The most common electrocardiograph (ECG) abnormalities are non-specific ST changes, supraventricular or ventricular arrhythmias. These may be attributable to other causes such as hypoxia, hypotension, electrolyte abnormalities, and head trauma. There are also autopsy reports of patients with significant myocardial contusion with no demonstrable ECG abnormalities before demise, and so this is not an absolute test for this condition.[4] Low ECG voltages may prompt one to rule out significant pericardial effusion especially in the presence of cardiomegaly on the chest radiograph.

There is some debate over the utility of creatinine kinase-MB (CKMB) in the diagnosis of myocardial contusion. Radionuclide imaging has been shown to be unhelpful. Most centres use ECG and CKMB (> 6% total CK) judiciously to diagnose myocardial contusion.

Chest radiography may be normal or there may be cardiomegaly or pulmonary oedema. Cardiomegaly may result from haemopericardium or ventricular dilatation from myocardial contusion. There may also be pneumopericardium or displaced heart borders in patients with pericardial injury. There may be bowel shadows within the cardiac borders if there is rupture of the diaphragmatic part of the pericardium. Mediastinal widening and significant haemothorax may also be suspicious of significant cardiac or great vessel injury.

Echocardiography can diagnose myocardial contusion with demonstration of haemopericardium, abnormal segmental wall motion abnormalities, haematoma of the myocardium and valvular dysfunction or pathology. The presence of septal akinesia is especially ominous as complete heart block may occur in the recovery period causing sudden collapse.[3] The specificity of echocardiography in the diagnosis of haemopericardium in the presence of significant haemothorax/pleural effusion has been questioned. Quality of echocardiography in patients with chest trauma and availability of echocardiography on a 24-hour basis in the trauma service are issues that may need to be considered.

Management

The unstable patient

The unstable patient with blunt cardiac injury and cardiovascular collapse (or haemorrhagic shock unresponsive to resuscitation) requires an *immediate* anterolateral thoracotomy in the Emergency Room. In most series of patients with survivors from blunt cardiac trauma, the diagnosis (73%) of cardiac or pericardial rupture is made on thoracotomy. In most series of patients there were no survivors after thoracotomy in patients who arrived without vital signs, whereas mortality was about 52% for patients who arrived with vital signs.[5] It has been noted that patients who sustain a witnessed arrest in the Emergency Room have the same survival as those who have not, if they were treated expediently. Patients may not survive the five to 10 minute transport to the operating theatre. This pre-arrest period represents a narrow window of surgical opportunity to salvage the patient.

Rapid initiation of treatment with the ABCs of resuscitation is essential. Intubation and setting of large bore intravenous lines for volume resuscitation and an arterial line for blood pressure monitoring, should be performed. Chest tubes are inserted for haemo/pneumothoraces expediently. If cardiac arrest occurs after intubation and positive pressure ventilation, the diagnosis of tension pneumothorax or coronary air embolism should be considered. Coronary air embolism occurs in patients with any air leak from either lung parenchyma or tracheobronchial injury and a torn pericardium with atrial or pulmonary vein tears. Immediate anterolateral thoracotomy has to be performed, and the patient placed in head down or left lateral decubitus position to localise the air in the left ventricular apex, and open cardiac massage performed with aspiration of air from the cardiac chambers. Haemorrhage from the atrium or ventricle can be controlled digitally, and the laceration repaired directly or with felt or pericardial pledgets. It is important that the process of metabolic resuscitation also takes place with correction of acidosis and anti-arrhythmic medication administration as necessary. If there is pericardial rupture with cardiac herniation with torsion of the great vessels, the laceration should be repaired. If there is a lack of space in the pericardium to replace the oedematous heart, equine pericardium or synthetic (Marlex®) mesh can be used to patch the pericardial defect after restoring the heart to its proper position. When the cardiac rupture or pericardial rupture is repaired and the patient is stabilised, the patient can then be brought to the operating theatre for formal exploration, cleansing and closure of the wound or for other required surgical procedures. Cardiopulmonary bypass is rarely utilised in these repairs (10%). Coronary artery bypass may be required in patients who have acute occlusion of coronary vessels which supply large areas of myocardium and present in cardiogenic shock. Arteriovenous (arteriocameral) fistulas or coronary left ventricular fistulas with steal syndrome may occur, requiring urgent repair.

Patients who present with new cardiac murmurs and controllable cardiac failure require urgent echocardiography and cardiac catheterisation. Acute valvular regurgitation may result in damage to the valve leaflets or tensor apparatus (Table 1). The aortic, mitral and tricuspid valves may be involved in that order of frequency. Parmley's series reported 9% of valvular damage in patients with blunt cardiac trauma.[6] Valvuloplasty or valve replacement may be carried out under cardiopulmonary bypass. Atrial or ventricular septal defects may also occur and require repair. If the patients with these trauma-induced valvular regurgitation or shunt lesions are stable, it is reasonable to wait for the acute trauma to settle and operate in an elective situation.

The mortality in this group of patients is higher than patients with penetrating cardiac trauma. In a large trauma centre, cardiac herniation was associated with a survival of 33%, cardiac chamber injury (40%), pericardial injury (67%), and combined atrioventricular injuries (0%).[5] Outcomes may ultimately be determined by cerebral status as young age, brief periods of cerebral hypoxia, lack of major intracardiac injuries, are positive prognostic factors.[3] Only expedient pre-hospital transport and surgery can improve outcomes in this group of patients.

The stable patient

Patients who are haemodynamically stable on admission but diagnosed with significant myocardial contusion, should be admitted to an Intensive Care Unit and also assessed by a cardiologist/cardiothoracic surgeon. The management is summarised below:

Monitoring in the intensive care unit

Electrocardiograph, arterial and central venous pressure monitoring for optimal fluid and electrolyte management, are mandatory. Early intubation and ventilation in respiratory distress, especially in the presence of decreased cardiac output, should be considered. Pulmonary artery catheter insertion should be performed for optimal cardiac management in seriously injured patients.

Myocardial support

There may be decreased cardiac output in patients with a severely contused myocardium. The anteriorly placed right ventricle may fail acutely. Inotropes will be required in this setting if there is adequate filling of the heart. An intra aortic balloon pump has also been used to augment cardiac output. Pulmonary oedema will have to be treated with diuretics. Pericardial effusions causing a tamponade will have to be ruled out. Significant pericardial effusions in the acute setting may require formal surgical exploration via median sternotomy. If there is evidence of myocardial ischaemia, coronary angiography may have to be considered, as coronary thrombosis with coronary occlusion may occur. The use of anticoagulants and thrombolytic agents is usually contraindicated in acute trauma.

Arrhythmia management

Arrhythmias may occur in this group of patients, and should be treated with anti-arrhythmic agents. Electrical cardioversion may be required for ventricular fibrillation or supraventricular tachycardia with hypotension. Emergency pacing may be required for heart block.

Those patients with significant myocardial contusion may have to undergo operations for other injuries and will require close monitoring.

The period of bed rest and monitoring for patients with significant myocardial contusion has not been well defined. The management is broadly similar to that of acute myocardial infarction. Such monitoring should continue for 48 to 72 hours after the acute trauma, or until the patient is asymptomatic.

The prognosis for patients who recover after blunt cardiac trauma is good. Significant contusion often heals without any other cardiac sequlae. If there is persistent or new cardiac symptoms, repeat echocardiographic assessment and/or cardiac catheterisation is required as there can be delayed presentation of cardiac pathologies caused by blunt trauma (Table 1).

References

1. Symbas PN (1989). Contusion of the heart. In *Cardiothoracic Trauma.* WB Saunders Company.
2. SGH Trauma Registry Database 2002.
3. Westaby S, Odell JA (2000). Blunt cardiac trauma. In *Cardiothoracic Trauma.* Edward Arnold.
4. Blair E, Topuzulu C, Davis JH (1971). Delayed or missed diagnosis of cardiac damage in blunt chest trauma. *J Trauma* **11**, 129.
5. Fulda G, Brathwaite CE, Rodriguez A, Turney SZ, Dunham CM, Cowley RA (1991). Blunt traumatic rupture of the heart and pericardium: a ten year experience (1979–1989). *J Trauma* **31**(2), 167.
6. Parmley LF, Manion WC, Mattingly TW (1958). Non-penetrating traumatic injury of the heart. *Circulation* **18**, 371.

11

Aortic Trauma

Kenny Yoong-Kong Sin
Yeow-Leng Chua

Introduction

The most common injury to the aorta is blunt trauma from direct impact or deceleration, usually from motor vehicle accidents or falls from height. The incidence varies from 12% to 23% of deaths from blunt trauma, and has increased in direct proportion to the number of high velocity motor vehicle accidents.

It is unusual for patients to present with an isolated aortic rupture. The presence of other injuries has to be excluded and, if present, prioritised in urgency of management before subjecting the patient to surgery. It has been estimated that half of such patients will succumb to associated injuries even in the absence of aorta disruption.[1,2] Besides skeletal trauma, concussion, cardiac and lung contusion, lacerated abdominal or retroperitoneal organs comprise 25% of such patients.[3]

Pathogenesis

The descending thoracic aorta is fixed at the isthmus. A combination of direct impact followed by deceleration produces traction stress between the mobile and fixed portions causing the classical tear just distal to the isthmus. This laceration involves the intima and part of the media, and may be circumferential or spiral in nature. The patient survives due to containment within the adventitia or mediastinal structures. However in autopsy series the aorta is usually completely transected, with the edges separated by several centimetres.

Tears of the ascending aorta are caused by cardiac displacement, while those of distal descending thoracic or abdominal aorta by hyperextension and vertebral injuries.

Natural History

Nearly 90% of patients with aortic rupture die onsite. Of patients who reach the hospital, about 10% survive beyond six hours.[1,4] In patients where aortic repair was delayed due to other injuries, treatment with beta blockade and vasodilators with blood pressure maintained between 100 to 120 mmHg until definitive surgery, did not produce any mortality during the delay.[5,6] Accurate assessment and prioritisation of treatment sequences are essential in managing such polytrauma patients.

In patients where the injury was missed, and self-selection allowed chronic traumatic aneurysm development, long term survival was 66% at ten years and 62% at 20 years. Twenty-two per cent were symptomatic at one year, 42% at five years, and 58% at ten years. One third died of late rupture. The majority of these aneurysms were located at the aortic isthmus.[7]

Clinical Presentation

In the backgound of polytrauma, especially where severe impact or deceleration is present, the possibility of a ruptured aorta should be suspected. Symptoms vary from the non-specific to that of chest pain, interscapular pain, hoarseness, dyspnoea, dysphasia and paraplegia. Examination findings include multiple rib fractures, sternal fractures, seat-belt or steering wheel imprint, and occasionally differential upper and lower limb pressures. Neurology should be documented, and any associated cervical spine injury should be actively excluded.

The initial management of the patient should follow established protocols which emphasises resuscitation and attention to airway, breathing and circulation before an expeditious but reasonably thorough physical examination. A chest X-ray is also performed, in addition to other indicated X-rays, which may provide the first indication of a ruptured aorta.

Diagnostic Studies

A widened mediastinum is present in more than 80% of patients with a ruptured isthmus who reach the hospital alive (Fig. 1). A supine film may show a normal wider mediastinum, especially with an anterior-posterior projection. Other features present on a plain chest X-ray include tracheal deviation, depression of the left main bronchus, obliteration of the aortic knob, loss of the aortic-pulmonary window, an apical cap, deviation of an oesophageal nasogastric tube, and a left hemithorax. A suggestive plain chest X-ray with a history of deceleration injury warrants further investigation.

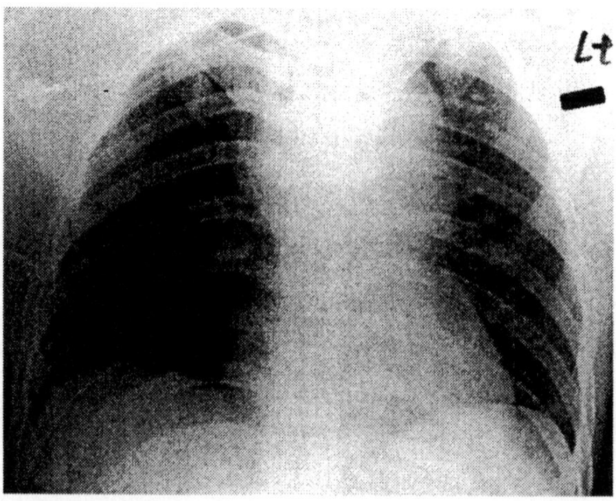

Fig. 1 Chest X-ray showing a widened mediastinum with loss of the aortic knob and deviation of the trachea.

Aortography has been the traditional gold standard. However, this procedure is time-consuming and is associated with exsanguination and death in the angiography suite, and may contribute to the development of renal failure in patients with shock. Up to 90% of aortograms performed to exclude aortic injury are negative. The false negative rate of aortography is low, and may be due to thrombosis of the laceration, inadequate views or inadequate contrast. False positives are caused by atheroma or ductal diverticula.

Computerised axial tomography (CT) is non-invasive, widely available and is the preferred imaging to exclude the diagnosis of ruptured aorta in patients with a widened mediastinum (Figs. 2 and 3). This modality is invaluable for assessing intra-cranial, intra-abdominal, pelvic and retroperitoneal structures. High speed spiral scanning coupled with contrast enhancement has yielded high sensitivity and specificity, and has superseded aortography as the definitive imaging in many centres.[8,9]

Magnetic Resonance Imaging (MRI) provides excellent views but is hampered by the risk of managing a critically injured patient in an inaccessible space. However, it is a useful tool in stable patients where there is an element of doubt despite normal conventional imaging.

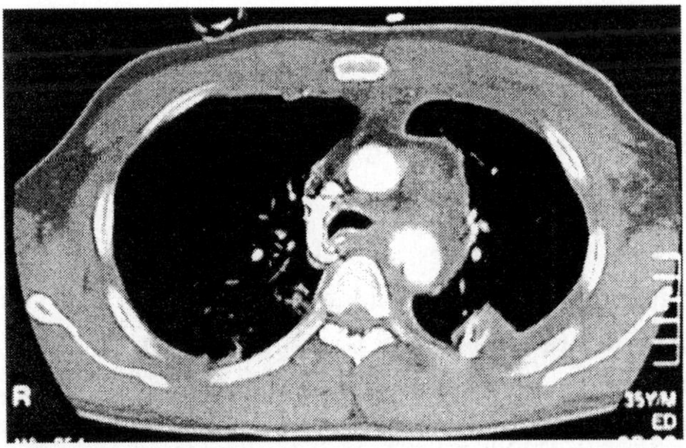

Fig. 2 CT scan image of the same patient demonstrating contrast leaking from a ruptured proximal descending thoracic aorta, with an extensive haematoma collection and deviation of the trachea.

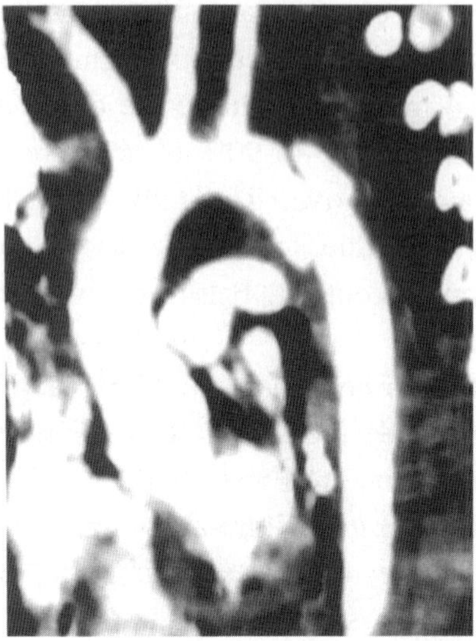

Fig. 3 Sagittal CT reconstruction of the same patient demonstrating the classical location of an aortic tear which is just distal to the isthmus, with a pseudoaneurysm formation. At surgery, the aorta was found almost completely transected; post-repair, the patient recovered with no neurological deficits.

Trans-oesophageal echocardiography images almost the entire thoracic aorta and is more sensitive and specific than transthoracic echocardiography. It is useful as an intra-operative adjunct, and to assess myocardial or valvular injury in addition to the presence of pericardial tamponade. The limitation is that the accuracy and speed are operator dependent, and the procedure is contra-indicated in patients with maxillofacial, esophageal or cervical spine injuries.

Emergency Room Management

Ninety-five per cent of patients with aortic trauma who reach hospital alive have associated injuries. Initial management follows established trauma protocols with establishment of the ABC's of resuscitation. Once ventilation and circulation is secured, and secondary survey has excluded other life-threatening injuries, the patient should have a CT scan performed to establish diagnosis prior to transfer to the operating room. CT of the abdomen should be included routinely to exclude any missed intra-abdominal injury.

The presence of other life-threatening injuries may mandate their immediate management before definitive aortic repair is performed. Such conditions include patients with compromised ventilation, serious head injuries, or haemodynamic instability from overt or covert bleeding. In some instances, unstable patients may require immediate transfer to the operating room for both diagnostic and therapeutic manoeuvres to take place simultaneously.

In patients where there is no active bleeding from a disrupted aorta, and associated injuries contra-indicate the use of partial cardiopulmonary bypass, the risk of rupture must be balanced against the risk of spinal cord compromise during aortic repair. In such instances, consider the use of beta blockade and vasodilators to control blood pressure until surgery can be safely affected.

Pre-operative Preparation of the Patient for Emergency Surgery

If the patient is haemodynamically stable, a double lumen endotracheal tube is inserted. Invasive monitoring includes a right radial artery line; a central venous pressure catheter; a large-bore venous cannula for transfusion, usually a haemodialysis catheter which provides two large lumens for transfusion via a rapid infusion system; rectal temperature probe; and transurethral catheterisation for urine output. Non-invasive monitoring includes electrocardiographic and pulse oximetry measurements. If time permits, a lumbar drainage catheter is inserted for cerebrospinal fluid (CSF) drainage as an adjunct for spinal cord monitoring. Where available, electroencephalographic and somatosensory evoked potential monitoring should be used to monitor spinal cord function.

Blood must be present in the operating room before the procedure. A minimum of six to ten units of blood and one litre of fresh frozen plasma is required at the start, while more blood is being matched at the blood bank. A rapid infusion system coupled with a cell-saver apparatus should be prepared and primed in readiness for large volume exchanges. In the absence of a rapid infusion system, pressure infusion bags should be placed and ready to use.

Intraoperative Procedures

The patient is positioned in a right lateral decubitus position with a slight thoracoabdominal tilt, and draped to allow bilateral femoral access if necessary. The left femoral vessels are exposed to allow cannulation for distal aortic perfusion, and for cardiopulmonary bypass if necessary.

A generous posterolateral incision is used with extension across the costal margin in the direction of the umbilicus (a modified thoracoabdominal incision). The left hemi-thorax is entered by resecting the sixth rib with the corresponding costal margin. The left lung is isolated and deflated and the aorta proximal and distal to the disruption is dissected for control. The left lower pulmonary vein and left common femoral artery are cannulated in preparation for left heart bypass and distal aortic perfusion; a cell-saver is prepared for use.

The isthmus is invariably distorted with a large haematoma, and should not be manipulated before proximal control is obtained. Finger dissection is used to encircle the aortic arch between the left common carotid and left subclavian artery, to gain adequate proximal aortic control without disrupting the haematoma. The distal descending aorta is easily dissected at some convenient point distal to the aortic rupture, but should not be excessively distal to the point of compromising spinal cord perfusion.

Once dissection is complete and sufficient for placement of cross-clamps, left heart bypass is commenced and the cross clamps placed simultaneously to prevent excessive after-load on the heart. The lower body is perfused at a rate of between 500 and 2000 ml/min to achieve a normotensive upper body blood pressure. If a lumbar drain is inserted, the cerebrospinal fluid pressure is monitored and maintained below 10 cmH_2O by drainage of the fluid.

Upon proximal and distal cross-clamp administration, the intervening aorta is palpated to ensure no pulsation and hence adequate proximal cross-clamping. The aorta is incised longitudinally and the area of disruption identified. A proximal and distal cuff of aorta is then prepared and dissected free of the adjacent esophagus, and a gelatin impregnated woven dacron graft is then sutured with continuous 4 O Prolene®, reinforced with interrupted pledgetted sutures in the posterior wall. The graft size is usually estimated pre-operatively by measurement of the normal aorta on the CT scan, and can be confirmed by intra-operative measurement. Once the proximal anastomosis is completed, the graft is clamped, and the proximal cross-clamp released to ensure adequate haemostasis before the distal anastomosis is performed.

Upon completion of the anastomosis, left heart bypass is terminated and heparinisation is reversed with protamine. Further pledgette reinforcement is performed if necessary, and the chest closed in layers after two large-bore chest drains are inserted.

Spinal cord protection

Upon cross-clamping, the perfusion pressure of the spinal cord diminishes and CSF pressure increases, further decreasing spinal cord blood flow akin to compartmental syndrome. The adjunctive use of CSF drainage to lower the compartmental pressure, coupled with distal aortic perfusion to optimise collateral flow, has been shown to reduce the incidence of paraplegia following aortic surgery.[10] The use of somatosensory evoked potential monitoring provides an early predictor of spinal cord compromise.

Management of the ruptured aorta

In the event of a free rupture, a single lumen endotracheal tube is placed, and a rapid thoracotomy is performed with the aim of an expeditious proximal and distal aorta dissection and cross-clamp administration. If the bleeding is contained, left heart bypass is established before opening the haematoma over the rupture. If the aorta is freely ruptured, the "clamp and sew" method is employed without lower body perfusion. Direct repair or an interposition graft is performed as expeditiously as possible while blood pressure resuscitation is being carried out.

Torn left subclavian artery

In the event that the left subclavian artery is involved, the proximal clamp is shifted to partially occlude the left common carotid artery and the proximal anastomosis performed with later inclusion of the subclavia artery either by direct anastomosis or with an interposition graft. Left carotid occlusion can be tolerated for ten to 15 minutes, and the clamp is moved distally upon completion of the suture line.

Ascending or arch laceration

In the uncommon event of a laceration of the ascending aorta or arch, blood pressure control should be instituted, and a full evaluation of associated injuries performed before aortic repair using full cardiopulmonary bypass and hypothermic circulatory arrest.

Early Post-operative Care of the Patient

Surgery for associated injuries can be performed as indicated once the aorta is repaired. Otherwise, the post-operative care is similar to patients who have undergone major cardiac or lung surgery. The patient is commonly hypothermic and coagulopathic, and will require blood product support and rewarming in the intensive care. In isolated aortic injuries, the patient can be weaned off the ventilator within 24 hours of surgery. However, extubation is often delayed due to impaired neurology and poor gas exchange related to associated head and lung trauma, and occasionally adult respiratory distress syndrome (ARDS).

Neurological monitoring is essential to diagnose late-onset paraplegia. The CSF drain is left for three days with intermittent drainage, to maintain a pressure of less than 10 cmH_2O before removal. In the event where no CSF drain was inserted and paraplegia develops, drainage can be instituted post-operatively to attempt to reverse or limit the degree of neurological impairment.[11]

Chest drains are left *in situ* with underwater seal suction of 15 cmH_2O, and removed when the drainage is serous in nature and less than 100 ml per day. Prophylactic antibiotics are maintained until the CSF and chest drains are removed.

Renal failure is not an uncommon occurrence after successful aortic repair, and may be related to hypotension, aortic clamp time, and the use of contrast in diagnostic studies. A proportion of patients may require acute haemodialysis, but return to normal renal function may be expected with time.

Vocal cord palsy and left phrenic nerve injury may be evident, and can be managed at a later stage after recovery. In patients who develop respiratory compromise from diaphragmatic paralysis, application may be necessary to assist in weaning the patient from ventilator dependancy.

Summary

Acute traumatic aortic rupture must be excluded in polytrauma patients, especially in association with high velocity and deceleration forces. Up to 90% of these patients succumb onsite, and the survival of the remaining 10% depends on the skill and judgement of the cardiothoracic surgeon and multidisciplinary team involved in the care.

Recognition of associated injuries and prioritisation of management is essential and must be individualised for each patient. Surgical management has evolved from the "clamp and go" technique, followed by the use of passive proximal to distal aortic shunts (Gott shunt), to the current use of left heart bypass for distal aortic perfusion. These various techniques are still in use today depending on the circumstance.[12,13]

Minimally invasive surgery in the form of endovascular stent grafting is evolving into a credible therapeutic option.[14] However, long term concerns regarding the development of late onset endoleak and rupture, especially in the setting of young trauma patients, remains unaddressed. In the meantime, open repair using left heart bypass for distal perfusion remains the technique of choice in this challenging group of patients.

References

1. Parmley L, Mattingly T, Manion W (1958). Nonpenetrating traumatic injury of the aorta. *Circulation* **17**, 1086.
2. Greendyke RM (1966). Traumatic rupture of aorta. *JAMA* **195**, 119.
3. Kodali S, Jamieson WRE, Leia-Stephens M, Tyers GFO (1991). Traumatic rupture of the thoracic aorta. *Circulation* **84**(Suppl. 3), III–40.
4. Dosios TJ, Salemis N, Angouras D, Nonas E. Blunt and Penetrating Trauma of the Thoracic Aorta and Aortic Arch Branches: Autopsy Study. *J Trauma* **49**(4), 696–703.
5. Hilgenberg A, Vlahakes G, Akins C, Torchiana D (1992). Blunt injuries of the thoracic aorta. *Ann Thorac Surg* **53**, 233.
6. Akins CW, Buckley MJ, Daggett W *et al.* (1981). Acute traumatic disruption of the thoracic aorta: a ten year experience. *Ann Thorac Surg* **31**, 305.
7. Finkelmeier BA, Mentzer RM Jr, Kaiser DL *et al.* (1982). Chronic traumatic thoracic aneurysm. Influence of operative treatment on natural history: an analysis of reported cases, 1950–1980. *J Thorac Cardiovasc Surg* **84**, 257.
8. Scaglione M, Pinto A, Pinto F, Romano L, Ragozzino A, Grassi R (2001). Role of contrast-enhanced helical CT in the evaluation of acute thoracic aortic injuries after blunt chest trauma. *Eur Radiol* **11**(12), 2444–2448.
9. Parker MS, Matheson TL, Rao AV, Sherbourne CD, Jordan KG, Landay MJ *et al.* (2001). Making the transition: the role of helical CT in the evaluation of potentially acute thoracic aortic injuries. *Am J Roentgenol* **176**(5), 1267–1272.

10. Estrera AL, Miller CC (III), Huynh TT, Porat E, Safi HJ (2001). Neurologic outcomes after thoracic and thoracoabdominal aortic aneurysm repair. *Ann Thorac Surg* **72**, 1225–1231.
11. Azizzadeh A, Huynh TT, Miller CC (III), Safi HJ (2000). Reversal of twice-delayed neurologic deficits with cerebrospinal fluid drainage after thoracoabdominal aneurysm repair: a case report and plea for a national database collection. *J Vasc Surg* **31**(3), 592–598.
12. Szwerc MF, Benkart DH, Lin JC, Johnnides CG, Magovern JA, Magovern GJ Jr, Magovern Sr (1999). Recent clinical experience with left heart bypass using a centrifugal pump for repair of traumatic aortic transection. *Ann Surg* **230**(4), 484–490.
13. Razzouk AJ, Gundry SR, Wang N, del Rio MJ, Vatrnell D, Bailey LL (2000). Repair of traumatic aortic rupture: a 25-year experience. *Arch Surg* **135**(8), 913–918.
14. Fujikawa T, Yukioka T, Ishimaru S, Kanai M, Muaoka A, Sasaki H *et al.* (2001). Endovascular stent grafting for the treatment of blunt thoracic aortic injury. *J Trauma* **50**(2), 223–239.

12

Acute Arterial Disease

Ming-Keng Teoh

Introduction

Limb ischaemia can be acute or chronic. The former is an emergency. Every doctor — whether in primary care or hospital practice — should be familiar with the presentation and management of limb ischaemia.

Clinical Presentation

Limb pain is the main symptom. The other classical features are limb pallor, coldness and pulselessness and when severe, paraesthesia and paralysis as given below. While the usual presenting complaint of chronic leg ischaemia is intermittent claudication, the acutely ischaemic limb may present without such a history.

In acute arterial occlusion, such as an acute embolus or thrombosis, the limb is painful, pale, cold and pulseless. It is commonly described as a limb which has "gone dead". In severe ischaemia there is also parasthesia — the limb feels numb — and paralysis ("**P**ain, **P**allor, **P**ulselessness, **P**erishing cold, **P**araesthesia, **P**aralysis"). The veins are empty and "guttered".

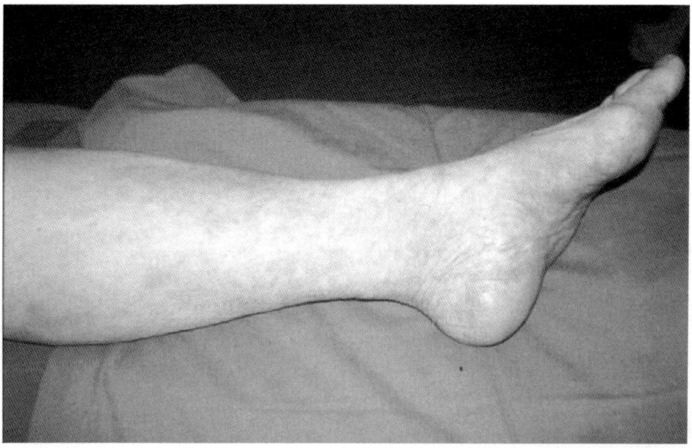

Fig. 1 Irreversible changes in an acutely ischaemic limb: note the fixed skin staining, early dermal gangrene and muscle turgidity.

It is important to recognise irreversible changes in long-standing severe ischaemia such as fixed skin staining or mottling, muscle rigidity, skin necrosis and gangrene (Fig. 1). When widespread, these changes indicate a limb that cannot be salvaged.

In chronic arterial insufficiency, the patient's pain, usually in the calf, (or the calf, thigh and buttocks in aorto-iliac disease) comes on after walking a predictable distance and disappears within a few minutes of resting: this is intermittent claudication. He may complain of numbness and a cold foot. In claudicants with mild disease, the pulses may be palpable at rest and the skin normal, so claudication may be difficult to distinguish from other causes of pain. Venous claudication is typically described as "bursting" pain occurring after walking, and is relieved by elevation of the leg.

Investigations

Doppler ultrasound assessment of the pulses can be performed at the femoral, popliteal and ankle arteries. The audible signals are a crude estimation of blood flow in the vessel. The ratio of the ankle-to-arm systolic pressures (Ankle-Brachial Pressure Index or ABPI) is a fairly reproducible estimate of the severity of arterial disease, except that calcified vessels will give a higher than expected reading (Fig. 2). Colour duplex scanning is non-invasive and is nowadays the standard method of assessing the arterial system.[1] It not only assesses the

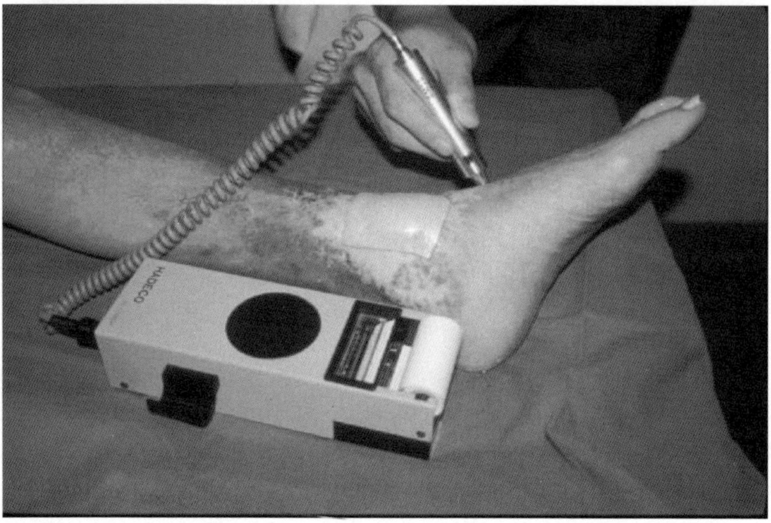

Fig. 2 Measuring the Ankle-Brachial Pressure Index using a hand-held Doppler on the dorsalis pedis artery.

Table 1 Assessment of Limb Ischaemia

Clinical: pulses, ischaemic changes, general
Doppler: ABPI, post-exercise ABPI, recovery time
Colour duplex scanning
Angiography

ECG, chest X-ray
Full blood count, ESR
Renal profile, urinalysis, glucose, lipid profile

In young patients, raised ESR:
Antinuclear factor, DNA binding, rheumatoid factor, immunoglobulins
SL70, cold agglutinin, cryoglobulins

severity but also provides an anatomical road-map of the arterial disease in the limb. Angiography is only used preoperatively when colour duplex scanning is inadequate for treatment planning, or when an intervention such as angioplasty or thrombolysis is anticipated (Table 1).

Acute Limb Ischaemia: An Emergency

Introduction

Acute limb ischaemia is the most common vascular emergency, and is often treatable if diagnosed early. However, it is often diagnosed late and/or inadequately treated. Morbidity and mortality rates for acute arterial occlusion remain stubbornly high today, both in Asia as well as in established units in the West. Literature review shows an amputation rate of 12% to 22%, and a mortality rate of 20% to 40%. The high mortality rate is attributable to underlying cardiac and generalised disease in these elderly patients.[2]

Aetiology

Most acute arterial occlusions are thromboembolic in origin, and most sources of emboli are from the heart (Table 2). The diagnosis of

Table 2 Aetiology of Acute Arterial Occlusion

Personal series of 101 consecutive patients (125 limbs), 1988–1992
Average age 57.6 years (range 10–90 years), Sex ratio 61M:40F

Embolus:		73 patients
	Myocardial infarction	19
	Atrial fibrillation	21
	Valvular lesions	3
	Injective endocarditis	2
	Aortic aneurysms	4
	Trauma	2
	No obvious source	22
Thrombosis:		28 patients

embolus is based on either angiography or the following clinical criteria: obvious source of emboli (recent myocardial infarction or arrhythmia), absence of claudication and short history of ischaemia especially in a younger person.

Clinical picture

Most patients complain of a sudden onset of pain, paralysis and numbness, and on examination the limb is cold, pale and pulseless. When ischaemia is severe there is paralysis and parasthesia. Gangrene, blisters and ulcers are a feature of late presentation. There is a wide spectrum of clinical scenarios ranging from a sudden arterial occlusion in a previously normal limb, typically from an embolus, to acute deterioration in a limb with previous claudication, typical of acute thrombosis in a severely diseased atherosclerotic limb. It is important to recognise the differences between a mildly ischaemic limb; a threatened but salvagable limb; and an irreversibly threatened ischaemic limb (Fig. 1).

Important management points for acute limb ischaemia

Early anticoagulation — The patient should be started on heparin therapy the moment a diagnosis of an acute arterial occlusion is made. An intravenous bolus of 3000–5000 international units (IU) followed by an infusion of 1000 IU of heparin per hour is administered with the aim of preventing both retrograde and antegrade propagation of thrombosis from the point of occlusion. Once extensive thrombosis of the side branches has occurred the prognosis is poor even if a successful embolectomy of the main trunk artery can be accomplished, because the revascularised main artery with poor distal vessel run-off will thrombose again.

Early referral to a vascular surgeon — This is most important lack of awareness amongst patients and health care personnel is frequently the cause for a late referral. The significant limb loss rate can only be reduced by earlier diagnosis and treatment[3,4] (Table 3).

Table 3 Outcome of Acute Limb Ischaemia Following Delay

		Period of Delay		
		< 24 hr	24–48 hr	> 48 h
Outcome	Salvaged	6	9	17
	Amputation	–	1	15
	Death	–	2	6

Table adapted from Teoh (1991).[3]

Investigations — Very few tests are really necessary, and these should not delay surgery. Preoperatively, the most important are electrocardiogram, chest X-ray, blood gas and serum electrolyte assays. Distinguishing between embolus and thrombosis is essential, as the prognosis is worsened when embolectomy is performed for thrombosis. As such, preoperative angiography is useful when the diagnosis of embolus or thrombosis is in doubt. An on-table angiogram is useful if the result of embolectomy is uncertain or if acute thrombosis is suspected at exploration. Postoperatively, once the diagnosis of embolus has been confirmed, a search for the source of emboli should be made using echocardiography of the heart, or Duplex ultrasound scan of the aorta and proximal arteries. In younger patients when spontaneous arterial thrombosis is suspected, the possibility of deficiency of antithrombin III, protein C or protein S must be investigated.

The embolectomy operation — Using a Fogarty balloon catheter here is well known, and remains a most elegant and effective procedure (Fig. 3). It is however only effective if the diagnosis of embolus is correct. Ischaemic limbs with acute thrombosis and widespread atheroma need vascular reconstructive surgery. Primary amputation is needed for limbs with late, irreversible ischaemia.

Local anaesthesia is adequate for most straightforward unilateral embolectomy. A general anaesthetic is advisable if acute thrombosis is suspected or when a fasciotomy is thought to be necessary.

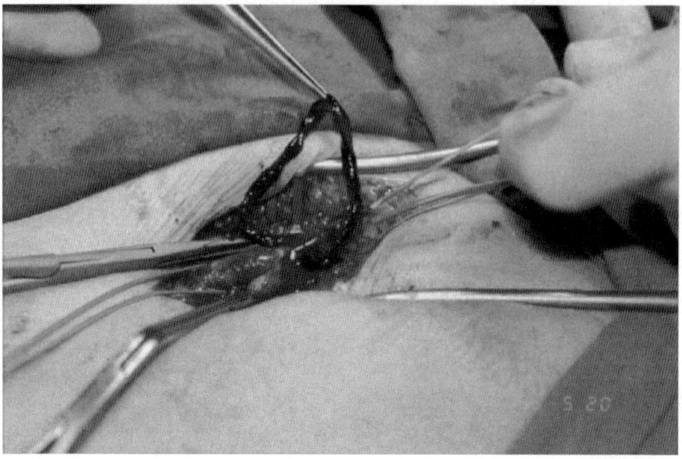

Fig. 3 Embolectomy: picture shows a large thrombus being pulled out by a Fogarty balloon catheter from the femoral artery.

Regional thrombolysis — This involves placing an intra-arterial catheter into the thrombus under flouroscopy with continuous infusion of either streptokinase or urokinase. This is continued until there is complete resolution of thrombus, or until there is no further improvement on angiogram. In practice most thrombolysis is completed within 12 to 24 hours. It is particularly useful in clearing thrombus occluded bypass grafts and in acute thrombosis in diseased arteries. It is also a treatment option for the more distal arterial embolic occlusion such as in infrapopliteal sites, where the side branches and smaller arteries are inaccessible to the embolectomy catheter.

Summary

When the patient has acute arterial ischaemia, correct aetiological diagnosis with minimum delay, early anticoagulation and the appropriate surgical management will reduce the high morbidity and mortality from this condition. Indeed, both primary care physicians and hospital doctors play a very important role here.

Aortic Aneurysms

Introduction

It is increasingly recognised that in the development of an aortic aneurysm, family history, as well as collagen and elastin metabolism, play an important role. No longer is the condition simply regarded as a degenerative disease brought about by atherosclerosis.

The incidence of abdominal aortic aneurysms is rising in the West. Data from the Mayo Clinic showed a rise from 12.2/100,000 in 1951, to 36.2/100,000 in 1980.[5] A rising incidence with age, peaking at an incidence of 5.9% at the age of 80, was reported in a Swedish study.[6] In the United States 40,000 aortic reconstructions for aneurysms were performed in 1988.[7] That translates into approximately 500 a year for a Singapore-size population, approximately ten times the actual number done annually. Although reliable local data is not yet available, the true incidence in Asians may be higher than is suggested by popular perception.

Clinical presentation

Most abdominal aortic aneurysms are picked up during routine clinical examination, when a pulsatile abdominal mass is palpated. Frequently they present with complications such as abdominal pain, back pain,

Table 4 Clinical Features of Abdominal Aortic Aneurysms

Clinical features
Pulsatile mass
Abdominal pain, backache
Compression ureter, IVC, bowel
Limb ischaemia: thrombosis, emboli
Inflammation: retroperitoneal fibrosis
Infection: mycotic aneurysm
Aorto-duodenal fistula, aortocaval fistula
Rupture: peritonitis, shock

acute arterial occlusion from peripheral emboli, or shock with peritonitis from aneurysm rupture (Table 4).

Important management points for aortic aneurysms

If a ruptured abdominal aneurysm is suspected, there should be no further investigation and the patient should be transferred immediately to the operating room. However if the patient is haemodynamically stable, or the diagnosis is in doubt, a CT scan is the best modality to confirm the leak and delineate the anatomy. Angiography is only needed preoperatively in an acute situation when the aneurysm is to be excluded by endovascular stenting.

Emergent inlay graft repair is the procedure of choice for all leaking or symptomatic aneurysms. Endovascular stenting for ruptured aneurysms is still under evaluation.

The mortality for emergency repair is much higher than for elective repair. In the U.K., up to 30% of sudden deaths in men are caused by ruptured abdominal aortic aneurysms.[8] The mortality rate for emergency repair is 50% but for elective repair it is less than 5%.[7] The true mortality from ruptured aneurysms is even higher when we consider that 50% of these patients die even before they reach the hospital.

The current state of affairs, therefore is: all aneurysms should be referred to a vascular surgeon for assessment, since any aortic aneurysm greater than 5 cm should be repaired electively. If the aortic aneurysm is less than 4 cm in diameter the patient should be followed up with a repeat ultrasound scan every six months.

References

1. Davies AH, Willcox JH, Magee TR, Currie I, Cole SE, Murphy P, Lamont PM, Baird RN (1995). Colour duplex in assessing the infrainguinal arteries in patients with claudication. *Cardiovasc Surg* **3**(2), 211–212.

2. The Vascular Surgical Society of Great Britain and Ireland (1995). Critical limb ischaemia: management and outcome. Report of a national survey. *Eur J Vasc Endovasc Surg* **10**, 108–113.
3. Teoh MK (1991). Acute arterial occlusion: management and prognosis for late presentation. *Asian J Surg* **14**(4), 178–183.
4. Teoh MK (1995). Acute arterial occlusion — Can results be improved? *SGH Procs* **4**(3), 87–90.
5. Bickerstaff LK, Hollier LH, van Peenen HJ, Melton LJ III, Pairolero PC, Cherry KJ (1984). Abdominal aortic aneurysms: the changing natural history. *J Vasc Surg* **1**, 6–12.
6. Bengtsson H, Bergqvist D, Sternby N (1992). Increasing prevalence of abdominal aortic aneurysms: a necropsy study. *Eur J Surg* **158**, 19–23.
7. Ernst C (1993). Abdominal aortic aneurysm: current concepts. *N Engl J Med* **328**(16), 1167–1172.
8. Dent A, Kent S, Young T (1986). Ruptured abdominal aortic aneurysm. What is the true mortality? *Br J Surg* **73**, 318.

13

Vascular Trauma

Mathew G Sebastian

This complex topic is itself the subject of several textbooks. A detailed account of the diagnosis and management of the various injuries that can manifest in the vascular system is beyond the scope of this chapter. What will be presented are the principles of management of common vascular injuries sustained as a result of either penetrating trauma (such as stab or gunshot wounds) or blunt trauma (such as motor vehicle accidents). A brief account of iatrogenic vascular injuries will complete the picture.

Triage and Pre-intervention Considerations

After the ABCs of trauma resuscitation, patients with vascular injuries can be triaged into one of three groups:

(1) Life threatening injuries or unstable patients that require immediate operation.
(2) Obvious vascular injuries but stable vital signs that permit arteriography.
(3) Injuries whose proximity to vascular structures require evaluation.

Table 1 Signs of Arterial Injury

Hard Signs	Soft Signs
Pulsatile or expanding haematoma	Unexplained shock
Pulsatile bleeding	Proximity to major vessels
Bruit or thrill	Stable haematoma
End-organ ischaemia	Injury to adjacent nerve
	Questionable history of arterial bleeding

Signs of arterial injury are as given in Table 1. Palpable pulses do not exclude a significant arterial injury. Ankle-brachial index (the ratio of blood pressure at the ankle over the blood pressure in the upper arm) of < 0.9 (absolute value) or > 0.1 less than the unaffected extremity is usually indication for arterial evaluation. Digital subtraction angiography is the gold standard evaluation and should be performed whenever possible.

Control of external haemorrhage is most effectively achieved by direct digital pressure. Use of tourniquets should be avoided, and blind placement of clamps should never be practised. Embedded weapons should not be removed; haematomas should not be disturbed until the patient is in an operating theatre, and proximal control can be established expeditiously.

Extension of the surgical approach may be necessary, and the patient should be prepared as such. In dealing with lower extremity trauma, both legs should be prepared in case a saphenous vein graft is necessary. The chest should be prepared in any truncal injury in case of thoracic vessel injury, or to facilitate cross clamping of the descending thoracic aorta in cases where control of intra-abdominal bleeding cannot be achieved from a laparotomy.

Surgical management consists of establishing proximal and distal control before exposing the injury. Thorough debridement must be performed, especially in high-velocity injuries in which the tissues may be damaged well beyond the margins of visible injury. The type of repair depends on the nature and extent of the injury. Some injuries can be repaired by direct suture or by vein patch angioplasty but the majority usually requires an interposition graft. This may be a saphenous vein or prosthetic graft, usually expanded polytetrafluoroethylene (ePTFE); which for some centres is the preferred conduit.[1] Completion arteriography is recommended since distal pulses may not be palpable in the presence of spasm, hypothermia and hypovolaemia.

Specific Vascular Injuries

Injury to the thoracic aorta

Penetrating injuries of the aortic arch or thoracic aorta by gunshot or stab injuries are mostly fatal at the scene of injury. Those that survive the initial event will need left anterior thoracotomy or median sternotomy for exposure, and repair usually involves cardiopulmonary bypass.

By far the most common injury involving the thoracic aorta is aortic transection resulting from sudden deceleration, as in a motor vehicle accident, for example. This may be diagnosed by an aortogram or by a multi-detector helical CT scan with reconstruction showing a "step" or an intimal tear in the aorta, usually at the isthmus. Traditional open techniques of repair include "clamp and sew techniques", repair under atrio-femoral bypass with perfusion of large intercostals as well as the use of shunts. Newer techniques involve the use of endovascular stent-grafts that can be deployed precisely over the injury site to exclude the injury from the bloodstream. These have been found to give good short and medium-term results with lower morbidity and mortality than open repair.[2,3]

Extracranial Vascular Trauma

Carotid and jugular injuries

Penetrating injury of the carotid artery is more common and easily diagnosed whereas blunt injuries resulting from a direct blow or hyperextension may be more subtle. Such injuries include intimal or medial tears that result in dissection, stenosis or thrombosis of the carotid, with neurologic sequelae that may present several hours post injury.

Airway management is of primary importance in penetrating carotid injuries with expanding neck haematomas. Pressure may also affect cranial nerves IX-XII, all of which course through the neck. Arteriography is of paramount importance in root-of-neck injuries as well as injuries above the angle of the mandible, in order to plan surgery. The chest should also be prepared for entry to obtain proximal control. Most penetrating carotid injuries can be managed by direct suture or by end-to-end anastomosis. Saphenous vein or external carotid artery grafts are suitable conduits if interposition grafting is needed. Isolated external carotid injury should be treated by primary ligation as should internal jugular vein injury unless it is bilateral, in which case at least one of the internal jugular veins should be reconstructed.

Neurological deficit has a significant bearing on intervention. Carotid injuries in a neurologically intact patient should be repaired.[4] Those who have a mild deficit or a severe deficit with maintenance of antegrade flow should be repaired. Severe neurological deficit with concomitant absence of flow is best treated by carotid ligation.

Vertebral artery injuries

The vast majority of thesc are from penetrating trauma. Neurologic symptoms are rare because of the dual blood supply to the basilar artery, but severe haemorrhage can occur. Operative therapy consists of proximal and distal ligation unless the opposite vertebral is occluded or diseased, in which case transposition to the common carotid artery is indicated. More recent advances include the use of endovascular techniques to occlude the injured vertebral artery, but this requires experienced interventionalists.

Proximal brachiocephalic injuries

Injury to the brachiocephalic, subclavian and common carotid arteries require immediate intervention to control haemorrhage. Chest tube insertion is necessary for pneumothorax or haemothorax. The patient is prepared for all possible approaches, including median sternotomy, left anterior thoracotomy or a "trap-door" approach.[5] Repair by direct suture or autogenous patch is possible most of the time.

Extremity Vascular Injuries

These can be complicated and even masked by the associated bone, muscle and nerve injury. Arteriography is mostly necessary to establish the diagnosis, and to define the extent of the lesion.

Upper extremity injuries

Subclavian artery injuries are often associated with concomitant brachial plexus injury (either directly by bullet or blade, or indirectly by blast injury or compression by haematoma). These determine the functional outcome of the repair; which is almost always successful in re-establishing flow to the extremity. Proximal injuries may require a thoracotomy for left-sided injuries and median sternotomy for right-sided injuries.

Brachial artery injury must always be suspected and excluded when dealing with elbow dislocations or fractures about the elbow. The lesion is almost invariably a distraction injury resulting in intimal disruption and thrombosis of the brachial artery. Treatment involves resection of the disrupted segment with interposition graft placement, usually saphenous vein. This artery can also be injured at the elbow by knife or glass lacerations; which also usually involve the neighbouring median nerve. Immediate simultaneous repair by cutting back the edges of the lacerated artery and nerve followed by end-to-end anastomosis, gives the best functional outcome.

Injuries to the radial artery at the wrist are usually of no consequence due to the dual blood supply of the hand. If the cut radial artery displays pulsatile bleeding from both ends, it can be ligated. If, however, the palmar arch is incomplete and the backbleed is inadequate, the radial artery will have to be repaired in an end-to-end fashion with interrupted sutures utilising microsurgical techniques.

Lower extremity injuries

Penetrating injuries of the lower extremity such as stab wounds or gunshot wounds usually involve the superficial femoral artery, and may present with an exsanguinating bleed or more commonly, a pulsatile haematoma. Arteriography is useful but probably not mandatory if the groin is not involved. The surgical approach is as for femoral-popliteal bypass, with resection of the injured segment and placement of an interposition graft. Associated bone, soft tissue and nerve injury may be the final determinants of limb preservation.

Missile wounds at the trifurcation (the division of the popliteal artery into the three tibial vessels) are technically the most demanding injuries as they demand reconstruction by femoro-crural bypass, which is a more extensive and tedious procedure. There might also be compromise of the popliteal vein as well as the tibial and peroneal nerves, in which case re-establishment of circulation may be a pointless exercise as the limb will be functionally useless.

Blunt injuries of the lower extremity vasculature are usually associated with posterior dislocation of the knee, or long bone fractures, in particular those about the knee.[6] Most of these result from motor vehicle accidents as well as from sporting injuries, particularly high velocity sports such as skiing and wakeboarding. Hyperextension with intimal disruption or subintimal haematoma results in occlusion, and reconstruction has to be undertaken after stabilisation of the associated bony injuries. If the bony injuries are extensive and stabilisation is expected to take enough time to compromise already ischaemic tissues, temporising measures (such as the use of artificial shunts) can restore circulation and buy time before definitive repair can be carried out. Saphenous vein grafts should be harvested from the contralateral limb to avoid further compromise of venous drainage from the injured limb. Four-compartment fasciotomy should always be carried out post reconstruction or even pre-reconstruction if the situation demands it. When there is also extensive venous injury, consideration should be given to venous reconstruction to enable venous drainage and prevent gross limb swelling; with or without distal arteriovenous fistula creation to prevent re-thrombosis. Finally, soft tissue cover over the reconstructed vessels is mandatory, if necessary by rotation or myocutaneous advancement flaps.

Injury to the abdominal aorta and visceral arteries

These injuries are usually the result of penetrating trauma. Two problems present themselves; control of haemorrhage and containment of contamination. The mortality quoted in most series dealing with penetrating intra-abdominal aortic trauma ranges from 50% to 90%. Principles of management include rapid establishment of proximal control at the diaphragmatic hiatus, followed by identification of the injury and expeditious repair. The Mattox manoeuvre (medial visceral rotation) may be necessary to expose the visceral segment of the aorta. Direct suture of the injury is seldom possible but prosthetic patch repair or an interposition graft are acceptable options in the absence of contamination, or if there is limited contamination and the graft can be shielded from it. If there is major contamination, a safer option than *in situ* reconstruction is aortic ligation and extra-anatomical bypass. More recently described techniques for *in situ* reconstruction (in the presence of infection) such as composite superficial femoral vein grafts, are not appropriate in this setting due to the need to be expedient.

Blunt abdominal trauma can also result in vascular injuries, usually by avulsion of bowel mesentery or laceration of solid organs involving the vascular pedicle. Mostly, these can be adequately managed by resection or direct suture without having to resort to complex reconstructions. Endovascular options also exist to control intra-abdominal haemorrhage, although these do not preclude eventual laparotomy.

Whatever the aetiology of injury, and irrespective of the vessels involved, the principles of abbreviated laparotomy or staged laparotomy[7] should be observed with bailout options such as packing, temporary interruption of vessels, shunt placement, and so forth, allowing for the operation to be terminated, and resuscitation, rewarming and reversal of coagulopathy to continue in the intensive care unit with planned re-operation, for definitive reconstruction once the patient's altered physiology has been corrected.

Iatrogenic Vascular Injury

These include the traditional vascular injuries caused by inexperienced or overly aggressive surgeons, external iliac or common femoral artery injury during hernia repairs, superior mesenteric artery injury during right hemicolectomy, or portal vein injury during the posterior approach to the liver being examples of these, as well as a whole host of injuries resulting from the explosion of percutaneous coronary and peripheral vascular interventions.[8] These include access site complications such as overt external bleeding; groin and retroperitoneal haematomas; dissection, occlusion and thrombosis; vessel disruption and pseudoaneurysm formation, as well as target vessel complications such as rupture, dissection, thrombosis and embolism.

Most access site injuries can be managed non-surgically by compression, restoration of normal coagulation parameters, thrombin injection for pseudoaneurysms, and so on. Occasionally, surgical repair of the arterial injury has to be performed with evacuation of the haematoma.

Endovascular salvage is the first choice for dissections and ruptures by stent or stent graft placement with surgery reserved for endovascular failures. Thrombosis with distal ischaemia can be treated with percutaneous mechanical aspiration, thrombolysis, a combination of both or surgery; which is the bailout option when all else has failed.

Target vessel injuries can also often be managed by percutaneous interventions although surgery may be required more than in access problems. Surgery may involve direct repair, patch angioplasty, interposition graft or bypass depending on the site and extent of target vessel injury. As the scope of endovascular interventions widens (as is happening at the present time), more iatrogenic injuries are to be anticipated, and recognition of high risk situations as well as good peri-procedural monitoring and care, will help to reduce adverse outcomes.

References

1. Feliciano DV, Mattox KL, Graham JM, Bitondo CG (1985). Five-year experience with PTFE grafts in vascular wounds. *J Trauma* **25**(1), 71–82.
2. Thompson CS, Rodriguez JA, Ramaiah VG, DiMugno L, Shafique S, Olsen D, Diethrich EB (2002). Acute traumatic rupture of the thoracic aorta treated with endoluminal stent grafts. *J Trauma* **52**(6), 1173–1177.
3. Hoffer EK, Karmy-Jones R, Bloch RD, Meissner MH, Borsa JJ, Nicholls SC, So CR (2002). Treatment of acute thoracic aortic injury with commercially available abdominal aortic stent-grafts. *J Vasc Interv Radiol* **13**(10), 1037–1041.
4. Brown MF, Graham JM, Feliciano DV, Mattox KL, Beall AC Jr, DeBakey ME (1982). Carotid artery injuries. *Am J Surg* **144**(6), 748–753.
5. Graham JM, Feliciano DV, Mattox KL, Beall AC Jr (1982). Innominate vascular injury. *J Trauma* **22**(8), 647–655.
6. Bishara RA, Pasch AR, Lim LT, Meyer JP, Schuler JJ, Hall RF Jr, Flanigan DP (1986). Improved results in the treatment of civilian vascular injuries associated with fractures and dislocations. *J Vasc Surg* **3**(5), 707–711.

7. Burch JM, Ortiz VB, Richardson RJ, Martin RR, Mattox KL, Jordan GL Jr (1992). Abbreviated laparotomy and planned re-operation for critically injured patients. *Ann Surg* **215**(5), 476–483.
8. Ricci MA, Trevisani GT, Pilcher DB (1994). Vascular complications of cardiac catheterisation. *Am J Surg* **167**(4), 375–378.

Further Reading

Wolfe JHN (1992). ABC of Vascular Disease. *Br Med J.*

14

Penetrating Trauma to the Chest

Chong-Hee Lim
Thirugnanam Agasthian

Introduction

Penetrating chest injuries are relatively uncommon in Singapore. According to the trauma database of the Singapore General Hospital, 449 patients with thoracic trauma were treated between January 1998 and December 2001. Penetrating chest trauma constituted 21.6% (97) of these cases. This averages to about 24 cases per year. Of these, 96% were males. Mean age was 29.7 years. Almost all of the cases were from stabbing (96/97). There was one case of gunshot injury. Overall in-hospital mortality was 7% (7/97).

The low incidence of penetrating trauma is tied to our strict local laws and harsh punishments, restricting ownership of firearms and keeping violent crimes at a low level. The majority of open chest injuries result from domestic violence and gang fights among youths. Occasionally, gunshot wounds occurred from accidents during military live-firing exercises may be encountered.

This chapter reviews the types of wounds; the surgical principles of managing penetrating chest wounds; and the prioritisation of management. Guidelines and indications for open thoracotomy in the emergency room will be discussed.

Types of Wounds

Penetrating chest injuries[1] are divided into the following three broad types of wounds based loosely on the offending weapon.

(1) *Stab wound*

This is by far the most common penetrating injury seen at local emergency departments. Severity of the injury is based on the area of the chest injured, the angle of entry and depth of penetration.

Danger areas are:

- median areas where the heart is situated
- the neck and the thoracic inlet where large vessels and the trachea are at risk
- the lower lateral aspects of the chests where the spleen and liver may be injured on the left and right flanks, respectively.

(2) *Gunshot wound*

The severity of injury is evaluated by the type of gun used, which can be classified into low or high velocity bullet wound injury types. Intuitively, the higher the velocity of the bullet on penetrating a body cavity, the greater the damage. Collateral damage from the rapid deceleration or cavitation effect of the offending bullet often results in a much greater injury than expected. Delayed complications such as Acute Respiratory Distress Syndrome (ARDS) should be anticipated.

For gunshot injuries, a thorough search for the exit site of the bullet must be performed. This can provide clues to the potential damage to the organs in the bullet's path.

(3) *Impalement*

This form of insult often results from a dramatic accident, and is usually fatal. If the person survives the initial injury, the offending weapon is still in place. In these cases, the instrument is displacing or only partially injuring the underlying organ.

Principles of Management

A patient with an open chest wound is in critical condition, and all efforts are made to expedite management. Diagnosis and treatment often have to be performed simultaneously.

Initial management is based on current and established protocols[1] outlined in the Advanced Trauma Life Support® (ATLS) programme.[2] The primary survey includes assessments of airway, breathing and circulation. Vital signs are measured and monitored. A short but thorough history is taken from the patient or accompanying witnesses, including information on the type of weapon, angle of directed injury, and position of the patient on impact. A keen physician should be able to reconstruct the trajectory of the offending weapon. The wound is examined in both inspiration and expiration, in search of a "sucking" chest wound which occurs when air is drawn in and out of the chest cavity (open pneumothorax) during the respective phase of the respiratory cycle. All stab injuries are considered serious until proved otherwise. A small and seemingly innocuous external wound may be deep with cardiac penetration and could lead to rapid exsanguination.

Two large-bore intravenous lines are inserted into the antecubital veins on both arms. If there is suspected injury to the large veins in the neck, access should be via the femoral or long saphenous veins.

Imaging

In a haemodynamically stable patient, upright chest and abdominal radiographs are preferred. In the multiply injured, supine X-rays are often obtained but interpretation may be difficult. Mediastinal air, pneumothorax, haemothorax, and subcutaneous emphysema are indicative of airway or lung injuries. A widened mediastinum suggests to aortic or great-vessel injury.

A contrast computed axial scan of the chest does not usually provide additional information that will help in the diagnosis in penetrating chest injuries, but may be useful in blunt trauma, in assessing aortic injury. It is also useful in abdominal and brain injuries.

Suspected concomitant injury in the abdomen may be investigated with computed tomography scans and barium studies.

Priority of Management

Patients may be prioritised into three categories based on their clinical status on evaluation:

(1) *Almost normal*

In this group of patients, the wound is cleaned and sutured but must be monitored closely in a high dependency area.

(2) *Unstable*

The patient in this category is critical and urgently requires therapeutic intervention. Usually the poor haemodynamic state is due to bleeding or pneumothorax. Fluid resuscitation and haemostasis, or a chest tube thoracostomy are usually sufficient to stabilise the patient.

(3) *Near collapse (shock, coma, asphyxia)*

In this category, the following causes have to be considered:

- cardiac perforation with exsanguination or tamponade
- uncontrolled intrathoracic haemorrhage with severe hypovolaemia
- tension pneumothorax
- intra-abdominal haemorrhage
- massive air embolism from an open central vein

The need for immediate or urgent thoracotomy in the emergency room is to be considered in these situations.

Role of Emergency Room Thoracotomy

Emergency room thoracotomy (ERT) is often dramatic and potentially life saving in a small but well defined group of patients. In large volume trauma centres where this procedure can be performed in a sufficiently expedient manner, survival rates of up to 57% can be achieved for penetrating trauma.[4] In most other centres, however survival is limited to 3–15%.[5,6] In our setting, its role is particularly difficult to define. Cases of penetrating cardiac injuries are far too few for our emergency room physicians to gain sufficient surgical experience. Delay in diagnosis, haemodynamic deterioration, and a pre-collapse state often from exsanguination or tamponade, are factors contributing to poor outcome. In what situations can we balance the overall low survival rates has to be considered and balanced against the risk of exposing emergency room personnel to blood and potential contamination.

Indications:

(1) Patients with stab wounds to the "cardiac box" (the area defined between the nipples laterally, the sternal notch superiorly to the xiphoid inferiorly) presenting to the ER, with initial relatively stable haemodynamic status but suddenly deteriorate.
(2) Patients with a penetrating chest wound with features of cardiac tamponade.

    Note: these patients may have a palpable pulse but no measurable blood pressure

Contraindications:

(1) Blunt trauma — this is often associated with a much greater injury and poor outcome if presented with haemodynamic collapse.
(2) Patients without a palpable pulse.
(3) Unstable haemodynamics from associated severe injuries, for example, intracranial haemorrhage, intra-abdominal injuries.

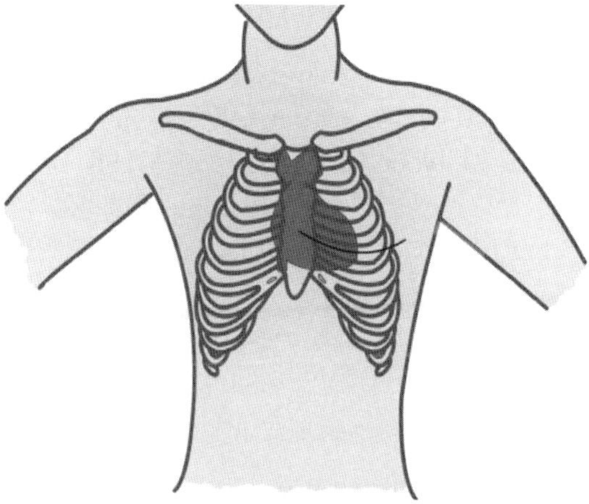

Fig. 1 Incision made deep cutting the skin, subcutaneous tissues and muscle layers.

Emergency Room Thoracotomy

Emergency room thoracotomy[3] (ERT) is performed only if the airway is secured with an endotracheal tube. Large bore venous access (> 16G) must be available, preferably through the femoral veins. Swan Ganz sheaths (8.5F) are particularly useful for rapid transfusion. Urine output should be monitored via a urinary catheter.

A large curved incision is made in the fifth interspace on the left side. The skin, subcutaneous tissue and pectoralis muscle are incised to reach the intercostal muscles (Fig. 1). The intercostal muscles are then carefully but expediently divided, usually starting more laterally. The left pleural space is entered and the entire intercostal space is then divided with a pair of straight Mayo scissors, laterally and medially (Fig. 2). A large Finochetto® chest retractor is placed and spread opened. Fluid in the left chest is aspirated. Identify the left phrenic nerve to avoid injuring it. The pericardium is then incised with a No. 15 blade anterior to the phrenic nerve and the incision is carried upwards with a pair of scissors. Evacuate any clots. If there is tamponade, haemodynamics will improve correspondingly. If there is excessive bleeding, efforts are made to identify the source. Usually, this is from the right ventricle.

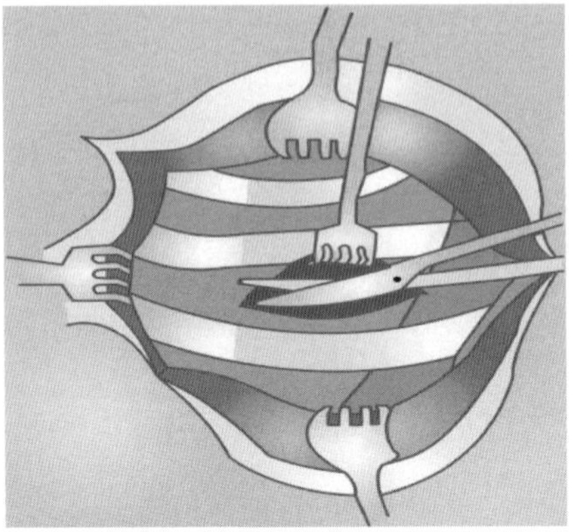

Fig. 2 After entering the pleural cavity, the incision is extended lateral and medially with a pair of scissors.

Visibility is often poor in the emergency room setting. If so, extend the incision by dividing the costal cartilages superiorly. This allows the retractor to open wider. If the cardiac laceration is small, do not attempt to repair it at the emergency room. The laceration will get larger as it tears through with each cardiac contraction. It is safer to compress the laceration with a large piece of gauze. This will sufficiently reduce the bleeding and with simultaneous resuscitation with emergency blood, the patient can be stabilised. Transfer the patient to the operating room when he or she is more stable, for definitive repair.

Cardiorrhaphy

Putting a stitch on the beating heart is never easy. If the laceration is small, avoid doing it. It is often better to apply digital pressure over a piece of gauze on the laceration to stop the bleeding. Wait for help to arrive.

If the bleeding cannot be controlled, and the patient is in danger of exsanguination, a 3.0 polypropylene stitch with large Teflon felt pledgets may be used (Fig. 3). The heart in this setting is often

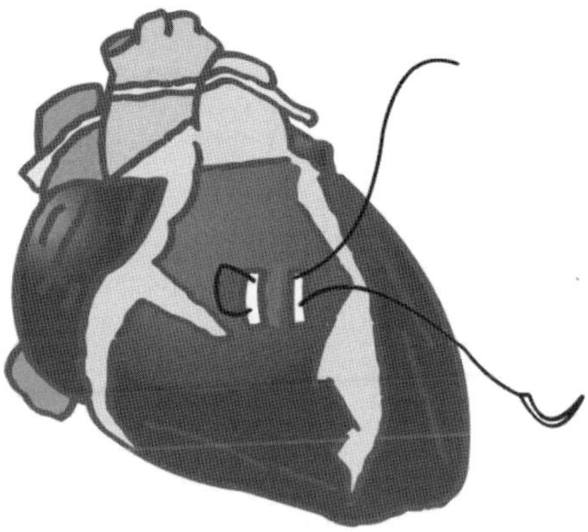

Fig. 3 Cardiorrhaphy is done with a 3.0 polypropylene stitch reinforced with large Teflon® pledgets.

oedematous and prone to tearing. A useful adjunctive technique of inducing transient asystole with intravenous adenosine has been described.[7] The transient arrest of the heart allows accurate placement of sutures and haemostasis.

If ventricular fibrillation occurs during the open resuscitation cardiorrhaphy is performed before attempts at defibrillation. This controls further loss of blood and makes the defibrillation easier and more likely to succeed.

Defibrillation

Two types of defibrillation are available, with external pads and internal paddles. In the emergency room, internal paddles are not readily available. One external pad is placed on the right chest and the other over the left back.

Standard ATLS® defibrillation techniques are used as in closed cardiopulmonary resuscitation (CPR). It is important for the team leader in the CPR effort to communicate with the surgeon when defibrillation is taking place, to avoid injury to personnel.

If internal paddles are used, the charged energy need not exceed 10 J.

The paddles in contact with the epicardium should be wet with saline to reduce burns on the heart.

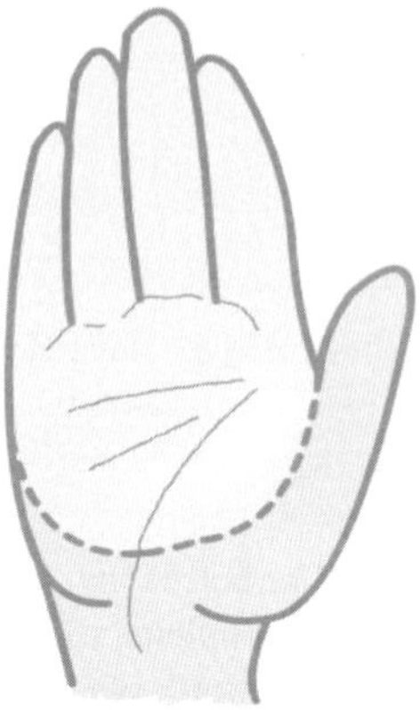

Fig. 4 The flat part of the hand is used for open cardiac massage.

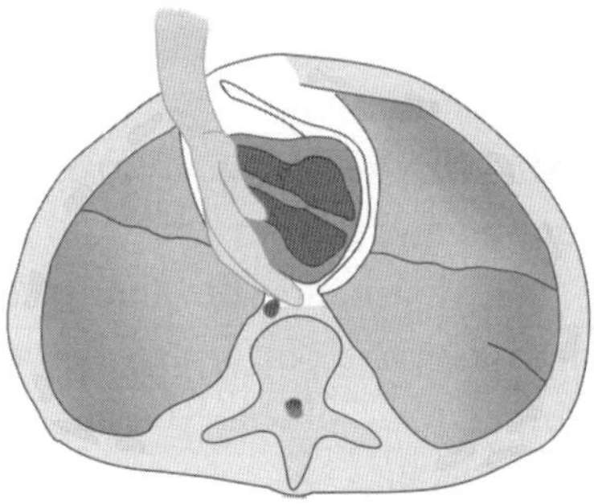

Fig. 5 A gentler open massage method done against the spine.

Open Cardiac Massage

More often than not, after opening the pericardium, the heart fibrillates. This is due to prolonged periods of hypotension and myocardial ischaemia. Though open cardiac massage is said to be more effective than closed massage, some degree of experience is necessary to maintain adequate cerebral perfusion and to avoid cardiac injuries.[8]

Open massage is done with the flat part of the hand (Fig. 4), against the back of the sternum. This can be dangerous as cardiac rupture can occur when pushed against the sharp edge of the divided costal cartilage (Fig. 5). An alternative approach is placing the flat palmar surface of the hand over the right ventricle and pushing the heart against the spine (Fig. 6). This may be safer but is more demanding.

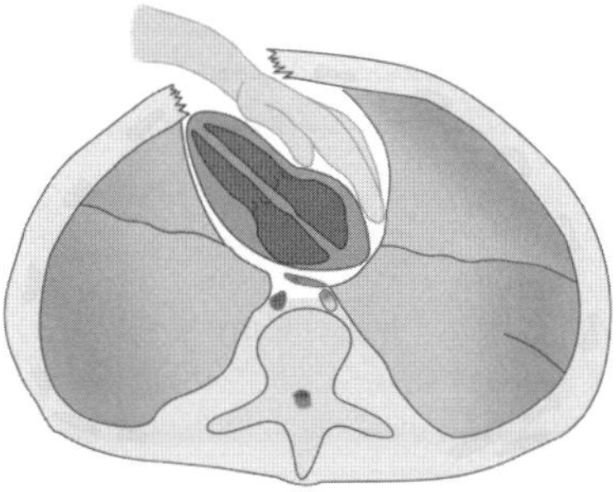

Fig. 6 Open massage done against the back of the sternum, cardiac injury may result from force against the sharp bone edges.

During the entire period of internal cardiac massage, efforts are made to convert the cardiac rhythm back to sinus, both pharmacologically and by defibrillation.

Disadvantages of the ERT

Overall poor results of ERT lies with the inavailability of trained staff at time of the haemodynamic collapse which necessitates the urgency of the procedure. ERT is often done too late to have an impact on patient survival.

Poor lighting in the emergency room, poor access to the entire heart via the anterior thoracotomy, and consequently, ineffective CPR and defibrillation, are limiting factors for a successful outcome.

In general, if the patient's condition allows it, efforts should be made to transfer the patient to the operating room for a definitive procedure.

Elective Thoracotomy/Thoracoscopy

In a stable patient with penetrating injury, chest tube thoracostomy may not be sufficient to evacuate the haemothorax. Significant blood clots in the chest should be evacuated in the operating room on an elective setting. Most cases can be performed via thoracoscopy which allows excellent visualisation of the entire chest cavity. All clots should be removed. Warm distilled water lavage of the pleural

Table 1 Disadvantages of the ER Thoracotomy

Ineffective CPR
Untrained staff in ER
Poor lighting
Difficult defibrillation
Poor access to the entire heart with left anterior thoracotomy
Ineffectiveness in more severe injuries
Lack of suitable vascular clamps in ER

cavity helps with visualisation. Definitive repair of the lung is rarely necessary. Pulmonary decortication via a thoracotomy may sometimes be necessary to re-expand areas of lung trapped by fibrin clots.

Conclusion

Serious penetrating chest injury is uncommon in Singapore. Mortality depends on the type of injury, and the offending weapon, with most deaths occurring in the field. Expedient and efficient management of the patient with signs of life, reduces mortality and morbidity. Emergency room thoracotomy when appropriately executed, may be life-saving. All other urgent thoracotomy procedures, where required, should be performed in the operating room to allow for definitive repair of the injured organs and achieve a more efficient resuscitation of the wounded patient.

References

1. Besson A, Saegesser F (1982). *A Colour Atlas of Chest Trauma and Associated Injuries.* Wolfe Medical Publications, Vol. 1.
2. Committee on Trauma (1989). *American College Advanced Trauma Life Support Course for Physicians*. Chicago: American College of Surgeons.
3. Mattox KL (1989). Indications for thoracotomy: deciding to operate. *Surg Clin North Am* **69**(1), 47–58.

4. Tavares S, Hankins JR, Moulton AL, Attar S, Ali S *et al.* (1984). Management of penetrating cardiac injuries: the role of emergency room thoracotomy. *Ann Thorac Surg* **38**(3), 183–187.
5. Boyd M, Vanek VW, Bourguet CC (1992). Emergency room resuscitative thoracotomy: when is it indicated? *J Trauma* **33**(5), 714–721.
6. Washington B, Wilson RF, Steiger Z, Bassett JS (1985). Emergency thoracotomy: a four year review. *Ann Thorac Surg* **40**(2), 188–191.
7. Lim R, Gill IS, Temes RT, Smith CE (2001). The use of adenosine for repair of penetrating cardiac injuries: a novel method. *Ann Thorac Surg* **71**(5), 1714–1715.
8. Arai T, Dote K, Tsukahara I, Nitta K, Nagaro T (1984). Cerebral blood flow during conventional, new and open-chest cardio-pulmonary resuscitation in dogs. *Resuscitation* **12**(2), 147–154.

Section IV

Gastrointestinal Tract Emergencies

15

Management of the Acute Abdomen

Melissa Teo
Kee-Chee Soo

Introduction

The complaint of abdominal pain is a common one at the Accident and Emergency Department. A patient is described as having an acute abdomen when the presentation is that of a recent or sudden onset of unexpected abdominal pain, of less than one week in duration. The acute abdomen is interesting from the point of view of being a diagnostic challenge. In the derivation of a correct diagnosis, the importance of careful history taking and longitudinal assessment of subtle changes in significant signs, cannot be emphasised enough. There is a narrow window of opportunity for some acute abdominal conditions, after which any delay may initiate an irreversible course of events[1] (Fig. 1).

A compilation of the work done in a surgical audit of 1190 emergency admissions,[2] and that performed in the Acute Abdominal Pain Survey[3] on 10,682 patients revealed several common causes of acute abdominal pain (Table 1).

In spite the extensive list of causes (the mentioned causes in Table 1 is far from exhaustive), early diagnosis is of utmost importance

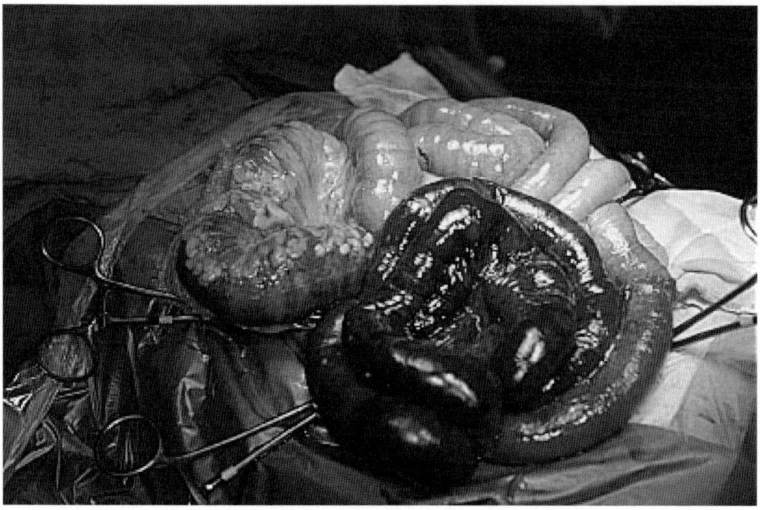

Fig. 1 Ischaemic bowel.

Table 1 Common Causes of Acute Abdominal Pain

Non-specific abdominal pain (NSAP)	33%
Acute appendicitis	24%
Intestinal obstruction	11%
Acute cholecystitis	9%
Acute gynaecological disorders	4%
Acute pancreatitis	3%
Renal colic	3%
Perforated peptic ulcer	2%
Abdominal trauma	2% (variable)
Abdominal malignancy	2%
Diverticular disease	2%
Miscellaneous (e.g. acute medical conditions like inferior myocardial infarction, lobar pneumonia, diabetic ketoacidosis and acute porphyria)	5%

in the management of the acute abdomen. Knowledge of the anatomy of the abdomen will be useful in the process of coming to a diagnosis.

Anatomy of the Peritoneum

The peritoneum comprises two components that have separate nerve supplies. The visceral peritoneum is innervated by the autonomic nervous system, and pain is triggered by inflammation, ischaemia, distension, traction and pressure. Visceral pain is usually dull and poorly localised, and may not necessarily indicate a need for surgical intervention. The parietal peritoneum is innervated by somatic nerves that supply the abdominal wall, and pain is usually triggered by an inflammatory process with chemical or bacterial peritonitis.

The main site of the pain at onset relates to the embryologic origin of the affected organ. Foregut-derived structures (from the stomach to the second part of the duodenum (D2), the hepatobiliary system, the spleen and the pancreas) commonly present with epigastric pain. Midgut-derived structures (from D2 to the proximal two-thirds of the transverse colon) present with periumbilical pain; and hindgut-derived structures (up to the anal verge) present with suprapubic pain.

The pain results from central neural pathways in the spinal cord that are common to both somatic nerves and visceral organs. For example, diaphragmatic irritation (innervated by the phrenic nerves C3 to C5) from a subphrenic abscess may present with pain referred to the ipsilateral shoulder.

With a complete patient history and thorough physical examination, a correct diagnosis can usually be made in 80% of patients with acute abdomen. Failure to obtain or perform either often results in delayed diagnosis and performance of unnecessary investigations.

History

Careful consideration of the onset, character and distribution of pain is mandatory. The acuteness of the onset gives some indication of

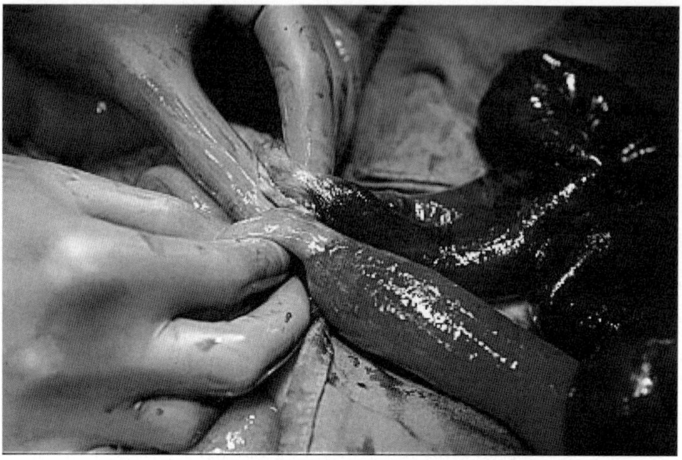

Fig. 2 Volvulus resulting in ischaemic bowel.

the severity of the lesion. A sudden onset (occurring within seconds) suggests perforation of a viscus, or the presence of blood in the peritoneum (for example, secondary to a leaking aortic aneurysm, or a ruptured ectopic pregnancy), acute mesenteric ischaemia or acute volvulus (Fig. 2) or intussusception (Fig. 3). Pain of gradual onset can be a result of colic (as experienced in intestinal) ureteric or biliary obstruction; or an inflammatory condition, such as cholecystitis, appendicitis or pancreatitis.

The main site of pain at onset gives an idea of the origin of pathology, either from the foregut, midgut or hindgut. The subsequent radiation of the pain suggests the anatomical location of the pathology, as the underlying inflamed peritoneum gives rise to the radiating pain.

The character of the pain can be described as colicky or persistent, with or without an increase in severity and intensity. Colic occurs as a result of hyperperistalsis of smooth muscle, and is experienced in intestinal, ureteric obstruction. Classically, colic is described as exacerbations of pain with relatively pain-free intervening periods. The exception is biliary colic, which is neither separated by pain-free intervals, nor located at the expected site (the right hypochondrium) — it is situated at the epigastrium.

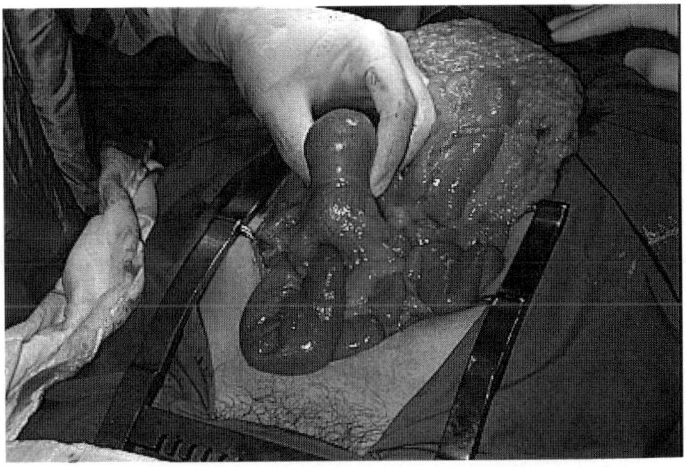

(a)

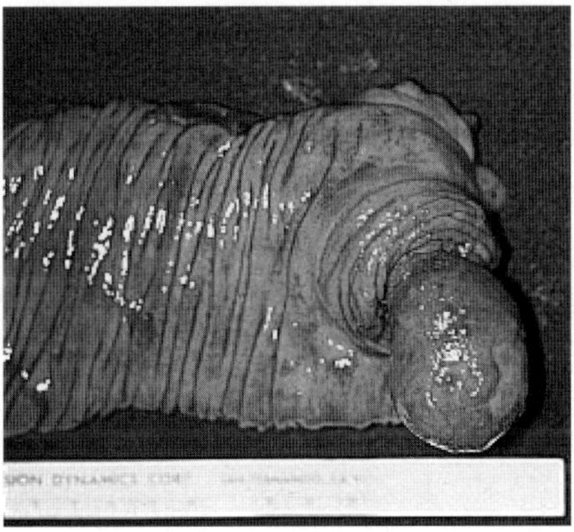

(b)

Fig. 3 Intusussusception.

Persistent pain suggests an inflammatory or infective process. The location and radiation of the pain may point towards the diagnosis, especially when it is site-specific; for example, at the right iliac fossa in acute appendicitis, and at the right hypochondrium in acute cholecystitis. But, this may not always be the case. Radiation of the pain may be classical, such as to the back (for retroperitoneal structures like the pancreas and abdominal aorta), and to the inferior angle of the right scapula in bilary colic.

Pain from diffuse peritonitis may be ameliorated by stillness. Inflammation of the gallbladder may inhibit inspiratory effort, as movement of the diaphragm exacerbates pain.

Associated symptoms of fever and chills suggest an inflammatory or infectious process. Nausea and vomiting may be present, and the sequence of events with regard to emesis and pain is important. In sudden and severe stimulation of the peritoneum, vomiting occurs early, as in ureteric or bile duct obstruction. In appendicitis, the pain usually precedes the vomiting by a few hours. The length of time before vomiting ensues in intestinal obstruction, gives some indication of where the obstruction is proximally situated. The content of the vomitus (presence or absence of bile, blood and faeces) should be noted. Reflex vomiting secondary to pain should be distinguished from vomiting as a consequence of obstruction due to reactive peristalsis. The volume and content of the vomitus is different, and vomiting relieves the pain achieved in the latter situation.

Anorexia is common in acute peritonitis and hence is always significant, especially if the history is deficient, for example, when being recorded from a child or a demented elderly.

There can be a recent change in bowel habit. This can be ominous especially if it is associated with a loss of weight and/or appetite, and presence of blood in the stools.

Menstrual history should always be sought in any woman of child-bearing age, with inquiry into the date of the last menstrual period, and probing for any history of amenorrhoea. Query for the presence of monthly abdominal pain (suggesting dysmenorrhoea — as in endometriosis), and the presence of vaginal discharge.

A sexual history should also be obtained. The history can be completed by asking about previous abdominal surgery (intestinal obstruction secondary to adhesions is a common cause of colicky abdominal pain); other medical co-morbidities; drug and alcohol intake; and smoking history. A special mention should be made about steroid therapy as it diminishes the symptoms produced by inflammation. It may result in a difficult assessment that ultimately necessitates surgical intervention in ambiguous situations. Steroid therapy also predisposes a patient to peptic ulcer disease, as does non-steroidal anti-inflammatory drug (NSAID) therapy.

Physical Examination

The general appearance of the patient will furnish valuable evidence of the seriousness of the nature of the pain. The restlessness of those suffering from severe colic, contrasts sharply with the immobility of those with diffuse peritonitis. The latter group is likely to lie quietly and may have their knees drawn up to their chest to relax the abdominal tension and to bring a slight reprieve from their pain and discomfort. Of special mention is the extreme distress and restlessness of patients with mesenteric ischaemia, that is often accompanied by a paucity of abdominal signs. Patients with pain of pancreatic or retro-peritoneal origin may prefer a sitting to a recumbent position. The patient may also be lethargic, with an alteration in the mental status that may be secondary to sepsis or electrolyte imbalance.

Vital signs are important indicators of the patient's overall condition. Fever suggests the presence of inflammation or infection, but may be blunted in the elderly and the immuno-compromised. Tachycardia and/or hypotension should be alerting signs, and may indicate hypovolaemia or sepsis.

The abdominal examination should be systematically conducted. Inspection for distension, surgical scars and of all hernial orifices (including the femoral canal) should be performed. Limitation of movement on respiration may hint at the site of pathology.

On palpation of the abdomen, it is preferable to begin with a point most remote from the site of pain. Gentleness is essential to success. Palpation determines the extent and intensity of the muscular defence or rigidity (voluntary or involuntary), locates any tenderness, and determines the presence of any swelling. It should be noted if the swelling moves well with respiration, can be felt all around (especially if it is adjacent to the subcostal margin or the pelvis) and whether it is dull or tympanic to percussion (bowel loops overlying the mass will result in a tympanic percussion note). Rebound tenderness occurs on the release of a palpating hand over an inflamed focus. Bimanual palpation of the loins may reveal a palpable renal or adrenal mass, and tenderness is elicited by performance of a renal punch.

Auscultation may reveal the high-pitched, tinkling bowel sounds of obstruction; the absence of bowel sounds may be due to ileus from diffuse peritonitis.

Percussion of the patient's abdomen is useful for delineating localised tenderness and peritoneal irritation (and may be better accepted by a child if performed before palpation). It may also reveal the fluid shift characteristic of ascites.

An abdominal examination is incomplete without a pelvic examination. Per-vaginal examination is conducted to look for cervical excitation, adnexal masses or tenderness and cervical discharge. A per-rectal examination is extremely important and informative. It may reveal a stricture of the rectum due to carcinoma or fibrosis; bulging of a pelvic abscess against the anterior rectal wall, or carcinomatosis implants on Blummer's shelf. Tenderness elicited with pressure applied laterally may be due to an inflamed or swollen appendix, abscess in the lateral pelvic wall, or an adnexal lesion. Lastly, the glove is checked for the presence of blood, pus or mucus on the stool.

The cardiac, respiratory and neurological systems should also be thoroughly examined.

Investigations

Laboratory evaluations include the following.

Complete blood count with cell count differential

A raised white cell count may indicate an infectious source. An elevated haematocrit may be a result of haemoconcentration, while a low haematocrit may signify blood loss.

Serum urea and electrolytes concentrations

Derangements may be seen with vomiting and diarrhoea (hypokalaemia, hypochloraemia), and dehydration may be reflected in raised serum urea and creatinine concentrations.

Liver function tests

Elevated serum bilirubin and alkaline phosphatase concentrations point towards an obstructive cause. Derangements are seen in cholangitis and may be present in pancreatitis and cholecystitis.

Serum amylase concentration

This is usually elevated in acute pancreatitis, but is neither highly sensitive nor specific.

Diagnostic Imaging

These would include:

Erect chest film

Free air under the diaphragm, without recent abdominal surgery, indicates a perforated viscus. However, this sign may be absent in up to 20% of patients with such a condition. Insufflation of air, or a lateral decubitus film, may improve the sensitivity of the chest X-ray in such a scenario. It is also useful for exclusion of lobar pneumonia.

Supine abdominal X-ray

The abdominal X-ray may show abnormal bowel pattern (dilatation of bowel loops in obstruction (Fig. 4), presence of a sentinel loop adjacent to inflamed organ due to localised ileus), soft tissue masses, and calcification in 90% of urinary stones, 15% of gallstones and in some cases of chronic pancreatitis. A psoas shadow may also be seen occasionally. Presence of gas in the portal and mesenteric venous system, and intramural gas in the gastrointestinal tract are ominous signs. Aerobilia may occasionally be seen in gallstone ileus (Fig. 5) and anaerobic cholangitis, but is seen most commonly following surgery or endoscopic retrograde cholangiopancreatography (ERCP).

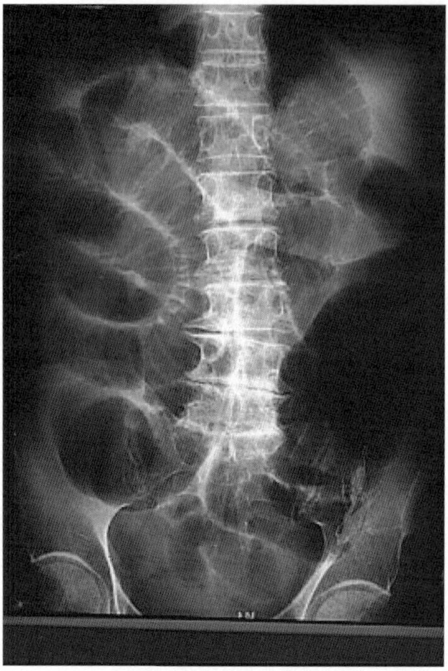

Fig. 4 Dilated small bowel loops.

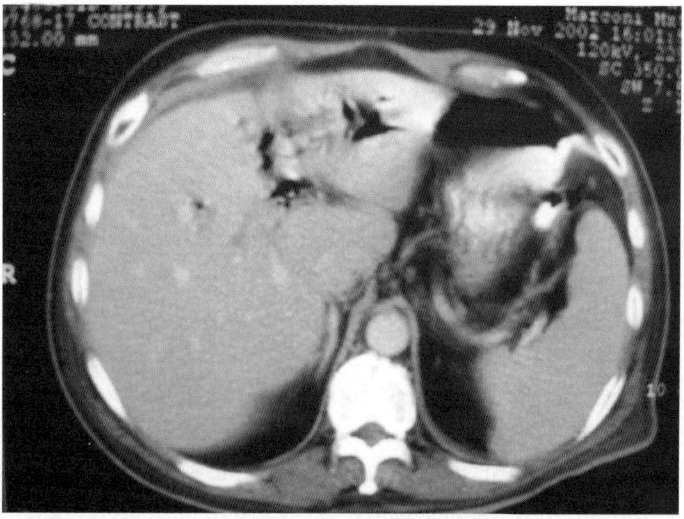

Fig. 5 Aerobilia.

Erect abdominal film

This is less useful but may reveal multiple air-fluid levels, confirming intestinal obstruction.

Ultrasonography

This modality has the advantage of being portable, inexpensive and free of radiation. It is useful in acute biliary disease, detecting gallstones in up to 95% of patients. Acute cholecystitis can usually be diagnosed with evidence of gallbladder wall thickening, pericholecystic fluid, sonographic Murphy's sign, and occasionally a stone in the neck of the gallbladder, or a dilated common bile duct of more than 1 cm. It can also be helpful in evaluating pelvic pathology; for example, ruptured or twisted ovarian cyst, ectopic pregnancy; and for determining the presence of an abdominal aortic aneurysm and the presence of intraperitoneal free fluid or abscess.

Computed tomography

This is performed with oral and intravenous contrast, and is useful in (1) patients with worrisome abdominal pain but without definitive signs of peritonitis; (2) the evaluation of retroperitoneal structures;

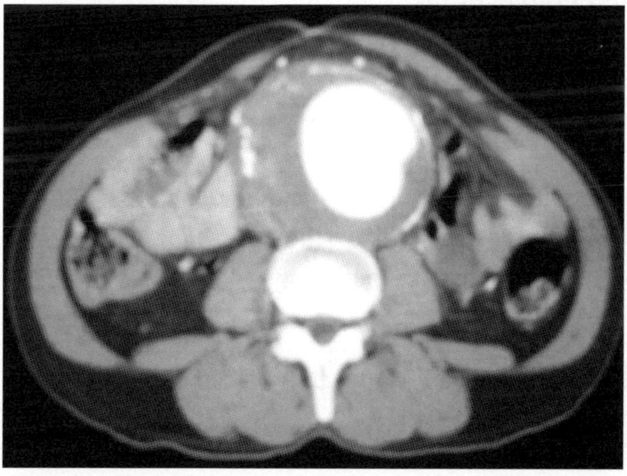

Fig. 6 Leaking abdominal aortic aneurysm.

for example, stable patients with suspected leaking abdominal aortic aneurysm (Fig. 6); (3) patients with a history of intra-abdominal malignancy; (4) patients with acute abdominal pain in the presence of chronic illness, for example, Crohn's disease; and (5) patients who cannot give a complete and accurate history.

Hydroxy indole-diacetic (HIDA) scan

This modality can be used to evaluate filling and emptying of the gallbladder in suspected acute cholecystitis, if the condition cannot be diagnosed by ultrasonography. Absence of filling four hours after dye injection may indicate acute cholecystitis. It is especially useful for diagnosis of acalculus cholecystitis.

Radioisotope-labelled red or white blood cell scans can be performed for delineating sites of bleeding and focus of inflammation, respectively.

Angiography can be used to diagnose suspected mesenteric arterial occlusion and acute gastrointestinal bleeding (if the rate of bleeding is greater than 1 ml per second). For gastrointestinal bleeding, therapeutic procedures such a embolisation can be performed at the same time.

Other investigations:

Electrocardiograph (ECG)

Besides excluding a differential diagnosis of an inferior myocardial infarction, the ECG will serve as a preoperative assessment as well.

Urinalysis

A sample of urine should be obtained for bacterial culture, to exclude a urinary tract infection, and to look for the presence of haematuria that would suggest a urinary aetiology.

Common Causes of Acute Abdomen

Upper abdomen

Perforated peptic ulcer, acute cholecystitis, acute pancreatitis.

Lower and mid-abdomen

Acute appendicitis, acute diverticulitis, intestinal obstruction, mesenteric ischaemia, ruptured abdominal aortic aneurysm.

Other causes

(1) Gynaecological — Pelvic inflammatory disease, ectopic pregnancy, ruptured or twisted ovarian cyst; (2) urological — Nephrolithiasis, pyelonephritis; and (3) acute medical conditions — Inferior myocardial infarction, lobar pneumonia, diabetic ketoacidosis.

Treatment of acute surgical abdomen

(1) *Supportive*

- Nil by mouth.
- Adequate rehydration with balanced salt solutions while monitoring the urine output.
- Cross-match blood and blood transfusion if necessary.
- Insertion of nasogastric tube (for both diagnostic as well as therapeutic measures, to decompress the stomach and for conservative management).
- Intravenous antibiotics, after obtaining a sample of blood for appropriate bacterial culture and test for sensitivity to antimicrobial agents.

(2) *Symptomatic*

- Analgesia after having obtained the diagnosis.

(3) *Specific*

- Therapy directed at underlying disease process.

Acute Appendicitis

Variation in the anatomical position of the appendix may result in atypical signs and symptoms. Diagnosis can be difficult in the very young, the elderly or the pregnant woman. There is frequently a history of indigestion or abdominal discomfort a few hours or a day before the onset of the pain. The classical presentation is that of peri-umbilical pain that migrates to the right iliac fossa over a 24–48 hour period. It may be associated with a fever, nausea and vomiting, diarrhoea or constipation and some patients may even have urinary symptoms or testicular pain. Anorexia is common and a ravenous patient is unlikely to have acute appendicitis. Right iliac fossa tenderness and focal peritoneal signs are usual, with or without psoas, obturator or Rovsing's signs and rectal tenderness or mass. Perforation of the appendix may result in diffuse peritonitis.

Formation of an appendiceal mass may occur with later presentation and can be managed conservatively. Acute appendicitis is usually associated with leukocytosis, and the definitive treatment is an appendicectomy. The diagnosis may be more difficult in females, and it is important to consider gynaecological causes of lower abdominal pain.

Perforated Peptic Ulcer

There may be history of peptic ulcer disease, or of steroid, NSAID or traditional Chinese medication ingestion, and the patient presents with a dramatic and sudden onset of epigastric pain. It is one of the most easily diagnosed acute abdominal conditions, provided that the symptoms are known and appreciated. Prompt surgical intervention is essential. Peri-operative mortality in patients with a perforated peptic ulcer is related to preoperative hypovolaemic shock, severe concurrent medical disease or a delay in treatment exceeding 24 hours after the perforation. In this centre, it was found that the presence of one of these risk factors resulted in a mortality of 10%; if two were present, the mortality was 46%, and the presence of all three brought about a mortality[1] of 100%. Mortality is higher in the elderly and those with significant co-morbidities. It should be borne in mind that "silent" perforations may occur in patients who have sustained a head or burn injury, in comatose or moribund patients or in those on steroid therapy. Diffuse abdominal tenderness, guarding and peritoneal signs are detected on physical examination, and white cell count and serum amylase concentration may be elevated. Free gas in seen on erect plain films although it may be absent in up to 20% of patients. Other causes of free gas under the diaphragm include ruptured large intestine, usually from an obstructing carcinoma (at the tumour site, due to stercoral ulceration just proximal to the tumour or at the caecum), perforated appendix or ruptured intra-abdominal abscess (due to gas-forming organisms).

An exploratory laparotomy should be performed as soon as possible once the diagnosis of a perforated peptic ulcer or viscus is made (refer to Chapter 17).

Acute Cholecystitis

An antecedent history of biliary colic may be present (steady non-paroxysmal pain, frequently in the epigastrium) that gradually subsides within four to six hours. It returns after an interval, to the right hypochondrium, and is characterised by a constant ache that is secondary to that of peritoneal irritation of an inflamed organ. It may be associated with nausea and vomiting. Fever is usually present, while jaundice is not always a constant feature. Examination reveals right hypochondrial tenderness with a positive Murphy's sign. Occasionally, a distended gallbladder may be palpated. Leukocytosis is seen, and may be accompanied by a derangement of the liver function test.

Ultrasonographic findings of a thickened gallbladder wall, pericholecystic fluid, sonographic Murphy's sign with or without gallstones, are consistent with the diagnosis of acute cholecystitis. A trial of conservative management with institution of intravenous antibiotics may be attempted for 24 hours with the aim of performing an interval laparoscopic cholecystectomy. However, failure to resolve, or a worsening of signs and symptoms, would warrant an immediate surgical exploration. Common bile duct stones causing obstruction, with evidence of ascending cholangitis, should be removed either via ERCP or by surgery, especially if ERCP is unsuccessful (refer to Chapter 19).

Acute Pancreatitis

Alcohol consumption and an ageing population with a high incidence of gallstones are major contributing factors to this condition. The remaining 10% of aetiological factors of acute pancreatitis can be attributed to trauma, hyperlipidaemia, hyperparathyroidism and drugs such as thiazide diuretics.

Acute pancreatitis typically presents with excruciating epigastric pain that radiates to the back. The proximity of the celiac plexus accounts for the severity of the pain. Occasionally, the pain is felt in the left scapular region or the left supraspinous fossa. Hypovolaemia manifesting as tachycardia, and shock or impending shock, usually accompany the pain. A fever may also be present.

Examination often reveals an acutely ill patient with cold extremities, sweating skin and a weak pulse depending on the severity of the shock. A patient who appears to be relatively well may deteriorate rapidly with the onset of systemic inflammatory response syndrome (SIRS). Epigastric tenderness is a common finding, and may or may not be accompanied by guarding. Grey Turner's sign of discolouration around one or both loins, and Cullen's sign of discolouration around the umbilicus, are not a constant feature and if present signify a rather severe form of the disease. Severity of the attack is determined by various prognostic indicators (Ranson's criteria).

Raised serum amylase and lipase concentrations and/or abnormal liver function test while consistent with the diagnosis, is not an absolute requirement. Ultrasonography for confirmation of diagnosis can be conducted, noting also the presence of gallstones and their location. Computed tomography with intravenous contrast is indicated if the condition is severe or deteriorating, to determine the presence of pancreatic necrosis or fluid collection (refer to Chapter 19).

Small Bowel Obstruction

This most commonly is secondary to adhesions from previous abdominal surgery. Other causes include hernias, carcinoma, intussusception, and volvulus. Bezoars causing intestinal obstruction should also be considered, especially in patients who have had previous gastric surgery or a vagotomy and pyloroplasty (unpublished institution data). Patients with intestinal obstruction normally present with sharp, crampy, peri-umbilical pain with intervening pain-free periods, associated with nausea and vomiting. The patient may be restless in between the paroxysms of pain.

Examination may reveal a distended abdomen with peristalsis occasionally seen through the abdominal wall, or borborygmi heard on ascultation.

A plain abdominal film may reveal dilated loops of small bowel, air-fluid levels and paucity of colonic gas. When severe pain assumed to be due to intestinal colic persists for more than three to four hours, the condition generally requires surgical intervention.

Large Bowel Obstruction

This is relatively common but usually less prostrating than that resulting from small bowel colic. The pain is usually referred to the hypogastrium, and may be due to a stricture from carcinoma, diverticulae, impacted faeces or volvulus. The presenting symptoms include constipation, abdominal distension, and varying degrees of abdominal pain. If severe and prolonged enough, the patient may also complain of vomiting of initially gastric, then bilious, and eventually, faeculent material. In patients with competent ileocaecal valves, there is a closed loop obstruction, and in such situations, large bowel obstruction will need earlier surgical intervention.

Plain abdominal films may reveal colonic dilatation, a tense distended caecum, and a paucity of small bowel shadows. The risk of caecal perforation increases significantly when diameters of 12 cm and beyond are present (Fig. 7).

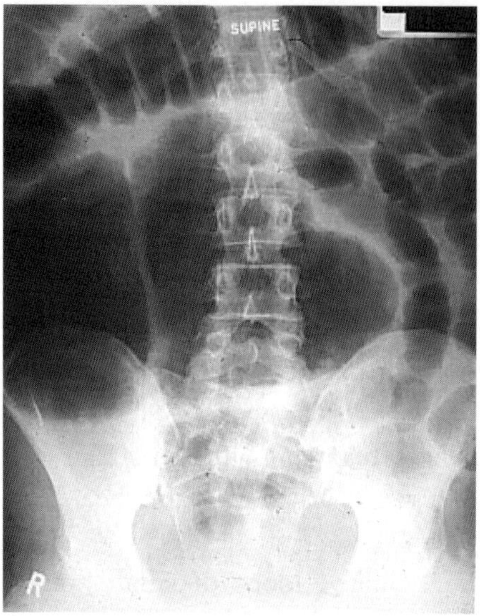

Fig. 7 Dilated caecum with impending perforation.

Conservative management may be attempted, resting the bowel and decompressing the gastrointestinal system whilst correcting the fluid and electrolyte imbalances. A colonoscopy or sigmoidoscopy should be attempted after a digital rectal examination. Impending caecal perforation, deterioration of the patient's condition, or failure to resolve within 12–24 hours necessitates an exploratory laparotomy (refer to Chapter 16).

Mesenteric Ischaemia

Superior mesenteric artery thrombosis or occlusion secondary to atherosclerosis or embolism may give rise to this condition. It may also occur in the hypotensive patient who had been receiving high doses of inotropic agents to maintain cardiac output and blood pressure. There is a sudden onset of severe, constant pain that can be associated with vomiting and diarrhoea. Pain out of proportion to physical findings is the usual comment on examination of patients with mesenteric ischaemia. Leukocytosis and acidosis are consistent. Presented with such symptoms and signs, the index of suspicion has to be high. Confirmation of the diagnosis may be obtained on angiography and sometimes, CT.

Ruptured Abdominal Aortic Aneurysm

There is usually a history of atherosclerotic disease with its associated risk factors of hypertension, diabetes, smoking, positive family history and hyperlipidaemia. Sudden onset of abdominal pain with radiation to the flank or back is the common complaint, and the patient will rarely survive if free intra-abdominal rupture occurs. Abdominal examination may reveal a tender, pulsatile mass in the abdomen and may be associated with unequal pulses in the limbs. Computed tomography is the gold standard, but it can only be performed in haemodynamically stable patients. Immediate surgery is the treatment for a persistently hypotensive patient with a known aneurysm (refer to Chapter 12).

Conclusion

The abovementioned list is by no means exhaustive, but represents the more common causes of an acute abdomen seen at the hospital. In the management of any patient who presents with acute abdominal pain, resuscitation is a priority. A patent airway, adequate ventilation, and stable haemodyamic status are the foremost aims. The next step endeavours to obtain an early diagnosis by taking a complete history and performing a thorough physical examination.

It is prudent to bear in mind that at the extremes of life, more precautions have to be taken. The elderly may present to the hospital late, or give an incomplete or inaccurate history. They are often without the classical physical signs, and have multiple co-morbidities resulting in less reserve should there be a delay in diagnosis. On the other hand, children may present earlier but may not have developed the typical manifestations expected of a diagnosis.

An exploratory laparotomy is mandatory in any patient in whom a surgically correctable cause of acute abdomen is suspected. Early intervention is advocated when the following situations are diagnosed.

(1) Diffuse peritonitis, such as resulting from a perforated viscus.
(2) Ischaemic or gangrenous bowel.
(3) Acute high-grade intestinal obstruction.

In the event that a diagnosis is uncertain, review of the patient at regular intervals to allow for the diagnosis to unfold, and to ensure that deterioration has not occurred, is essential.

In all cases of acute abdomen, or in patients with abdominal pain severe enough to warrant admission, early surgical assessment is essential, and ideally, longitudinal monitoring of symptoms and signs should be conducted by the surgical team in the ward.

References

1. Chan WH, Wong WK, Khin LW, Soo KC (2000). Adverse operative risk factors for perforated peptic ulcer. *Ann Acad Med Singapore* **29**(2), 164–167.
2. Irvin TT (1989). Abdominal pain: a surgical audit of 1190 emergency admissions. *BJS* **76**(11), 1121–1125.
3. de Dombal FT (1988). Acute abdominal pain survey by the research committee of World Organization of Gastroenterology. *Scand J Gastroenterol* **144 (Supp.)**, 35–42.

Further Reading

1. Silen W (1991). *Cope's Early Diagnosis of the Acute Abdomen*, 18th Ed. New York: Oxford University Press.
2. Spirt, MJ (1998). *Acute Care of the Abdomen*, 1st Ed. Baltimore, MD: Williams and Wilkins.
3. Doherty GM *et al.* (1997). *The Washington Manual of Surgery*. Department of Surgery, Washington University School of Medicine, St. Louis Missouri. Boston: Little Brown.

4. De Dombal FT (1980). *Diagnosis of Acute Abdominal Pain*, 1st Ed. Edinburgh: Churchill Livingstone.
5. Kriestin GP, Choyke PL, Becker C *et al.* (1996). *Acute Abdomen: Diagnostic Imaging in the Clinical Context*, 1st Ed. Stuttgart: Georg Thieme-Verlag, Thieme Medical Publishers.
6. Beyer D, Modder U, Benz G *et al.* (1988). *Diagnostic Imaging of the Acute Abdomen: A Clinico-radiologic Approach*, 1st Ed. Berlin: Springer-Verlag.
7. Taylor MB, Gillan JL, Steer ML, Wolfe MM (1996). *Gastrointestinal Emergencies*, 2nd Ed. Baltimore, MD: Williams and Wilkins.

16

Management of Intestinal Obstruction

Choong-Leong Tang
Francis Seow-Choen

Introduction

From the management viewpoint, intestinal obstruction may be grouped into either large intestinal or small intestinal in origin. The level of obstruction in the small intestines may be situated proximally in the jejunum, or distally in the ileum. Proximal obstruction is characterised by significant vomiting and fluid loss without much abdominal distension. Indeed, some patients may even continue to pass small amounts of stool. In contrast, aetiologies in the lower small intestines and large intestines are characterised by abdominal distension, colicky pain and absence of bowel opening. In colonic obstruction, there may be an antecedent history of change in bowel habits, with the preponderance of frequent loose stool from luminal narrowing, bleeding per rectum, or reduction in stool calibre. The common aetiologies of intestinal obstruction are shown in Table 1.

Table 1 Aetiology of Intestinal Obstruction

Small Intestine Obstruction	Colonic Obstruction
Within the lumen	*Within the lumen*
Gall-stone	Faecal impaction
Bozoar	Inssipated barium
Foreign body	Gall-stone
	Foreign body
Within the wall	*Within the wall*
Tumours especially carcinoma	Carcinoma
Lymphoma	Lymphoma
Polyps	Inflammation — Diverticulitis (stricture)
Crohn's disease	Crohn's disease
Tuberculosis	Tuberculosis
	Congenital — Adult Hirschsprung disease
	Ischaemic stricture
	Radiation stricture
	Anastomotic stricture
	Intussusception
Outside the wall	*Outside the wall*
Bands and adhesion	Bands and adhesions
External hernias	External hernias
Internal hernias	Internal hernias
Tumours of adjacent organs or lymph nodes	Tumours of adjacent organs or lymph nodes
Abscesses	Abscesses
Volvulus	Volvulus
Post-operative paralytic ileus	Pseudo-obstruction

Assessment of Intestinal Obstruction

A good clinical history is important, and often gives a clue to the cause of the obstruction. A previous history of a laparotomy makes postoperative adhesions a likely aetiology; a history of an intra-abdominal malignancy makes intra-peritoneal disseminated disease likely until proven otherwise. In the early post-operative period, prolonged return of bowel activity may be due to metabolic causes, early fibrinous adhesions or even occult subclinical intra-abdominal sepsis such as an abscess or an anastomotic dehiscence. An antecedent history of an abdominal trauma raises the possibility of a visceral rupture or traumatic pancreatitis leading to intestinal ileus. Similarly, a history of alcohol consumption or gallstone disease may lead to pancreatitis and subsequent ileus. Very often, an acute appendicitis presents as intestinal obstruction due to either localised suppuration leading to distal ileal ileus, or a pelvic abscess with obstruction due to intestinal "walling off".

Clinical examination is required to assess the degree of dehydration. Generally, third space loss as well as loss from reduced intake or through vomiting may easily amount to several litres. Postural hypotension is often the first and only sign. In addition, the examination should be focused on the abdomen for ingunial and femoral hernias, and surgical scars when an obstructing incisional hernia is suspected. Tenderness, localised or diffused, must be established. Often when localised, it usually signifies a tense loop of intestine with impending perforation. This may be in the area under an abdominal scar or over the right iliac fossa where a severely distended caecum with mural ischaemia may have occurred. Acute appendicitis may also present with localised tenderness in the right iliac fossa. Surgery should be arranged without delay. Likewise, generalised peritonitis mandates surgery. Per rectal examination often yields valuable information. An obstructing tumour may be felt. The rectum may be loaded with impacted stool and "obstruction" may be due to faecal loading, which is not uncommon in the elderly bed-ridden. Pelvic tenderness and "bogginess" on per rectal examination may alert the examiner of a pelvic abscess.

Investigations

A plain supine abdominal radiograph may give a clue to the diagnosis and aetiology. A clear cut-off may be visible in the distal colon. A distended, isolated loop of small intestine may signify either a closed-loop obstruction or localised ileus such as in mild pancreatitis (sentinel loop). The absence or paucity of "bowel shadows" does not exclude intestinal obstruction, as the intestine may be filled with fluid with no air in it to act as a contrast. Sometimes, the "string of beads" sign may be visible, signifying prolonged obstruction with re-absorption of the luminal air leaving small amounts trapped in between the plicae circulares.

A computed tomography (CT) with oral, intravenous and enema contrast is more sensitive than a plain radiograph in diagnosing the obstruction, and may also shed light on the aetiology as well. However, the scan is only good if the lesion causing the luminal obstruction is large (greater than 1 cm in extent) and is certainly inefficient in diagnosing a band or a kink if that was the cause of the obstruction. Very often, interpretation of a CT may be difficult, as a mural lesion is sometimes indistinguishable from luminal contents. In contrast, free perforations are easily detected. Findings of pancreatitis, intra-abdominal abscesses, inflammatory changes and mass lesions are often possible on the scan. Patients must be properly resuscitated with crystalloids before any intravenous contrast is given in order to minimise the risk of acute renal failure.

A phosphate enema given on admission is helpful in stimulating bowel movement to overcome critical narrowing in the intestines, clear impacted stool and prepare the lower large intestines for a diagnostic endoscopy. This may be followed by a colonic washout with either olive oil or enema saponis. Enemas should be avoided if abdominal sepsis is suspect. The presence of fever or an elevated total white cell count with predominant polymorphs usually suggests an infective aetiology or the presence of infective complications. A gentle diagnostic colonoscopy is the most informative investigation. Through a colonoscopy, colonic pathology, which is by far the more common in accounting for intestinal obstruction, may be established. If formed stools are seen during the examination despite an adequate washout, then there is no proximal organic large bowel obstruction. However, proximal colonic screening is still essential. If the colon is normal up to the caecum, the obstruction then lies in the small intestines. A complete examination of the colon is useful in planning of surgery, as lesser colonic lesions are more easily diagnosed intra-luminally than at laparotomy.

It is important to measure the serum amylase concentration in order to rule out pancreatitis. This condition is better treated supportively than by laparotomy. Other tests include those in preparation for laparotomy, such as the full blood count, the serum urea and electrolytes concentrations, chest X-ray, electrocardiography, group and cross-matching of blood, arterial blood gases (for those above 70 years old) and serum carcinoembryonic antigen concentration.

Initial Management

Adequate fluid resuscitation is important. A litre of saline may easily be infused over the initial one to two hours. Subsequent infusion should be based on urine output, and normal saline (0.9%) solution is favoured over dextrose 5% solution, as serum sodium concentration is almost always low in the patient with intestinal obstruction. In patients where fluid replacement is difficult and critical to assess, a central venous catheter should be inserted once sufficient fluid has been infused to increase the venous filling pressure for the procedure. The serum sodium concentration should not be aggressively treated with hypertonic saline (either 3% or 30%) solution, as hyponatraemia is usually due to loss from vomiting or reduced intake and should be corrected with normal saline. Serum potassium replacement is not essential initially until normal urine output is observed. As tissue acidosis corrects, a persistently low serum potassium concentration will require correction. Measured acidosis in the arterial blood gas often corrects with hydration. Only very rarely is correction of serum bicarbonate concentration required in severe acidosis, and this should alert the surgeon of possible bowel ischaemia secondary to distension. Early intervention is required. Similarly, intra-abdominal sepsis should be suspected in the presence of persistent hypotension despite adequate fluid resuscitation. In the elderly patients, central venous pressure monitoring during resuscitation is extremely useful and should be initiated early. Furthermore, the central venous catheter may be used post-operatively for nutritional supplementation if paralytic ileus is prolonged.

An enema is helpful in stimulating bowel movement, and may be effective in relieving a subacute obstruction; or an obstruction arising from the use of paralytic drugs such as hyosine, which is frequently administered for the treatment of abdominal colicky pain. Placement of a nasogastric tube helps to decompress the stomach and upper small intestines, and thus reduces the risk of pulmonary aspiration. However, it does not contribute much to decompression of the colon, even in the presence of an incompetent ileo-caecal valve. Bowel preparation by oral lavage should be avoided in suspected intestinal obstruction.

Indications for Surgery

The indications for surgery are as follows:

- Unresolving small intestinal obstruction after 48 hours of treatment with intravenous fluid and naso-gastric decompression. This is particularly in the case of a post-operative abdomen. The lack of progress may present with a persistently high volume of nasogastric aspirate, progressive abdominal distension (may be measured by increase in abdominal girth) and the absence of bowel movement. The threshold for surgery in small intestinal obstruction in an abdomen without previous surgery is lower. Prior colonoscopy before surgery is preferred.
- Clinical evidence of obstructing external hernia such as an obstructed inguinal hernia, incisional hernia or a femoral hernia.
- Obvious or suspected intra-peritoneal sepsis or abscesses that cannot be drained percutaneously.
- Progressive localised tenderness. The common area of localised tenderness is in the right iliac fossa over the caecum.

- Colon or rectal mass lesions or strictures diagnosed at endoscopy.
- Mass lesions seen on CT of the abdomen and pelvis.
- Recurrent colonic volvulus with or without megacolon.

Surgery should be avoided in pseudo-obstruction. Hypothyroidism must be excluded.

Surgical Treatment and Options

Small intestines

This should be treated according to the pathology. Adhesion bands should be lysed if this is the cause of the obstruction. Small intestinal tumours must be resected together with wide margins and lympho-vascular clearance. Strictures in the small intestines are a common cause of bowel obstruction. This may commonly be due to Crohn's disease or tuberculosis, where this disease is endemic. Isolated ileo-colic Crohn's disease may be resected, and many of these patients would remain symptom- and disease-free after that. Multiple strictures in Crohn's disease may be better treated by stricturoplasty. This can be done either by cutting the stricture lengthwise and closing the opening breadth-wise for short segment strictures, or by creating a side-to-side anastomotic opening in the proximal and distal ends of the narrowing for longer segment strictures. Resection of one of the strictures is important for initial histopathological diagnosis. Tuberculous strictures may also be similarly treated. Extensive resection is not necessary in these conditions, as the mainstay is medical. The margins of any resection may remain positive and will not significantly affect healing. It is common for lymphoma, either arising murally or from the mesenteric lymph nodes, to cause intestinal obstruction. Adequate tissue must be taken for diagnosis or typing. The disease responds well to chemotherapy.

Resection and primary anastomosis is generally easy to perform in the small intestines. In conditions affecting multiple sites in the small intestines, such as Crohn's disease or tuberculous strictures, a policy of maximal conservation must be adopted to reduce risks of short-gut syndrome.

Colon and rectum

This may be subdivided into right-sided lesion, left-sided lesion or low rectal lesion.

(1) Right-sided lesion

This may range from a large caecal lesion (which rarely obstructs); an ileo-caecal valve lesion; an ascending colon lesion; a lesion in the hepatic flexure or the proximal transverse colon. Resection and primary anastomosis is safe, and may be done after decompression of the proximal bowel. A stapled anastomosis (functional end-to-end anastomosis using a linear cutter stapler) avoids the size discrepancy problem of a handsewn end-to-end anastomosis. The cut ends of the bowel should be cleaned with a tumouricidal agent such as plain chlorhexidine prior to creation of the anastomosis. This is to reduce the risk of tumour implantation and local recurrence. Closure of the mesenteric window after anastomosis is not mandatory, although this may minimise loops of intestines sliding underneath leading to obstruction. In some centres, the use of the "no-touch" technique in resection is preferred, although no significant survival advantage in terms of local and distant recurrence has been demonstrated. In the small group of patients with an angio-invasive component in the tumour, such a technique has been shown on subset analyses to be potentially useful in reducing recurrence. This technique essentially involves (1) luminal isolation using proximal and distal ties around the colon; (2) lympho-vascular isolation and division at their origins before mobilisation of the tumour (achieved by opening the medial leaf of the root of the mesentery to expose the origin of the right colic from the ileocolic vessel); and (3) wide resection of the tumour with adequate margins.

Assessment of resectability is an important skill in the management of locally advanced right-sided tumour, especially those affecting the hepatic flexural area. Gentle rocking of the tumour mass may give a fair idea of the extent of attachment to deeper structures (such as the pancreas, aorta or vertebral column). Attachment to such structures may preclude resection or even if it is possible, resection of the tumour is associated with high morbidity or mortality. Opening the medial leaf of the small intestinal mesentery will provide a good view and assessment of possible involvement of the superior mesenteric vessels. If these are not involved, structures lateral to these vessels may usually be safely resected. Assessment of invasion to the head of the pancreas and duodenum may be done by doing the Kocher's manoeuvre, palpation from the top through the lesser sac of the stomach, and by mobilisation of the small bowel mesentery all the way to the duodeno-jejunal (D-J) junction. Tumour, with invasion through the duodenum, may be resected together with a duodenal cuff, and primary anastomosis of the duodenum performed, while care is taken not to injure the opening of the common bile duct. Finally, a gastroduodenoscopy may give definite evidence of invasion.

A "trial of mobilisation" must be avoided, as cutting into tumour planes will only disseminate the disease and may very well speed up recurrence. A by-pass should be done followed by neo-adjuvant chemo-irradiation with a view to subsequent laparotomy and resection, after the tumour shrinks.

(2) Left-sided lesion

This usually includes lesions located anywhere from the distal transverse colon to the rectum. The colon proximal to the site of obstruction contains considerable faecal matter and may be severely distended, leading to an increase in the mural tension, and reduction of the venous flow. Venous congestive ischaemia may result. In the more severe instances, there is reduction of the arterial flow leading to patchy transmural ischaemia and perforation. In the initial laparotomy, careful assessment of the viability of the caecum and the transverse colon is important in the planning of surgical options. Very often, the initial assessment of the caecum may show congestion and venous stasis with a bluish tint, leading the operator to diagnose non-viability. However, following decompression of the colon, it may resume the normal appearance, saving the need for more extensive resection. An obviously "black" or ischaemic caecum mandates resection. A perforation which may be pin-point in nature is better treated by resection than by merely excising the ischaemic edges with primary closure. The transverse colon may have mucosal ischaemia proximal to the point of obstruction, but may not be evident from the serosa. Thus, it is mandatory for inspection of the mucosa of the proximal end of the transected colon for congested and thickened, ischaemic or even ulcerated mucosa prior to anastomosis.

Colonic decompression

After the initial assessment, the next maneouvre is to try and decompress the colon. This would facilitate subsequent resection. This is not necessary if the distension is not severe, and is localised mainly in the proximal colon or small intestines. Decompression may be achieved through several means. A large-bore light-weight tubing, such as a tubing taken from the "circle" anaesthetic breathing system, may be used for this purpose. The sigmoid colon or the descending colon proximal to the point of obstruction is first mobilised sufficiently to allow attachment of one end of the tubing. The other (distal) end of the tubing is placed into a disposable bag on the floor with the opening of the bag tied around the tube. The proximal end of the tube is placed into a decompressed and isolated segment of colon in-between clamps and secured. The grooves on the tubing allow for securing, either with nylon tape or several strong silk ties to prevent slippage. Once secured, the clamps may be released, and the faecal contents may be expediently milked out via the tubing into the bag. Towel packs are used to isolate this part of the colon from the rest of the peritoneum in case of spillage.

Alternative methods of decompression include dividing the colon and milking the contents into a dish. This is a particularly useful approach if the faecal matter is semi-solid or firm, making passage through a tubing difficult. Care must be taken to avoid spillage. Small intestinal content may also be milked via the colon into the anaesthetic tubing. Another alternative is to use a sheathed suction tip placed through an enterotomy in the distal ileum, and decompressing the colon via the caecum and the small intestines in turn. This has the disadvantage of frequent suction channel blockage due to the more solid contents of the colon. If the colonic distension is largely gaseous, quick and convenient decompression may be achieved by placing a large-bore needle (14 gauge) into the transverse colon with the hub connected to the suction tubing. The pinpoint perforation from the needle should be closed with a stitch and included in the resected colon if possible. The different methods may be used in combination. For example, initial decompression of the colonic gas with a large-bore needle may facilitate mobilisation of the colon for further decompression through an anaesthetic tubing.

In the presence of proximal colonic non-viability:

(i) Performance of a subtotal or total colectomy with a ileo-sigmoid anastomosis or an ileo-rectal anastomosis.[1] This procedure involves mobilisation of the entire colon up to the rectosigmoid region, or even lower if the rectum is involved. The total operative time is often not more than required in segmental resections with decompression or irrigation. Indeed, the advantage lies in dispensing with the need for decompression or irrigation.[2] Although post-operative function is manageable, the patient will inevitably have frequent bowel movements that may need long-term or life-long anti-diarrhoeal agents. The added advantage is the removal of synchronous cancers or polyps not detectable at the time of surgery, and also reduction in the future risks of metachronous colorectal cancer by reducing the length of the at risk colon.

(ii) Performance of a localised limited ileo-colic resection and a left-sided segmental resection as per tumour location. This is aimed at conserving colonic length, which will translate into improved function post-operatively. The criticism of this approach is the presence of two colonic anastomoses, each with its own attendant risks of dehiscence. This is obviously not suitable in the presence of transverse colonic ischaemia.

In the absence of proximal colonic non-viability:

(i) Colonic decompression and primary anastomosis. This is a one-stage process and does not require on-table colonic irrigation. Colonic irrigation is more time consuming than decompression alone and may result in possible changes in body temperature, and fluid and electrolytes shifts.[3] The Scottish trials have shown that colorectal anastomosis may be safely performed without an increase in risks of anastamotic dehiscence even if the bowel was not prepared in elective surgery. Case-controlled trials in an emergency setting have shown similar results.

(ii) Colonic decompression and on-table colonic irrigation with primary anastomosis.[4] This procedure involves performing either an appendicostomy or an ileal enterotomy, followed by insertion of a large-bore 21 French Foley catheter into the caecum for irrigation with warm saline. Usually, at least four to six litres of irrigant are required before the effluent is relatively clear. Mobilisation of the hepatic and splenic flexures are not always necessary prior to the washout. Naturally, the procedure would be easier if these were mobilised.

(iii) Colonic decompression with on-table irrigation and a defunctioning loop ileostomy or colostomy. The creation of the temporary stoma will reduce the impact of faecal peritonitis should a leak occur. The use of a colostomy located nearer to the site of the anastomosis would translate into a shorter length of distal bowel that needs to be irrigated. Irrigation may be done either before creation of the anastomosis, or after, with the help of a proctoscope inserted anally.

(iv) Subtotal or total colectomy with an ileo-rectal anastomosis.[1] This has been discussed in the foregoing section.

(v) Resection and colostomy (for example, the Hartmann's Procedure). This is perhaps the quickest way of performing the surgery and removing the tumour.[5] The distal rectal stump is closed off while the proximal end is brought out into a stoma. This procedure is a good option in the very ill patients, or if the surgeon is technically not confident for other procedures. While theoretically possible, re-anastomosis at a later date is often not easily achievable because of the medical status of the patient, and even if attempted, may fail, due to dense adhesions.

(vi) Defunctioning colostomy only, and staged procedures. This is simple and quick and allows for decompression of the obstruction. The duration of anaesthetic risk is kept short, and risk from extensive surgical resection is avoided. After decompression of the colon, more time is available for optimisation of the medical status of the patient before embarking upon subsequent definitive resections. The second stage involves resection of the tumour with resection of the colostomy or ileostomy (two-staged) or with the later closure of the stoma after healing of the anastomosis (three-staged). The Large Bowel Cancer Project has shown that these two- or three-staged procedures do not improve overall morbidity or mortality rates compared to a single procedure, and this is at the expense of a longer hospital stay and increased healthcare costs.[6] The rate of bowel leakage after a primary anastomosis in an acutely obstructed patient is however reduced (18% versus 6% in the Large Bowel Cancer Project).[7]

In the presence of free colonic perforation with faecal peritonitis, most surgeons would avoid performing an anastomosis. Even if one is done, there is usually a defunctioning colostomy as the risk of an anastomotic dehiscence is greater in these instances. Alternatively, a Hartmann's procedure may be undertaken. Mortality is usually greater than 50% following gross faecal peritonitis.

(3) Low rectal lesions

These are lesions situated below the peritoneal reflection, and consequently, anastomoses created here after resections are at increased risk of dehiscence. Defunctioning is often favoured in such lesions, and distal limb irrigation is necessary. In locally advanced rectal lesions where resection is deemed unsuitable, a defunctioning sigmoid loop colostomy followed by neo-adjuvant chemo-irradiation with the view to subsequent resection is preferred.

Colonic Stenting

In recent years, development of an intra-colonic self-expanding stent has made it possible to decompress the colon if placement across the stricture is possible.[8] This may be done under colonoscopic guidance and/or fluoroscopic guidance. A guide wire is firstly manipulated across the tumour. If fluoroscopy is used, instillation of a small volume of water-soluble enema will show the tract better. The closed self-expanding stent is then deployed across the stricture and slowly opened up. It provides immediate relieve of the obstruction if successfully deployed, and delays the need for urgent surgery, thereby allowing time for optimisation. In patients with advanced metastatic disease, the stent is sufficient palliation for the obstruction, but not for bleeding. Deployment of the stent is most successful if the lesion is located in the left colon, and not across a bend such as the rectosigmoid junction or the splenic flexure. Low rectal lesions are not suitable for stenting, as the distal end of the stent is likely to protrude out of the anal canal causing severe discomfort.

Post-operative Management

Fluid and electrolyte replacement should be continued, and a central venous catheter placed intra-operatively will assist tremendously in the management. The central venous catheter may also be used for supplemental parental nutrition if ileus persists beyond the fifth post-operative day. Due consideration should be given to post-operative ventilatory support if the abdominal distension and diaphragmatic splinting is significant. The patient with severe septicaemia will most likely require ventilatory support as well as inotropic support. There are no trials to support the continued use of post-operative antibiotics, although pre-operative antibiotics have been shown in numerous trials to reduce the incidence of wound infection, but not anastomotic leaks. Certainly, if there was intra-operative peritoneal soilage, it is only prudent to continue treatment. Prophylaxis against deep vein thrombosis prophylaxis should be started, and this may take the form of low molecular weight heparin[9] or the use of sequential mechanical compression, as patients with cancer and pelvic surgery are at moderate risk of deep venous thrombosis.

Anastomotic dehiscence may occur anytime from the second post-operative day onwards for up to two weeks. While easily detected if there are catastrophic signs with peritonitis, prolonged ileus or persistent diarrhoea should lead the surgeon to suspect a leak in patients with lesser symptoms. If a drain was left in the pelvis, it will show faeculant content by this time and may effectively control the sepsis without the need for another laparotomy. Serial erect chest radiographs in the postoperative period are useful in the defection of anastomotic dehiscence. The increase in free gas under the diaphragm, or the re-emergence of free gas, would signify a possible leak.[10] Persistence of free gas under the diaphragm is, however, not always correlated with an anastomotic dehiscence.

References

1. Nyam DC, Leong AF, Ho YH, Seow-Choen F (1996). Comparison between segmental left and extended right colectomies for obstructing left-sided colonic carcinomas. *Dis Colon Rectum* **39**(9), 1000–1003.
2. Eu KW, Lim SL, Seow-Choen F, Leong AF, Ho YH (1998). Clinical outcome and bowel function following total abdominal

colectomy and ileorectal anastomosis in the Oriental population. *Dis Colon Rectum* **41**(2), 215–218.

3. Nyam DC, Seow-Choen F, Leong AF, Ho YH (1996). Colonic decompression without on-table irrigation for obstructing left-sided colorectal tumours. *Br J Surg* **83**(6), 786–787. (Erratum in: *Br J Surg* **83**(8), 1159.)
4. Seow-Choen F, Eu KW (1993). Intraoperative irrigation for acute distal colonic obstruction caused by carcinoma. *Br J Surg* **80**(4), 516.
5. Heah SM, Eu KW, Ho YH, Leong AF, Seow-Choen F (1997). Hartmann's procedure versus abdominoperineal resection for palliation of advanced low rectal cancer. *Dis Colon Rectum* **40**(11), 1313–1317.
6. Fielding LP, Phillips RK, Hittinger R (1989). Factors influencing mortality after curative resection for large bowel cancer in elderly patients. *Lancet* **1**(8638), 595–597.
7. Phillips RK, Hittinger R, Fry JS, Fielding LP (1985). Malignant large bowel obstruction. *Br J Surg* **72**(4), 296–302.
8. Morino M, Bertello A, Garbarini A, Rozzio G, Repici A (2002). Malignant colonic obstruction managed by endoscopic stent decompression followed by laparoscopic resections. *Surg Endosc* **16**(10), 1483–1487.
9. Ho YH, Seow-Choen F, Leong A, Eu KW, Nyam D, Teoh MK (1999). Randomized, controlled trial of low molecular weight heparin versus no deep vein thrombosis prophylaxis for major colon and rectal surgery in Asian patients. *Dis Colon Rectum* **42**(2), 196–202. (Discussion, pp. 202–203.)
10. Tang CL, Yeong KY, Nyam DC, Eu KW, Ho YH, Leong AF, Tsang CB, Seow-Choen F (2000). Postoperative intra-abdominal free gas after open colorectal resection. *Dis Colon Rectum* **43**(8), 1116–1120.

17

Management of Upper Gastrointestinal Bleeding

Wai-Keong Wong

Introduction

Upper gastrointestinal (UGI) bleeding is one of the common admissions to surgical wards. It can be life threatening if not managed appropriately and expediently. The mortality rate ranges from 10% to over 50% depending on the cause of bleeding and associated risk factors. Peptic ulcer is the most common cause of upper GI bleed and it accounts for 50% to 60% of the cases. Mortality rate of over 10% for peptic ulcer was reported in the recent U.K. study, and the risk is highest in elderly patients over 60 years of age.[1] Mortality from peptic ulcer bleeding commonly results from the associated co-morbidity and complications following emergency surgery for bleeding ulcers.[1,2] The next common cause is variceal bleeding secondary to portal hypertension. The in-hospital mortality rate for the first bleed is in the region of 50%, and worst in the re-bleeding cases.[3] Early re-bleeding occurs in 30% to 50% of patients, usually within the first five days after initial bleeding. Other causes are gastric erosions, Dieulafoy lesions, Mallory-Weiss tear, stomach cancer and others.

Although hospitalisation rates for uncomplicated ulcers have dropped over the last two to three decades, the number of patients admitted for bleeding peptic ulcers has remained steady. The proportion of all bleeding patients with duodenal ulcer or gastric ulcer has also remained relatively unchanged.

The outcome of UGI bleed depends on prompt resuscitative measures, early endoscopic assessment and therapy, and timely surgical intervention when endoscopic therapy fails. Close monitoring of patients is essential in every step of management.

Risk Factors of Bleeding Ulcers

Non-steroidal anti-inflammatory drugs (NSAIDs)

The use of NSAIDs is probably the most important cause of bleeding in patients with peptic ulcer disease. The relative risk for the development of peptic ulcer disease among NSAID users was 4:1 compared with non-users, and the risk increased with higher doses of NSAID used.[4] NSAID causes gastric and duodenal mucosal damage by inhibiting the synthesis of prostaglandins. There are two distinct enzymes (cyclo-oxygenase) involved in the production of prostaglandins, COX 1 and COX 2. COX 1 is responsible for producing gastric prostaglandins required for normal mucosal defence, and COX 2 is produced in response to inflammatory stimuli. The use of aspirin is reported to be associated with an increased risk of upper gastrointestinal bleeding regardless of its dose used. Enteric-coated aspirin does not reduce the risk of UGI bleed. However concomitant use of low dose aspirin and NSAIDs puts patients at higher risk of UGI bleeding.[5,6]

Helicobacter pylori

There is a high association between *Helicobacter pylori* (*H. pylori*) infection and peptic ulcer disease. However, the association between *H. pylori* and peptic ulcer bleeding is less clear. The prevalence of

H. pylori in bleeding ulcers is lower than in uncomplicated ulcer disease. Several studies reported that eradication of *H. pylori* infection is associated with reduced recurrent bleeding.[7,8] Another controversial area is the relation between *H. pylori* and NSAID in the pathogenesis of peptic ulcer disease and ulcer bleeding. Whether their relationship is independent, synergistic or antagonistic remains controversial. Recent meta-analysis reported increased risk of ulcer bleeding in *H. pylori* infected patients and NSAID users, and the risk of ulcer bleeding increased six-fold when both factors were present.[9]

Corticosteroids

By itself, corticosteroid is not associated with increased risk of ulcer or bleeding. However, the concomitant use of both steroids and NSAID is associated with an almost ten-fold increase in the risk of upper gastrointestinal bleeding.[4,10]

Alcohol and smoking

A large population-based cohort study of over 26,000 subjects revealed a four-fold increase in the risk of ulcer bleeding with excessive drinking, and smoking of more than 15 cigarettes per day increased the risk of ulcer perforation more than three-fold.[11]

Clinical Presentation

Patients with UGI bleed present with melena or haematemesis or both. Some may present with symptoms of anaemia such as giddiness, especially with sudden postural change. In patients with profuse bleeding, they may present with haematochezia mimicking lower GI bleeding. In the extreme case, they may present in a state of shock.

In the case of variceal bleeding, it is important to obtain any history of alcohol drinking, hepatitis infection and other causes of liver cirrhosis.

Resuscitation

Immediate resuscitation is crucial in the management of patients who present with upper GI bleeding.

Clear airway

First a clear airway must be maintained, and patients intubated (if necessary) to prevent aspiration, especially in patients who are drowsy. This is particularly true in patients who have variceal bleeding, where bleeding can be profuse.

Assessment of haemodynamic status

Pulse rate, blood pressure and respiratory rates must be taken immediately and monitored at close intervals.

Fluid resuscitation

In patients who are haemodynamically stable, maintenance intravenous crystalloid infusion is given. If the patients are hypotensive, this should be corrected with rapid transfusion of plasma expander (Gelofundin®, Haemaccel®) for the first hour until blood is available. "Emergency" blood (O negative) should only be given when the patient is exsanguinating.[12]

There is no threshold haemoglobin level for initiating blood transfusion in acute blood loss. This must be taken based on clinical parameters, amount of blood loss and associated co-morbidity, particularly in patients with ischaemic heart disease. In general, the haemoglobin level for patients with coronary artery disease should be topped up to 10 g/L.

In patients who receive massive blood transfusion (defined as transfusion of more than 10 units of packed red blood cells in adults, or replacement of more than one blood volume in 24 hours), fresh frozen plasma (FFP) and platelets must be given, as stored blood is deficient in clotting factors and functional platelets. In general, two units of FFP are given for every 10 units of blood transfusion.[12]

Oxygen supplementation

With low haemoglobin level and hypovolaemic state, oxygen delivery to the tissues will be severely affected. Oxygen supplementation must be given to the patients either by nasal cannula or facemask. Oxygen saturation should be maintained above 97%.

Investigations

While the patient is being resuscitated and assessed, the following baseline investigations must be carried out:

- haemoglobin and haematocrit levels
- platelet count
- clotting profile (PT, PTT levels)
- urea and electrolytes, glucose
- CXR
- baseline ECG
- Group and Cross Match
- liver function test particularly in cirrhotic patients.

Monitoring

The following parameters should be monitored:

- hourly pulse rate, blood pressure, respiratory rate
- hourly urine output to assess the adequacy of resuscitation
- central venous pressure particularly in elderly patients with massive GI bleed (while it is essential to replace the blood, it is equally important to avoid overtransfusion to prevent cardiac failure and pulmonary oedema)

- pulse oximetry for arterial haemoglobin oxygen saturation
- serial haemoglobin and haematocrit levels to help guide the amount of blood transfusion.

In patients who are unstable, continuous monitoring of vital signs and ECG is advisable.

Bleeding Peptic Ulcer

Role of medical treatment (anti-secretory medication)

Even though histamine$_2$ (H_2) antagonists and proton pump inhibitors are commonly used in patients with acute UGI bleeding, there is lack of strong evidence in the literature to support their role in the control of a bleeding ulcer.[13,14] A recently published meta-analysis of the efficacy of intravenous H_2-receptor antagonists showed that there was no beneficial effect on bleeding duodenal ulcers, and only mildly beneficial effects in a bleeding gastric ulcer.[15] Another meta-analysis evaluated the role of both H_2-receptor antagonists and proton pump inhibitors in UGI bleeding.[16] The results showed a significant reduction in re-bleeding and surgery rates. There was no difference in mortality rates. The beneficial effect of acid suppression was attributed to modification of mucosal fibrinolytic activity, which is increased in the setting of UGIB, and decreased with acid suppression.[17]

In light of the above evidence, it is reasonable to initiate intravenous anti-secretory medications when patients with UGI bleeding are admitted. Proton pump inhibitors are preferred, and this should be started as soon as possible.

Endoscopy

Endoscopy is able to diagnose the cause of bleeding in more than 98% of the cases with acute UGI bleeding. However, one must be aware of the difficult sites which often result in failure to diagnose the source of bleeding.

These are high lesser curve, anastomotic line and the junction of the first and second part of duodenum.[18]

The role of endoscopy in the treatment of UGI bleeding is well established. Early endoscopy and therapy has been shown to reduce risk of re-bleeding, requirement for blood transfusion, hospital admission and the need for surgery.[19]

Indication for emergency endoscopy

Patients who are actively bleeding or are at high risk of re-bleeding should have emergency endoscopy done as soon as possible. The indications are:

- shock with blood pressure < 100 mmHg and pulse rate > 100 per minute
- fresh haematemesis or nasogastric suction of fresh blood
- fresh melena.

Apart from above indications, endoscopy can be carried out within 12 hours of admission. At endoscopy, in addition to identifying the cause of bleeding, it is important to note the presence or absence of evidence of stigmata of recent haemorrhage (ESRH), size of ulcer and location of ulcer, as these have prognostic significance with regard to the risk of re-bleeding. The ESRH determines whether the ulcer requires endoscopic treatment. The classification of ESRH was originally described by Forrest.[20] Table 1 summarises the prevalence and outcome of bleeding ulcers according to ESRH.[10]

Indications for endoscopic haemostasis

Ulcers at a high risk of re-bleeding should receive endoscopic therapy. These are ulcers with active bleeding, visible vessels and adherent clots.

Table 1 Prevalence and Outcome of ESRH in Bleeding Ulcers

Endoscopic Characteristics	Forrest's Classification	Prevalence % (Range)	Re-bleeding % (Range)	Mortality % (Range)
Clean base	III	42 (19–52)	5 (0–10)	2 (0–3)
Flat spot	IIC	20 (0–42)	10 (0–13)	3 (0–10)
Adherent clot	IIB	17 (0–49)	22 (14–36)	7 (0–10)
Visible vessel	IIA	17 (4–35)	43 (0–81)	11 (0–21)
Active bleeding	I	18 (4–26)	55 (17–100)	11 (0–23)

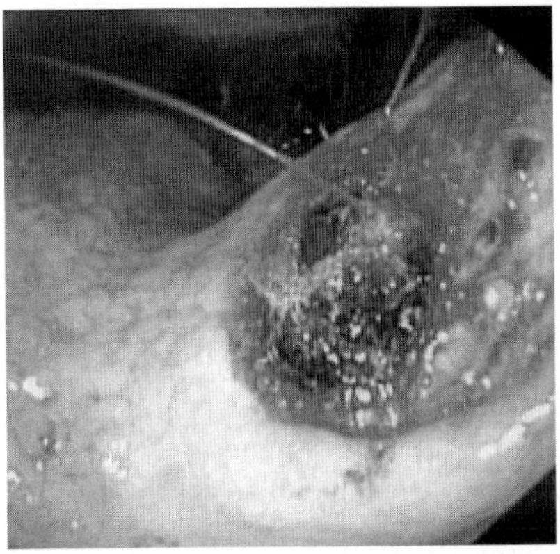

Fig. 1 Large gastric ulcer with active bleeding.

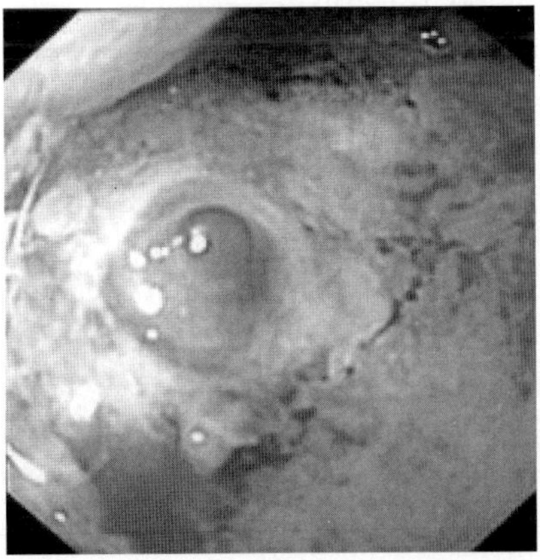

Fig. 2 Large duodenal ulcer with visible vessel.

Endoscopic haemostatic technique

Various endoscopic haemostatic techniques are used. This can be broadly classified under:

(1) Injectional — for example, adrenaline (1:10,000 dilution), sclerosant
(2) Thermal therapy — for example, bipolar coagulation, heater probe, laser
(3) Mechanical — for example, clips
(4) Combination therapy — for example, adrenaline injection and heater probe.

Injection with adrenaline is the most widely used, as it is cheap, easily available and effective. All other techniques are equally effective.

Risk of re-bleeding after initial endoscopic haemostasis ranges from 10% to 20%. One of the reasons for this is the resolution of clots overlying the ulcers. High dose omeperazole has been shown to achieve an intra-gastric pH level to above 6, which helps to facilitate platelet aggregation and prevent lysis of clots.[21] Several studies have shown that in high risk ulcers, endoscopic therapy followed by high dose omeperazole (80 mg bolus followed by 8 mg/hour infusion) for at least three days was associated with lower re-bleeding rates, less blood transfusion and less need for surgery.[22–24] On current available evidence, it is reasonable to initiate high dose proton pump inhibitors with a continous infusion regime for at least three days in patients with high risk ulcer after endoscopic therapy.

Prognostic risk factors for mortality

Despite the progress made in the endoscopic therapy, the risk of re-bleeding is still significantly high. Re-bleeding is an important risk factor for mortality. Therefore, all attempts must be made to prevent re-bleeding. Other adverse prognostic risk factors for mortality are concomitant medical illness, age over 60, blood transfusion of more than 5 units, and ulcer size > 1 cm.[25]

Indications for surgery

The success in therapeutic endoscopy has resulted in fewer patients requiring surgery.[19] Whilst it is true that most bleeding ulcers can be successfully treated by endoscopic treatment, it is important to identify those that are likely to benefit from early surgical intervention. Re-bleeding occurs in 10% to 20% of patients after endoscopic therapy. Traditionally, surgical intervention is indicated for recurrent bleeding. However, with improved endoscopic expertise, repeat endoscopic treatment for re-bleeding ulcers is practised in some centres. Its role, however, remains controversial. A recent prospective randomised study showed that repeat endoscopic treatment for re-bleeding reduced the need for surgery without increasing the risk of death, and was associated with fewer complications than surgery. Multivariate analyses of risk factors showed that hypotension at the time of re-bleeding, and ulcer size of 2 cm or more, were predictors of failure with endoscopic re-treatment.[26] However it must be stressed that such excellent results can only be achieved in centres with experienced and competent endoscopists.

Other significant risk factors predictive of re-bleeding are ulcer size more than 2 cm, location of ulcers on high lesser curve and posteroinferior bulb of the duodenum.[27]

The indications for surgery are:

(1) Primary failure of endoscopic therapy

When endoscopic therapy fails to stop the bleeding, it is important to bring the patient to the operating theatre.

(2) Re-bleeding after endoscopic therapy in patients with high risk factors:

- patients who are hypotensive at time of re-bleeding
- ulcer size more than 2 cm

- large high lesser curve gastric ulcers and posteroinferior duodenal ulcers.

Bleeding Gastro-oesophageal Varices

The primary pathology leading to gastric and oesophageal variceal bleeding is portal hypertension, liver cirrhosis being the most common cause. Common aetiological factors leading to liver cirrhosis are chronic alcohol intake and chronic hepatitis infection.

The principles of treating an acute variceal bleeding are:

- resuscitation
- control of bleeding
- prevention of complications
- prevention of early re-bleeding.

Role of pharmacotherapy in the control of bleeding

Vasoactive drugs

Early pharmacotherapy using *vasoactive* drugs like *somatostatin* or somatostatin analogue and terlipressin have been shown to improve initial control of bleeding and increase the efficacy of endoscopic treatment.[28–30] It also reduces the risk of early re-bleeding. Early re-bleeding is a common occurrence often associated with significant mortality. Early administration of this drug also results in reduction in blood transfusion requirements and the need for rescue therapy. Therefore, in patients who are suspected of having variceal bleeding on clinical grounds, early administration of *somatostatin* or its analogue is recommended.

Vasoconstrictive drugs

Vasoconstrictive drugs like vasopressin are effective but these are associated with a high incidence of side effects like angina and abdominal pain. These must be used in combination with nitrates.

Antibiotics

Sepsis is a common complication in patients with variceal bleeding. Therefore early administration of intravenous antibiotics is essential to prevent septic complication. Wide spectrum antibiotics are used. In addition, gut decontamination using lactulose and neomycin to prevent hepatic encephalopathy should be carried out.

Emergency endoscopy

Oesophageal varices

Emergency endoscopy should be carried out as soon as adequate resuscitation has been instituted. Either band ligation or injection sclerotherapy may be used depending on the endoscopist's experience. Both are equally effective, although band ligation has been shown to have significantly fewer complications.[31]

When pharmacologic and endoscopic therapy fail to control oesophageal variceal bleeding, balloon tamponade is used as an interim measure. Repeat second therapeutic endoscopy is performed 24 hours later.

When all measures fail to control bleeding, the transjugular intrahepatic portosystemic shunt (TIPSS) or surgical shunting must be considered as the next line of treatment.

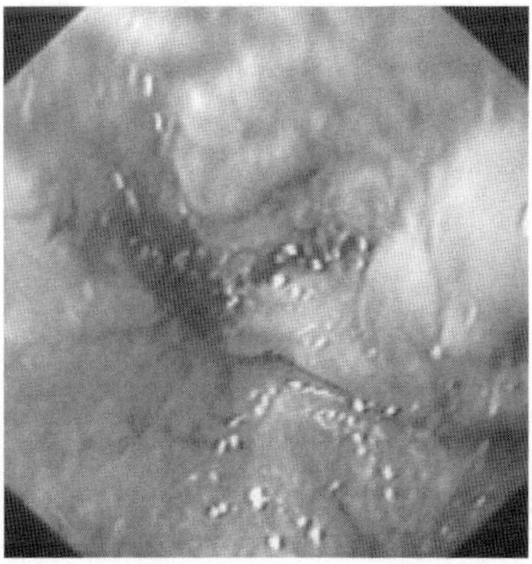

Fig. 3 Bleeding oesophageal varices.

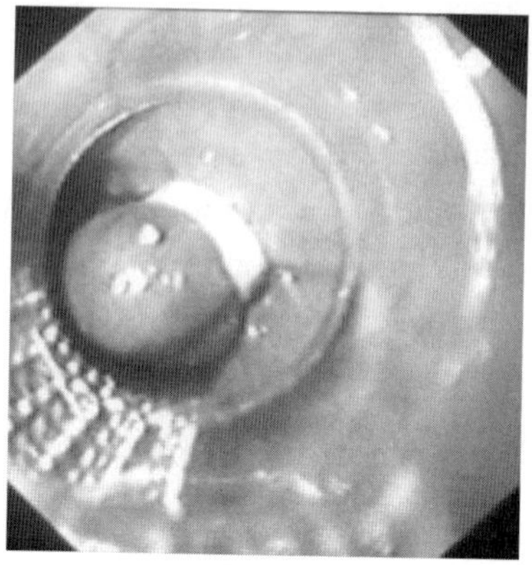

Fig. 4 Oesophageal varix after endoscopic banding.

Gastric varices

Gastric varices are less common but they are associated with more profuse bleeding and higher mortality. Initial resuscitative management is similar to oesophageal varices. However, the endoscopic treatment of choice is injection sclerotherapy using cyanoacrylate glue (Histoacryl®) or commonly called "super glue". Cyanoacrylate polymerises and solidifies rapidly within 20 seconds in a physiological milieu and instantaneously upon contact with blood.[32] To prevent rapid solidification of the glue, it is necessary to dilute with an oily contrast agent like Lipiodol® in dilution ratio of 0.5 ml of glue to 0.8 ml of Lipiodol®.

Despite its widespread use, there remains some controversies regarding its safety and long term outcome.[33] Pulmonary embolisation from the glue is the biggest concern. This can be prevented by limiting the amount of cyanoacrylate-Lipiodol® mixture per injection of not more than 1.3 ml. High re-bleeding is another concern and this is due to incomplete obliteration of the varix.[32] It is therefore essential to obliterate the varix completely in the same session.

Prevention of re-bleeding

After initial haemostasis, patients are at risk of re-bleeding in the first five days. It is recommended that vasoactive drugs be continued for five days.

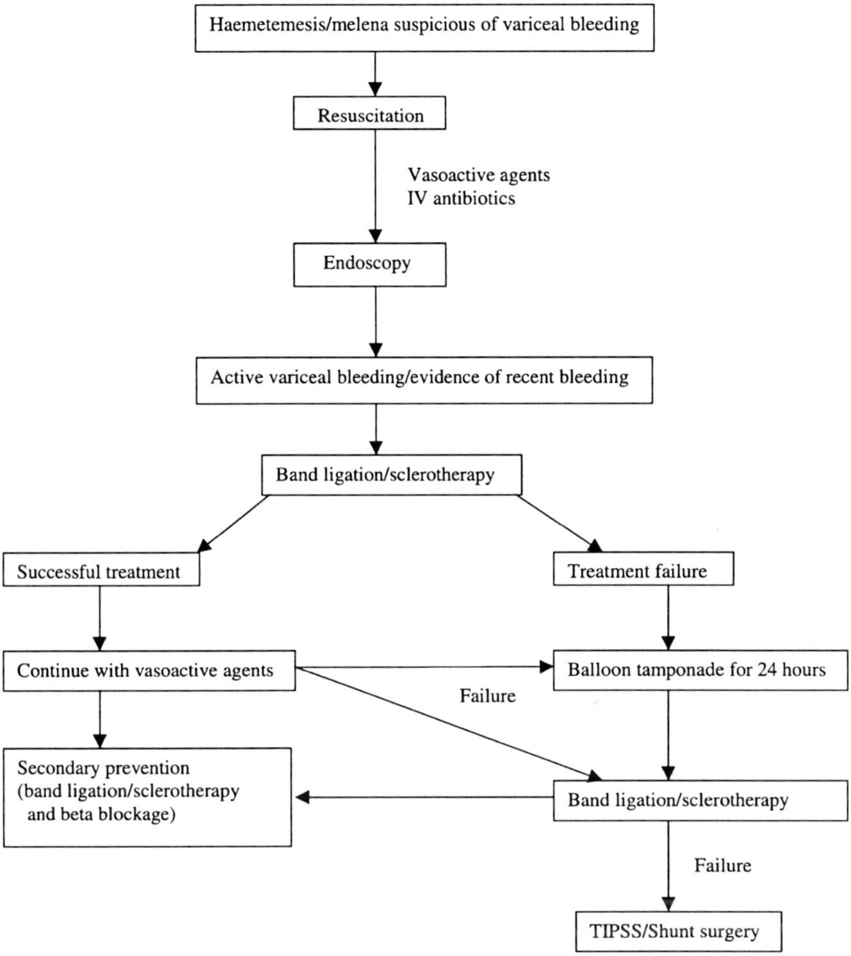

Fig. 5 Algorithm for the management of oesophageal varices.

For long term prevention of re-bleeding, either band ligation or sclerotherapy is equally effective. The addition of a beta-blocker (propanolol) to endoscopic therapy helps to reduce the re-bleeding rate.

Summary

Improved medical and endoscopic treatment in the last few decades have resulted in better outcome for patients with acute UGI bleeding. Immediate resuscitation is essential in the initial management of patients. In peptic ulcer bleeding, endoscopic therapy is now the accepted first-line treatment. However re-bleeding remains a major problem as it is associated with increased morbidity and mortality. The introduction of proton pump inhibitor particularly given in high dose and in continuous infusion after endoscopic therapy has shown in some studies to reduce re-bleeding rate. In patients with re-bleeding after initial endoscopic therapy, repeat endoscopic treatment may be attempted in selected cases. The role of surgery is now reserved for those who fail endoscopic therapy and in patients with high risk ulcers like large ulcers in high lesser curve and ulcers located at posteroinferior aspect of duodenum. All patients should be tested for *Helicobacter pylori* infection, regardless of NSAIDs usage. Eradication of *H. pylori* decreases the risk of recurrent bleeding.

In oesophageal variceal bleeding, band ligation is the preferred endoscopic treatment because of the lower complication rate; whereas in gastric varices, cyanoacrylate glue is the therapy of choice. Early use of vasoactive agents like somatostatin has been shown to decrease re-bleeding and facilitate endoscopic treatment.

References

1. Rockall TA, Logan RFA, Devlin HB, Northfield TC (1995). Incidence of and mortality from acute upper gastrointestinal haemorrhage in the United Kingdom. *Br Med J* **311**, 222–226.
2. Hunt PS (1984). Surgical management of bleeding peptic ulcer. A 10-year prospective study. *Ann Surg* **199**, 44–50.
3. Graham DY, Smith JL (1981). The course of patients after variceal haemorrhage. *Gastroenterol* **80**, 800–809.
4. Griffin MR, Piper JM, Daugherty JR, Snowden M, Ray WA (1991). Non-steroidal anti-inflammatory drug use and increased risk for peptic ulcer disease in elderly persons. *Ann Int Med* **114**, 257–263.
5. Sorensen HT, Mellemkjaer L, Blot WJ, Nielsen GL, Steffensen FH, McLaughlin JK, Olsen JH (2000). Risk of upper

gastrointestinal bleeding associated with use of low-dose aspirin. *Am J Gastroenterol* **95**(9), 2218–2224.

6. Garcia Rodriguez LA, Hernandez-diaz S, de Abajo FJ (2001). Association between aspirin and upper gastrointestinal complications: systematic review of epidemiologic studies. *Br J Clin Pharmacol* **52**(5), 563–571.
7. Graham DY, Hepps KS, Ramirez FC, Lew GM, Saeed ZA (1993). Treatment of *Helicobacter pylori* reduces the rate of re-bleeding in peptic ulcer disease. *Scand J Gastroenterol* **28**, 939–942.
8. Rokkas T, Karameris A, Mavrogeorgis A, Rallis E, Giannikos N (1995). Eradication of *Helicobacter pylori* reduces the rate of re-bleeding in ulcer disease. *Gastrointest Endosc* **41**, 1–4.
9. Huang JQ, Sridhar S, Hunt RH (2002). Role of *Helicobacter pylori* infection and non-steroidal anti-inflammatory drugs in peptic ulcer disease: a meta-analysis. *Lancet* **359**, 14–22.
10. Laine L, Peterson WL (1994). Bleeding peptic ulcer. *N Engl J Med* **331**, 717–727.
11. Andersen IB, Jorgensen T, Bonnevie O, Gronback M, Sorensen TI (2000). Smoking and alcohol intake as risk factors for bleeding and perforated peptic ulcers: a population-based cohort study. *Epidemiology* **11**, 434–439.
12. Guidelines for Red Blood Cell and Plasma Transfusions for Adults and Children (1997). Report of the expert working group. *Can Med Assoc J* **156**(Suppl. 11), S1–S23.
13. Walt RP, Cottrell J, Mann SG, Freemantle NP, Langman MJS (1992). Continous intravenous famotidine for haemorrhage from peptic ulcer. *Lancet* **340**, 1058–1062.
14. Daneshmund TK, Hawkey CJ, Langman MJS, Logan RFA, Long RG, Walt RP (1992). Omeperazole versus placebo for acute upper gastrointestinal bleeding: randomised double blind controlled trial. *Br Med J* **304**, 143–147.
15. Levine JE, Leontiadis GI, Sharma VK, Howden CW (2002). Meta-analysis: the efficacy of intravenous H2-receptor antagonists in bleeding peptic ulcer. *Aliment Pharmacol Ther* **16**(6), 1137–1142.

16. Selby NM, Kubba AK, Hawkey CJ (2000). Acid suppression in peptic ulcer haemorrhage: a "meta-analysis." *Aliment Pharmacol Ther* **14**, 1119–1126.
17. Vreeburg EM, Levi M, Rauws EA *et al.* (2001). Enhanced mucosal fibrinolytic activity in gastro-duodenal ulcer haemorrhage and the beneficial effect of acid suppression. *Aliment Pharmacol Ther* **15**, 639–646.
18. Chung YFA, Wong WK, Soo KC (2000). Diagnostic failures in endoscopy for acute upper gastrointestinal haemorrhage. *Br J Surg* **87**, 614–617.
19. Cook DJ, Guyatt GH, Salena BJ, Laine LA (1992). Endoscopic therapy for acute non variceal upper gastrointestinal haemorrhage: a meta-analysis. *Gastroenterology* **102**, 139–148.
20. Forrest JAH, Finlayson NDC, Shearman DJC (1974). Endoscopy in gastrointestinal bleeding. *Lancet* **2**, 394.
21. Green FW Jr, Kaplan MM, Curtis LE, Levine PH (1978). Effect of acid and pepsin on blood coagulation and platelet aggregation: a possible contributor prolonged gastroduodenal mucosal haemorrhage. *Gastroenterology* **74**, 38–43.
22. Schaffalitzky de Muckadell OB, Havelund T, Harling H *et al.* (1997). Effect of omeperazole on the outcome of endoscopically treated bleeding ulcers. Randomized double-blind placebo-controlled multicentre study. *Scand J Gastroenterol* **32**, 320–327.
23. Lin HJ, Lo WC, Lee FY, Perng CL, Tseng GY (1998). A prospective randomized comparative trial showing that omeperazole prevents re-bleeding in patients with bleeding peptic ulcer after successful endoscopic therapy. *Arch Intern Med* **158**, 54–58.
24. Lau JYW, Sung JJY, Lee KKC *et al.* (2000). Effect of intravenous omeperazole on ecurrent bleeding after endoscopic treatment of bleeding peptic ulcers. *N Engl J Med* **343**, 310–316.
25. Branicki FJ, Coleman SY, FokPJ *et al.* (1990). Bleeding peptic ulcer: a prospective evaluation of risk factors for re-bleeding and mortality. *World J Surg* **14**, 262–270.
26. Lau JYW, Sung JJY, Lam YH *et al.* (1999). Endoscopic retreatment compared with surgery in patients with recurrent bleeding

after initial endoscopic control of bleeding ulcers. *N Engl J Med* **340**, 751–756.

27. Brullet E, Campo R, Calvet X, Coroleu D, Rivero E, Simo Deu J (1996). Factors related to the failure of endoscopic injection therapy for bleeding gastric ulcer. *Gut* **39**, 155–158.
28. Levacher S, Letoumelin P, Pateron D, Blaise M, Lapandry C, Pourriat JL (1995). Early administration of terlipression plus glyceryl trinitrate to control active upper gastrointestinal bleeding in cirrhotic patients. *Lancet* **346**, 865–868.
29. Avgerinos A, Nevens F, Raptis S, Fevery J, and the ABOVE Study Group (1997). Early administration of somatostatin and efficacy of sclerotherapy in acute oesophageal variceal bleeds: the European Acute Bleeding Oesophageal Variceal Episodes (ABOVE) randomised trial. *Lancet* **350**, 1495–1499.
30. Cales P, Masliah C, Bernard B *et al.* (2001). Early administration of vapreotide for variceal bleeding in patients with cirrhosis. *N Engl J Med* **344**, 23–28.
31. Stiegmann GV, Goff JS, Michaletz-Onody DY *et al.* (1992). Endoscopic sclerotherapy as compared with endoscopic ligation for bleeding oesophageal varices. *N Engl J Med* **32**, 1527–1532.
32. Seewald S, Sriram PVJ, Naga M, Fennerty MB, Boyer J, Oberti F, Soehendra N (2002). Cyanoacrylate glue in gastric variceal bleeding. *Endoscopy* **34**, 926–932.
33. Sheikh RA, Trudeau WL (2000). Clinical injection of endoscopic injection sclerotherapy using N-butyl-2-cyanoacrylate for gastric variceal bleeding. *Gastrointest Endosc* **52**, 142–144.

18

Massive Lower Gastrointestinal Bleeding

Kong-Weng Eu
Kok-Sun Ho

Introduction

Massive lower gastrointestinal bleeding (LGIB) accounts for less than 2% of surgical emergencies. By definition, any bleeding distal to the ligament of Trietz, in other words, from the beginning of the jejunum, is considered LGIB.

The cause of the bleeding can be determined only in about 80% to 90% of the time. Most cases are self-limiting and stop spontaneously. In 10% of patients, the bleeding is ongoing and needs urgent intervention. In another 5% the bleeding is intermittent and may pose a diagnostic challenge.

Not all patients presenting with LGIB requires surgical intervention. The principles of management would involve resuscitation, localisation of the lesion, and therapeutic intervention if required (Fig. 1).

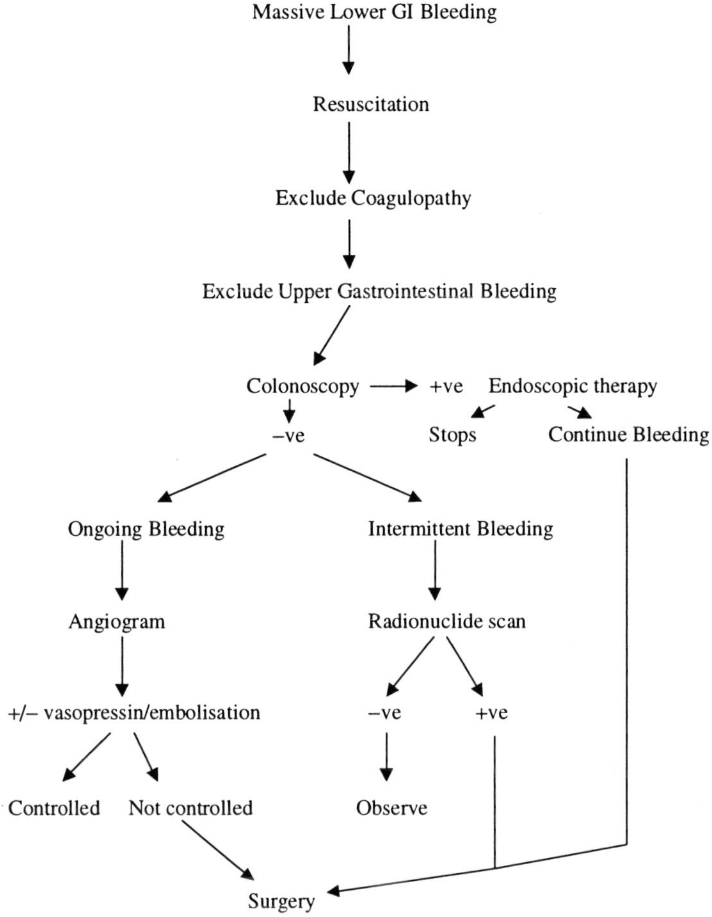

Fig. 1 Management algorithm for massive lower gastrointestinal bleeding.

Resuscitation

Resuscitation follows the basic principles of ABC — Airway, Breathing and Circulation. Patients require two large-bore intravenous cannulas. Haemodynamic instability should be corrected with intravenous fluids and blood. Patients are to be monitored in at least a high dependency area. Urine output and vital signs are monitored hourly. Central venous pressure and invasive intra-arterial blood pressure monitoring may be required if the patient is unstable.

Aetiology

In massive LGIB, the colon is the source of bleeding in about 85% of the cases. Small bowel bleeding and upper gastrointestinal bleeding accounts for 5% and 10% respectively.[1] Systemic coagulopathy may also present as LGIB.

Colonic Causes

Although colonic bleeding can occur from a number of lesions, the two commonest causes of massive bleeding are diverticular disease and angiodysplasia.

Diverticular disease is the presumptive cause of bleeding in 42% to 55% of studies, though only one in five cases has been validated. Seventy-six per cent of diverticular bleeding stops spontaneously. Angiodysplasia is an incidental finding in 1–2% of colonoscopies, and accounts for about 3–12% cause of LGI bleeding.[2]

Non-steriodal anti-inflammatory drugs (NSAIDs) and aspirin are also increasingly recognised as a contributory cause in LGIB. Up to 92% of patients with diverticular bleeding were taking NSAIDs or aspirin.

Other causes of LGIB include neoplasia (2–26%), which includes polyps (5–11%) and carcinoma (21%); post-polypectomy bleeding (2–6%); inflammatory and infectious conditions (6–30%) and ischaemic colitis (3–20%). However, these do not commonly cause massive bleeding.

Other less common causes of bleeding include colonic endometriosis, which may present with cyclical bleeding, vasculitis and aorto-colonic fistula.

Anorectal Causes

Anorectal bleeding may also present with LGIB. Causes[3] include haemorrhoids, fissures, solitary rectal ulcer syndrome, stercoral ulcer, portal colopathy and varices, proctitis, especially after radiation, and Dieulafoy lesion.

Small Bowel Causes

This includes Meckel's diverticulum, which usually presents in a younger age group; other types of small bowel diverticulum; small bowel tumours; as well as radiation enteritis, infection, angiodysplasia and Crohn's disease.

Localisation of Bleeding Source

Localisation of the bleeding source is the most important step in the correct management of LGIB. It is not uncommon that a definite source of bleeding cannot be identified, and a pathological lesion is a presumed source of bleeding. Up to 9% of these lesions can be a false positive, and in up to 50%, there can be more than one bleeding source.

Colonoscopy

Colonoscopy is the main modality of investigation for patients with LGIB. Most patients with LGIB usually stop bleeding spontaneously. This allows time to stabilise the patient and for bowel preparation. Two litres of polyethylene glycol are given to cleanse the colon. This is usually adequate to clear the colon of residual blood and faeces. Some people believe that since blood in the colon acts as a cathartic, a rectal enema is adequate preparation prior to colonoscopy. However, in our experience, the colon commonly remains coated with stale blood, and mucosal lesions such as angiodysplasia or diverticular disease can easily be missed unless the colon is actively bleeding at the time of colonoscopy.

It is also common to find that the rectum may be filled with blood clots, making colonoscopy difficult. The clots and/or faeces can easily be removed via a proctoscope and a large suction catheter. Once the rectum is cleared, the proximal colon is usually quite clean and allows clear visualisation.

With proper bowel preparation, failure to intubate the caecum occurs in less than 2% of patients. If no definite bleeding site is identified, the terminal ileum should be intubated to exclude bleeding from small bowel.

Colonoscopy can allow therapeutic measures[4] as well. Haemostatic measures include adrenaline injection, diathermy coagulation and argon plasma coagulation. These measures are usually adequate to stop the bleeding, though rebleeding rates are highly variable.[5,6]

Radionuclide Scan

Radionuclide scans are for diagnosis only, and have no therapeutic role. These are usually used when the rate of bleeding is very slow or intermittent, and colonoscopy has failed to identify a presumptive cause.

There are actually two types of radionuclide scans: 99m-Tc sulphur colloid and 99m-Tc-labelled RBC scan. The sulphur colloid scan requires less preparation time, and is rapidly cleared from the circulation. The imaging time is about 10 minutes. It detects the bleeding site by picking up a travelling area of activity. This has a disadvantage in that there must be ongoing active bleeding at the time of imaging. In addition, the sulphur colloid is taken up by the liver and spleen and can obscure bleeding in both colonic flexures.

The more commonly used scan is the 99m-Tc-labelled RBC (tagged RBC scan). It can detect bleeding rates as slow as 0.5 ml/min, and activity can be detected for up to 24 hours. It is thus useful for slow intermittent bleeding. The disadvantage of the tagged RBC scan is that it requires labeling of the patients' blood, as well as a need for repeated imaging.

Radionuclide scans are highly sensitive for bleeding. However, they offer only approximate localisation of the bleeding point, and there can be a false localisation rate of up to 45%.[7,8]

Angiogram

Angiogram is another technique that allows detection of active bleeding. It needs a bleeding rate of at least 1 ml/minute. One disadvantage is that it does not detect venous bleeding. It is also not without complications, which include haematoma formation, femoral artery thrombosis, renal failure, contrast reaction and transient ischaemic attacks.

The angiogram also offers an option of therapy if active bleeding is seen. Selective injection of vasopressin[9] can cause vasospasm and stop bleeding. However, this has a re-bleeding rate of 40%, and as vasopressin can get into the systemic circulation, it is not suitable for patients with ischaemic heart disease.

Transarterial embolisation[10] of the bleeding vessel is also successful in more than 80% of cases. However, there is a 20% rate of colonic infarction and rebleeding.

Currently, transarterial embolisation is used only as a temporary measure. The angiogram catheter is left in place until surgery. The catheter can be felt intra-operatively, and dye can be injected via the catheter to act as a guide to locating the source of bleeding.

Intraoperative Procedures

Surgery is only offered if the patient has recurrent or repeated episodes of bleeding. If the bleeding source is localised, the aim of surgery would be a directed segmental resection as opposed to a subtotal colectomy, as rebleeding rates are similar.

In cases of diverticular bleeding, the extent of surgery would depend on the accurate localisation, as well as the extent of diverticular disease. In the presence of extensive diverticular disease, the operation of choice is a total colectomy even if bleeding is localised to one side. This is to prevent further bleeding from diverticular disease from the remaining colon.

When the bleeding source cannot be localised, a total colectomy would be the operation of choice, rather than a blind segmental colectomy. The rebleeding rates are much lower after a total colectomy, though the morbidity and mortality for the two procedures are similar.[11]

The patient is placed in the Lloyd-Davies position for laparotomy. At laparotomy, the stomach, duodenum, entire small and large bowel are inspected gently for any gross pathology. It is important to handle the bowel gently to avoid petechial haemorrhage on the surface of the bowel, as this may cause confusion with the offending lesion. On-table gastroscopy, colonoscopy and enteroscopy may be required to inspect the mucosal surface for the source of bleeding. Dimming the operation theatre lights and viewing the bowel with the aid of transillumination helps to detect small lesions in the bowel wall.

For on-table colonoscopy, if the colon is filled with blood, antegrade lavage may be useful. An appendicectomy is performed and a large-bore Foley's catheter is introduced into the appendiceal stump. A proctoscope is inserted into the anus to allow fluid to run out. Normal saline is then run through the colon until the effluent from the anus is clear. The colonoscope is then inserted through the anus and passed up.

Early Postoperative Care of the Patient

Most of these patients are usually quite ill and require monitoring in high dependency units, if not intensive care.

Early post-operative care is centred upon maintenance of adequate blood volume and haemodynamic stability. Feeding is usually progressed slowly upon evidence of return of bowel function.

Conclusion

Massive lower gastrointestinal bleeding requiring urgent surgical intervention is relatively uncommon. A proper understanding of the different roles of the investigative modalities are important in the proper management of the patient.

References

1. Levinson SL, Powell DW, Callahan WT *et al.* (1981). A current approach to rectal bleeding. *J Clin Gastroenterol* **3**(Suppl. 1), 9–16.

2. Zuckermann GR, Prakash C (1999). Acute lower intestinal bleeding, part 2: etiology, therapy and outcome. *GI Endoscopy* **49**(2), 228–235.
3. Leong AFPK, Seow-Choen F (1997). Lower gastrointestinal bleeding. In *Surgery of the Colon and Rectum*. Nicholls RJ, Dozois RR (eds.) New York: Churchill Livingstone, pp. 765–778.
4. Jensen DM, Machicado GA, Jotabha R, Kovacs TOG (2000). Urgent colonoscopy for the diagnosis and treatment of severe diverticular haemorrhage. *N Engl J Med* **342**, 78–82.
5. Prakash C, Chokshi H, Walden DT, Aliperti G (1999). Endoscopic haemostasis in acute diverticular bleeding. *Endoscopy* **31**(6), 460–463.
6. Savides TJ, Jensen DM (2000). Therapeutic endoscopy for non-variceal gastrointestinal bleeding. *Gastroenterol Clin N Am* **29**(2), 465–485.
7. Zuckermann GR, Prakash C (1998). Acute lower intestinal bleeding, part 1: clinical presentation and diagnosis. *GI Endoscopy* **48**(6), 606–616.
8. Gutierrez C, Mariano M, Laan TV, Wang A, Faddis DM, Stain SC (1998). The use of technetium-labeled erythrocyte scintigraphy in the evaluation and treatment of lower gastrointestinal haemorrhage. *Am Surgeon* **64**, 989–992.
9. Lefkovitz Z, Cappell MS, Kaplan M, Mitty H, Gerard P (2000). Radiology in the diagnosis and therapy of gastrointestinal bleeding. *Gastroenterology Clin N Am* **29**(2), 489–509.
10. Luchtefeld MA, Senagore AJ, Szomstein M, Fedeson B, van Erp J, Rupp S (2000). Evaluation of transarterial embolisation for lower gastrointestinal bleeding. *Dis Colon Rectum* **43**, 532–534.
11. Farner R, Lichliter W, Kuhn J, Fisher T (1999). Total colectomy versus limited colonic resection for acute lower gastrointestinal bleeding. *Am J Surg* **178**, 587–591.

19

Surgical Emergencies of the Hepato-Pancreato-Biliary System

Pierce Chow

Introduction

Surgical emergencies involving the hepato-pancreato-biliary (HPB) system comprise a large proportion of emergency laparotomies for acute abdomen. In a prospective study of consecutive non-trauma emergency laparotomies carried out in the Singapore General Hospital, 32% of the cases involved the HPB system.[1] This study excluded emergency laparoscopic cholecystectomy for acute cholecystitis, which would have increased the proportion of emergency surgery for HPB conditions to 40% of the total cases of emergency abdominal surgery.

A number of HPB surgical conditions are significantly more prevalent in Southeast Asia than in the West. Examples of these are pyogenic liver abscess, recurrent pyogenic cholangitis, and the acute rupture of hepato-cellular carcinoma. Detailed discussions of the management of these conditions are currently only found in sub-specialty textbooks. These are, however, conditions that surgical staff on-call are routinely confronted with, in Singapore and elsewhere in the region.

Acute Surgical Conditions of the Biliary Tree

Brown or pigment gallstones have traditionally been perceived to be the predominant type of gallstones in Southeast Asia, but there is evidence to suggest that Western-type cholesterol stones are becoming more prevalent. In a recent series of 484 cases in Singapore, cholesterol stones comprised 46% of the cases; black pigment stones comprised 30.5% and brown stones 13%.[2] This implied change in the epidemiology reflects the emergence of gallstone disease of the Western type, but there is no data to suggest that this necessarily implies a decrease in the traditional pigmented type of gallstones.

Pigment stones reportedly form 60% of gallstones in Japan, and only 25% of gallstones in the United States of America.[3] Bacteria, especially those that produce B-glucuronidase, are believed to play an important role in the pathogenesis of pigmented stones and these bacteria are more often associated with sepsis and stasis. Primary ductal stones are overwhelmingly pigmented in type. Cholesterol stones are due to hyper-saturation of bile, and are associated with obesity.

Acute cholecystitis

This remains the most common acute surgical condition of the biliary tree. More than 80% of acute cholecystitis are associated with impaction of stone in the cystic duct (Hartman's pouch) and about 10% are acalculous. Acalculous cholecystitis is associated with systemic illness, and generally has a worse prognosis.

Patients typically present with right hypochondral pain and fever. There is usually leucocytosis (which may be mild) and sometimes elevation of serum bilirubin. Jaundice may be found in a small proportion of patients. Elicitation of Murphy's sign on clinical examination clinches the diagnosis. Although ultrasonography remains the most sensitive and cost effective investigation for acute cholecystitis, it is however, operator-dependent. The diagnosis of acute cholecystitis should still be made when Murphy's sign is positive, and other clinical features are consistent with acute cholecystitis, even if the ultrasonographic report is equivocal.

Other important causes of upper abdominal pain need to be considered in a patient with a presumptive diagnosis of acute cholecystitis. An erect chest X-ray to look for free gas is useful as the surgical approach to a perforated viscus is significantly different from that for acute cholecystitis. Grossly elevated serum amylase concentration suggests the presence of pancreatitis although this does not exclude concomitant acute cholecystitis.

Surgery remains the mainstay of treatment in acute cholecystitis. Although acute cholecystitis resolves in about 60% of patients with conservative management (withholding oral feeds, starting antibiotic therapy, and providing analgesia), up to 20% experience recurrent attacks before interval cholecystectomy can be carried out. In addition, mortality in the group of patients with failed medical treatment (and who require surgery) is high.[4–6] The general medical consensus is that cholecystectomy (and preferably laparoscopic cholecystectomy) should be performed within the first few days.[7] Cholecystectomy is mandatory if fever does not resolve within 24 hours, or if there is evidence of gangrene or perforation. The author has adopted a policy of surgery within the same admission for all cases of acute cholecytitis unless they have been treated conservatively elsewhere and their symptoms have resolved by the time they are admitted.

Pre-operative management

Once diagnosis is established (either clinically or by imaging) the patient should be fasted, and an intravenous infusion of fluid started. Broad-spectrum antibiotics, including coverage for anaerobes, should be started at the same time. Blood should be sent for analysis for a full blood count, and serum urea and electrolytes concentrations. Although routine emergency cholecystectomy does not require blood to be grouped and crossed-matched, typing the patient's blood is advisable. Chest X-rays and electrocardiographs are mandatory.

Surgery

(1) *Laparoscopic cholecystectomy*

Patients who present with acute cholecytitis within 48–72 hours of the onset of symptoms are candidates for laparoscopic cholecystectomy.[8] Pre-operative indicators of successful laparoscopic surgery in acute cholecystitis are: minimal oedema or peri-cystic fluid on pre-operative imaging; leucocytosis of less than 14.0×10^9/L; and surgery within 72 hours of onset of symptoms.[9,10] Contra-indications are the presence of jaundice or any suspicion regarding the presence of ductal stones. Pre-operative imaging is thus mandatory in this group of patients as laparoscopic surgery does not allow the surgeon to adequately assess the extra-hepatic biliary tree.

Laparoscopic surgery in acute cholecystitis should only be carried out by experienced surgical staff because there is greater risk of damage to the extra-hepatic biliary tree. There should also be a lower threshold for conversion to open surgery if intra-operative conditions are not favourable. When successful, reported outcomes of laparoscopic cholecystectomy are good.[8] These patients enjoy the same benefits of elective laparosopic cholecystectomy and can expect to ambulate quickly and be discharged in one or two days.

(2) *Open cholecystectomy*

Open surgery should be carried out for patients who present after 72 hours, for those with suggestion of ductal stones, and for complications such as perforation and gangrene, and for those who do not meet the criteria for laparoscopic surgery (see above). This generally represents a more ill group of patients. It is advisable to leave an intra-abdominal drain (Radivac® or tube-drain) and if fever does not resolve within 24 hours of surgery, active measures should be taken to look for sources of sepsis. This is especially relevant in higher risk patients such as those with diabetes mellitus and those on steroid therapy for whatever indication.

(3) *Cholecystotomy*

In a small group of very ill and poor-risk patients with acute cholecystitis, percutaneous or open cholecystotomy helps to tide them through the acute episode until definitive surgery can be contemplated. Examples of such patients would be those who have had an acute myocardial infarction or a stroke (cerebrovascular event) within the preceding few days, and in whom the operative mortality would be extremely high.

Cholecystotomy can be performed as a percutaneous image-guided procedure by interventional radiologists especially when the gallbladder is very distended and is seen to be immediately adjacent to the anterior abdominal wall during imaging. Open cholecystotomy can otherwise be carried out through a small incision under local anaesthesia, and the gallbladder drained with a large-bore Foley's catheter (at least 24 French) and secured with an inkwell type closure of the gallbladder incision. The author's experience with cholecystotomy in this group of ill patients is consistent with that reported in the literature, and is favourable.[11] Post-procedure, the patient should be continued on antibiotics and all other supportive measures, including care in the intensive care unit. The drainage from the gallbladder should be checked twice a day, and if there is suggestion that the tube could be blocked, this should be gently irrigated with small amounts of heparinised saline.

Empyema of the gallbladder

This is a serious complication of acute cholecystitis and is potentially life-threatening. Empyema of the gallbladder occurs with unresolved acute cholecystitis and obstruction of the cystic duct. The gallbladder undergoes suppuration and becomes a bag of pus with subsequent risk of perforation. The clinical presentation is classically described as spiking high fever, chills and rigours (temperature 39–40°C) and leukocytosis greater than 15.0×10^9/L.

However, a significant number of patients with empyema of the gallbladder may only have few physical signs.[12,13] This is collaborated by a retrospective study on atypical presentations of empyema of the gallbladder in the Singapore General Hospital [unpublished data]. These patients are generally elderly with diabetes mellitus who have received broad-spectrum antibiotics and anti-pyretic therapy in the outpatient setting. They are admitted when their symptoms do not completely resolve. Diagnosis is made intra-operatively in these patients when frank pus is found within the gallbladder and a subsequent pathology report confirms suppuration. A high index of suspicion is thus important in this group of patients. Open emergency surgery is mandatory in empyema of the gallbladder.

Perforation of the gallbladder

This serious complication of acute cholecystitis may take one of three forms; localised perforation with pericholecystic abscess (usually sealed off by omentum), free peritoneal perforation with peritonitis and perforation into an adjacent hollow visus, and formation of a fistula. Generally, the first two types present as acute abdomen.

Pericholecystic abscess presents as acute cholecystitis, and the management is the same except that if laparoscopic surgery is attempted it should be converted to open surgery because the associated oedema obscures the anatomy and increases the risk of laparoscopic surgery. The outcome in this group of patients is generally good.

Free perforation generally occurs early in the disease when localised gangrene and perforation occur before there is time for adhesions to be formed. Pre-operative diagnosis of perforation is difficult. Strenuous efforts to obtain a precise pre-operative diagnosis when laparotomy is warranted, are unnecessary and may be counter-productive.

The patient presents with sudden onset of severe pain. This together with signs of guarding and tenderness, clearly point towards the need for immediate emergency laparotomy. Although the reported mortality rate in acute perforation of the gallbladder is approximately

28.6%[14] the experience in Singapore General Hospital is somewhat better, possibly due to a policy of immediate surgery for patients with signs of peritonitis. In a retrospective analysis of 23 patients with free perforation of the gallbladder during the period 1998–2001 in the Singapore General Hospital, the mortality was 5% [unpublished data].

At emergency laparotomy, choleystectomy is carried out followed by copious saline lavage. A large-bore tube-drain should be left *in situ* and post-operatively the patient may require management in an intensive care or high-dependency setting.

Acute cholangitis

Cholangitis is an acute bacterial infection of the biliary tree, and is associated with increased ductal pressure, and bacterial proliferation and transduction into the systemic circulation. Cholangitis has traditionally always signified ductal obstruction (either complete or partial), commonly by stones or strictures, both benign and malignant. A biliary stone causing obstruction may primarily arise from the duct itself due to stasis and obstruction, or secondarily, after having passed into the duct from the gallbladder. Cholangitis develops in less than 15% of patients with neoplastic obstruction.

Another variant of cholangitis is found in coastal East and Southeast Asia, including Singapore. This is known as recurrent pyogenic cholangiohepatitis (RPC) or Oriental cholangitis. The main features are recurrent infection of the biliary tree, formation of strictures and the presence of primary pigmented ductal stones and biliary sludge. Intrahepatic stones and strictures are common, and tend to involve the left lobe of the liver more than the right.

The symptoms of cholangitis are referred to as Charcots' Triad, and consist of upper abdominal pain, jaundice and chills and rigours. The complete triad is found in 70% of patients with cholangitis. There is leucocytosis, elevated serum bilirubin and alkaline phosphatase.

Patients with acute cholangitis can be severely ill and in endotoxaemic shock. The immediate management of patients with acute cholangitis consists of fluid resuscitation, intravenous broad-spectrum antibiotics, oxygen therapy, and close monitoring in a high-dependency ward setting. The important differential diagnoses are acute cholecystitis, empyema of the gallbladder, hepatic abscess and acute viral hepatitis. The correct diagnosis is crucial as further management of the patients in acute cholangitis and the first three differential diagnoses is interventive in nature and urgent. Imaging studies are mandatory when a diagnosis of acute cholangitis is considered. Urgent ultrasonography of the hepatobiliary system should be carried out looking specifically for evidence of biliary tract dilatation.

Unless the patient responds rapidly to antibiotic therapy, urgent decompression of the biliary system must be arranged, and this is best carried out by emergency endoscopic sphincterotomy followed by definitive surgery when the patient recovers from the acute episode of illness. Data from both the Queen Mary Hospital in Hong Kong[14] and the Singapore General Hospital[16] show that emergency open surgery and common bile duct exploration carried a mortality of greater than 30% in the absence of prior endoscopic decompression of the biliary tree.

Acute Non-trauma Surgical Conditions of the Liver

Pyogenic liver abscess

Pyogenic liver abscess is relatively more common in Southeast Asia than in the West. In a review of 296 patients treated for pyogenic liver abscess in the Singapore General Hospital over a five-year period (1995–2000),[17] the offending organism was found to be of the *Kleibsella* species in the majority of cases. Patients classically presents with spiking fever and may be associated with chills, rigours and occasionally jaundice. There is usually significant leucocytosis but derangement of the liver function tests may be mild. The sensitivity of ultrasonography in hepatic abscess is between 85–90% whereas the sensitivity of a CT scan is 95%. Amoebic liver abscess is an important differential diagnosis (see below), as is necrotic metastatic malignancy.

In the management of pyogenic liver abscess, consideration of the underlying cause of the abscess is important, and a systematic search for cholecystitis, cholangitis, acute appendicitis and diverticultis is crucial in order not to miss these potentially life-threatening conditions. A significant number of patients with pyogenic liver abscess have co-morbidities, especially diabetes mellitus, and in these patients it is important to achieve early successful treatment.

The results of minimally-invasive management of pyogenic liver abscess, such as percutaneous aspiration or drainage of the abscess and antibiotics therapy, or even antibiotic therapy alone, vary widely. Non-operative management generally results in a longer duration of hospital stay and resolution of symptoms as well as a second procedure (usually surgical drainage) in a significant number of patients.

Patients with a clinical diagnosis of pyogenic liver abscess should be started on broad-spectrum (including anaerobe) antibiotic cover. The further management of pyogenic liver abscess requires precise knowledge of the number, size, location and physical nature of the abscesses, and an urgent computed tomography (CT) should be carried out. A CT is also invaluable in excluding other diagnoses as well as other associated pathology.

Open surgical drainage of pyogenic liver abscesses is recommended in the following groups of patients:

(1) Patients in whom a co-existing surgical pathology is either shown to exist on the CT, or is suspected to exist.
(2) Patients with multi-septated abscesses especially if these are more than 5 cm in diameter. Percutaneous drainage in this group of patients is less likely to be successful.
(3) Immuno-compromised patients in whom successful resolution of the infection must be rapidly achieved.
(4) Patients with a location of abscess in the liver that precludes an appropriate percutaneous access route. This typically refers to abscesses located in segments VII and VIII of the liver.
(5) Patients who have had minimally-invasive techniques to bring about resolution of the abscess, but failed treatment.

The types of pyogenic liver abscesses amenable to antibiotic therapy alone include multiple small abscesses of less than 3 cm in diameter.

The surgical approach to drainage of pyogenic liver abscess is identical to that for liver resection. While the approach to abscesses located in segments V and VI of the right lobe and most parts of the left lobe is relatively straightforward, safe drainage of abscesses in segment VII and VIII requires formal mobilisation of the right lobe of the liver, and should be carried out by experienced surgical staff. During open drainage, a biopsy specimen should routinely be obtained from the abscess wall to exclude an underlying malignancy. It is also good practice to carry out cholecystectomy and a cystic duct cholangiogram, as well as to inspect the large bowel and the appendix. A large-bore drain similar to that used for a chest tube should be left to drain the abscess cavity. This can easily be removed in the ward when the patient's condition resolves.

Most patients with open drainage of pyogenic abscess are discharged within a week of the procedure. Outpatient colonoscopy to exclude underlying large bowel pathology four to six weeks later is recommended.

Endogenous endophthalmitis is a devastating complication of pyogenic liver abscess, and the onus is on the clinical staff to exclude this and document its absence.[17,18] Delayed diagnosis and treatment can lead to permanent loss of sight.

Amoebic liver abscess

In contrast to pyogenic liver abscess, the mainstay of management in amoebic liver abscess is non-surgical. In Singapore, this is relatively less common than pyogenic abscesses, and the offending agent is a protozoa, *Entamoeba histolytica*. Transmission of cysts is via the orofaecal route, and trophozoites are released into the lumen of the intestine. The liver is the major extra-intestinal site.

Patients tend to be younger, and are either manual workers or have a history of travel to endemic regions. There is, however, no good clinical method to differentiate between amoebic and pyogenic abscess, and a serology test is necessary. The aspirate is classically described as anchovy paste-like (reddish brown) and gives a negative Gram stain.

The mainstay of treatment is metronidazole (750–1000 mg tds). Defervescence is expected within 48–72 hours of the commencement of metronidazole therapy. Rupture into the thoracic cavity or into the pericardium are known complications of amoebic abscess. These, together with rupture into the peritoneal cavity, mandate surgical intervention.[19]

Acute rupture of hepatocellular carcinoma

Hepatocellular carcinoma (HCC) is endemic to East and Southeast Asia, and is associated with viral hepatitis, especially Hepatitis B and C. Hepatocellular carcinoma is significantly less common in the West. Acute rupture of an HCC into the peritoneal cavity is a devastating event, and patients present with sudden onset of abdominal pain with or without hypovolaemic shock. Ruptures are usually spontaneous in nature, and occur when an enlarging tumour has caused necrosis through the liver capsule, although ruptures are also known complications of trans-arterial chemo-embolisation (TACE) therapy. The incidence in Asia ranges from 5–15 % of HCC[20,21] but appears to be less in the West (2.7%).[22] The differential diagnoses are perforated viscus or a ruptured abdominal aortic aneurysm.

The abdomen is guarded and rigid, and clinical examination will reveal pallor (which can be marked) and evidence of stigmata of chronic liver disease in most cases. The immediate management is aggressive resuscitation with crystalloids and blood, and an urgent CT with intravenous contrast as soon as the patient can be stabilised.

The further management of ruptured HCC is determined by the haemodynamic stability of the patient, the underlying functional reserve of the liver and the pathological stage of the tumour.[23] If the patient is stable after resuscitation, but the underlying liver function is poor (Child-Pugh B or C) or the tumour is inherently inoperable, management is conservative. If this poor-stage patient shows evidence of continual bleed, then angiographic embolisation is carried out to stop the bleed. Angiographic embolisation is successful in stopping the bleeding in the majority of the patients.

A good-stage patient with operable tumour who remains stable after resuscitation will be offered elective resection of the tumour. If he shows evidence of continual bleed, immediate laparotomy will be carried out for haemostasis and resection. Pre-operative angiographic embolisation will only be carried out if it can be speedily arranged.

Surgical Management in Acute Pancreatitis

Acute pancreatitis is relatively uncommon in Singapore when compared to the West. In the United Kingdom, acute pancreatitis accounts for 3% of all cases of abdominal pain admitted to the hospital.[24] The aetiology of acute pancreatitis in Southeast Asia also appears to be ethnic-based and is different from that in Western countries.[25]

The natural history of acute pancreatitis varies widely. While approximately 80% of these patients present with mild and self-limiting disease, a significant number develop serious life-threatening complications with multi-organ failure and death as common end-points. The overall death rate of acute pancreatitis is around 10–15%.[26] The mortality from necrotising pancreatitis is however around 30–40%.[27] It is thus important to prognosticate patients with pancreatitis, and to allocate resources to the group of patients who most need the resources. In addition, many of the therapeutic and monitoring procedures that may be helpful to patients with acute pancreatitis are themselves associated with morbidity. The Ranson score, the Imrie score and the APACHE score are widely used prognostic tools in this respect.

Patients classically present with severe acute upper abdominal pain following a large meal or a drinking bout. The pain radiates to the back, is unrelenting and associated with nausea and vomiting. Patients may also be in hypovolaemic shock. Abdominal signs may be non-specific and a clinical diagnosis can be difficult. Important differential diagnosis such as perforated viscus or bowel infarction must be entertained. Serum amylase concentrations that exceed four times the upper limit of normal (or serum lipase concentration that is twice above upper limit of normal) are characteristic, but not diagnostic, and other abdominal pathology must be excluded. There is no direct correlation between the concentration of serum amylase and the severity of pancreatitis. In cases where there is acute pancreatitis over a background of chronic pancreatitis, serum amylase concentrations may be normal. The presence of hyperlipidaemia interferes with the assay for amylase, and values can be spuriously low.

The clinician must also be aware that another acute abdominal condition, such as mesenteric ischaemia, can co-exist with acute pancreatitis. Measurement of urinary diastase concentration and serum C-reactive protein concentration is occasionally useful. The diagnostic dilemma in acute pancreatitis is the complete exclusion of other reversible pathology in which laparotomy is mandatory.

The diagnosis and stratification of acute pancreatitis should be made within 48 hours of admission.[28] Acute pancreatitis is defined as severe when there is evidence of organ failure and/or complications such as necrosis, infection, formation of pseudocyst or abscess (Atlanta definition).[29] The dynamic CT scan has become established as the single most reliable tool in the diagnosis and evaluation of pancreatitis, and if not already done for diagnosis, should be done within three to ten days of admission.[27] Reduced or absent perfusion of the pancreas indicates pancreatic necrosis. Ultrasound of the abdomen may be useful in the initial diagnosis of pancreatitis, but the gland is poorly visualised in 25–50%.[28]

The mainstay of treatment in acute pancreatitis are: analgesia, restriction of oral intake, fluid resuscitation (as there can be significant third-space loss) and close monitoring of haemodynamic parameters and tissue oxygenation. Acute respiratory distress syndrome is an important complication and can occur between 48–72 hours after the onset of the attack, and also later following established sepsis. Acute respiratory distress syndrome should be managed in the intensive care unit.

There is currently no proven pharmacological means to halt the onset of pancreatitis although there has been suggestion that somatostatin and its analogues may be useful.[30] The role of endoscopic intervention is uncertain, and should only be applied when clear evidence of impacted gallstone is present. Broad-spectrum antibiotics are commonly used in severe pancreatitis as a means of prophylaxis.

The management of the majority of patients with acute pancreatitis is thus supportive and non-surgical. Around 20% of patients will have severe pancreatitis, and 95% of the mortality occurs in this group.[26] Patients with severe pancreatitis should be managed by a surgical specialist team.[28] There are clear surgical roles in the management of a small group of patients with complicated acute pancreatitis. These surgical indications may be divided into four categories:[31]

(1) To establish diagnosis and exclude other pathology: the diagnosis of acute pancreatis can be arrived at in most patients by a combination of clinical, biochemical and radiological assessment, but in approximately 5% of patients, other life-threatening extrapancreatic pathology that mandates immediate surgery, cannot be excluded by non-operative means.
(2) To interrupt the pathogenesis of complications: important examples are pancreatic resection, debridement and lavage.
(3) To treat complications arising from acute pancreatitis: for example, to drain an infected pseudocyst.
(4) To prevent recurrent pancreatitis: for example, cholecystectomy to remove the source of gallstones before the patient is discharged.

Summary

Pathology involving the HPB system constitutes a large proportion of emergency abdominal surgery. This chapter describes common conditions in some detail, especially those conditions which, though common in Southeast Asia, are less common elsewhere and are thus not well described in general textbooks. A good understanding of these conditions is, however, crucial to junior surgical staff here as these are conditions that they will be confronted with in their daily duties.

References

1. Chuwa WL, Tan YM, Khin LW, Chow PK, Soo KC (2001). Does ASA correlate with surgical outcomes in emergency abdominal surgery? *Asian J Surg* **24**(2), S130.
2. Ti TK, Wong CW, Yuen R, Karunanithy R (1996). The chemical composition of gallstones: its relevance to surgeons in Southeast Asia. *Ann Acad Med Singapore* **25**(2), 255–258.
3. Way LW (1994). Biliary tract. In *Current Surgical Diagnosis and Treatment*, 10th Ed. Way LW (ed.) East-Norwalk: Appleton and Lange, pp. 537–566.
4. Lahtinen J, Alhava EM, Aukee S (1978). Acute cholecystitis treated by early and delayed surgery. A controlled clinical trial. *Scand J Gastroenterol* **13**(6), 673–678.
5. Jarvinen H, Hastbacka J, Turunen MI (1979). The treatment of acute cholecystitis. A series of 497 consecutive patients. *Acta Chir Scand* **145**(6), 399–404.
6. Cameron IC, Chadwick C, Phillips J, Johnson AG (2002). Acute cholecystitis — room for improvement? *Ann R Coll Surg Engl* **84**(1), 10–13.
7. Clark ML, Kumar PJ (1998). Liver, biliary tract and pancreatic disease. In *Clinical Medicine*, 4th Ed. Kumar PJ, Clark ML (eds.) Edinburgh: Saunders, pp. 287–351.
8. Lo CM, Liu CL, Fan ST, Lai EC, Wong J (1998). Prospective randomized study of early versus delayed laparoscopic cholecystectomy for acute cholecystitis. *Ann Surg* **227**(4), 461–467.
9. Rattner DW, Ferguson C, Warshaw AL (1993). Factors associated with successful laparoscopic cholecystectomy for acute cholecystitis. *Ann Surg* **217**(3), 233–236.
10. Teixeira JP, Saraiva AC, Cabral AC, Barros H, Reis JR, Teixeira A (2000). Conversion factors in laparoscopic cholecystectomy for acute cholecystitis. *Hepatogastroenterology* **47**(33), 626–30.

11. Gagic N, Frey CF (1975). The results of cholecystostomy for the treatment of acute cholecystitis. *Surg Gynecol Obstet* **140**(2), 255–257.
12. Thornton JR, Heaton KW, Espiner HJ, Eltringham WK (1983). Empyema of the gall bladder — reappraisal of a neglected disease. *Gut* **24**(12), 1183–1185.
13. Chow WC, Ong CL, Png JC, Rauff A (1993). Gall bladder empyema — another good reason for early cholecystectomy. *J R Coll Surg Edinb* **38**(4), 213–215.
14. Tsai CJ, Wu CS (1991). Risk factors for perforation of gallbladder. A combined hospital study in a Chinese population. *Scand J Gastroenterol* **26**(10), 1027–1034.
15. Lai EC, Mok FP, Tan ES, Lo CM, Fan ST, You KT, Wong J (1992). Endoscopic biliary drainage for severe acute cholangitis. *N Engl J Med* **326**(24), 1582–1586.
16. Koh JS, Chow PK, Chung FAY, Ooi LP, Wong WK, Fook-Chong S, Soo KC (2003). Outcomes of emergency common bile duct exploration: impact of preoperative endoscopic decompression. *ANZ J Surg* **73**(6), 376–380.
17. Tan YM, Chee SP, Chow PK, Soo KC (2001). The association between pyogenic liver abscess and endogenous bacterial endopthalmitis: a devastating complication. *Asian J Surg* **24**(2), S135.
18. Tan YM, Chong CK, Chow PK (2001). Pyogenic liver abscess complicated by endogenous endophthalmitis. *ANZ J Surg* **71**(12), 744–746.
19. Pitt HA (1990). Surgical management of hepatic abscesses. *World J Surg* **14**(4), 498–504.
20. Nagasue N, Inokuchi K (1979). Spontaneous and traumatic rupture of hepatoma. *Br J Surg* **66**(4), 248–250.
21. Chen MF, Hwang TL, Jeng LB, Jan YY, Wang CS (1988). Surgical treatment for spontaneous rupture of hepatocellular carcinoma. *Surg Gynecol Obstet* **167**(2), 99–102.
22. Kew MC, Dos Santos HA, Sherlock S (1971). Diagnosis of primary cancer of the liver. *Br Med J* **4**(784), 408–411.

23. Leung KL, Lau WY, Lai PB, Yiu RY, Meng WC, Leow CK (1999). Spontaneous rupture of hepatocellular carcinoma: conservative management and selective intervention. *Arch Surg* **134**(10), 1103–1107.
24. de Dombal F (1991). The acute abdomen: definitions, diseases and decisions. In *Diagnosis of Acute Abdominal Pain*, 2nd Ed. de Dombal F (ed.) London: Churchill Livingston, pp. 19–30.
25. Kandasami P, Harunarashid H, Kaur M (2002). Acute pancreatitis in a multi-ethnic population. *Sing J Med* **43**(6), 284–288.
26. Mann D, Hershman M, Hittinger R (1994). Multicentre audit of death from acute pancreatitis. *Br J Surg* **81**, 890–893.
27. Thompson JS, Bragg LE, Hodgson PE, Rikkers LF (1988). Postoperative pancreatitis. *Surg Gynecol Obstet* **167**(5), 377–380.
28. United Kingdom Guidelines for the Management of Acute Pancreatitis (1998). British Society of Gastroenterology. *Gut* **42**(Suppl. 2), S1–S13.
29. Bradley EL, 3rd (1993). A clinically based classification system for acute pancreatitis. Summary of the International Symposium on Acute Pancreatitis, Atlanta, 11–13 September, 1992. *Arch Surg* **128**(5), 586–590.
30. Dervenis C, Bassi C (2000). Evidence-based assessment of severity and management of acute pancreatitis. *Br J Surg* **87**(3), 257–258.
31. Ranson JH (1997). Acute pancreatitis. In *Maingot's Abdomial Operations*, 10th Ed. Zinner MJ, Schwartz SI, Ellis H (eds.) New York: Appleton and Lange, pp. 1899–1915.

20

Abdominal Trauma

Allen Yeo

Introduction

Abdominal trauma remains one of the commonest reasons for preventable deaths in any trauma system.[1] Despite recent advances in diagnostic tests, some injuries continue to elude attempts at early diagnosis. However, basic management principles have been established that allow us to manage this group of patients in a more organised way and help reduce the number of missed injuries. In this chapter, the various modalities for assessing the abdomen will be discussed, and a suggested approach to the workup of these patients will be provided. The management of specific injuries will not be covered.

Assessment of the Abdomen

Abdominal injury can be broadly divided into two groups, based on the mechanism of injury — blunt or penetrating. Penetrating injury can further be subdivided into those due to stab wounds or gunshot wounds. This division is necessary because the management principles are unique to each group.

Patients who sustain major trauma tend to have multiple injuries. This is especially so when the mechanism of injury is blunt. There is a need to identify and prioritise these injuries. As outlined in the Advanced Trauma Life Support (ATLS)® protocol, the management of the airway, breathing and circulation during the primary survey must always take precedence.[2] Only after these are secured, can the assessment of the rest of the body proceed as described in the secondary survey.

The various components in the assessment of the abdomen are discussed below.

Clinical evaluation

The history of the injury is often incomplete, either because the patient is unconscious, or because of the lack of eyewitnesses. Whenever possible, the "AMPLE" history (Allergies, Medication, Past illnesses, Last meal, Events and environment) as recommended in the ATLS protocol, should be obtained. In the majority of cases, the mechanism of injury is usually known, and is a good guide to

Table 1 Mechanism of Injury and the Associated Injury Pattern

Mechanism	Injury Pattern
Fall from height	Pelvic fracture, bladder, abdominal solid organ Spine and calcaneal fracture, aortic transection
Bicycle handle-bar	Bowel, pancreas
Sporting injury	Spleen, kidney
Seat belt	Small bowel, duodenum, pancreas Chance fracture spine
Vehicular frontal impact	Head, chest, abdominal solid organ Lower limb fracture dislocation
Vehicular lateral impact	Pelvic fracture, liver, spleen Rib fractures, lung contusion

the likelihood of intra-abdominal as well as other associated injuries. Specific injury patterns occur as shown in Table 1.

Clinical examination of the abdomen is important, as the presence of peritonitis is an absolute indication for laparotomy. The presence of localised abdominal pain or tenderness should increase the suspicion of intra-abdominal injury. In a study by Velmahos, 23% of patients with the "seat belt sign" had significant intra-abdominal injury.[3] Figures 1(a) and (b) show a patient with the "seat belt

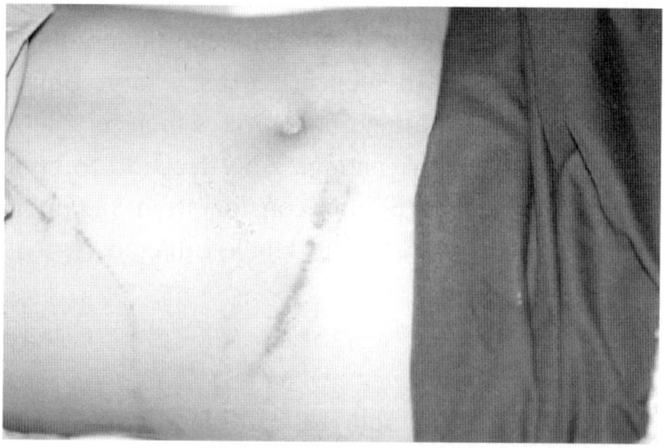

Fig. 1(a) Motor vehicle accident patient with "seat belt sign".

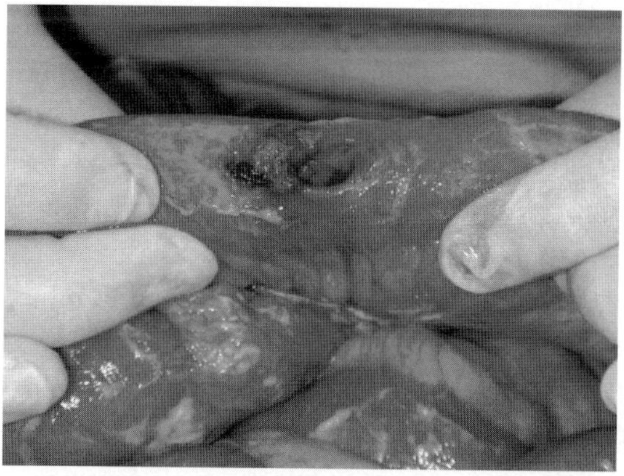

Fig. 1(b) Bowel perforation at laparotomy in a patient with "seat belt sign".

sign" who had a small bowel perforation at laparotomy. Even if the initial examination is negative, serial examination (especially in penetrating injury) can detect the evolution of signs that eventually point to the presence of significant intra-abdominal injury. However, there are recognised limitations. For example, the patient's response to the presence of haemoperitoneum varies widely — some patients do not even complain of any abdominal pain. In addition, clinical examination may be difficult in uncooperative patients, and is often unreliable in patients with head or spinal cord injury, alcoholic intoxication or other distracting injuries. In others, serial clinical examination may not be possible, for example, in those who are undergoing surgery for a prolonged period of time. In such instances, a more objective assessment should be attempted, the choice of which is dictated by the haemodynamic stability of the patient. The decision to continue monitoring the patient has to take into consideration the morbidity of a negative laparotomy versus that of a delayed diagnosis.

Laboratory tests

No single laboratory test is able to confidently make or exclude a diagnosis of intra-abdominal injury. Other than its importance as a baseline, it may sometimes raise the possibility of these injuries. The admission haemoglobin may not accurately reflect the degree of blood loss, and should be repeated a few hours later. A raised total white cell count is a common finding immediately after trauma, but a rising trend may signify the onset of sepsis. Arterial blood gas analysis is important as it provides information regarding the respiratory status, and the base deficit reflects the state of hypoperfusion. Deranged liver function tests may indicate the presence of liver injury, while an elevated serum amylase may suggest pancreatic injury. However, it is important to realise that the serum amylase may be normal even in the presence of significant pancreatic injury. Blood for alcohol or toxicology should be done if clinically necessary. Urine pregnancy tests or serum beta-HCG are mandatory in all females of reproductive age group. While pregnancy should not dissuade one from essential tests, it may influence our choice of screening investigations. The presence of microscopic haematuria after blunt trauma requires further evaluation only in the presence of hypotension, or if haematuria is persistent. Gross haematuria should always prompt assessment of the kidney and bladder with computed tomography (CT) and cystography.

X-rays

The three mandatory X-rays in a multi-trauma patient are the cross-table lateral cervical spine, chest and pelvis. A chest X-ray showing the presence of free intra-peritoneal air or a ruptured diaphragm would mandate laparotomy. Pelvic X-rays are essential, as pelvic fractures can result in significant retroperitoneal bleeding — an occult source of hypotension. The abdominal X-ray is of limited use in blunt abdominal trauma. CT is the imaging modality of choice in suspected intra-abdominal injury. However, in penetrating trauma, the abdominal X-ray is helpful for predicting the trajectory as well as document the presence of any retained foreign body. The one-shot intravenous urogram (IVU) has been advocated to determine the function of both kidneys in the emergent setting.

Diagnostic peritoneal lavage (DPL)

First described by Root and colleagues in 1965, the diagnostic peritoneal lavage proved to be a very sensitive test for intra-abdominal bleeding.[4] It is best used in the setting of a hypotensive patient to exclude intra-abdominal bleeding. The only absolute contra-indication to DPL is a definite indication for laparotomy. Relative contra-indications include a scarred abdomen from previous surgery or trauma, advanced pregnancy and coagulopathy. Diagnostic peritoneal lavage is not contra-indicated in pelvic fractures although modifications in technique are necessary.

Diagnostic peritoneal lavage is done using either the open or Seldinger technique.[5] Complications arising from trocar insertion (resulting in vessel or bowel injury) are low, at 1%.[6] The incision is made in the sub-umbilical region. In patients with pelvic fracture, a supra-umbilical incision is used to avoid entering the pelvic haematoma. The catheter is then advanced into the pelvis. The aspiration of gross blood or bowel contents is considered positive by gross criteria. Otherwise one litre of saline is infused, and the return fluid is sent for microscopy. A positive microscopic criterion is met when more than 100,000 rbc/mm^3 or 500 wbc/mm^3 are detected. It only takes 20–30 ml of blood (in a patient with normal haemoglobin) diluted in one litre of saline to achieve this positive criterion.

A positive lavage in a hypotensive blunt-trauma patient mandates laparotomy. In patients with pelvic fractures where extravasation of blood from the retroperitoneum may give a false positive result, only the gross criteria is accepted as being positive. With the growing realisation that many solid organ injuries can be successfully managed conservatively, DPL was felt to be too sensitive, with an unacceptably high rate of non-therapeutic laparotomies. If DPL is done in a stable patient and found to be positive, it might increase the pressure on the surgeon to operate. Therefore, if the haemodynamic stability can be restored, CT is preferable. This may demonstrate an isolated solid organ injury that may then be managed conservatively. Diagnostic peritoneal lavage has also been used to confirm the diagnosis of bowel injury when the white blood cell count exceeds 500/mm^3. The result may be spuriously negative if done early, because the migration of white blood cells only occurs after a few hours. Leaving the catheter and repeating it in a few hours may be useful.[7] Some authors have suggested that the white cell count to red cell count ratio (more than 150:1) is a more sensitive indicator of bowel perforation, as the absolute white cell count can be elevated as a result of the haemorrhage alone.[8] Diagnostic peritoneal lavage can also fail to detect diaphragmatic, pancreatic and other retroperitoneal injury. In penetrating injuries, a reduced red blood cell count would increase the sensitivity of DPL in detecting diaphragmatic injury.[9]

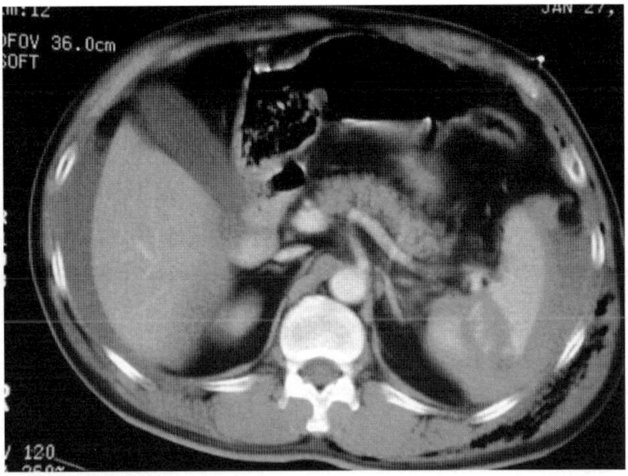

Fig. 2 CT showing splenic rupture with haemoperitoneum.

Computed tomography (CT)

The increased utilisation of CT since the 1980's has changed the way we manage abdominal injury. For the first time, surgeons know with a high degree of accuracy the specific intra-abdominal injury even before laparotomy is performed. It permitted the safe conservative management of solid organ injuries by allowing the grading of its severity, as well as the exclusion of other concomitant injuries (Fig. 2). It is able to assess the retroperitoneal organs, an area missed by DPL and ultrasound. In addition, advances in technology have resulted in newer generations of high-speed CT scanners that can even demonstrate active bleeding.[10,11] This is seen as a contrast blush and is often amenable to angiographic embolisation, as illustrated in Figs. 3 and 4.[12]

Computed tomography, when done for suspected abdominal injury, should include both the abdomen and pelvis. It is necessary to include the latter as it is a dependent area of the abdomen where free fluid from a bowel perforation can accumulate. The scan should be enhanced with both intravenous and preferably oral contrast.

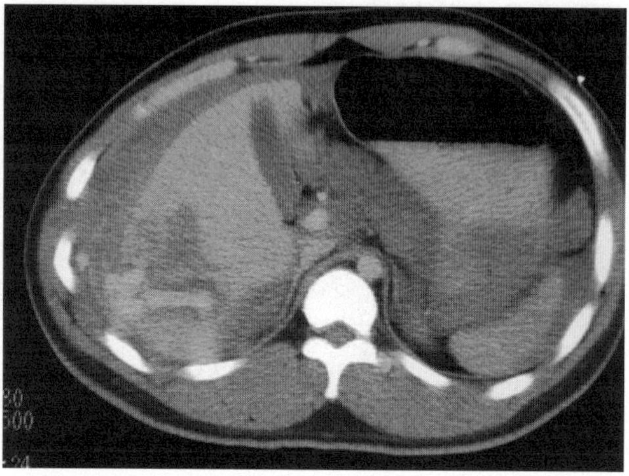

Fig. 3(a) CT showing liver laceration with contrast blush suggesting active bleeding into the free peritoneal cavity.

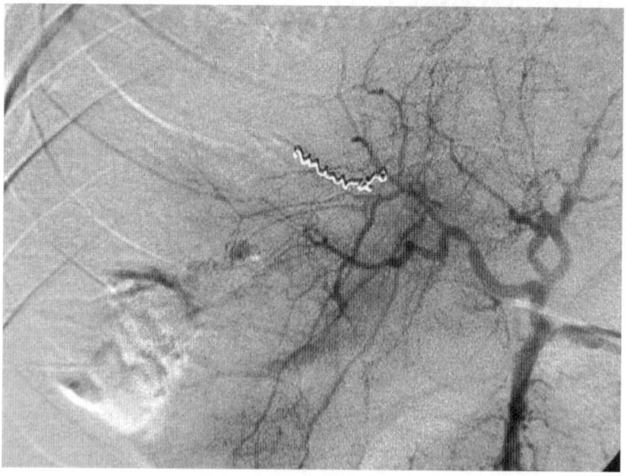

Fig. 3(b) Angiogram with embolisation of the bleeding vessel.

The "lung windows" on the upper cuts may occasionally reveal an occult pneumothorax (Fig. 5). This may require the placement of a chest tube, especially if the patient is to undergo positive pressure ventilation subsequently. In addition, the detection of a para-aortic

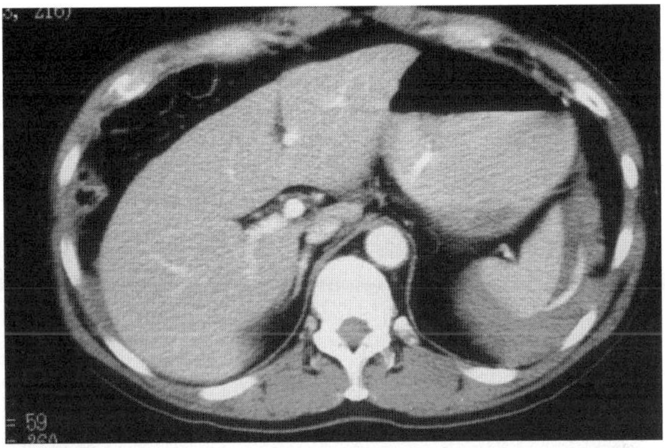

Fig. 4 Active bleeding from spleen on spiral CT.

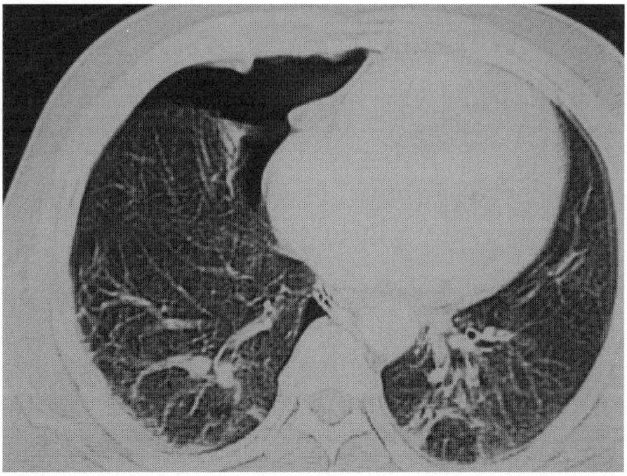

Fig. 5 Occult pneumothorax discovered on upper cuts of an abdominal CT.

haematoma in the upper abdominal views may suggest the existence of a traumatic aortic transection higher up in the chest. The CT has replaced the need for intra-venous urogram (IVU) to assess the kidneys. Bladder injuries can only be confidently excluded by CT if it is adequately filled up with the retrograde administration of contrast via a Foley catheter (CT cystogram).

Patients who are haemodynamically unstable, or require rapid on-going transfusion, should not undergo CT as they may collapse during the scan. There is a potential but small risk of allergy to intravenous contrast and aspiration from administration of oral contrast. While

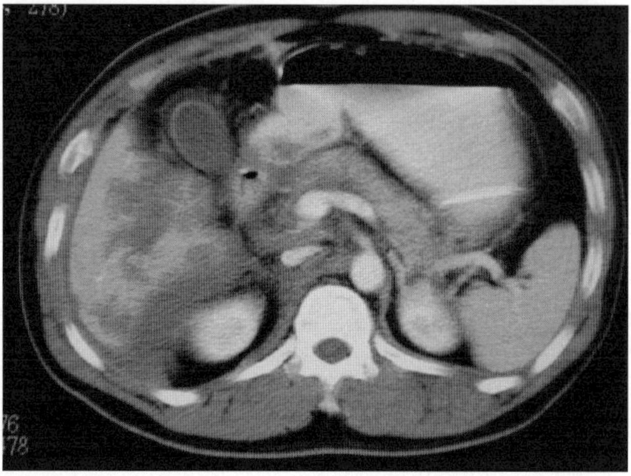

Fig. 6(a) CT showing liver laceration with adjacent haemoperitoneum.

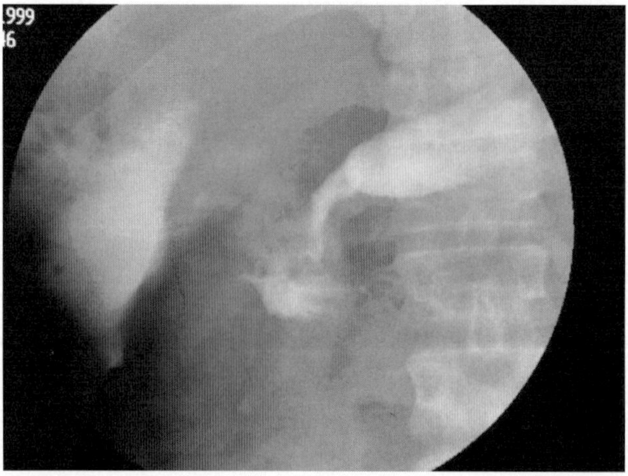

Fig. 6(b) Contrast study in the same patient showing extravasation of contrast from duodenum outlining the inferior surface of liver. This was not obvious on CT.

intravenous contrast is essential, oral contrast may be omitted in patients at risk of aspiration. The use of oral contrast provides a road map for the radiologist but does not appear to improve the detection rate of bowel perforation.

Injury to the bowel, pancreas or diaphragm, may not be easily detected by CT. This is more likely if the CT is obtained soon after the injury. Indirect signs of bowel injury include the presence of free air, bowel wall thickening, streaking or haematoma of the mesentery, and the presence of unexplained free fluid.[13,14] A review by Rodrigues suggested that 27% of patients with unexplained free fluid had therapeutic laparotomies.[15] Occasionally contrast studies are necessary to demonstrate duodenal injuries if the clinical suspicion is strong [Figs. 6(a) and (b)].

Computed tomography has a limited role in penetrating abdominal injury except in the region of the back and flank when it is used to demonstrate the proximity of the track to vital organs.[16–18] Figure 7 shows a patient with a flank stab wound showing a superficial track on CT scan. Patients with scans showing the track in proximity to bowel may require laparotomy to exclude bowel injury.

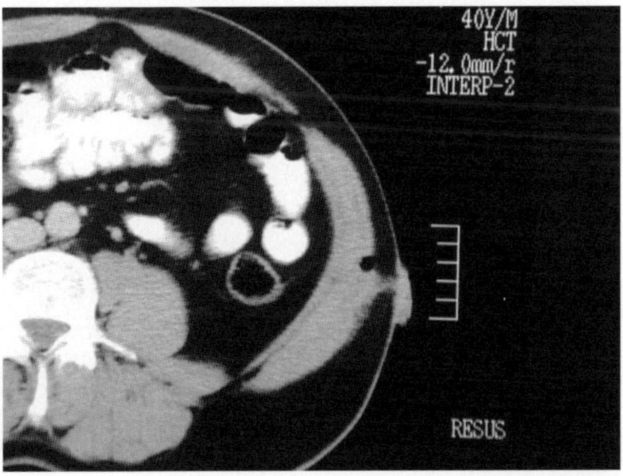

Fig. 7 CT of patient with a stab wound to the flank showing a track involving only the abdominal wall.

Ultrasonography (FAST)

Ultrasound has until recently not been deemed useful in the assessment of trauma patients. Since 1980, a more focused use of ultrasound in trauma was advocated, and the results have since been validated in large series of patients.[19,20] This has been termed the Focused Assessment by Sonography in Trauma examination (FAST). It is a focused search for blood in the pericardium and three dependent areas of the abdomen (hepatorenal pouch, splenorenal space and the pouch of Douglas). An example of free fluid in Morrison's pouch is shown in Fig. 8. FAST is a rapid and simple technique, and can be learnt after undergoing a concise introductory course incorporating didactic instructions and hands-on training. There is a short learning curve, and proficiency should be documented before depending on its results.

In trained hands, it can be performed in under two minutes at the bedside of an unstable patient. It is important to realise that both blood and ascitic fluid appears anaechoic on the ultrasound. However, in the setting of a hypotensive trauma patient, the presence of free

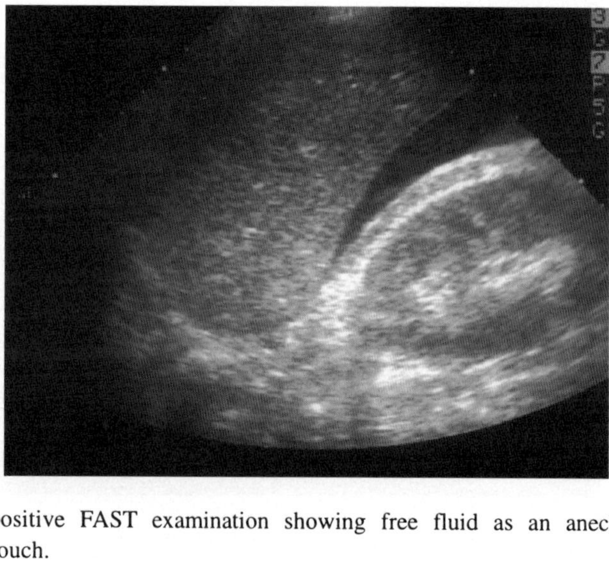

Fig. 8 A positive FAST examination showing free fluid as an anechoic rim in Morrison's pouch.

intra-abdominal fluid is presumptive evidence of haemoperitoneum and would warrant a laparotomy. It has the same indications as DPL, but its advantage lies in its non-invasiveness and repeatability. FAST has replaced DPL in some centres in North America, and has also been used as a screening tool in blunt abdominal trauma.[21,22] FAST does not assess the retroperitoneal structures, and solid organ injuries that are not associated with haemoperitoneum may be missed.[23] The procedure may be difficult to perform in obese patients, and often impossible in patients with subcutaneous emphysema.

Laparoscopy

Laparoscopy has not been popular in the assessment of the trauma patient. It is an invasive investigation and requires a general anaesthetic. The problem lies in the small but real risk of missing bowel injury even though it is possible to run the bowel laparoscopically. It is best used selectively in penetrating trauma to rule out diaphragmatic injury, and to confirm the tangential trajectory of a gunshot wound in the asymptomatic patient.[24,25] In experienced hands, it may reduce the non-therapeutic laparotomy rate in penetrating abdominal trauma.[26]

Endoscopy

Endoscopy has limited use in blunt abdominal trauma except perhaps to evaluate the oesophagus in suspected rupture. In penetrating injuries to the gluteal region, sigmoidoscopy is used to demonstrate rectal injury. Contrast studies can be used as a complementary test when the results of endoscopy are equivocal.

Approach to Blunt Abdominal Trauma

The management of blunt abdominal trauma is often complex because of its association with other injuries. The most important decision the surgeon needs to make is to decide whether there is sufficient evidence of intra-abdominal injury to warrant laparotomy. The exact diagnosis itself is "good" to know, but not essential.

The two absolute indications for laparotomy are the presence of shock and peritonitis.

(1) Shock

The management of a patient in shock is challenging. Concurrent with resuscitation, the physician needs to rapidly determine the source of bleeding. Patients who remain unstable (transient-responders or non-responders to resuscitation) should undergo laparotomy if the abdomen is obviously the cause of the hypotension (such as a distended abdomen with evidence of tire marks on the surface). A cautionary note: the abdomen is able to accommodate a significant volume of blood without appearing distended. In addition, up to 50% of patients with hypotension have an extra-abdominal cause of bleeding. In order to confidently rule out intra-abdominal injury, DPL or FAST should be expediently performed during the primary survey.

(2) Peritonitis

Although this may seem simple enough, the threshold for labelling a tender abdomen as having peritonitis varies from surgeon to surgeon. Sometimes it is clear-cut, for example when the whole abdomen is board-like with rebound tenderness. The surgeon should not attribute this to voluntary guarding from abdominal wall contusion. Whenever there is any doubt, further imaging or serial examination by the same surgeon will usually establish the diagnosis.

In the absence of shock or peritonitis, further work-up (imaging studies) may be necessary in the following circumstances:

(1) Equivocal examination

This is usually the result of injury to adjacent body regions, for example, tenderness over the upper abdomen associated with lower rib fractures or lower abdominal tenderness with pelvic fractures. Some patients may have abdominal wall contusion that may or may not be associated with intra-abdominal injury.

(2) Unreliable examination

The abdominal examination may be unreliable in the presence of spinal cord injury, head injury or the intoxicated patient. The use of morphine in trauma patients may dull the subjective sensation of pain but does not usually take away the abdominal signs.

(3) Inability to perform serial abdominal examination

Some patients may need to undergo surgery under general anaesthesia and should be properly assessed regarding the need for imaging studies beforehand.

(4) Significant associated injuries

The presence of significant associated injuries would heighten the possibility of intra-abdominal injuries. Examples include lower rib fractures, pelvic fractures, chance fracture of the vertebrae, seat-belt sign and gross haematuria.

In the group of patients with no shock or peritonitis, CT is the imaging modality of choice. A normal scan should not lull the clinician into believing everything is fine. Serial abdominal examination is still necessary as bowel or pancreatic injury may not be detectable by CT, especially if performed soon after the injury. DPL has no role in the stable patient except possibly to exclude bowel injury. In a low risk patient, FAST can be used as a screening test. This is especially useful in a mass disaster situation to rapidly triage patients on arrival in the hospital.[27]

The decision to further work-up a patient need to be individualised for each patient. For example, a haemodynamically stable head-injured patient with a large extradural haematoma requiring emergent craniotomy, should proceed straight from the CT facility to the operation theatre. Abdominal assessment can be done subsequently by performing FAST or DPL. Another option would be to perform CT of the abdomen after craniotomy.

The algorithm for the management of blunt abdominal trauma is outlined in Fig. 9.

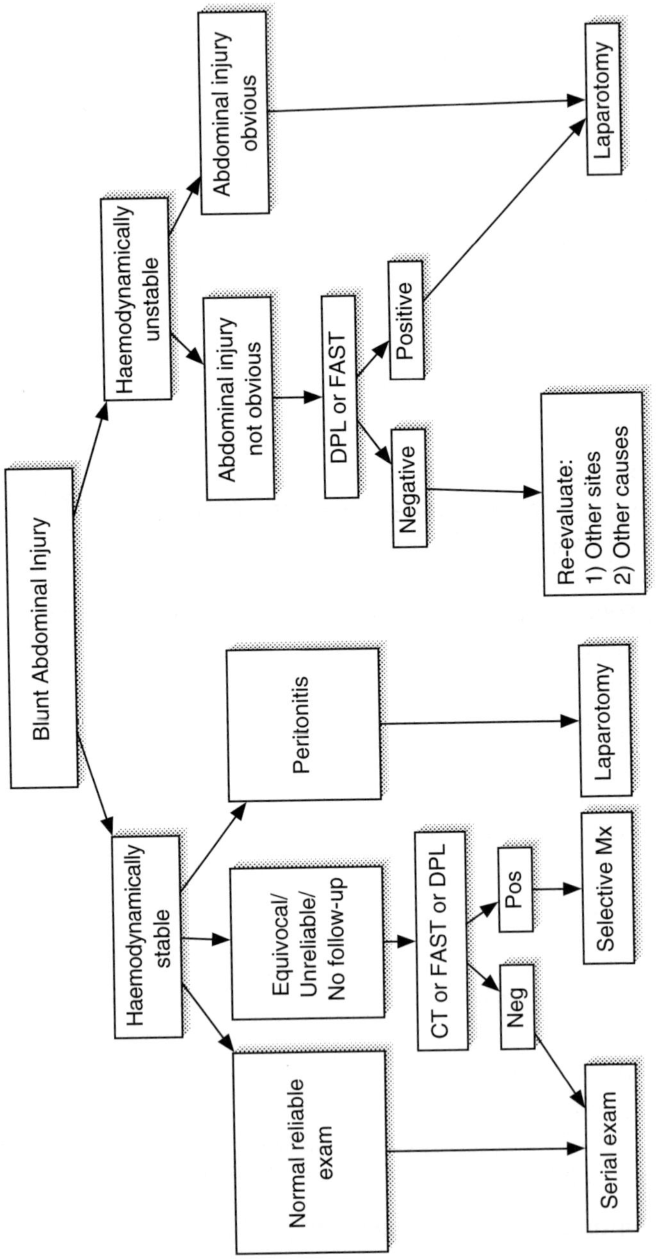

Fig. 9 Algorithm for management of blunt abdominal trauma.

Approach to Penetrating Abdominal Trauma

Penetrating abdominal trauma is in some ways easier to assess and manage. The presence of a skin breach would automatically raise the suspicion of underlying injury. It can be broadly divided into two categories — stab wounds and gunshot wounds. This division aids in defining the work-up for the patient. It is important to realise that haemodynamically unstable patients should not have an extensive work-up. Resuscitative measures and plain X-rays are all that are required before sending the patient to the operating theatre.

There are six indications for laparotomy in penetrating abdominal trauma:

(1) Peritonitis

Generalised tenderness and guarding would mandate exploration. One should not mistake localised tenderness from the penetrating wound as peritonitis. Tenderness in a quadrant away from the wound should raise the suspicion of intra-abdominal injury. A negative initial examination should prompt serial assessment as abdominal signs may evolve over time. Unevaluable patients should be presumed to have intra-abdominal injury and need appropriate work-up.

(2) Shock

This suggests the presence of significant intra-abdominal bleeding, and would warrant laparotomy. When there is profound shock, there is usually an associated abdominal vascular injury.

(3) Evisceration

Evisceration of bowel or omentum through the wound is an indication for laparotomy as it is associated with significant injury in 78% of patients.[28] In high volume centres, some surgeons have advocated reducing non-significant evisceration, closing the wound and following up with serial abdominal examination.[29,30] The practice is not universally accepted.

(4) Free air

The presence of free air on X-rays imply the breach of abdominal hollow viscera. However, it is not uncommon to see a small amount of air if an abdominal CT is done. This may not be significant, as air may have entered the abdominal cavity from the wound itself.

(5) Blood in tubes or orifices

This may present as blood in the naso-gastric tube or Foleys catheter, or as blood on digital rectal examination. This finding implies injury to the relevant hollow abdominal viscera.

(6) Retained implement

The presence of a retained knife would necessitate laparotomy for removal under direct vision so as to avoid uncontrolled bleeding if a vessel had been penetrated.

All other patients who do not have an immediate indication for laparotomy, come under the asymptomatic stable group. This group of patients needs to be worked up for potential injuries depending on the mechanism of injury — stab versus gunshot wounds.

Stab Wounds

The management of stab wounds to the abdomen when there is no immediate indication for laparotomy, is dependent on the site. The abdomen can be divided into four regions:

(1) Anterior abdomen

This area is defined as lying between the subcostal margin superiorly, pubic symphysis inferiorly and anterior axillary lines laterally. Not all stab wounds in this region penetrate the peritoneum, and not all wounds that penetrate the peritoneum result in significant injury. The risks of significant intra-abdominal injury are summarised by the "rule of thirds" — a third never penetrates the peritoneum, a third penetrates the peritoneum without causing significant intra-abdominal injury, and a third penetrates the peritoneum and results in intra-abdominal injury requiring a laparotomy. Performing local wound exploration (LWE) and looking for penetration of the anterior fascia would exclude those with non-penetration. The depth of the injury can be visualised by extending the wound under local anaesthesia. The anterior fascia is used as a reference as it is difficult to demonstrate actual peritoneal penetration beyond that layer. Patients with non-penetration could be safely discharged home. The remaining two-thirds of patients would have wounds that have penetrated the peritoneum. Mandatory laparotomy for all patients in this group would result in approximately a 50% non-therapeutic laparotomy rate. This is clearly not an acceptable option as even negative laparotomies are associated with significant morbidity.[31] Balanced against this is the fear of delaying the diagnosis of intra-abdominal injury with its attendant morbidity and mortality. To allow earlier diagnosis, DPL can be performed. A positive lavage using similar criteria as for blunt trauma would prompt a laparotomy. Also established is the role of selective conservative management using serial examination alone.[29,32] This region of the abdomen should manifest signs of peritonitis early if there is bowel injury. Such a conservative approach has been shown to be safe but necessitates careful serial clinical examination performed by the same surgeon. This is clearly only an option if there is 24-hour availability of surgeons, anaesthesiologists and operating theatres.

(2) Flank and back

The flank is defined as the area between the anterior and posterior axillary lines from the costal margin to iliac crest. The back lies between the posterior axillary lines. This area of the abdomen has thick abdominal musculature, and stab wounds are less likely to result in penetration. However, injury to the adjacent retroperitoneal organs is less likely to present with early signs. These include injury to the retroperitoneal duodenum, colon, pancreas and kidneys. Triple-contrast CT (oral, intra-venous and colonic contrasts) has been used to define the proximity of the track to vital structures, and allows classification of wounds into low and high risk groups.[16–18] Laparotomy should be considered in the high risk group. This would obviate the problem of severe retroperitoneal sepsis from delayed diagnosis of bowel injury.

(3) Thoraco-abdominal

This area is defined as the area lying below the nipple anteriorly, or the tip of scapular posteriorly, until the costal margin inferiorly. Injury in this zone can potentially involve two cavities. In a hypotensive patient, inserting chest tubes and performing a DPL can quickly point to the responsible cavity. A FAST examination can reveal pericardial fluid, and a subxiphoid pericardial window may then be necessary to confirm the presence of haemopericardium. The difficulty lies in the exclusion of diaphragmatic injury as the defect is often small and not detectable on the chest X-ray. Forty-two per cent of stab wounds to the left thoraco-abdominal region is associated with diaphragmatic injury, and this is occult in 26%.[33] Diagnostic peritoneal lavage has been used taking a reduced red blood cell count to detect diaphragmatic penetration.[9] However, laparoscopy or thoracoscopy remains the most reliable way of diagnosing these injuries.[24,25,34,35] Thoracoscopy should preferably not be employed in the acute setting, as it does not permit the exclusion of intra-abdominal injury. Herniation is less common on the right side (especially posteriorly) because of the buttressing effect of the liver.

(4) Gluteal injuries

Penetrating injuries to this region can result in damage to the pelvic vasculature and viscera (bladder and rectum). The patient may not be hypotensive because of the tamponading effect of the retroperitoneum, and abdominal examination may be misleadingly normal because of the absence of intraperitoneal irritation. The presence of blood in the urine or blood on digital rectal examination should suggest significant injury to these viscera. Sigmoidoscopy should be performed if the wound is near the rectum.

Gunshot Wounds

The bullet from a gunshot wound tends to cause more damage compared to that by a stab wound. It travels a longer distance and can be deflected or fragmented in its path. It also results in higher energy

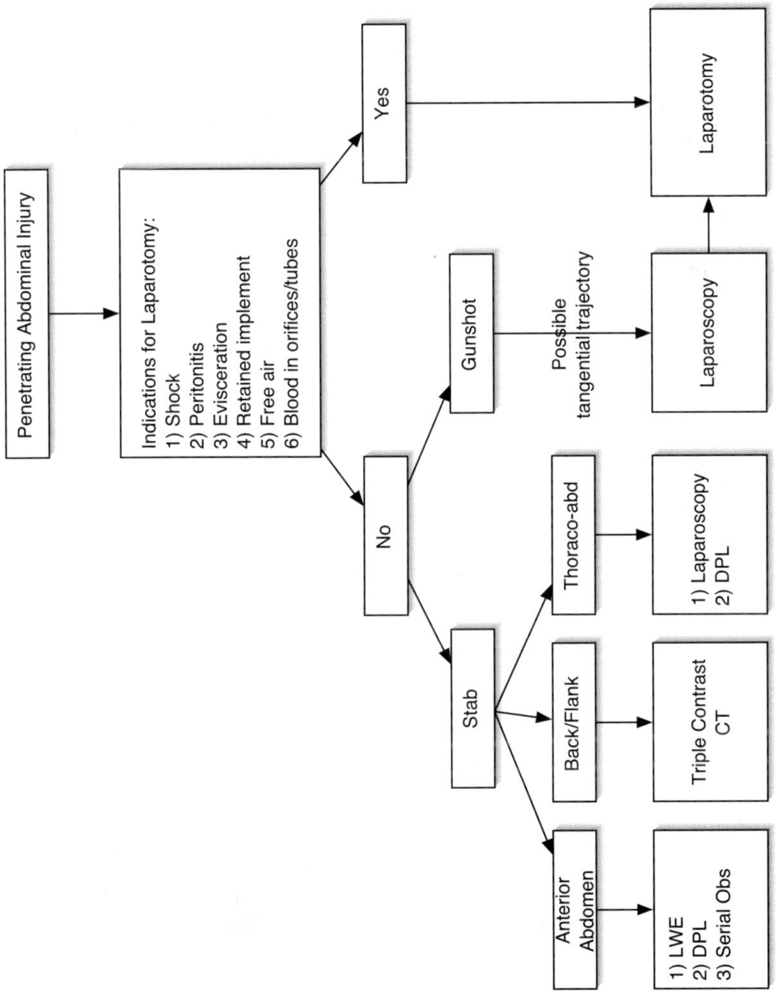

Fig. 10 Algorithm for management of penetrating abdominal trauma.

transfer to the tissues, resulting in greater damage along its trajectory. While clinical examination and X-rays help predict trajectory, it is not always reliable in determining the need for surgery. Whilst the majority of patients will require laparotomy, a small number will present in a stable asymptomatic condition. In this group, diagnostic laparoscopy can confirm the tangential trajectory by demonstrating the absence of peritoneal penetration. However once peritoneal penetration occurs, there is a high rate (over 90%) of significant organ injury and laparotomy is indicated. In gunshot wounds, there is always a small possibility of missile embolus or migration. The "even rule" which states that the sum of external wounds plus the number of bullets seen on X-rays must always be an even number, helps to establish this. An odd number should prompt one to scrutinise the body for missed wounds, and order additional X-rays to document the site of bullet embolus or migration.

Some authors have advocated selective non-operative management of gunshot wounds to the abdomen.[36,37] However, this concept is still controversial.

Shotgun wounds are managed differently depending on the distance from which the rounds were fired. A close-range shotgun wound (less than 3.5 metres) is similar to a wound caused by a high velocity missile. The massive destruction and contamination of soft tissue will require debridement. At longer ranges (more than six metres), the round behaves like a low velocity missile that is less likely to penetrate the abdominal wall.

The algorithm for the management of penetrating abdominal trauma is outlined in Fig. 10.

Summary

The abdomen is often likened to a "black box" as there is no perfect diagnostic investigation, and an injury is sometimes only obvious on opening the abdomen. Clinical examination has to be combined with the judicious use of diagnostic tests chosen based on the patient's haemodynamic status and the mechanism of injury. One has to always balance the morbidity of unnecessary laparotomies with the risk of delayed diagnosis and missed injuries when selective observation is practised.

References

1. West JG, Trunkey DD, Lim RC (1979). Systems of trauma care: a study of two counties. *Arch Sur* **114**(4), 455–460.
2. American College of Surgeons, Committee on Trauma (1997). *Advanced Trauma Life Support.*
3. Velmahos GC, Tatevossian R, Demetriades D (1999). The "seat belt mark" sign: a call for increased vigilance among physicians treating victims of motor vehicle accidents. *Am Surg* **65**(2), 181–185.
4. Root HD, Hauser CW, McKinley CR (1965). Diagnostic peritoneal lavage. *Surgery* **57**, 633–637.
5. Hodgson NF, Stewart TC, Girotti MJ (2000). Open or closed diagnostic peritoneal lavage for abdominal trauma? A meta-analysis. *J Trauma* **48**(6), 1091–1095.
6. Powell DC, Bivins BA, Bell RM (1982). Diagnostic peritoneal lavage. *Surg Gynecol Obstet* **155**(2), 257–264.
7. Henneman PL, Marx JA, Moore EE *et al.* (1990). Diagnostic peritoneal lavage: accuracy in predicting necessary laparotomy following blunt and penetrating trauma. *J Trauma* **30**(11), 1345–1355.
8. Otomo Y, Henmi H, Mashiko K, Kato K, Koike K, Koido Y *et al.* (1998). New diagnostic peritoneal lavage criteria for diagnosis of intestinal injury. *J Trauma* **44**(6), 991–999.
9. Nagy KK, Roberts RR, Joseph KT, Smith RF, An GC, Bokhari F *et al.* (2000). Experience with over 2500 diagnostic peritoneal lavages. *Injury* **31**(7), 479–482.
10. Yao DC, Jeffrey RB, Mirvis SE, Weekes A, Federle MP, Kim C (2002). Using contrast-enhanced helical CT to visualize arterial extravasation after blunt abdominal trauma: incidence and organ distribution. *AJR Am J Roentgenol* **178**(1), 17–20.

11. Willmann JK, Roos JE, Platz A, Pfammatter T, Hilfiker PR, Marincek B *et al.* (2002). Multidetector CT: detection of active hemorrhage in patients with blunt abdominal trauma. *AJR Am J Roentgenol* **179**(2), 437–444.
12. Velmahos GC, Konstantinos GT, Pantelis V, Sarkisyan G, Chan LS, Hanks SH *et al.* (2002). A prospective study on the safety and efficacy of angiographic embolisation for pelvic and visceral injuries. *J Trauma* **52**(2), 303–308.
13. Malhotra AK, Fabian TC, Katsis SB, Gavant ML, Croce MA (2000). Blunt and mesenteric injuries: the role of screening computed tomography. *J Trauma* **48**(6), 991–1000.
14. Butela ST, Federle MP, Chang PJ, Thaete FL, Peterson MS, Dorvault CJ *et al.* (2001). Performance of CT in detection of bowel injury. *AJR Am J Roentgenol* **176**(1), 129–135.
15. Rodriguez C, Barone JE, Wilbanks TO, Rha CK, Miller K (2002). Isolated free fluid on computed tomograpic scan in blunt abdominal trauma: a systematic review of incidence and management. *J Trauma* **53**(1), 79–85.
16. Kirten OC, Wint D, Thrasher B, Windsor J, Echenique A, Hudson-Civetta J (1997). Stab wounds to the back and flank in the hemodynamically stable patient: a decision algorithm based on contrast-enhanced computed tomography with colonic opacification. *Am J Surg* **173**(3), 189–193.
17. Albrecht RM, Vigil A, Schermer CR, Demarest GB 3rd, Davis VH, Fry DE (1999). Stab wounds to the back/flank in hemodynamically stable patients: evaluation using triple-contrast computed tomography. *Am Surg* **65**(7), 683–688.
18. Phillips T, Sclafani SJ, Goldstein A, Scalea T, Panetta T, Shaftan G (1986). Use of contrast-enhanced CT enema in the management of penetrating trauma to the flank and back. *J Trauma* **26**(7), 593–601.
19. Rozycki GS, Ballard RB, Felciano DV, Schmidt JA, Pennington SD (1998). Surgeon-performed ultrasound for the assessment of truncal injuries: lessons learned from 1540 patients. *Ann Surg* **228**(4), 557–567.

20. Dolich MO, McKenney MG, Varela JE, Compton RP, McKenney KL, Cohn SM (2001). 2576 ultrasounds for blunt abdominal trauma. *J Trauma* **50**(1), 108–112.
21. Brown MA, Casola G, Sirlin CB, Patel NY, Hoyt DB (2001). Blunt abdominal trauma: screening US in 2,693 patients. *Radiology* **218**(2), 352–358.
22. McKenney KL, Nunez DB Jr, McKenney MG, Asher J, Zelnick K, Shipshak D (1998). Sonography as the primary screening technique for blunt abdominal trauma: experience with 899 patients. *AJR Am J Roentgenol* **170**(4), 979–985.
23. Shanmuganathan K, Mirvis SE, Sherbourne CD, Chiu WC, Rodriguez A (1999). Hemoperitoneum as the sole indicator of abdominal visceral injuries: a potential limitation of screening abdominal US for trauma. *Radiology* **212**(2), 423–430.
24. Zantut LF, Ivatury RR, Smith S, Kawahara NT, Porter JM, Fry WR *et al.* (1997). Diagnostic and therapeutic laparoscopy for penetrating abdominal trauma. *J Trauma* **42**(5), 825–831.
25. Ivatury RR, Simon RJ, Weksler B, Bayard V, Stahl WM (1992). Laparoscopy in the evaluation of the intrathoracic abdomen after penetrating injury. *J Trauma* **33**(1), 101–109.
26. Simon RJ, Rabin J, Kuhls D (2002). Impact of increased use of laparoscopy on negative laparotomy rates after penetrating trauma. *J Trauma* **53**(2), 297–302.
27. Sarkisian AE, Khondkarian RA, Amirbekian NM, Bagdasarian NB, Khojayan RL, Oganesian YT (1991). Sonographic screening of mass casualties for abdominal and renal injuries following the 1988 Armenian earthquake. *J Trauma* **31**(2), 247–250.
28. Nagy K, Roberts R, Joseph K *et al.* (1999). Evisceration after abdominal stab wounds: is laparotomy necessary? *J Trauma* **47**, 622–626.
29. Demetriades D, Rabinowitz B (1987). Indications for operation in abdominal stab wounds. A prospective study of 651 patients. *Ann Surg* **205**(2), 129–132.
30. McFarlane ME (1996). Non-operative management of stab wounds to the abdomen with omental evisceration. *J R Coll Surg Edinb* **41**(4), 239–240.

31. Renz BM, Feliciano DV (1995). Unnecessary laparotomies for trauma: a prospective study of morbidity. *J Trauma* **38**(3), 350–356.
32. Nance FC, Wennar MH, Johnson LW, Ingram JC Jr, Cohn I Jr (1974). Surgical judgement in the management of penetrating wounds to the abdomen: experience with 2201 patients. *Ann Surg* **179**(5), 639–646.
33. Murray JA, Demetriades D, Cornwell EE 3rd, Ascensio JA, Velmahos G, Belzberg H *et al.* (1997). Penetrating left thoraco-abdominal trauma: the incidence and clinical presentation of diaphragmatic injuries. *J Trauma* **43**(4), 624–626.
34. Ochsner MG, Rozycki GS, Lucente F, Wherry DC, Champion HR (1993). Prospective evaluation of thoracoscopy for diagnosing diaphragmatic injury in thoracoabdominal trauma: a preliminary report. *J Trauma* **34**(5), 704–710.
35. Martinez M, Briz JE, Carillo EH (2001). Video thoracoscopy expedites the diagnosis and treatment of penetrating diaphragmatic injuries. *Surg Endosc* **15**(1), 28–33.
36. Demetriades D, Velmahos GC, Cornwell EE *et al.* (1997). Selective non-operative management of gunshot wounds to the anterior abdomen. *Arch Surg* **132**, 178–183.
37. Velmahos GC, Demetriades D, Foianini E *et al.* (1997). A selective approach to the management of gunshot wounds of the back. *Am J Surg* **174**, 342–346.

Section V

Gynaecological Emergencies

21

Female Genital Bleeding

Sun-Kuie Tay
Ann Tan

Introduction

Bleeding from the female genital tract is a common encounter in emergency medicine. The patients range from young infants to elderly women, and the pathology includes a wide spectrum of diseases. In this chapter, emergency treatment for common disorders presenting with genital tract bleeding are presented. Ectopic pregnancy is discussed in a separate chapter.

Bleeding from the genital tract can originate from the uterine cavity, cervix, vagina, or vulva. The aetiology of genital bleeding varies according to the age of the patient, and whether she is pregnant (Table 1).

Initial Evaluation

History

In a female patient, bleeding from the genital tract can be confused with bleeding from the urinary tract or intestinal tract. The importance

Table 1 Causes of Bleeding from the Female Genital Tract

1. Pre-menarchal girls
   - Estrogen withdrawal in neonatal life
   - Foreign bodies in the vagina
   - Vulvar, hymenal or vaginal injuries from accident or sexual assault
   - Tumours

2. Reproductive-age women

(a) Non-pregnant state
- Menstrual disorders
- Cervical or endometrial polyps
- Cervical ectropion or erosion
- Benign uterine tumours
- Malignant tumours of the uterus, cervix, vagina or vulva
- Genital tract injuries from consented and unconsented sex

(b) Pregnant state
- Threatened abortion
- Abortion and its complications
- Hydatidiform moles
- Ectopic pregnancy
- Antepartum haemorrhage
- Other causes as in the non-pregnant state

3. Post-menopausal women
   - Atrophic vaginitis and/or cervicitis
   - Genital tract malignancy
   - Trauma

of a good and comprehensive history cannot be over emphasised, and should specifically include the following points:

- date of the last normal menstrual period
- regularity of menstrual cycles
- method of contraception, if she is sexually active
- any associated pain in the lower abdomen, genital parts, or tips of shoulders

- any symptoms of urinary tract disease or pelvic inflammation
- any history of trauma
- any history of medication which could influence menstrual flow.

Clinical examination

A general examination and cardiovascular assessment are important in evaluating the severity and impact of the bleeding. A complete abdominal examination should always be followed by a genital examination which includes a careful inspection of the external genitalia, a speculum examination of the vagina and the cervix, and a digital examination of the pelvis. Discretion should be carefully exercised in the examination of children and virginal women. Parental consent is mandatory when examination of a child is contemplated. A rectal examination should also be performed for completeness of assessment of the pelvis, and for detection of ano-rectal diseases.

Investigations

A few simple and valuable investigations are now readily available in the office setting for evalution of the possible cause(s) and severity of genital tract bleeding.

These have, in many instances, become an extended part of clinical examination that most physicians would perform on the patients.

(1) Urinary pregnancy test — *B*-hCG urinary assay is sensitive for detection of the beta subunit of human chorionic gonadotrophin level of 25 iu per litre. This allows an early pregnancy (either intra- or extra-utrine) to be detected. As many women are uncertain of their last menstrual dates, or have irregular ovulation patterns such that an early pregnancy may be unexpected, all women at a reproductive age should have a urinary pregnancy test performed when they present with genital tract bleeding.

(2) Pelvic ultrasound scan — A detailed transvaginal or transabdominal ultrasound scan is now a *de rigeur* in the clinical work-up of women with genital tract bleeding but with no source of bleeding on the cervix, vagina or vulva. The scan may direct the gynecologist's focus to the most likely cause of the bleeding; for example, an ectopic pregnancy compared to a threatened abortion.

(3) Office hysteroscopy and endometrial sampling — Bleeding from the uterine cavity may arise from endometritis, endometrial polyps, submucous leiomyoma, or malignancy. An office hysteroscopy allows the condition of the uterine cavity to be clearly visualised. Any pathology encountered can be biopsied for histopathological assessment. In the absence of an obvious lesion, the endometrium can be sampled with one of the many available samplers for cytological or histological assessment to exclude endometritis, endometrial hyperplasia or malignancy. These procedures have greatly reduced the need for formal dilatation and currettage.

(4) Laparoscopy — The abdomen and pelvis can easily be accessed with a laparoscope. When an accurate diagnosis of the genital tract bleeding is uncertain, and the clinical condition warrants it, an emergency laparoscopy may have to be performed for an exact diagnosis, such as an ectopic gestation, to be made.

Management of Common Genital Tract Bleedings

Early pregnancy related vaginal bleeding

More than 20% of pregnancies are lost before eight weeks of gestation; another 20% of pregnancies are complicated by vaginal bleeding during the first trimester, and 1% of pregnancies are ectopic in location. The differential diagnosis is outlined in Tables 2 and 3. A common presenting symptom of all these conditions is vaginal bleeding. A good menstrual history often helps in the diagnosis of pregnancy but

Table 2 Differential Diagnoses for Bleeding in Early Pregnancy

Threatened abortion
Complete abortion
Incomplete abortion
Blighted ovum
Molar pregnancy
Ectopic pregnancy

Table 3 Typical Clinical and Sonographic Findings of Different Types of Abortion

Term	Clinical Signs	Serial HCG Levels	Ultrasound Findings
Threatened abortion	Vaginal bleeding, Closed cervix	Normal exponential rise	Embryo with cardiac activity
Complete abortion	Complete passage of embryo and gestational tissue	Rapid fall	Empty uterus
Incomplete abortion	Incomplete passage of gestational tissue	Slow fall or rapid plateau	Typically thickened and irregular endometrium or fluid within endometrial cavity
Inevitable abortion	Bleeding often with clots and uterine cramps	Variable, usually plateau	Gestational sac in process of expulsion
Embryonic demise	Lack of uterine growth, absent foetal heart tones	Variable, initial normal rise then plateau or fall	Discrete embryo lacking cardiac activity
Blighted ovum	Lack of uterine growth, absent foetal heart tones	Variable, initial normal rise then plateau or fall	Discrepancy in gestational sac development and embryonic development with little or no embryonic remnant

absence of a period of amenorhoea does not exclude a pregnancy. Indeed, all women in the reproductive ages and who had a recent sexual exposure, should be considered pregnant until proven otherwise.

Pain is not a reliable discriminatory indicator of diagnosis of genital tract bleeding in women, although an uncomplicated threatened abortion is generally pain free; an inevitable or incomplete abortion tends to be associated with a cramp-like lower abdominal pain. Ectopic pregnancies may manifest with an excruciating abdominal pain as often as without any pain. However, abdominal tenderness on clinical examination, particularly rebound tenderness, is generally absent in abortions or threatened abortions, but notable in ectopic pregnancies. On speculum examination, bleeding from the uterine cavity can be ascertained and, sometimes, product of conception in the cervical os or vagina will declare the right diagnosis. On digital and bimanual examination, dilatation of the cervical os; uterine size; presence of pelvic masses; and tenderness, are all important signs for an accurate diagnosis.

Transvaginal sonography (TVS) permits visualisation of early gestations with immense detail of the gestational sac, yolk sac and embryo. The accuracy of diagnosis hinges on the operator's understanding of the natural development of the gestational sac, and knowing when it can be visualised with certainty, and being aware of the expected sizes of the gestational sac, foetal pole and yolk sac (Table 4).

The early gestational sac must be differentiated from a decidual reaction seen in the presence of an ectopic pregnancy. There is a characteristic echogenic "double decidual sac" which is normally sited to one side of the mid-endometrial echo at the uterine fundus. Once visualised, the gestational sac grows at a fairly constant rate of 1 mm per day.

The presence of a yolk sac is the earliest sign that the pregnancy is progressing well. The yolk sac gradually increases in size from 3.4 mm to 5.4 mm. Early detection of foetal heart activity is possible as the foetus is connected to the yolk sac until 8 weeks (Fig. 1). Threatened abortion is confirmed when the viability of the foetus is

Table 4 Sonographic Detection of Embryonic Landmarks Related to Gestational Sac Size

Sonographic Landmark	Age at Detection (weeks)	Gestational Sac Size (mm)
Gestational sac	4.5	5
Yolk sac	5	10
Embryo	6	18
Foetal heart pulsations	6	18

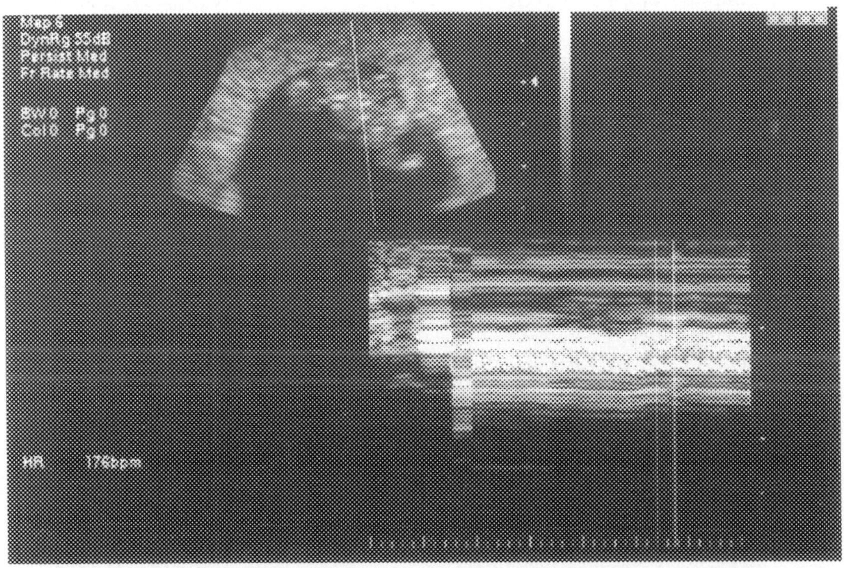

Fig. 1 A transvaginal sonograph showing an embryo of 8 weeks and 1 day gestation. The viability of the embryo is demonstrated on the B-mode display.

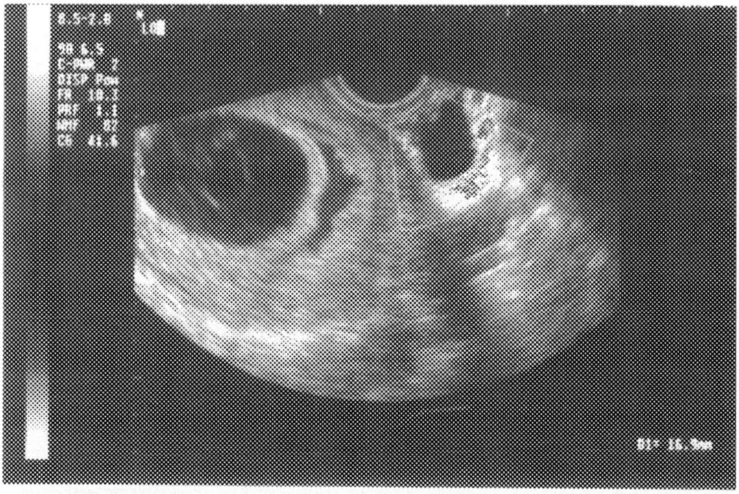

Fig. 2 A transvaginal sonograph from a case of threatened abortion. The gestational sac with a viable embryo is shown on the left of the photograph. On the right-hand side of the sac is a blood clot measuring 1.6 cm in diameter.

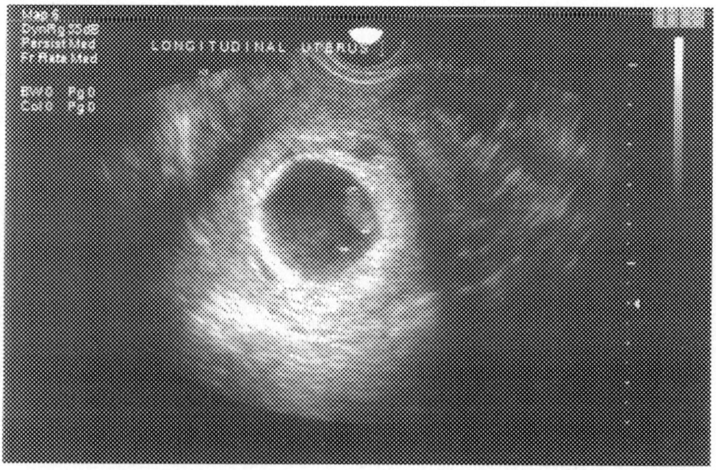

Fig. 3 A transvaginal sonograph showing a missed abortion. The embryo had no detectable heart pulsation.

demonstrated on the scan.[1] Sometimes, presence of an extra-amniotic blood clot may be seen on the scan (Fig. 2). Absence of heart pulsation in an embryo is diagnostic of a missed abortion (Fig. 3).

Transabdominal ultrasound is less sensitive in the early diagnosis of pregnancy, as the visualisation through the multiple layers of skin, muscles, and bladder attenuates the picture of the uterine contents greatly. Generally speaking, the embryonic landmarks described above seem to be detectable a week later than the transvaginal sonography.[2]

Management of Threatened Abortion

In the presence of a viable foetus, threatened abortion is a self-limiting disease, and spontaneous recovery can be expected in the great majority of cases. Curtailed physical activity during the active bleeding phase may shorten the duration of bleeding manifestation. Hospital admission is not necessary. Hormonal therapy with progestogens is widely practised, although evidence of luteal insufficiency is rarely observed, and objective benefits are not seen in clinical trials.[3]

Management of Abortions

Complete abortion as evidenced by diminishing vaginal bleeding and an empty uterus on ultrasound scan can be managed expectantly. Vaginal bleeding generally ceases within a week, and the normal menstruation cycle resumes with no delays.

Anembryonic pregnancy and missed abortion in the first 10 weeks of gestation usually abort spontaneously. Complete abortion occurs in more than 75% of cases. The duration of vaginal bleeding may be prolonged for up to two weeks, which is significantly longer than surgical evacuation of the uterus. The patient can opt for conservative management or an evacuation of the uterus.[4]

Incomplete abortions are usually complicated by heavy vaginal bleeding and uterine contraction pain. Surgical evacuation is indicated. Evacuation of the uterus is mandatory in septic abortion.

Evacuation of Uterus

Pre-operative management

The patient must be assessed clinically for suitability for general anaesthesia. Appropriate laboratory tests must be performed, most notably, a full blood count and ABO and Rhesus blood group determination.

While awaiting surgery, the patient's vaginal bleeding maybe controlled with intra-muscular or intra-venous ergometrine administration. Coagulopathy is uncommon, and routine coagulation profile investigation is not indicated.

Intra-operative management

Gravid uterus is usually very soft and easily perforated by the insertion of a Hegar dilator or currette, particularly in cases with the uterus in acute anteversion or retroversion. Judicious care is needed.

The amount of blood loss during evacuation of the uterus is closely related to the time taken to empty the uterine cavity. Expeditious evacuation can be achieved with a suction currette. Excessive dilatation and curretage should be avoided, as it can result in Asherman's syndrome with formation of uterine synechie within the cavity, causing iatrogenic amenorrhoea.[5] Currettings should be sent for histology as a rule, to confirm the diagnosis and to exclude hydatidiform mole.

Late Pregnancy Complications: Antepartum Haemorrhage

The second trimester of pregnancy traditionally denotes the period between the 14th and 28th weeks of gestation, before a foetus is viable extra-uterine. With the recent improvement in neonatal intensive therapy, newborns of 24 weeks gestation or of body weight above 500 g at birth have a reasonable chance of surviving nowadays. This change effectively redefines threatened abortions as vaginal bleeding in pregnancies of less than 24 weeks gestation.[6] Vaginal bleeding after the 24th week is considered antepartum haemorrhage. In both conditions, the management of vaginal bleeding should be done in an obstetric unit.

Antepartum haemorrhage can be caused by placenta praevia, abruptio placentae or other incidental bleeding from lesions on the cervix, vagina or vaulva.

Placenta praevia

Placenta praevia is defined as implantation of the placenta in the lower uterine segment, below the foetal presenting part. Classification is based on the location of the placenta relative to the cervical os. Placenta praevia is described as either major or minor, depending on whether the internal os is covered by the placenta.

The incidence of placenta praevia occurs in 1 in 200 to 250 pregnancies. The incidence is lower in nulliparous women, and higher in older and multiparous women. Ten per cent of placenta praevia occur after a previous lower segment caesarean section in a preceding pregnancy.

Diagnosis is made in with certainty through ultrasound in the third trimester. Transvaginal ultrasound is more accurate when a posterior praevia is suspected. Clinical suspicion should be aroused by the classical presentation of painless vaginal bleeding.

The management is largely dictated by the maternal condition. The first priority is to stabilise the haemodynamic state of the pregnant woman. The subsequent management is determined by gestational age, severity of the bleeding and foetal condition.

After 37 weeks of gestation, the patient should be prepared for a caesarean section with adequate grouped and cross-matched blood on standby. A paediatrician should also be on hand to receive the baby in cases where a significant blood loss from the baby is anticipated.

Between 34 and 37 weeks, there is no real necessity to wait for further maturity of the foetus as most neonatal facilities are able to support the neonatal period with little morbidity and mortality. If the antepartum haemorrhage is of significant severity to require blood transfusion, delivery of the foetus by caesarean section is indicated.

Between 24 and 34 weeks gestation, patients should be managed expectantly to "buy" time for foetal maturity as long as the patient and foetus are in a stable haemodynamic condition. Tocolytics may be used to suppress labour, while steroids are given to enhance foetal lung maturity. The patient's haemoglobin level should ideally be maintained at greater than 11 g/dl, and group and crossed matched blood should be readily obtainable at any time.

Abruptio placenta

Abruptio placenta is defined as premature separation of a placenta, which is implanted in the upper segment of the uterus, from the uteirne wall. Abruptio placenta occurs in approximately one in 120 pregnancies. Perinatal mortality is four in 1000 affected pregnancies.

Increased incidence of abruptio placenta is associated with advanced maternal age and multiparity, poor nutrition, maternal hypertension and chorioamnionitis. A rapid contraction of an over-distended uterus, as seen in the delivery of a multiple gestation or singleton with polyhydramnios. It can also occur as result of blunt trauma to the abdomen, as in a seat belt injury. Abruptio placenta has a recurrence rate of 5% to 17% after one affected pregnancy, and 25% after two affected pregnancies.

Abruptio placenta tends to be sudden in onset, and is associated with uterine contraction pain and tenderness. Eighty per cent of affected patients experience external vaginal bleeding. Maternal blood pressure and heart rate, foetal heart rate pattern and uterine tone are important diagnostic clues on physical examination.

Ultrasound should be used to exclude placenta praevia, determine the foetal lie, and obtain an estimate of the foetal weight. It is, however, unreliable as a diagnostic tool.

The management depends on the severity of the bleed and the maturity of the foetus. If the foetus is more than 34 weeks gestation and the mother is stable, induction of labour with a view to a vaginal delivery can be attempted. An emergency caesarean section should be performed in cases of foetal distress or maternal haemorrhage, and for traditional obstetric indications.

Other placental complications

Placenta accreta is adherence of placenta to the uterine wall without the usual intervening decidua basalis. Placenta increta is placenta accreta that invades the myometrium, and placenta percreta is placenta accreta that penetrates the entire uterine wall. Whenever any of these complications is anticipated, the mother and her spouse should be informed of the risk of severe post-partum haemorrhage and the possibility of a caesarean hysterectomy.

Vasa praevia is vaginal bleeding secondary to the rupture of a foetal blood vessel — usually a velamentous cord insertion. Foetal mortality is high, and the foetus usually presents itself with evidence of distressed foetal heart rate pattern on electronic heart rate monitoring. An emergency caesarean section is indicated.

Post-partum Haemorrhage

Post-partum haemorrhage is defined as a loss of more than 500 ml of blood during the first 24 hours after a vaginal delivery. It still contributes significantly to maternal mortality in the developing world. In Singapore, this condition presents itself to the emergency department only if the delivery occurs precipitately at home or on the way to hospital. These cases are immediately transferred to obstetricians for management. In the emergency room, basic principles of resuscitation to maintain an adequate circulatory function, and to prevent cardiopulmonary collapse, should be exercised.

Uterine atony is the main cause of post-partum haemorrhage. Predisposing factors include multiparity; overdistension from multiple gestation or polyhydramnios; chorioamnionitis or prior use of tocolytic agents. Instrumental delivery also increases the risk of severe haemorrhage.

Management

Bimanual massage of the uterus with one hand in the vagina and the other hand rubbing up the uterus per abdomen, must be the first manoeuvre while oxytocic agents are given either intravenously, intramuscularly or directly into the myometrium to cause a sustained uterine contraction.

When interventional radiology facility is available, uterine arterial embolisation provides a good alternative to surgical ligation of uterine arteries or internal iliac arteries.[7] The embolisation procedure should be considered early while the patient remains stable in the haemodynamic condition.

Fatality from post-partum haemorrhage due to uterine atony is usually attributed to delay in definitive surgery. If the uterus fails to respond to medical treatment, the patient should, after stabilising of the haemodynamic state, undergo an emergency laparotomy. If preservation of the uterus is requested by the patient, the internal iliac arteries should be ligated bilaterally. In all other cases, emergency hysterectomy is indicated.[8]

Should the bleeding persist despite good uterine contraction, other causes of post-partum haemorrhage, for example, vaginal or cervical lacerations, and retained products of conception, must be considered and excluded.

Lacerations

Lacerations should be suspected if an operative delivery was technically difficult. Most commonly, lacerations involve the cervix or vagina. In women with previous caesarean section or uterine surgery, rupture of the uterus can occur. The diagnosis must be ascertained by a thorough vaginal examination with adequate exposure of the cervix and the entire vagina under good illumination, and if necessary, in an operating theatre. The bleeder should be identified, and the laceration repaired. In cases of uterine ruptures, an emergency hysterectomy may be life saving.

Non-pregnant Causes of Female Genital Bleeding

In dealing with a patient of reproductive age who complains of an abnormal vaginal bleeding, one must always bear in mind that she may be pregnant. A history of a period of amenorrhoea is suggestive, but absence of history of amenorrhoea does not preclude a pregnancy. Appropriate measures, including a urinary pregnancy test with sensitive beta-subunit human chorionic gonadotrophin, must be carried out. After exclusion of a pregnancy, the physician's attention is directed towards making a diagnosis which includes trauma, tumour, inflammatory conditions and dysfunctional uterine bleeding. A detailed history of the complaint and meticulous abdominal and pelvic examination, often allow an accurate diagnosis to be reached.

Trauma

Lacerations can occur on the cervix, vaginal fornices, hymen or labia. This may be caused by both consensual and unconsensual sexual intercourse, and with or without the use of sexual aids. Foreign bodies and instrumentation in the vagina can also cause trauma to the genital tract and bleeding.

Bleeding from trauma in the genital tract manifests as bright red fresh blood. It can be brisk and severe, depending on the site and size of lacerations. Adequate exposure of the entire genital tract for inspection with a bright light source is mandatory, and the diagnosis is evident. Immediate repair of the trauma under anaesthesia is needed.[9]

Benign tumours and pseudo-tumours

These are common on the cervix, most notably the polyps and leiomyomata. Condylomata acuminata or genital warts are sometimes found as "tumours" on the vulva, vagina or cervix (Figs. 4 and 5).

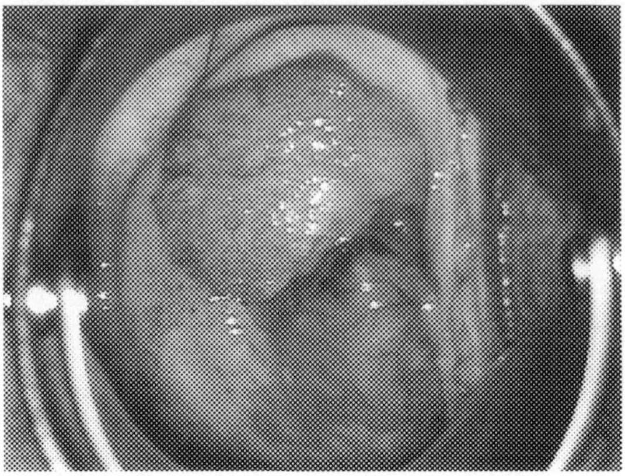

Fig. 4 A colpohotograph of a large condyloma acuminatum (wart) on the cervix.

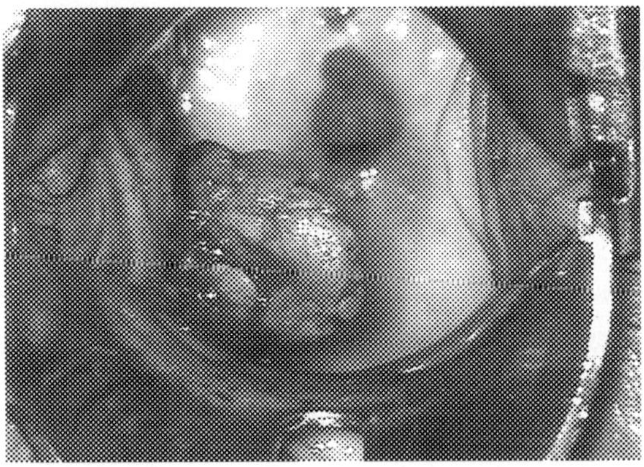

Fig. 5 A colphotograph of large condylomata acuminata in the vagina.

Endometrial polyps/cervical polyps

An endometrial polyp sometimes protrudes from the cervical os to appear as a red polypoid lesion on the cervix. Not uncommonly, the lesion may extend to manifest outside the introitus as a red and fleshy tumour. Cervical polyps are classically cherry red polypoid lesions sessile on the cervix. Cervical polyps most often encountered in clinical practice have the stalk at the lower end of the endocervical

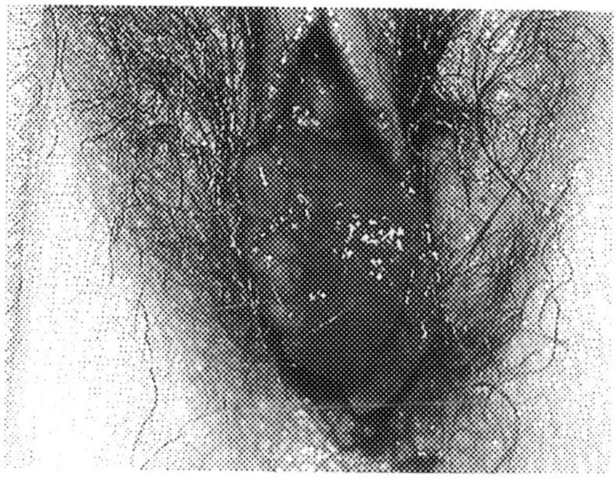

Fig. 6 A photograph showing a large endometrial polyp protruding through the introitus.

canal. These benign polyps are often asymptomatic, particularly the cervical polyp. However, symptomatic polyps usually present with intermenstrual bleeding or postcoital bleeding. The bleeding is typically painless (Fig. 6).

Generally, polyps can be treated at the bed-side by avulsion on speculum examination. Polyps with thick, vascular stalks are preferably treated in the operating theatre. The stalk of the polyp may be ligated before division, and the base of the stalk cauterised with electrocautery after avulsion. Under anaesthesia, the endometrial cavity can be further assessed with hysteroscopy to exclude other endometrial polyps concealed within the cavity.

Fibroids

Uterine leiomyoma can present as a polyp on the cervix, or extending from the cervix into the vagina. There is generally an antecedent history of menorrhagia. A fibroid polyp can be distinguished from an endometrial and cervical polyp by its firm to hard consistency on digital palpation. The uterus may be enlarged and irregular in contour to indicate the presence of other leiomyomata. An ultrasound scan is a useful evaluation tool.

If the presenting bleeding is not excessive, the patient can be treated electively with hysteroscopy and transcervical myomectomy. Women with multiple leiomyomata and menorrhagia may be offered a total hysterectomy as an option. Those with brisk bleeding from vascular fibroid polyps require an emergency polypectomy under general anaesthesia.

Malignant tumours

Gynaecological cancers are prevalent, accounting for 17% of all the cancers in women. In Singapore, carcinoma of the lower genital tract and, most notably, cervical cancer, accounts for 50% of all the gynaecological cancers. Endometrial cancer makes up another 20%.

Carcinoma of the vulva, vagina, cervix and uterus typically present with abnormal vaginal bleeding. Cervical cancer and endometrial cancer sometimes present at the emergency room with heavy vaginal bleeding. Spontaneous bleeding from these cancers is generally light while bleeding provoked by sexual intercourse can be very heavy. Careful inspection on speculum examination of the vulva, vagina and cervix will allow the diagnosis of the respective cancer. Endometrial cancer, on the other hand, requires a hysteroscopy for its detection.

When the bleeding is excessive, the patient should be admitted, and vascular access secured. If necessary, vascular support with intravenous fluid replacement, plasma expander or blood transfusion should be instituted without delay. Endometrial cancer most often presents in the early stage and can be treated with total hysterectomy, bilateral salpingo-ophorectomy and pelvic and para-aortic lymphadenectomy.

Cervical cancer, on the other hand, often presents late with parametrial and vaginal infiltration, precluding surgical options of treatment. Emergency hysterectomy is out of the question. The brisk bleeding can be treated with vaginal packing. If the bleeding persists, an emergency arterial embolisation by interventional radiology is recommended. Once the patient's condition is stable, a formal cancer staging with cystoscopy, sigmoidoscopy and parametrial and pelvic assessment under anaesthesia may be carried out, and appropriate definitive treatment with concurrent chemo-radiotherapy initiated.

Systemic Causes of Abnormal Uterine Bleeding

Women with disorders of coagulation can present with genital tract bleeding.[10] These include congenital clotting factor deficiency, anticoagulant therapy, and idiopathic or secondary thrombocytopenia. Acute thrombocytopenia from haemorrhagic dengue fever sometimes presents with excessive vagina bleeding. The treatment is supportive, and involves replacement of clotting factors with fresh frozen plasma, fresh blood or platelets.

Conclusion

Female genital tract bleeding is a common encounter in the emergency department. An precise diagnosis can be reached by a detailed history, clinical examination, aided by simple bedside investigations such as a urinary pregnancy test, transvaginal pelvic ultrasound scan, and office hysteroscopy and endometrial sampling. In a more critical situation, an emergency laparoscopy allows a thorough evaluation of the abdominal and pelvic cavity for a definitive diagnosis to be made. Treatment of genital tract bleeding depends on the aetiology.

Acknowledgements

We thank Mrs LC Cheow, Senior Ultrasonographer, Department of Obstetrics and Gynaecology for providing Figs. 1 to 3.

References

1. Ball RH (2000). The sonography of pregnancy loss. *Semin Reprod Med* **18**(4), 351–355.
2. Wong TW, Lau CC, Yeung A, Lo L, Tai CM (1998). Efficacy of transabdominal ultrasound examination in the diagnosis of early pregnancy complications in an emergency department. *J Accid Emerg Med* **15**(3), 155–158.

3. Gerhard I, Gwinner B, Eggert-Kruse W, Runnebaum B (1987). Double-blind controlled trial of progesterone substitution in threatened abortion. *Biol Res Pregnancy Perinatol* **8**(1), 26–34.
4. Wieringa-de Waard M, Vos J, Bonsel GJ, Bindels PJ, Ankum WM (2002). Management of miscarriage: a randomized controlled trial of expectant management versus surgical evacuation. *Hum Reprod* **17**(9), 2445–2450.
5. Schenker JG (1996). Etiology of and therapeutic approach to synechia uteri. *Eur J Obstet Gynecol Reprod Biol* **65**(1), 109–113.
6. American College of Obstetricians and Gynecologists (2002). ACOG Practice Bulletin: Clinical Management Guidelines for Obstetrician-Gynecologists: Number 38, September 2002. Perinatal care at the threshold of viability. *Obstet Gynecol* **100**(3), 617–624.
7. Tourne G, Collet F, Seffert P, Veyret C (2003). Place of embolization of the uterine arteries in the management of post-partum haemorrhage: a study of 12 cases. *Eur J Obstet Gynecol Reprod Biol* **110**(1), 29–34.
8. Roopnarinesingh R, Fay L, McKenna P (2003). A 27-year review of obstetric hysterectomy. *J Obstet Gynaecol* **23**(3), 252–254.
9. Fallat ME, Weaver JM, Hertweck SP, Miller FB (1998). Late follow-up and functional outcome after traumatic reproductive tract injuries in women. *Am Surg* **64**(9), 858–861.
10. Ewenstein BM (1996). The pathophysiology of bleeding disorders presenting as abnormal uterine bleeding. *Am J Obstet Gynecol* **175**(3 Pt 2), 770–777.

22

Ectopic Pregnancy

Hak-Koon Tan
Su-Ling Yu
Sun-Kuie Tay

Introduction

Ectopic pregnancy is defined as the implantation of a fertilised ovum outside the uterine cavity. It was first described in medical literature by Abulcasis in 936 AD.[1] Ectopic pregnancy is a major problem in gynaecology because it is often difficult to diagnose, is one of the main causes of maternal mortality, and is associated with impaired fertility among the survivors. The outcome of ectopic pregnancy depends on early diagnosis and appropriate prompt treatment.

Ectopic pregnancy is frequently seen in the emergency department. It complicates 1% of all pregnancies. The incidence has been increasing over the last few decades worldwide. This may be due to the increase in aetiological factors such as pelvic inflammatory disease, therapeutic abortions, promiscuity, and more widespread use of assisted reproductive techniques.

Classification

Ectopic pregnancy is defined as any pregnancy occurring outside the uterine cavity. Ninety-five per cent of ectopic pregnancies occur at the fallopian tube. The ampullary region of the fallopian tube is the commonest site of implantation of ectopic gestation. The rest of ectopic gestations are found in the isthmic, fimbrial or interstitial portions of the tube.

Ovarian ectopic pregnancy may occur when the fertilised ovum implants directly on the ovary or as a result of tubal abortion and re-implantation on the ovary. The incidence is reported to be between one per 2000 to one per 8500 deliveries. When the ectopic gestation implants on an abdominal structure, such as the omentum, mesentary or intestinal serosa, it is known as an abdominal ectopic pregnancy. This is very rare and is one of the very few conditions when ectopic gestation can survive the entire pregnancy. The other very rare location for ectopic implantation is the uterine cervix or the cervical ectopic pregnancy.

Heterotopic pregnancy is the combination of an ectopic pregnancy with an intra-uterine pregnancy. Naturally occurring heterotopic pregnancies are very rare, with an incidence of one per 30,000 deliveries. However, its incidence has increased significantly as a result of the introduction of intra-uterine transfer of multiple embryos in assisted reproductive treatment of infertility, such as *in vitro* fertilisation.

Aetiology

In a natural conception, the ovum is fertilised in the ampullary portion of the Fallopian tube. The gamete takes five to seven days to be transported into the endometrial cavity where implantation takes place. During the course of migration down the Fallopian tube, the gamete undergoes multiplication in the early embryo development. Any condition resulting in narrowing of the lumen of the Fallopian tube, or slowing down of the motility of the Fallopian tube, may lead to entrapment of the embryo in the Fallopian tube and cause an ectopic pregnancy. Several conditions are known to cause tubal damages or changes that increase the incidence of ectopic pregnancy. It is important to consider these conditions when evaluating the probability of the patient having an ectopic pregnancy.

Pelvic inflammatory disease

Pelvic inflammatory disease (PID) is widely regarded as the most important aetiological factor in ectopic pregnancy. Acute PID, most commonly resulting from an ascending infection from the lower genital tract, typically causes bilateral salpingitis, oophoritis and pelvic peritonitis. Neisserial gonorrhoea and chlamydia trachomatis are the two commonest organisms isolated in acute salpingitis. Other possible organisms include *Mycoplasma hominis* and *Mycobacterium tuberculosis*. The infection damages the endosalpingx with loss of the ciliated epithelium. This will impede the transportation of the gamete through the Fallopian tube. In more severe cases of infection, the fibrosis occurring as a result of healing of the Fallopian tube causes narrowing of the lumen, or formation of luminal synechae. A gamete can be lodged in one of these locations and then develop into an ectopic pregnancy.

Endometriosis

Endometriosis is defined as the presence of endometrial tissue outside the endometrial lining. Pelvic endometriosis or endometriotic cyst is associated with tubal and ovarian damage or adhesion formation. Alterations in tubal peristaltic action, and damage of ciliary motility within the tube, impede normal passage of fertilised ovum, thus predisposing to ectopic gestation.

Use of intra-uterine contraceptive devices

The use of intra-uterine contraceptive devices has been associated with an increase in ectopic pregnancy.[2] Several mechanisms have been proposed to explain the role of intra-uterine devices in the causation of ectopic pregnancies. The presence of intra-uterine contraceptive devices induces a low grade inflammatory response in the endometrium, with secretion of cytokines which are toxic to sperms and inhibit movement of sperms into the fallopian tubes. Intra-uterine contraceptive devices also slow down the motility of the fallopian tubes and impede sperm movement in the tubes. These are believed to be the main independent mechanisms responsible for the contraceptive effect in these women. If a small number of sperms do travel to the ampullary portion of the fallopian tube and fertilise the ovum, the gamete may not be able to implant in the endometrial cavity because of the hostile local environment. In some cases, the gamates may implant in the fallopian tubes because slow tubal motility delays transportation of the gametes into the endometrial cavity. The probability of becoming pregnant despite usage of intra-uterine contraceptive devices is approximately 2% annually. Of these pregnancies, 10% are ectopic pregnancies.

Tubal surgeries

Tubal ligation is a common method of permanent contraception among women. The common feature of all types of tubal ligation is local tissue crush injury which leads to scar formation. The scar tissues produce the permanent tubal blockade that prevents sperms from accessing the ovum. The probability of conceiving after tubal ligation is approximately two in 1000. The small defect in the scar through which some sperms traverse to fertilise the ovum may be too small to allow a gamete from passing. Consequently, an incidence of ectopic pregnancy as high as 50% has been reported in these women.

Similarly, tubal reconstruction is associated with an increased incidence of ectopic pregnancy. Microsurgical reconstruction may restore tubal patency but the loss of ciliary function from the initial cause of tubal obstruction predisposes to the risk of ectopic pregnancy in these women. Scars at the site of tubal reconstruction and re-anastomosis are responsible for some ectopic pregnancies in some women.

Assisted reproduction treatment

Fertility treatment with *in vitro* fertilisation techniques has been associated with increased chances of ectopic pregnancy. Two or more embryos may be transferred into the uterine cavity. Some embryos may gain access to the fallopian tubes as a result of either an inadvertant direct injection of embryos into the fallopian tube, or spontaneous migration of embryos from the uterine cavity to the fallopian tube. Other assisted reproduction methods involving direct placement of gametes or zygotes into the fallopian tubes, in procedures such as gamete intra-fallopian transfer (GIFT) or zygote intra-fallopian transfer (ZIFT), may further increase the risk of ectopic pregnancy.

Assisted reproduction treatments have gained wide acceptance by subfertile women during the last two decades. The high prevalence of these treatments has markedly increased the incidence of ectopic pregnancies.

Presentation

Ectopic pregnancy can present in a variety of ways. The most common symptoms are lower abdominal pain, a variable duration of amenorrhoea, and abnormal vaginal bleeding. The severity and mode of onset of the symptoms determine three clinical presentations of ectopic pregnancy:

Catastrophic presentation

Acute rupture of the fallopian tube causes massive intra-peritoneal haemorrhage, acute abdominal pain and cardiovascular collapse. There may be a short history of lower abdominal pain, shoulder tip pain or interscapular pain which usually evolves rapidly. A clinical picture of shock with hypotension and tachycardia is evident. Typically, the abdomen presents with a generalised rigidity and rebound tenderness. Bimanual pelvic examination is unsatisfactory because of exquisite tenderness.

Ectopic gestation in the isthmus or interstitial portion of the fallopian tube is more likely to present with a catastrophic clinical condition than ectopic pregnancy elsewhere. It usually occurs between six and eight weeks of amenorrhoea, and accounts for less than 10% of all ectopic pregnancies.

Active presentation

Ectopic pregnancy most frequently presents acutely with sharp lower abdominal pain with rebound tenderness and vaginal bleeding, but, with little cardiovascular changes such as a mild elevation of pulse rate. Sixty per cent of ectopic pregnancies occur in the right fallopian tube, but the maximum point of tenderness elicited during abdominal examination may not be localised to the side of the ectopic gestation. Bimanual examination elicits exquisite tenderness which precludes palpation of any adnexal masses.

Acute ectopic pregnancy may be the manifestation of a ruptured gestation in the ampullary portion of the fallopian tube, or distension of the fallopian tube by an unruptured gestation, or tubal abortion into the abdominal cavity.

Sub-acute presentation

Sub-acute presentation of ectopic pregnancy is common, and presents in a number of guises. It is often a diagnostic dilemma and requires a high index of suspicion in arriving at the right diagnosis. The patient complains of abdominal pain which may be localised to the iliac fossa, or experienced diffusely across the lower abdomen. The pain may be constant in nature, colicky, or vague and non-descriptive. It may mimic symptoms of constipation or urinary tract infection.

The amount and characteristics of vaginal bleeding is also variable, ranging from staining of blood to bleeding similar to that of menstruation. The period of amenorrhoea may be confused by the pattern of bleeding from ectopic pregnancy.

On bimanual examination, there may be localised tenderness at one of the fornices, and the cervical excitation test is positive. There may be a tender swelling in the adnexum.

Diagnosis and Investigations

Since the availability of beta-hCG sub-unit assay, the early diagnosis of pregnancy is now possible. Ectopic pregnancy must be differentiated from threatened abortion or incomplete abortion. The use of ultrasonography to exclude an intra-uterine pregnancy allows ectopic pregnancy to be diagnosed early in suspected cases.

Measurement of beta-hCG

Detection of beta-hCG in serum confirms the presence of trophoblastic tissue in 99–100% of cases. Beta-hCG can be detected in serum as early as seven to 10 days after ovulation or embryo transfer. Following the development of trophoblastic tissue, the serum concentration of beta-hCG increases exponentially, and has a doubling time of 48 hours. Subnormal rates of increase in serum concentrations of beta-hCG are indicative of an abnormal gestation, but not diagnostic of ectopic pregnancy. Nonetheless, the test is very useful when combined with a transvaginal ultrasound scan in the clinical management of suspected ectopic pregnancies.

Ultrasonography

The ultrasound scan has been widely used in the diagnosis of ectopic pregnancy since the time of Donald (1965). Demonstration of an ectopic gestation on a transvaginal ultrasound scan is occasionally possible, but more often, the role of ultrasound is to exclude an intra-uterine pregnancy. The presence of an intra-uterine gestational sac, in general, excludes an ectopic pregnancy, except in the presence of a heterotopic pregnancy.

Serum beta-hCG is detectable very early in pregnancy, whereas an intra-uterine gestational sac can only be visualised on the ultrasound scan 28 days after conception. Generally speaking, an intra-uterine gestational sac is detectable on the ultrasound scan when the serum beta-hCG concentration reaches 1000 IU/ml. Beyond this concentration of serum beta-hCG, absence of an intra-uterine gestational sac on a transvaginal ultrasound scan is highly suggestive of an ectopic pregnancy.

It is important to distinguish between a genuine sac of intra-uterine pregnancy and a pseudogestational sac of tubal pregnancy. A genuine sac displays a "double ring" feature which is not seen in a pseudogestational sac of decidual changes of ectopic pregnancy.

Diagnostic laparoscopy

Advances in laparoscopic techniques and their wide clinical application, permit early and accurate diagnosis of ectopic pregnancy. With the availability of laparoscopy, the majority of laparotomies can be avoided. Early diagnosis and treatment have resulted in a significant decrease in maternal morbidity and mortality.

Treatment

Immediate management of suspected ectopic pregnancy is summarised in the algorithm below:

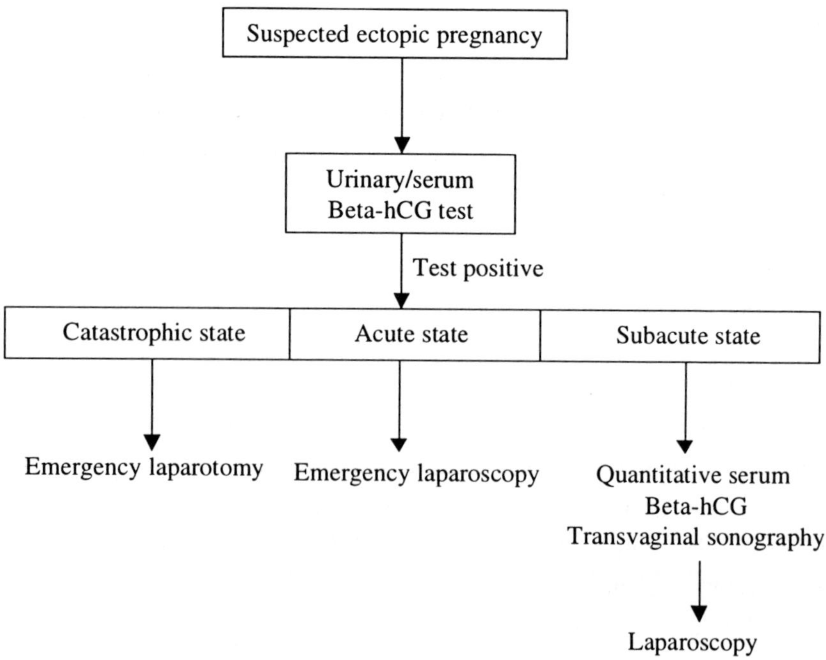

Recent developments in diagnostic procedures and laparoscopic techniques have resulted in early and more conservative management of ectopic pregnancies. Various important factors such as the site of ectopic pregnancy, the clinical presentation, and the desire for future fertility, must be taken into consideration in deciding the best modality of treatment.

Acute management

Patients presenting with acute cardiovascular collapse due to massive intra-peritoneal bleeding must be resuscitated. An intravenous access capable of rapid transfusion of blood must be set up, and blood product or colloid should be rapidly infused.

Immediate exploratory laparotomy must be performed to arrest the source of bleeding.

Salpingectomy

This procedure was first described by Tait in 1884.[3] It remains the life-saving treatment of ectopic pregnancy. It is particularly indicated in patients with ruptured tubal ectopic pregnancy, with severe tubal damage. It is also the preferred treatment for patients with failed conservative treatment of ectopic pregnancy, or for those with pre-existing tubal damage. Patients who have been previously sterilised and do not desire further pregnancy should also be treated with salpingectomy.

Conservative procedures

Partial or segmental salpingectomy with removal of the site of gestational implantation is an adequate treatment for unruptured ectopic pregnancy. It is performed for patients who wish to spontaneously conceive again. Tubal re-anastomosis of the remaining segments may be done at a later stage.

Conservation procedures such as salpingostomy without removing the segment of the tube have become widely practised with good results.[4,5] The anti-mesenteric border on the site of gestational implantation is opened with either a scalpel or electro-cautery, and the product of conception is gently removed. Haemostasis is secured with electrocoagulation. The salpingotomy may be closed or left open.

Microsurgical principles such as gentle handling of the tissues, avoidance of peritoneal damage, meticulous haemostasis, use of fine and non-absorbable sutures to avoid adhesion formation, must be applied during the procedures.

Laparoscopic techniques

The early diagnosis of ectopic pregnancy, and advancements in the field of laparoscopic instruments, have led to early and more conservative treatment of ectopic pregnancy. Patient selection is important for successful laparoscopic surgery. The patients should be haemodynamically stable, and the ectopic pregnancy should be small, preferably less than 6 cm in diameter. Most important of all, the surgeon must be well-trained in laparoscopic techniques. Salpingectomy, partial salpingectomy, and salpingostomy can all be performed laparoscopically. Laparoscopic treatment of ectopic pregnancy is associated with significantly less blood loss, lower analgesic requirement in the post-operative period, shorter hospital stay, faster post-operative recovery and lower overall health care cost. The subsequent reproductive outcome after laparoscopy is also very favourable.

Medical treatment

Methotrexate may be useful in the treatment of ectopic pregnancy, especially in cases where there is residual trophoblastic tissue after conservative surgery, or in cases of early ectopic pregnancy. Patients treated with methotrexate should be followed up with monitoring of serial serum beta-hCG concentrations, and for side effects. A small number of patients develop acute abdominal symptoms that necessitate surgical intervention.

Conclusion

Ectopic pregnancy is a common surgical emergency seen in early pregnancy. Some present with catastrophic symptoms, others with an acute abdomen, while some with less specific symptoms and signs and pose a diagnostic dilemma. The measurement of serum beta-hCG concentration and the use of a transvaginal ultrasound scan can improve diagnostic accuracy, but vigilance and prompt decisions are important to the successful management of ectopic pregnancy. The incidence of severe morbidity and mortality from ectopic pregnancy can thus be reduced.

References

1. Abulcasis [Abdul Qasim] 936–1013. *De chirrugia, Arabice et Latine cura Johannis Channing*, Vol. 3, Oxonii, e typ. Clarendoniano, 1778. Spink MS, Lewis GL (eds.) London: Wellcome Institute for the History of Medicine, 1973.
2. Ory HW and The Women's Health Study (1981). Ectopic pregnancy and intra-uterine contraception devices: new perspectives. *Obstet Gynecol* **57**, 137–144.
3. Tait T (1884). Five cases of extrauterine pregnancy operated upon at the time of rupture. *Br Med J* **1**, 1250–1251.
4. DeCherney AH, Maheux R, Naftolin F (1982). Salpingostomy for ectopic pregnancy in the sole patent oviduct: reproductive outcome. *Fertil Steril* **37**, 619–622.
5. Pouly JL, Manhes H, Mage G, Ganis M, Bruhat MA (1986). Conservative laparoscoic treatment of 321 ectopic pregnancies. *Fertil Steril* **46**, 1093–1097.

Further Reading

1. DeCherney AH, Boyers SP (1985). Isthmic ectopic pregnancy: segmental resection as the treatment of choice. *Fertil Steril* **44**, 307–312.

2. Gemzell L, Guillome J, Wang FC (1982). Ectopic pregnancy following treatment with human gonadotropins. *Am. J Obstet Gynecol* **143**, 761–765.
3. Westrom L, Bengtsson LPH, Mardh PA (1981). Incidence, trends and risks of ectopic pregnancy in a population of women. *Br Med J* **282**, 15–18.

23

Emergency Management of Ovarian Cysts

Sun-Kuie Tay

Introduction

Ovarian cysts are common gynaecological complaints in all age groups from infancy to the elderly. Some patients remain asymptomatic until the cysts reach a huge size. The common symptoms are vague abdominal bloatedness or distension. However, some ovarian cysts present with abdominal pain, which may be acute or chronic. There may be associated urinary or bowel symptoms which are confusing, and may delay the exact diagnosis. Not uncommonly, patients with ovarian cysts are attended to by doctors from a variety of specialties.

Emergency management of ovarian cysts is needed for patients who present with an acute abdomen arising from complications such as haemorrhage, torsion or leakage of cyst contents. Less frequently, acute abdominal pain results from a rapid growth or rupture of an ovarian malignancy. Ovarian cysts contribute to 10% of emergency laparotomy or laparoscopy, and present a challenge for diagnosis and treatment to accident and emergency physicians, general surgeons, urologists, colorectal surgeons, and gynaecologists. This chapter outlines the basis of clinical evaluation, investigation and emergency treatment of ovarian cysts. The primary objective is to provide a framework for accurate diagnosis of ovarian cysts and their complications, so that timely and appropriate treatments can be instituted for the best outcome, and in young patients, preservation of the endocrine and fertility functions of the ovaries.

Pathology of Ovarian Cysts

Ovaries are prone to the development of cysts. Clinically, the cysts can be classified according to the pathogenesis and pathology, into three main categories: functional cysts, inflammatory cysts and neoplastic cysts. Each of these cysts runs a characteristic natural course and dictates its own management approach.

The functional cysts

During the reproductive years, a woman's ovaries undergo a cascade of events in a 28-day cycle. The first two weeks constitute the follicular phase, during which the oocytes develop within follicles. After ovulation, the luteal phase ensues, with evolution of the Graffian's follicle into a corpus luteum. In the absence of a pregnancy, the corpus luteum undergoes the process of atresia which marks the end of the luteal phase. The control and regulation of the development and regression of Graffian's follicle and corpus luteum are complex and not well elucidated. Persistence of these follicles forms functional cysts.

Follicular cysts are simple, unilocular, clear cysts. The average diameter of these cysts is between 2–3 cm. Rarely, a follicular cyst can reach a size of 5 cm in diameter. The majority of follicular cysts are transient, lasting for less than three menstrual cycles.

Corpus luteum can give rise to a luteal cyst. These cysts are generally complex cysts with marked vascularity on blood flow studies on ultrasound scans. The cysts are 3–5 cm in diameter, and are most prominent in the third week of the menstrual cycle. Persistence of a corpus luteal cyst beyond three menstrual cycles is uncommon.

Inflammatory cysts

Pelvic inflammatory disease often involves the fallopian tubes and ovaries, causing tubo-ovarian abscesses which may present as ovarian swellings or cysts on clinical examination. In untreated cases, symptoms of pelvic inflammatory disease predominate the clinical picture and point to the correct diagnosis.

Ovarian endometriomas are the commonest inflammatory ovarian cysts in women during their reproductive age. Some endometriomas may persist for years after menopause. These vary in size, ranging from 1–15 cm in diameter, and are often bilateral. There may be a history of dysmenorrhea, dyspareunia, infertility and tenesmus. Pathologically, the cysts arise from invagination of ovarian endometriosis into the ovarian stroma, with the accumulation of altered blood thus forming cysts with chocolate-like content. These are often referred to as chocolate cysts. Leaking of the cyst content provokes an intense peritoneal inflammatory reaction, with severe pain and signs of peritonism.

Ovarian neoplasms

More than 90% of ovarian tumours are epithelial in origin, arising from the coelomic epithelial surface of the ovary. Others are germ cell tumours, sex cord tumours, stromal cell tumours, and rarely, tumours of the other constituent tissues of the ovary, such as fibroma, lymphoma and sarcoma. Ovaries are also a common site for secondary tumours, particularly, transcoelomic spread from tumours of the gastrointestinal tract.

The commonest benign tumour of the ovary is the epithelial cystadenoma. Serous papillary and mucinous cystadenomas are the most prevalent varieties. These occur in women during the reproductive age as well as in the elderly, particularly in the nulliparous or in women with low parity. Serous papillary cystadenoma has a mean diameter of 10 cm while a mucinous cystadenoma can attain a size of more than 30 cm, one of the largest tumours in human pathology. Most serous papillary cystadenoma are simple, unilocular clear cysts. Mucinous cystadenoma tend to be multiloculated, containing the characteristic viscous mucin.

Benign germ cell tumours are the commonest ovarian cysts in infancy and the teens. The majority of these cysts are mature teratoma or the dermoid cysts. These cysts contain the classical sebaceous material and skin appendages, typically hair. There may be other ectopic tissues such as teeth or cartilage. The cysts have a diameter of 8–10 cm on average, and are bilateral in 20% of cases.

Primary ovarian malignancy can occur in women of all ages. The incidence of epithelial adenocarcinoma rises rapidly after the fifth decade of life. The tumours can be predominantly cystic, or a mixture of cystic and solid materials. The size of the tumour varies greatly and is often bilateral. Most ovarian malignancy present late at stage III or IV when there are ascites and pleural effusions or other distant metastasis. There may also be constitutional symptoms such as loss of appetite, loss of weight, and change in urinary or bowel habits. In young women, malignant cysts are usually germ cell in origin — most frequently, dysgerminoma, immature teratoma and endodermal sinus tumour. These are rapidly growing tumours, particularly the endodermal sinus tumour, and may present with acute symptoms of pain and haemorrhage.

Acute Presentation of Ovarian Cysts

Ovarian cysts typically run a silent course. There maybe a history of vague symptoms of increased girth, abdominal bloatedness or constipation prior to acute manifestation. The most common presentation is abdominal pain. Acute symptoms occur with development of a complication in the cyst, regardless of the exact pathology of the cyst:

(1) *Haemorrhage:* Bleeding into a cyst causes a rapid rise in the pressure within the cyst. The increased tension in the capsule causes an intense pain over the ovary. This is felt mainly in the ipsilateral iliac fossa. For a cyst situated in the Pouch of Douglas, the pain may

be felt in both the iliac fossae. The point of maximum tenderness on abdominal palpation may not correlate with the side of the ovary harbouring the cyst. On pelvic examination, the cyst is tender.

Some ovarian cysts may bleed into the peritoneal cavity, with signs and symptoms of haemoperitoneum: tenderness, guarding and cardiovascular compromise or shock.

(2) *Torsion:* The ovary is suspended at the two poles, to the uterus medially, and at the pelvic side-wall laterally. These suspension ligaments lie in line with the long axis of the ovary. As the ovary enlarges to a size of between 5–10 cm in diameter, the ovary may rotate on its long axis. Torsion of the ovary may be partial or complete. Partial torsion occurs when rotation of the ovary is less than a full circle, and it corrects itself spontaneously when a counter-rotation occurs. This can recur, producing an intermittent partial torsion with intermittent pain. The pain is often described as an intense "twisting" pain on the ipsilateral iliac fossa. Complete torsion may involve more than one full rotation. The pain is "twisting" and persistent. The blood flow to and from the ovary is interrupted and the ovary becomes avascular after a while. Tissue necrosis ensues, with the associated acute inflammatory response. This is manifested as an increase in the intensity of pain locally. Subsequently, dissemination of exudate across the pelvis and peritoneal cavity produces a generalised peritonism. The intestinal tract is frequently involved in inflammation, producing diarrhoea or tenesmus. These are also constitutional symptoms and haematological and biological evidence of sepsis.

(3) *Leakage:* Perforation of the ovarian cyst capsule is usually spontaneous, occurring as a result of reduced tensile strength caused by inflammation. The clinical significance and presentation of leakage depends on the nature of the cyst content. Leaking of clear fluid from a serous papillary cystadenoma may produce little pain only. On the other hand, chocolate content of an endometrioma and sebaceous material of a teratoma are most irritating to the peritoneum. The chemical

peritonitis produces an acute abdominal pain indistinguishable from peritonitis of other aetiology.

(4) *Infection:* Ovarian cysts can be infected by either an organism ascending from the lower genital tract or haematogenous spread of a systemic infection. The resultant tubo-ovarian abscess causes local or generalised acute abdominal signs and symptoms of sepsis.

(5) *Ascites:* After running a silent course of a variable duration, ovarian neoplasms can rapidly produce a large volume of ascites through a process of transudation. There may be accompanying pleural or pericardial effusion. The patient experiences a sudden onset and rapidly worsening symptoms of abdominal distension, pain and shortness of breath. The presence of ascites and pleural effusions are easily detected by clinical examination.

Differential Diagnosis

Acute abdominal pain from an ovarian cyst must be differentiated from pelvic inflammatory disease, ectopic pregnancy, appendicitis, diverticulitis, and other surgical causes of acute abdomen.

Pelvic inflammatory disease is characterised by a history of prior gynaecological intervention or sexual contact with a partner with sexually transmitted diseases. There is usually an increase in the vaginal discharge, which may or may not be purulent. The cardinal clinical signs are locoregional peritonism in the lower abdomen. On pelvic examination, cervical excitation is marked. The ovarian swellings are ill-defined but tender.

Ectopic pregnancy must always be considered in women in the reproductive age presenting with sudden onset acute abdominal pain. The duration of amenorrhoea is an important tell-tale feature, although not an invariable history. There is almost always an associated vaginal bleeding, which may be scanty in amount and ignored by the patient herself, unless specifically enquired. In the presence of haemoperitoneum from a leaking or ruptured ectopic gestation, the patient may report a referred pain from the diaphram to the shoulder tips. Clinical examination may demonstrate mucosal pallor, tachycardia, and other signs of cardiovascular compromise. The abdominal pain varies from a pain localised to one iliac fossa, to a generalised tenderness with guarding and rebound tenderness. Pelvic examination is usually unsatisfactory because of excruciating tenderness in the pelvis. The patient is usually febrile. Thus, the adnexal swellings are often not palpable.

Acute appendicitis can occur in women of any age. Typically, the pain begins at the peri-umbilical region and, later, shifts to the right iliac fossa. There may be signs of local or generalised peritonism. The patient is febrile. Nausea, vomiting and diarrhoea may also be present.

Acute diverticulitis is encountered in older women. There may be a history of change of bowel habits, constipation or diarrhoea. The pain can be in either iliac fossa or in the lower abdomen generally. Pelvic examination is usually normal and without tenderness.

Acute abdomen from other surgical causes must be considered, depending on the presenting symptoms. Haemotoperitoneum from ruptured splenic artery is indistinguishable from haemorrhage within an ovarian cyst or a ruptured ectopic gestation. Urgent recourse to surgery is life saving.

Investigations

Ovarian cysts can be demonstrated on ultrasound (US) or computerised tomography (CT) scans. The ready availability of US scan makes it the most commonly employed investigation in the evaluation of ovarian masses. It is superior to the CT scan in distinguishing a cystic structure from a solid structure.

Pelvic ultrasound scan

Pelvic US scan can be done per abdomen or transvaginally. For ovarian cysts confined within the true pelvis, a transvaginal US scan is preferred to an abdominal scan for its better resolution. US scan has a high sensitivity in detecting cysts arising from ovaries, and differenting them from other structures, such as a distended urinary bladder.

In more than 90% of cases, haemorrhage in an ovarian cyst can be seen by its characteristic features of mixed hypoechoic and hyper-echoic areas on transvaginal US scans. There may be smooth septae of differing thickness. The property of Colour Doppler US in demonstrating the vascular status of a pelvic structure is particularly useful in differentiating a number of diagnoses. For example, inflammatory diseases such as acute appendicitis or salpingitis reveal localised increases in blood flow, while torsion is avascular.

CT scan

The CT Scan provides images of intra-abdominal, intra-pelvic and retroperitoneal anatomy and pathologies. It is a useful investigation tool for elucidation of masses of uncertain origins, and the extent of disease in the case of malignancy. Although it has been reported to reveal torsion and haemorrhagic complication of ovarian cysts presenting as an acute abdomen, its specificity is not as good as ultrasound scans.

Tumour markers

The serum concentrations of a number of tumour markers become elevated in patients with ovarian cysts. The most prevalent tumour marker is CA125, a glycoprotein found in as much as 80% of epithelial ovarian cancers. A moderately elevated serum concentration of CA125 is also encountered in women with endometriosis and ovarian endometrioma. A mild elevation of CA125 is detected in a large number of other pathology, including pelvic inflammatory disease, uterine fibroids and peritonitis. Serum concentration of CA125 in women during the reproductive age is too non-specific to be of clinical significance in the emergency management of an ovarian cyst.

Serum alpha-fetoprotein and human chorionic gonadotrphin concentrations are useful in evaluating ovarian cysts in younger women, particularly girls in the first and second decade of life. Ovarian cysts in these young women are often germ cell tumours, which may present with raised serum concentrations of these markers. In these women, ovarian preservation surgery instead of ovariectomy is the most appropriate treatment.

Emergency Operations

All patients presenting with an acute complication of an ovarian cyst should be managed as in-patients. They are fasted while adequate hydration is maintained with an intravenous infusion of dextrose (5%) saline solution (0.9%). Pain is treated with analgesia, including intramuscular injection of an opoid, such as pethedine.

Pre-operative investigations should be carried out: full blood counts, serum concentrations of urea and electrolytes, pelvic US scan, and cross matching of blood if haemorrhage is diagnosed. Patients are prepared for surgery under general anaesthesia.

Laparoscopy

Laparoscopy provides a clear view of the pelvis and abdominal cavity. Definitive diagnosis can be made in all women with acute lower abdominal pain of uncertain aetiology. It also provides therapeutic capabilities and prevents laparotomies in 80% of cases, including women who are in the first trimester of pregnancy.

Under general anaesthesia, the patient is placed in lithotomy position, cleaned and draped. The urinary bladder is emptied and, if the patient is not pregnant, a uterine manipulator or a Hegar dilator is passed into the uterine cavity for manipulation of the uterine cavity. A stab incision is made in the lower portion of the umbilicus through which a Verres needle is inserted into the peritoneal cavity. Pneumoperitoneum is created with two to three litres of carbon dioxide (CO_2) gas. An 11 mm trocar and canula is inserted through the same

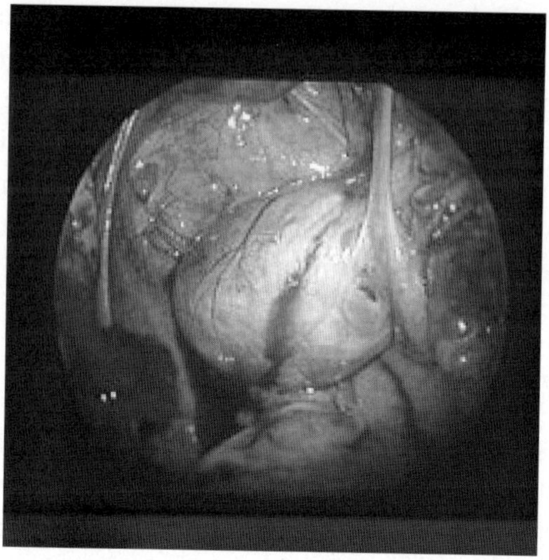

Fig. 1 Laparoscopic view of a right ovarian cyst. A serous cystadenoma of the right ovary.

umbilical incision into the peritoneal cavity. A 10 mm laparoscope is introduced through the canula into the pelvis. A video camera is attached to display the images onto a television monitor (Fig. 1). The entire pelvic and abdominal cavities should be carefully inspected. Samples of peritoneal fluid can be obtained for further investigations such as cytological assessment for the presence of malignant cells, or for bacteriological culture and antibiotic sensitivity test.

A second and third instrument can be introduced into the pelvis through canulae placed at the iliac fossae. This approach provides versatile operative capabilities to deal with a large number of pelvic and intra-abdominal conditions.

(1) *Ovarian cystectomy:* Benign ovarian cysts up to a size of 12 cm in diameter can be removed laparoscopically. For cysts adherent to the uterus, bowels or other adnexal structures, adhesiolysis should be performed before attempting ovarian cystectomy. A large ovarian cyst, with the exception of a dermoid cyst, maybe deflated by aspiration of the cyst content to facilitate surgical manoeuvre. A dermoid cyst

contains viscous sebaceous materials and hair which are difficult to aspirate completely. Spillage of these cyst contents into the pelvis and abdominal cavity can induce chemical peritonitis.

The ovarian capsule is incised at the anti-mesosalpingial border and deflected to reveal the cyst wall. The cyst wall is held with a grasping forceps, and the ovarian capsule dissected away from the cyst for a complete removal of the cyst. Haemostasis is secured with electrocauterisation. The ovarian capsule can be closed with a fine prolene suture or left open. The ovary maybe wrapped with an anti-adhesion preparation such as "Seprafilm®" to reduce adhesion formation.

A deflated cyst can be retrieved from the pelvis through one of the accessory ports. An intact cyst can be put into an endoscopic pouch for retrieval without spillage of the cyst content.

(2) *Ovarietomy (Figs. 2 and 3):* Preservation of the ovary may be inappropriate when its viability is compromised by severe torsion, or when an early cancer is suspected. Excision of the ovary can be performed safely, laparoscopically. It is prudent to open up the broad ligament to display the course of the ureter before the infundibulo-pelvic ligament is clamped and severed. This will avoid inadvertent

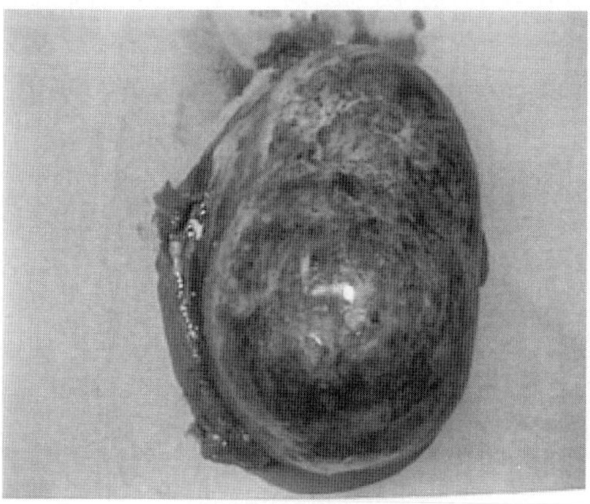

Fig. 2 A haemorrhagic ovarian cyst. The ovarian cyst is filled with blood.

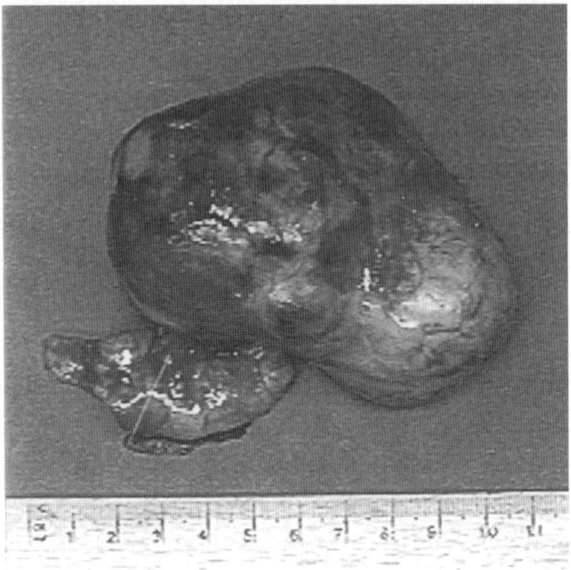

Fig. 3 Torsion in an ovary. The ovary is necrotic with evidence of acute inflammation.

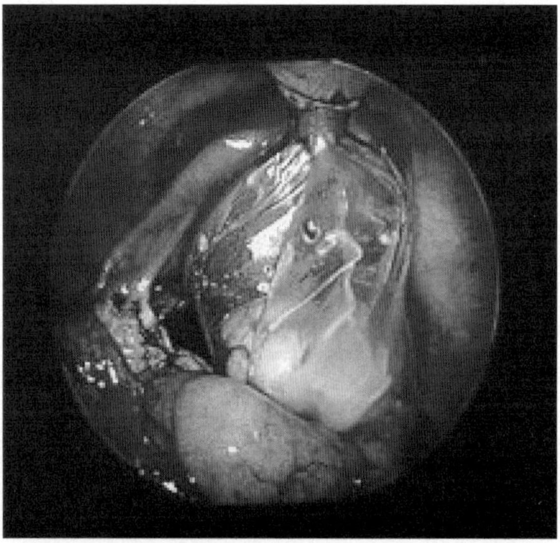

Fig. 4 An ovarian cyst retrieved with an endoscopic pouch.

injury to the ureter. The ovary is usually detached from the uterus together with the fallopian tube. The excised structures are then retrieved from the pelvis with the aid of an endoscopic pouch (Fig. 4).

(3) *Haemostasis:* Bleeding from a corpus luteum can be arrested with electrocautery or insertion of a haemostatic suture. Excision of a corpus luteum is unnecessary, even in the presence of haemoperitoneum.

(4) *Drainage of ovarian cyst:* Ovarian endometriomas in young women are preferably treated by aspiration alone. This is followed by medical treatment with an anti-oestrogen or gonadotrophin releasing hormone analogue. An elective laparoscopy is performed three or four months later for CO_2 laser ablation of the cyst wall. This will reduce loss of ovarian tissue and preserve reproductive function.

A tubo-ovarian abscess is also best treated with drainage and antibiotics.

Laparotomy

Laparotomy is the traditional surgical approach to all ovarian cysts, regardless of the exact pathological nature. With the popularisation of laparoscopy in recent years, laparotomy is viewed as a radical approach reserved for complex ovarian surgery for large ovarian cysts, malignant tumours, or when the diagnosis is uncertain and operation on other organs is contemplated.

In young patients in whom ovarian malignancy is uncommon, a Pfannenstiel incision is appropriate for the laparotomy. In older women, a midline incision is preferrable. Ovarian cystectomy, salpingo-oophorectomy, drainage of ovarian cyst or abscess can be done with the same techniques as in laparoscopy. Delivery of the ovarian cyst from the abdomen must be carried out carefully to avoid spillage of cyst contents onto the abdominal incision. Implantation of ovarian tumours or endometriotic cells in the incision wound is a well recognised and preventable complication of ovarian surgery.

Unexpected finding of an ovarian cysts

Despite careful pre-operative clinical evaluation and investigation, diagnosis of an ovarian cyst may remain obscure. Most commonly, a right sided abdominal pain is misdiagnosed as a sign of acute appendicitis. Appendicectomy is then performed through the classical grid iron incision. This is an inappropriate incision for pelvic surgery for an ovarian cyst. In this situation, the pelvis should be thoroughly inspected with a laparoscope introduced through the grid iron incision. If laparoscopic surgery is suitable, additional instruments can be introduced into the pelvis in the routine laparoscopic approach to accomplish the surgery. If the ovarian cyst is deemed unsuitable for laparoscopic excision, the grid iron incision should be closed in the routine manner and a conventional approach of laparotomy through an appropriate incision (Pfannenstiel or midline) should be made. This allows optimal pelvic surgery, and avoids the creation of an unsightly oblique extension of the grid iron incision across the lower abdomen.

Ovarian cancers

When an ovarian cancer is diagnosed during an emergency laparotomy, a gynaecological oncologist's assistance should be sought to ensure proper staging and optimal debulking of the tumour. In an older woman, a total hysterectomy and bilateral salpingo-oophorectomy, together with omentectomy and excision of tumour deposits on the peritoneum or other viscera, is the operation of choice. In a younger woman with a tumour confined to one ovary, a unilateral salpingo-oophorectomy and omentectomy should be performed. The contralateral ovary should be carefully inspected and palpated for an occult tumour. Any suspicious lesion on the contralateral ovary should be biopsied for histological assessment but routine bisecting of a normal sized contralateral ovary is unnecessary. Retroperitoneal lymphatic spaces should be carefully examined. If no lymph node enlargement is detected, an ipsilateral pelvic lymphadenectomy and para-aortic lymph node sampling should be performed to complete the staging procedure.

When a germ cell tumour is suspected in a teen or young woman, serum concentrations of tumour markers are a useful diagnostic aid, and intra-operative frozen section examination of the tumour is desirable. These tumours are highly chemo-sensitive. Fertility sparing surgery with excision of tumour deposits outside the reproductive organs is the recommended approach.

Complications of Emergency Operations for Ovarian Cysts

All operations carry a risk of complications. The magnitude of the rate of complication is closely related to the pathology of the cyst, the patient's constitutional makeup, and the surgical skill and experience of the surgeon.

Haemorrhage

Operative and peri-operative bleeding is always a concern to all surgeons. Pelvic adhesion requiring extensive adhesiolysis, enterolysis and ovariolysis significantly increases the incidence of operative bleeding. After ovarian cystectomy, the large potential space on the ovary is prone to haemorrhage. The most reliable preventive measures for these complications are none other than meticulous surgical technique and securing haemostasis during surgery.

Visceral injuries

The ureter enters the pelvis anterior to the bifurcation of the common iliac artery, and inferior to the infundibulopelvic ligament. It then courses along the pelvic side wall immediately posterior to the ovarian fossa, turns medially at the inferior border of the broad ligament, enters the ureteric tunnel below the uterine artery, before it approaches the bladder. Ligation of the infundibulopelvic ligament and dissection of the ovarian cyst from the ovarian fossa are the two most common sites where the ureter can be injured. Injuries can arise from sharp dissection, ligature or electric cauterisation.

Bowel injuries occuring with enterolysis are usually due to sharp incisions or lacerations. Extensive enterolysis can lead to devitalisation of the bowel with post-operative perforation and soilage of the peritoneal cavity. Delayed perforation of the bowels can also arise from thermal injuries from electric cauterisation. Adequate bowel preparation with purgatives prior to the surgery is helpful in the further management of these injuries.

Bladder injuries from perforation, incision, laceration and contusion can happen with laparoscopy or laparotomy. Pre-operative bladder catheterisation is imperative in reducing these injuries.

Vascular injuries can occur with laparoscopy during insertion of the Verres needle or trocar. The inferior hypogastric vessels are the most commonly injured vessels at the iliac fossa, but internal and external iliac vessels and abdominal aorta are sometimes injured by perforation.

Infection

Intra-abdominal sepsis is uncommon without concomitant complications, especially after bowel injury. Prophylactic antibiotics are recommended in cases where extensive enterolysis or appendicectomy has been carried out.

Lower urinary tract infection occurs in 5% of gynaecological patients. Due care must be exercised during catheterisation of the bladder perioperatively.

Appropriate intravenous antibiotic therapy should be instituted intra-operatively if any acute inflammatory process is encountered with the ovarian cyst.

Conclusion

Ovarian cysts and their complications are common causes of acute abdominal pain, demanding emergency medical attention and treatment. A carefully taken medical history and clinical examination may successfully diagnose and differentiate an ovarian cyst from other differential diagnoses such as acute appendicitis, pelvic inflammatory disease, ectopic gestation, diverticulitis or a malignancy. Pelvic US scan is the most useful investigation in confirming the diagnosis of an ovarian cyst. Other imaging technologies such as the CT scan may be necessary in complicated cases. When malignancy is suspected, obtaining tumour markers such as serum CA125, alpha-fetoprotein, and human chorionic gonadotrophin concentrations may be useful.

As much as 80% of ovarian cysts can be treated successfully via laparoscopy, with either ovarian cystectomy, salpingo-oophorectomy or cyst aspiration and cautery to secure haemostasis. Laparotomy is reserved for complicated ovarian cysts, or in patients deemed at high risk of complications for laparoscopy. Special consideration for fertility preservation is of paramount importance in young patients, even for management of a malignant ovarian cyst. When ovarian malignancy is encountered, assistance from a gynaecological oncologist should be sought.

A high standard of surgical skill and experience, and optimal preoperative preparation of the patients, including the use of appropriate antibiotics, may prevent some of the complications of emergency treatment of ovarian cysts.

Section VI

Urological Emergencies

24

Acute Non-traumatic Urological Emergencies

Weber Lau
Keong-Tatt Foo

Introduction

Most urological complaints are not emergencies. Although serious underlying pathology such as bladder, prostate, or renal cancer may be detected, rapid action is rarely required. On the other hand, not uncommonly, some urological conditions may present acutely and demand rapid diagnosis and immediate treatment. This chapter describes the management of the following non-traumatic urological emergencies:

- Acute urinary retention
- Torsion of testis } in male patients
- Paraphimosis } in male patients
- Priapism } in male patients
- Infected hydronephrosis

Acute Urinary Retention

The most common urological emergency is acute retention of urine.[1,2] It is the sudden inability to urinate. The most common causes are:

- Medications that inhibit bladder contractility (alcohol or anti-histamines), or cause a physiologic narrowing of the urethra (ipratropium bromide, albuterol, epinephrine)
- Impaired detrusor function from delaying urination for a long time, long period of inactivity or bed rest, spinal cord injury/nerve damage, other neurological disease, and after lower urinary tract, perineal, gynaecologic and anorectal surgery
- Urinary system obstruction (benign prostatic hyperplasia (BPH), kidney stones)
- Urinary tract infection
- Prolonged exposure to cold temperature
- Psychogenic causes (rare)

Clinical features

History taking should include the voiding pattern before retention, past urologic surgery, medications with anti-cholinergic side effects, and other common cold remedies containing nasal decongestants and anti-histaminic compounds.

Clinical examination should focus on the supra-pubic area to determine whether a distended bladder can be palpated or percussed. In acute urinary retention, the patient typically experiences distress associated with an uncomfortably distended bladder, and the inability to void normally. Pressure on the bladder during the examination will usually exacerbate the supra-pubic discomfort or pain. Catheter drainage brings prompt symptomatic relief. With chronic retention the patients may complain of frequency, poor urine flow, and a sensation of incomplete emptying. They hardly feel any discomfort from pressure on the distended bladder. Digital rectal examination should be done to evaluate the size of the prostate, and to exclude possible prostatic abscess or cancer.

Investigations

A computed tomography (CT) or magnetic resonance imaging (MRI) of the spine may be required if a neurogenic cause such as spinal cord compression is suspected to be the cause of the urinary retention.

Ultrasonography (US) of the kidneys and bladder may be useful to evaluate prostate size and configuration, or to exclude bladder stone.

Elective cystoscopy or urodynamic study may be indicated subsequently to examine the bladder, urethra, and prostate for abnormalities that can cause urinary retention.

Treatment

This condition is managed by insertion of a urethral or supra-pubic catheter. Insertion of catheters is a skill best learnt by bedside teaching, and the technique will not be discussed here. Frequently, catheterisation can be made difficult by the presence of urethral stricture, prostate enlargement, or prostate cancer. In the trauma patient with acute retention, the possibility of a ruptured urethra must be considered in patients with blood at the urethral meatus prior to an attempt at catheterisation.[3]

Problematic catheterisation

If a urethral catheter will not pass easily, then do not persist, but seek urological advice. Difficult catheterisations should be performed by those with more experience. The most likely cause is spasm of the external sphincter. Other differential diagnoses include urethral stricture, bladder neck contracture or hypertrophy. Prostatic enlargement rarely prevents the passage of a catheter, as the lobes of the prostate can be easily pushed aside by the catheter, especially one with a 22 Fr diameter. In patients with a known history or suspected urethral stricture, flexible cystoscopy should be carried out. Mild strictures can be dilated by the urologist. Otherwise percutaneous suprapubic cystostomy would be a good alternative for temporary relief of urine retention. If no stricture is evident, the urologist may insert a catheter using a catheter introducer or over a guide wire that is inserted under direct vision through flexible cystoscopy. The amount of urine drained on initial passing of the catheter (residual urine) should be noted. This gives a guide to the type of retention (acute or chronic) and may influence further management and prediction of outcome.

If one suspects that the patient may have a urinary tract infection, prophylactic antibiotics with an aminoglycoside such as gentamicin, or a third generation cephalosporin such as ceftriaxone may be required, as catheterisation can precipitate sepsis (usually Gram-negative). In patients with chronic retention, post-catheterisation diuresis can be a problem. If significant diuresis occurs (> 400 ml/hr), replacement with intravenous normal saline solution is required. A rough guide is to infuse 90% of the previous hour's volume of urine output. Syncope often follows rapid bladder decompression, and a patient with a chronically distended bladder may bleed. Seek advice from the urologist early, as the management of fluid balance in these patients can be challenging.

Torsion of the Spermatic Cord

Torsion of the spermatic cord happens when one or more of the blood vessels in the testicle twists back on it and cuts off the testicle's blood supply, creating a painful testicular mass with subsequent testicular necrosis and atrophy. The patient experiences the sudden onset of pain in the scrotum, which may also be felt in the lower abdomen or the groin.

This surgical emergency requires prompt diagnosis and immediate urological referral for rapid definitive treatment for salvage of the testicle. A salvage rate of 80–100% is found in patients who present within six hours of pain. After six to eight hours, the salvage rate markedly decreases to near 0% at 12 hours.

Testicular torsion can be classified broadly into two types:

(1) Extravaginal torsion: This happens in the neonatal period, and most commonly develops prenatally in the spermatic cord, proximal to the attachment of the tunica vaginalis. This is commonly associated with high birth weight. Approximately 5% of all torsions belong to this type. Up to 20% of bilateral cases happen synchronously, and 3% asynchronously.

(2) Intravaginal torsion occurs within the tunica vaginalis and happens mainly in older children, with a peak incidence at age 13 years. Intravaginal torsion is related to the bell-clapper anomaly (an anatomical abnormality in which the high insertion of the tunica vaginalis on the spermatic cord rather than on the lower pole allows for poor testicular fixation and extreme testicular mobility). This anomaly may be bilateral in 2% of the cases.

Reported incidence in males younger than 25 years is approximately one in 4000. The left testicle is more often involved. Although it has been seen from birth to 77 years of age, it is most often observed in males younger than 30 years. One peak age is around puberty, although a smaller peak also occurs during the first year of life. The differential diagnoses include strangulated hernia, trauma, torsion of a testicular appendage, and acute epididymitis or orchitis.

There are many pre-disposing factors such as:

- Undescended testis
- Ectopic testis
- High attachment of tunica vaginalis on the testis — "bell clapper" arrangement — this allows the testis to rotate freely
- Inverted or transverse position of testis in the scrotum — same mechanism as above
- Separation of epididymis from the body of the testis — enables rotation of testis separate from the epididymis
- In the neonatal age group, the testicle frequently has not descended into the scrotum and becomes attached within the tunica vaginalis. Additionally, this mobility of the testicle predisposes it to torsion

Clinical features

Characteristically, the pain is of sudden onset, severe, and usually felt primarily in the scrotum, but may radiate to the groin or lower abdomen. Nausea and/or vomiting are common associated symptoms. Patients may have a history of recurrent pain that is transient and resolves spontaneously.

Physical examination reveals an obviously uncomfortable patient with a swollen, severely tender, high-riding testis. He may be pale and diaphoretic, but usually is not febrile. If one can palpate the epididymis in an anterior location at this stage, the diagnosis of torsion is most likely. The absence of the cremasteric reflex in a patient with acute scrotal pain also supports the diagnosis of torsion.

The diagnosis of testicular torsion should be considered in any man presenting with an acute scrotum where testicular torsion cannot be definitely ruled out by history and physical examination. In that case, urgent scrotal exploration is indicated. The patient's age will provide a guide to the likely diagnosis. Children localise pain poorly, and it is recommended that the testicles always be examined in any child presenting with abdominal pain. It is often difficult to confidently exclude torsion, and most urologists will have a low threshold for performing a scrotal exploration. It is also important to remember that 10% of testicular tumours can present with acute testicular pain.

Imaging studies

Testicular torsion is a clinical diagnosis. Imaging studies are usually not necessary when the clinical suspicion is high. None of the investigations (ultrasonography, radionuclide scan, colour doppler) are absolutely accurate, and are time-consuming and do not provide reliable information as much as a thorough history and physical examination. Therefore, they should not be ordered as a matter of routine. Only surgical exploration will give a definitive diagnosis.[4] Sometimes, one might come across a testicular tumour presenting as a painful testicular mass. Ultrasonography would certainly help in making a diagnosis and altering the surgical approach.

Treatment

Emergency department care

Urgent and accurate diagnosis is needed, followed by prompt urologic referral, (for surgical exploration and detorsion of the testis), since time is critical in the salvage of the testicle.[5] Analgesia can be provided once testicular torsion has been diagnosed.

In the event that there is an unavoidable delay in transferring the patient to the operating room, an attempt may be made to manually detorse the testicle in the emergency department if it is within four hours of onset. Remember that the testes twist toward the midline as seen from the feet, in a lateral to medial fashion. Therefore, detorsion should be attempted initially in a medial to lateral motion similar to opening a book, with the right testicle being rotated counter clockwise and the left clockwise (Figs. 1 and 2). Two complete circles (72°) will probably be needed and a relief of pain is the end point of detorsion. As detorsion is a painful procedure, parenteral morphine or local anaesthesia injected around the spermatic cord may be required. Manual detorsion is successful in 30–70% of patients. If manual detorsion is successful, elective bilateral orchidopexy is indicated within the next few days.

Surgical treatment

If detorsion fails, immediate surgical exploration is indicated. If the presentation is between four hours and 24 hours after onset of pain, immediate surgical exploration, detorsion, and bilateral orchidopexy should be performed. If more than 24 hours have passed since onset of pain, surgical exploration is indicated — however, preservation of testicular function is unlikely. A non-viable testis should be removed in light of current information suggesting that the contralateral testis

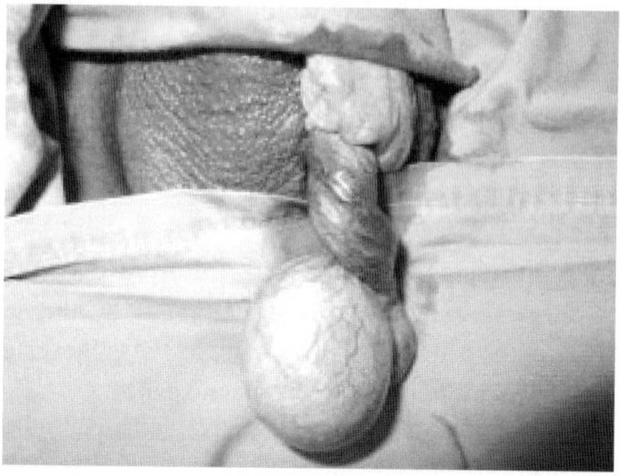

Fig. 1 Torsion of the spermatic cord on exploration.

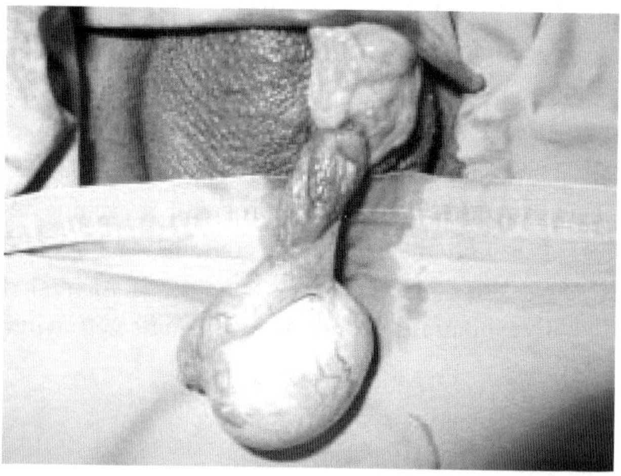

Fig. 2 Successful detorsion and salvage of the testis.

may be adversely affected by a retained damaged testis. This is possibly due to autoimmune injury to the contralateral testicle. Risk of malignancy in the dead testis, and prevention of infection, are other concerns as well.[6] A thorough explanation regarding the nature of the operation should be given to the patients and their parents. Consent should be obtained for orchidectomy if the testis is not viable. A testicular prosthesis might be considered to replace the removed non-viable testis.

Prognosis

The outcome depends much on the duration and degree of testicular torsion. Viability of the testis is only possible if there is no delay between the onset of symptoms and the time of surgical or manual detorsion.

Paraphimosis

Paraphimosis is another urologic emergency of the male patient and is often iatrogenic. It is particularly common in those with a urethral catheter *in situ*. The foreskin is retracted back over the glans to the corona following urologic procedures such as catheterisation or self-manipulation, causing a constriction around the corona that cannot be relieved (Fig. 3). The effects of paraphimosis may range from mild glandular and preputial oedema to severe ischemia and gangrene.

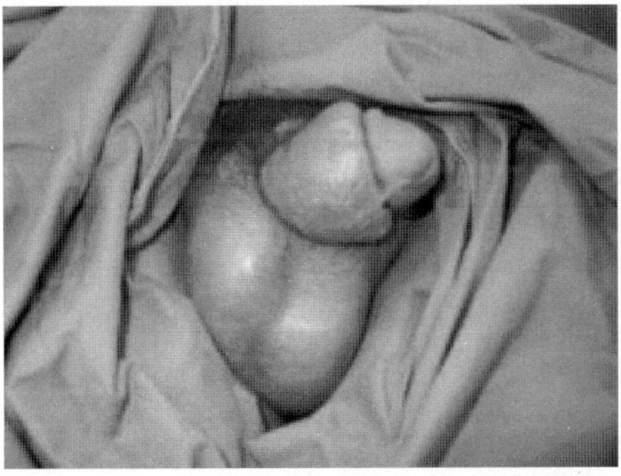

Fig. 3 Paraphimosis with swelling of the prepuce and glans penis.

Often the patient delays seeking help as he has been trying to "cure" the problem himself to avoid embarrassment. The prognosis is excellent if the condition is diagnosed and rapidly treated.

Treatment

Emergency department care

Attempts to reduce the paraphimosis must be performed after determining the absence of an encircling foreign body. Many techniques of paraphimosis reduction have been described.[7,8] The main goal of each method is to reduce the foreskin to its naturally occurring position over the glans penis by manipulating the oedematous glans and/or the distal prepuce. When necessary, reduction of the foreskin can be facilitated by the use of local anaesthesia or a penile block using lignocaine hydrochloride without epinephrine. The "puncture technique" using a hypodermic needle to puncture the oedematous foreskin at multiple sites, followed by gentle manual compression, has been described as well.[8] Occasionally, some patients require conscious sedation for this procedure.

Manual reduction of the prepuce over the glans can be achieved by placing both index fingers on the dorsal border of the penis behind the retracted prepuce, while placing both thumbs on the end of the glans. The glans is pushed back through the prepuce with the help of thumb pressure while the index fingers pull the prepuce over the glans. This technique may be facilitated by the use of hand compression on the foreskin, glans, and penis to help decrease the amount of oedema prior to manual reduction. This, as with all of the reduction techniques, requires a fair amount of patience, and cannot be rushed.

Surgical treatment

If the less invasive measures fail to reduce the paraphimosis, a urologic consultation is required. Dorsal incision of the constricting ring under local anaesthesia would usually be performed. Once the inflammation and edema have subsided (three to four days) elective circumcision is recommended. If gangrene has developed, treatment involves aggressive surgical debridement, cutting away of the infected and necrotic tissue, and appropriate antibiotic therapy.

Priapism

Priapism was first described by Tripe in 1845. It is a persistent, usually painful, erection of the corpora cavernosa of the penis, lasting for more than two to three hours; if it is prolonged (over four hours) the patient is at risk of developing permanent impotence. This process affects only the corpora cavernosa. The corpora spongiosum of the glans penis and around the urethra remain flaccid.

With the advent of intracavernosal injections, such as prostaglandin E1, papavarine, phentolamine and oral sildenafil for erectile dysfunction, patients with priapism are more frequently seen in the middle of the night in the emergency department.[9] Occasionally, priapism is associated with some systemic diseases. It can be broadly classified according to the aetiology:

(1) Primary (30% to 50% of cases)
(2) Secondary
  - Thromboembolic disorder: sickle cell trait or disease, thalassaemia thrombocytopenia and polycythaemia
  - Medications: many psychotropic medications, especially chlorpromazine, trazodone and thioridazine; intracavernosal injections (PGE1, papavarine and phentolamine); anticholinergic agents; oral sildenafil for erectile dysfunction; cocaine, marijuana and ethanol abuse[10]
  - Neurogenic: central nervous and spinal cord disorders, diabetic neuropathy
  - Cancer: leukaemia, lymphoma, bladder or prostate cancer[11]
  - Others: penile trauma, dialysis, total parenteral nutrition, especially after administration of 20% intravenous fat emulsion

Clinical features

Arterial high-flow priapism

Presentation may be delayed after the acute injury. The delay may be due to initial vasospasm, or to the formation of a clot that is gradually reabsorbed over a period of time. Priapism secondary to arterial causes is usually less tumescent, and may be significantly less painful than priapism due to venous congestion.[12,13]

Veno-occlusive priapism

Patients with veno-occlusive priapism present with a painful erection. Erection may have been present for hours to days.[13]

Physical finding of an erect or semierect penis, with a flaccid glans penis, confirms the diagnosis. Carefully examine for evidence of trauma to the genital region. Look out for evidence of concomitant disorders that may predispose the patient to priapism.

Laboratory investigations

A full blood count and coagulation profile is appropriate in order to identify the rare causes of priapism, such as leukaemia or sickle cell disease in patients with no known risk factors.

Imaging studies like elective penile angiography may be required in order to identify the site of the fistula in patients with high-flow priapism. Penile doppler testing may be necessary to differentiate high-flow from low-flow priapism.

Treatment

Emergency department care

The goal of treatment is detumescence with relief of associated pain, and preservation of potency. The duration of priapism has direct prognostic significance on the eventual outcome. With delayed presentation (more than 24 hours) the risk of permanent impotence rises to approximately 50% despite prompt treatment.[14] All patients should be warned of the possible poor outcome and this should clearly be documented in the case notes.

(1) *Medical therapy:* The use of medications such as alpha-agonists or methylene blue may be useful in some instances. Alpha-agonist agents counteract smooth muscle relaxation. However, there is risk of significant systemic hypertension. Methylene blue inhibits guanylate cyclase, and has a second messenger inhibitory effect; thus, it inhibits smooth muscle relaxation. The effect of methylene blue is rather short-lasting, and priapism may recur.[12,15,16] Other more common measures include application of ice packs or pressure dressings, administration of ice water, warm water enemas, sedatives and analgesics. However, none of these are particularly effective.

(2) Corporeal aspiration and injection with an alpha-adrenergic agonist: This forms the mainstay of initial treatment if the patient presents within 24 hours.[14] A penile nerve block is obtained by injecting 1% plain lignocaine at around the base of the penile shaft. Some form of sedation may be required as well. After the onset of anaesthesia is confirmed, the corpus cavernosum is punctured using a 19-gauge needle attached to a large syringe. Blood is aspirated and sent for blood gas analysis to evaluate the degree of ischaemia. This should be done through the shaft of the penis at the 2 O'clock or the 10 O'clock position, but not through the corpus spongiosum. Initially, 20–30 ml of blood should be aspirated. Milking the shaft of the penis will help to empty the corpora if necessary. Aspiration is usually required only at one or the other site because of the multiple communications from one corpus to the other. After detumescence is obtained, the penis should be dressed with an elasticised bandage to ensure continued emptying of the corpora, and to compress the puncture site.

If aspiration fails, intracorporeal injection of adrenergic agonists is indicated.[16] The drug of choice is phenylephrine, because of its high selectivity and potency in inducing vasoconstriction. It has a quick onset of action of less than one minute, and its duration of action is between seven to 20 minutes. The dose is 100–500 μg per dose, and up to ten doses may be administered. Preparation involves adding 10 mg (usually 10 mg per ml) of phenylephrine to 490 ml of saline 0.9% solution. This yields a solution of 20 μg/ml of phenylephrine. Use 10–20 ml of this solution for intracavernous injection every five to ten minutes. Other possible agents for consideration include intracavernous injection of either norepinephrine 20–80 μg or epinephrine 0.05–0.1 mg, or ephedrine 50–100 mg.

(3) Supportive treatment, such as administration of analgesics, warm or cold enemas and more specific measures may be required:

(i) Leukaemic infiltration of the corpora may respond to local radiation therapy of the penis and systemic chemotherapy.[17]

(ii) Priapism due to sickle cell disease may respond to hydration, alkalinisation, analgesia and hypertransfusion, and/or exchange transfusions to increase haemoglobin concentration to higher than 10% and decrease haemoglobin S to less than 30%. Red cell transfusion may be required. The aim is to reduce sinusoidal acidosis and sludging. In patients with sickle cell disease, priapism is often self-limited, therefore longer durations of conservative management may be appropriate.[18] Occasionally, intractable priapism may be managed with insertion of an inflatable penile prosthesis.[19]

Surgical treatment

Establishment of venous drainage from the engorged corpora cavernosa is indicated in patients with prolonged priapism of more than 24 hours or if detumescence does not respond to the above conservative measures. Shunting of the corpora cavernosa can be done in various ways.[16] The Winter procedure, first described in 1976, is a relatively easy and safe procedure to create a fistula between the glans penis and the corpus spongiosum.[20] A spring-loaded trucut biopsy needle is used for this procedure. The Al-Ghorab procedure involves the creation of a glans-cavernosum shunt by the removal of a small 5 mm diameter of tunica albuginea from each corpus, after making a 2 cm dorsal transverse incision in the glans penis 1 cm distal to the coronal sulcus.[21] Very seldom, more elaborate shunts may be required, such as saphenous vein-to-corpora, dorsal vein-to-corpora, or side-to-side cavernosum-spongiosum shunt.[22] Arterial high-flow priapism with a documented arterial-lacunar fistula would require selective embolisation by the interventional radiologist.[12,23]

Prognosis

The duration has direct prognostic significance on the eventual outcome. With delayed presentation (> 24 hours) the risk of permanent impotence rises to approximately 50% despite prompt treatment.

Infected Hydronephrosis

Infected hydronephrosis represents a continuum of disease, from upper urinary tract bacterial infection in the setting of hydronephrosis to frank pyonephrosis. Infected hydronephrosis may develop from bacterial infection either ascending via the urinary tract or from the haematogenous route. Usually, there is concomitant obstruction, such as from a urinary calculus, or sloughed papilla or stricture. This leads to collection of leucocytes, bacteria, and debris in the collecting system, and subsequently the development of pyonephrosis. Common pathogens involved are gram negative *Escherichia coli*, *Enterococcus* species, *Candida* species and other fungal infections. Immunocompromised states secondary to steroid therapy or disease (diabetes mellitus, AIDS) exaggerate the pathology.

Clinical features

Patients are usually septic with fever, chills, and flank pain. They may have a history of urinary calculi, infection, or diabetes mellitus. In some elderly patients, they may even be asymptomatic (15%). On clinical examination, the hydronephrotic kidney may be palpable as an abdominal mass. Tenderness is usually elicited at the renal angle of the affected side.[24]

Investigations

Laboratory investigations

Full blood count with a differential count, serum urea, electrolytes and creatinine concentrations, coagulation studies, urinalysis with culture, and blood cultures are indicated in the initial workup of a patient suspected of having infected hydronephrosis.

Imaging studies

(1) Plain radiograph

Kidney, ureter and bladder (KUB) X-ray may be useful to ascertain possible radiopaque urinary calculi or gas shadows from gas-forming pathogens.

(2) Ultrasonography

Renal sonography is the most useful and convenient investigation in this setting. In the presence of hydronephrosis, a fluid-debris level that shifts with patient positioning can often be demonstrated. If echogenic gas is demonstrated, the patient should be assumed to have a severe infection suggestive of emphysematous pyelonephritis.[24]

(3) Computed tomography (CT)

Advantages of CT include definitive delineation of the obstruction, the function of the kidney, and the severity of hydronephrosis as well as the presence of other abdominal pathologies such as metastatic cancer or retroperitoneal fibrosis that are not observed with ultrasonography. However, intravenous contrast should not be administered to patients with significant renal impairment.[25]

Treatment

Emergency management

The presence of infected hydronephrosis is a surgical emergency and requires immediate intervention. The patient should be aggressively resuscitated with crystalloid therapy, especially if dehydrated or in septic shock. Airway management may be indicated in critically-ill patients. Supplemental oxygen, intravenous access, and continuous cardiac monitoring may be necessary. Patients with poorly controlled diabetes mellitus should be quickly stabilised.

Initially, patients should be treated with appropriate intravenous antibiotics, consisting of a third generation cephalosporin (ceftriaxone). Depending on the clinical situation, additional anaerobic coverage with metronidazole may be needed. Be cognisant of the fact that patients may have fungal infection or tuberculosis. The use of antifungal or antibacterial agents depends upon culture results.

With the advent of ultrasonography, ultrasound-guided percutaneous drainage has become the mainstay of treatment.[26] It has low morbidity and mortality rates with an excellent outcome, resulting in renal preservation. The advantage is that this procedure can be performed with local anaesthesia, and is associated with minimal trauma or risk to the patient. Once the patient is stable, subsequent antegrade radiographic studies help with treatment planning

Retrograde decompression, or placement of a ureteral stent, should be avoided if possible because of the lack of antegrade access for radiologic studies, and the need for general anaesthesia. In addition, the risk of pyelovenous, pyelolymphatic, and pyelosinus backflow of infected urine into the systemic circulatory system always exists with retrograde manipulation. This may result in sepsis and decompensation of the patient.

Definitive treatment

The infectious process often resolves within 24–48 hours following drainage, and the patient usually improves significantly once this occurs. The patient should remain afebrile for one to two weeks after placement of a nephrostomy tube before any definitive evaluation and management of obstruction. An antegrade nephrostogram is extremely helpful in determining the aetiology of the obstruction, and in planning further treatment strategies. These are based on the type of obstruction, and clinical situation. Nephrectomy is occasionally needed in the case of a severely damaged kidney and a normal contralateral kidney.

If a definitive anatomic abnormality, such as a stone or tumour, cannot be determined, further imaging studies and tests may be needed to establish the aetiology of the infected hydronephrosis. These tests may include a voiding cystourethrogram to exclude vesicoureteral reflux, urodynamics to establish a possible neurogenic bladder with urine stasis, and serial renal ultrasounds to document resolution of hydronephrosis after treatment.

Definitive treatment of the cause of obstruction is only indicated after the infection has fully resolved. These are based on the type of obstruction and clinical situation.

Prognosis

If infected hydronephrosis is recognised and promptly treated, recovery of the affected renal unit, is rapid. Long-term complications are rare when the condition is promptly managed. Otherwise, abscess and fistula formation, and scarring of the renal unit, may occur if definitive therapy is delayed.

Conclusion

Not uncommonly, some non-traumatic urologic problems may present in the emergency department setting, which demand rapid diagnosis and immediate treatment. Knowledge of these problems and the appropriate initial assessment is obviously important to the eventual outcome. Early referral to the urologist may be required if there is uncertainty in the diagnosis, or on failure of initial management. Some of these patients will require immediate surgical therapy, while many others can be adequately managed in the emergency department and discharged. In this situation, appropriate outpatient follow-up with the urologist should be arranged.

References

1. Fontanarosa PB, Roush WR (1988). Acute urinary retention. *Emerg Med Clin North Am* **6**, 419–437.
2. Fuselier HA, Jr (1993). Etiology and management of acute urinary retention. *Compr Ther* **19**, 31–36.
3. Elkabir JJ, Patel A, Vale JA, Witherow RO (1999). Acute urinary retention in men. Management is more complex issue than was described. *Br Med J* **319**, 1004–1005.
4. Lupi A, Campobasso P, De Antoni MG (1993). Value and limits of testicular scintigraphy in paediatric acute scrotum. *J Nucl Biol Med* **37**, 207–212.
5. Corbett HJ, Simpson ET (2002). Management of the acute scrotum in children. *ANZ J Surg* **72**, 226–228.
6. Sanz Jaka JP, Villanueva JA, Garmendia Larrea JC, Mendivil DJ, Arocena LF (1989). Torsion of the spermatic cord. *Arch Esp Urol* **42**, 508–514.
7. Raveenthiran V (1996). Reduction of paraphimosis: a technique based on pathophysiology. *Br J Surg* **83**, 1247.
8. Fuenfer MM, Najmaldin A (1994). Emergency reduction of paraphimosis. *Eur J Pediatr Surg* **4**, 370–371.
9. Perimenis P, Athanasopoulos A, Geramoutsos I, Barbalias G (2001). The incidence of pharmacologically induced priapism in the diagnostic and therapeutic management of 685 men with erectile dysfunction. *Urol Int* **66**, 27–29.
10. Clayton DO, Shen WW (1998). Psychotropic drug-induced sexual function disorders: diagnosis, incidence and management. *Drug Saf* **19**, 299–312.

11. Morga Egea JP, Ferrero Doria R, Guzman Martinez-Valls PL, Navas Pastor J, Garcia Ligero J, Garcia Garcia F, Sempere Gutierrez A, Rico Galiano JL, Tomas Ros M, Fontana Compiano LO (2000). Metastasis priapism. Report of four new cases and review of the literature. *Arch Esp Urol* **53**, 447–452.
12. Colombo F, Lovaria A, Saccheri S, Pozzoni F, Montanaris E (1999). Arterial embolization in the treatment of post-traumatic priapism. *Ann Urol (Paris)* **33**, 210–218.
13. Harmon WJ, Nehra A (1997). Priapism: diagnosis and management. *Mayo Clin Proc* **72**, 350–355.
14. El Bahnasawy MS, Dawood A, Farouk A (2002). Low-flow priapism: risk factors for erectile dysfunction. *BJU Int* **89**, 285–290.
15. deHoll JD, Shin PA, Angle JF, Steers WD (1998). Alternative approaches to the management of priapism. *Int J Impot Res* **10**, 11–14.
16. Fernandez Arancibia MI, Martinez Portillo FJ, Musial A, Spahn M, Junemann KP, Alken P (2000). Diagnosis and therapeutic options for prolonged erection and priapism: up-date review. *Arch Esp Urol* **53**, 919–927.
17. Saikia T, Advani SH, Dinshaw KA, Gopal R, Nair CN, Chandwani IM (1984). Priapism complicating chronic myeloid leukaemia and its management. *J Indian Med Assoc* **82**, 294–296.
18. Mantadakis E, Ewalt DH, Cavender JD, Rogers ZR, Buchanan GR (2000). Outpatient penile aspiration and epinephrine irrigation for young patients with sickle cell anemia and prolonged priapism. *Blood* **95**, 78–82.
19. Upadhyay J, Shekarriz B, Dhabuwala CB (1998). Penile implant for intractable priapism associated with sickle cell disease. *Urology* **51**, 638–639.
20. Altebarmakian VK, Rabinowitz R, Rana SR, Ettinger LJ (1980). Transglandular cavernosum-spongiosum shunt for leukemic priapism in childhood. *J Urol* **123**, 287–288.
21. Falandry L (1999). Priapism: treatment and results. Personal series of 56 cases. *Prog Urol* **9**, 496–501.

22. Dawam D, Kalayi G, Nmadu PN (2000). Cavernosal spongiosium shunt in the management of priapism in Zaria, Nigeria. *Trop Doct* **30**, 31–32.
23. Bastuba MD, Saenz dT, I, Dinlenc CZ, Sarazen A, Krane RJ, Goldstein I (1994). Arterial priapism: diagnosis, treatment and long-term follow-up. *J Urol* **151**, 1231–1237.
24. St Lezin M, Hofmann R, Stoller ML (1992). Pyonephrosis: diagnosis and treatment. *Br J Urol* **70**, 360–363.
25. Fultz PJ, Hampton WR, Totterman SM (1993). Computed tomography of pyonephrosis. *Abdom Imaging* **18**, 82–87.
26. Camunez F, Echenagusia A, Prieto ML, Salom P, Herranz F, Hernandez C (1989). Percutaneous nephrostomy in pyonephrosis. *Urol Radiol* **11**, 77–81.

25

Renal and Ureteric Injury

Sidney Yip
Michael Wong

Introduction

Upper urinary tract injuries that are encountered are generally blunt injuries as a result of road traffic accidents, industrial accidents and occasionally, domestic events. Approximately 10% of the blunt abdominal injuries involve the genital-urinary tract — most commonly the kidney. The Acute Trauma Life Support Program[1] sets priority regarding airway, breathing, circulation, disability and exposure, as well as environment assessment (American College of Surgeons 1997). Attention to these areas is of utmost importance, especially in the early hours of injury. A well-organised team of specialists, preferably led by a trauma care surgeon, should manage a typical polytrauma patient. Many a times, while the primary survey of trauma patients evaluates life threatening injuries, it is during the secondary survey that genito-urinary trauma is revealed. In any event, urological assessment would contribute to the overall management of the patient. The key point is that many of the blunt renal traumas can be managed by a conservative (non-operative) approach.

Presentation and Assessment

The nature of injury should be assessed as far as possible. One of the most important piece of information to be obtained is the extent of deceleration involved. Rapid deceleration can cause injury to vessels, resulting in renal artery thrombosis, renal vein disruption or renal pedicle avulsion. With high velocity impact, multiple organ injury is likely to have occurred.

If the patient is conscious, history can be taken during physical examination, which should be complete and should cover all the body systems. In the polytrauma patient, resuscitation should be started. Immobilisation of the cervical spine is necessary until appropriate radiographs can safely exclude cervical spine injury. The abdomen, chest and back must be examined. Significant flank ecchymosis is suggestive of underlying renal trauma. Fractures of the ribs, and of the lower thoracic-upper lumbar spines, are often associated with renal injuries.

Haematuria is the best indicator of trauma to the urinary system. However, the degree of haematuria and the severity of the renal injury do not correlate consistently, especially for renal vascular injuries, where up to 36% do not have haematuria.[2] Gross haematuria, if present, is most likely associated with significant renal trauma. On the other hand, microscopic haematuria may be present with a wide range of significant renal injuries. When microscopic haematuria occurs concurrently with shock (systolic blood pressure < 90 mmHg at any time during evaluation and resuscitation) the incidence of significant renal injury increases.[3]

Classification

The Organ Injury Scale (OIS) was developed by the American Association for the Surgery of Trauma's Organ Injury Scale Committee, and is currently most widely used and accepted.[4] The renal injuries are graded from I to V in ascending order of severity (Table 1). The wide availability of computed tomography (CT) provides anatomical details that facilitate very accurate grading. One shortcoming is that the scale does not describe pelvic ureteric junction disruption as a

Table 1 American Association for the Surgery of Trauma Organ Injury Severity Scale for the Kidney

Grade	Description
I	• Renal contusion (cortical) • Perirenal haematoma
II	• Renal laceration (< 1 cm) • Perirenal haematoma
III	• Deep laceration (> 1 cm), or • Segmental arterial thrombosis without parenchymal laceration
IV	• Deep laceration involving collecting system
V	• Renal artery thrombosis • Avulsion of renal pedicle • Shattered kidney

separate category. In addition, there is some overlap in the Grade IV and V categories, which is also the group where surgical intervention often needs to be considered. For instance, main renal artery thrombosis with contained haemorrhage — implying an intimal flap disruption from blunt trauma — is classified by some as Grade IV vascular injury. A main renal vein injury with contained haemorrhage can also be classified as a Grade V injury. Despite these shortcomings, the system has established a common scale where the extent of renal injury can be classified. As there are other classification systems for the grading of renal injuries, it is important to specify the classification system employed when describing the severity of a certain renal injury.

Using the OIS, Miller and McAninch noted that significant injuries (Grades II to V of OIS) are found in only 5.4% of renal trauma cases.[5]

Imaging

Based on the extensive work of Miller and McAninch, it is recommended that all blunt trauma patients with gross haematuria, and patients with microscopic haematuria and shock (systolic blood pressure < 90 mmHg) should undergo renal imaging — usually CT with intravenous contrast.[5] Penetrating injury with any degree of haematuria[6] should be imaged. As for paediatric patients, liberal use of imaging studies should be considered, because shock is not a useful parameter in children to determine if imaging should be performed, since their sympathetic response may be able to maintain the blood pressure, at least transiently, despite major blood loss.[7]

The best method of evaluating renal trauma should elicit the most information in the quickest manner.[6] Thus, where 24-hour CT is available, it is the modality of choice. The value of the CT lies not only in the speed at which the information is acquired, but also often in the evaluation of other solid organs of the abdomen. It should be noted that the usual protocol for CT abdomen and pelvis only entails a single series of early post-contrast injection images (< two minutes). Contrast extravasation (signifying major laceration of renal parenchyma or breach of the collecting system) will often be missed if further images in the delayed excretory phase are not obtained. The managing clinician should be aware of this major disadvantage, and request for a modified CT protocol to incorporate a delayed series at about ten minutes after initial contrast injection, whenever renal injury is suspected. The findings that suggest major injury are as follows: (1) medial haematoma, suggesting vascular injury; (2) medial urinary extravasation, suggesting renal pelvis and ureteropelvic junction avulsion injury; and (3) lack of contrast enhancement of the parenchyma, suggesting arterial injury. In the event that such delayed films are not obtained, a plain kidney-ureter-bladder film after the contrast enhanced CT may be able to provide useful information regarding renal excretion and extravasation. However, a complete set of CT with delayed contrast films is still desirable.

Single-shot excretory urography is still valuable in the intra-operative setting, especially when patients are "rushed" to the operating room without proper imaging for exploration due to unstable haemodynamic status. It would confirm renal perfusion and demonstrate rupture of the pelvic-calyceal system. Well taken intra-operative films have resulted in the reduction of renal exploration by 32% in a series of 50 patients.[8] Ultrasonography can demonstrate the presence of perinephric haematoma (which are hyperechoeic, while urinoma is hypodense), but anatomical details are usually lacking. The role of magnetic resonance imaging for acute renal trauma has not been established at this juncture, except in cases of major renal insufficiency or contrast allergy. The use of angiography is limited to defining renal artery injuries that have been identified on CT; but CT with three-dimensional reconstruction provides excellent images without patients

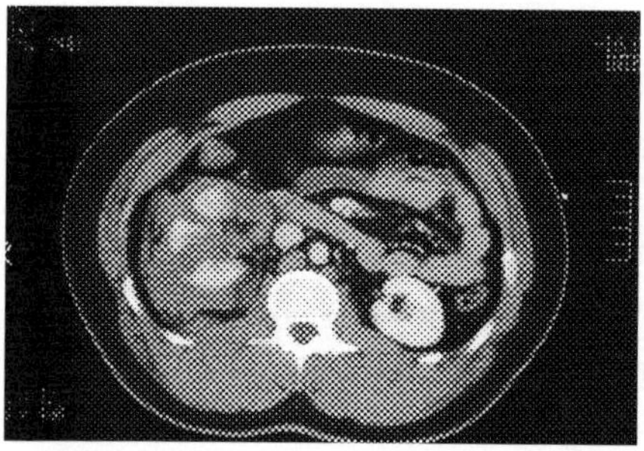

1(a)

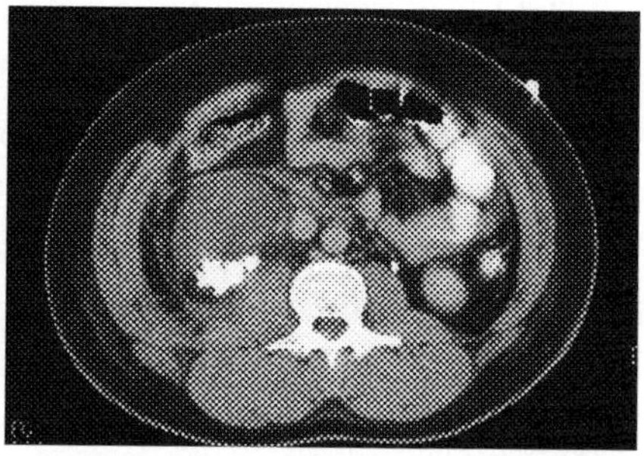

1(b)

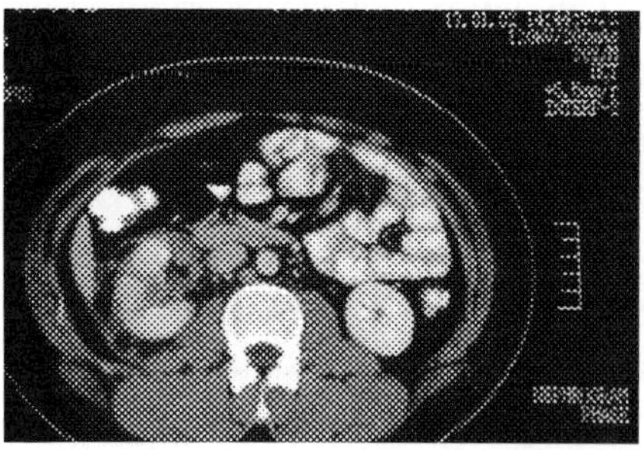

2(a)

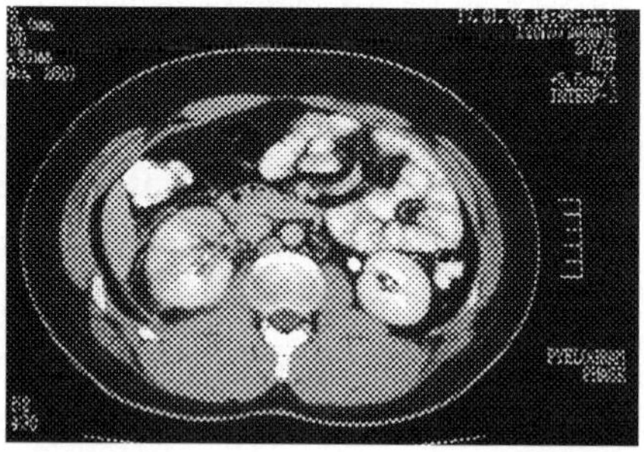

2(b)

Figs. 1(a) and (b), Figs. 2(a) and (b) A young motorcyclist was admitted with blunt renal injury after a road traffic accident. He had abdominal pain and gross haematuria. Clinical assessment showed that he was haemodynamically stable. Enhanced CT of the abdomen showed right renal laceration, perinephric haematoma, satisfactory perfusion, but extravasation in delayed contrast films [Figs. 1(a) and (b)]. In view of haemodynamic stability, decision was made for non-operative management. Follow-up enhanced CT scans after three weeks of conservative management [Figs. 2(a) and (b)] showed resolution of haematoma and sealing off of contrast leakage.

having to go through this invasive procedure. However, angiography does have a role in therapeutic embolisation to control bleeding.

Non-operative Management

A haemodynamically stable patient with an injury well staged by CT scan can usually be managed without renal exploration (Figs. 1(a) and (b), 2(a) and (b)). Indeed, 98% of renal injuries can be managed non-operatively. Grade IV and V injuries more often require surgical exploration, but even these high grade injuries can be managed without renal exploration if these have been carefully staged and identified.[9]

The majority of blunt injuries will heal with non-operative treatment. Only a small percentage of patients who sustain renal trauma with a devitalised segment and urine extravasation require endoscopic or percutaneous intervention. The presence of urinary extravasation, for instance, should not be the sole factor in the consideration for surgery.[10]

Operative Management

It is commonly agreed that for haemodynamically unstable patients, immediate surgery is recommended even in the absence of imaging studies. The absolute indications for renal exploration include (1) evidence of persistent renal bleeding, (2) expanding or pulsatile peri-renal haematoma, and (3) injury to the main renal vasculature. Relative indications include (1) urinary extravasation, (2) shattered kidneys with bulky non-viable tissue, (3) delayed diagnosis of arterial injury, (4) segmental arterial injury, and (5) incomplete staging. It is in this area that there remains some controversy in management. For instance, segmental renal artery injury with an associated renal laceration generally results in a substantial amount of non-viable tissue (usually > 20%). Such injuries should be managed with surgical reconstruction and tissue removal, as a high complication rate is associated with a conservative approach.[11]

In a series where renal exploration was performed in 195 patients (202 renal units or kidneys were involved), exploration alone was performed in 31, repair was performed in 145 and nephrectomy in 26 patients. The overall nephrectomy rate was 13%.[12] In no case was nephrectomy required as a complication of exploration or attempted repair. The report suggests that in properly staged patients undergoing early surgery for appropriate indications, the exploration itself is safe and would not unduly increase the rate of nephrectomy. However, it is important that the expertise, especially in the area of renal transplantation and reconstruction, be available before consideration of surgical exploration.

Renal Exploration and Reconstruction

The renal pedicles should be isolated before exploration, to allow for immediate vascular control if massive bleeding should occur following incision of the Gerota's fascia. While renal bleeding is a major cause of nephrectomy in renal trauma, obtaining early vascular control can decrease renal loss, and a salvage rate of 89% has been reported using this approach.[13]

The extent of renal injury is determined by complete renal exposure. Debridement of non-viable tissue, haemostasis by individual suture ligation of bleeding vessels, watertight closure of the collecting system, and coverage of the parenchyma defect, are to be performed meticulously. For polar injuries with significant tissue loss, partial nephrectomy is indicated.

Patients with reno-vascular injury represent a special group for whom prompt action is required to salvage the kidney. Involved vessels are repaired after application of vascular clamps. With deceleration injuries, tears of the arterial intima occur, and any thrombus formation will render the kidney ischaemic. With delayed diagnosis (> eight hours), the kidney typically cannot be salvaged.[2] In fact, Haas and associates found that revascularisation was seldom successful in the presence of renal artery thrombosis, and that 43% of these patients will subsequently develop hypertension.[14]

Indications for Nephrectomy

Nephrectomy should only be performed for shattered kidneys that cannot be reconstructed, or when attention to other life threatening intra-abdominal injuries prevents timely repair of the kidney. In fact, there remains a group of patients, whose unstable condition dictates that a nephrectomy be performed as the safest approach. In a review of the causes that led to renal trauma patients requiring nephrectomy, 77% were due to extensive parenchymal, vascular or combined injury.[12] In the remaining 23% of nephrectomies, although the kidneys were deemed to be reconstructable, nephrectomy was done as the patients were haemodynamically unstable.

Complications

Persistent urinary extravasation, especially in patients who are managed non-operatively, can lead to urinoma, perinephric infection and very infrequently, renal loss. However, with appropriate systemic antibiotics, endoscopic stenting and percutaneous drainage where appropriate, most extravasation can spontaneously resolve, and most renal units can be preserved.[10]

Long-term Follow-up

Patients with extensive injury who are managed conservatively, should be monitored by subsequent imaging. This is because healing by fibrosis may occasionally lead to pelvic ureteric junction obstruction, and hydronephrosis. The true incidence of post-trauma hypertension is debatable. On long term follow-up of patients managed non-surgically, an earlier report showed that these patients had a higher rate of developing hypertension or abnormal radiological findings compared with those managed by immediate surgery.[15] However, in a review of patients who developed post-traumatic hypertension, Monstrey *et al.* suggested that the rate may be over-estimated and that the event is actually rare.[16]

Even when the kidney can be successfully repaired, concurrent reno-vascular injury and severe injury to other organs, as well as extensive blood loss, may result in renal dysfunction. In a series of 59 patients who had renal scans after reconstructive surgery, a mean renal function of only 39% was demonstrated for the reconstructed kidney.[17]

Special Notes Regarding Penetrating Injury

The management of blunt and penetrating injuries must be considered separately. Penetrating renal injuries most often result from stab and gunshot wounds. Stab wounds are usually a result of assault. The upper abdomen, flank, and lower chest are common sites of entry resulting in renal injury. The dimensions of a recovered weapon may provide valuable information regarding the extent of injury. The extent of penetrating injury from a gunshot can be disproportionate to the external entry or exit wound, and in fact, is often misleading. Radiographs of the chest and abdomen may help to identify the presence of the metallic objects or fragments. As mentioned earlier, penetrating injuries with any degree of haematuria should be imaged (Fig. 3).

Due to the difficulty in assessing the extent of injury and the medicolegal implications, the surgeon tends to be more liberal in renal exploration for penetrating injuries. The repair of "sharp" renal

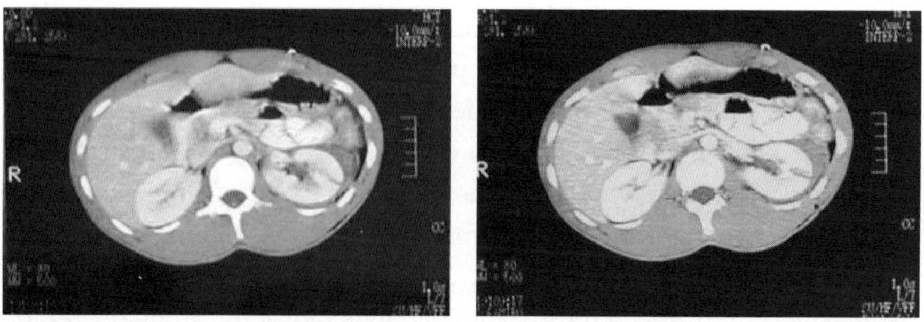

(a) **(b)**

Figs. 3(a) and (b) Enhanced CT showing well-defined penetrating injury to left kidney with small perinepheric collection.

injury is in fact often rather straightforward. During the renal exploration, any contamination from the foreign body can be managed appropriately. Thus, the general recommendation is to explore patients who sustained penetrating renal injury, even in the absence of haemodynamic disturbance. In view of the medicolegal implications, intra-operative photographs should be obtained. However, major trauma centres have also managed patients non-operatively after careful CT staging.[13] In the series from McAninch and associates, 55% of stab wounds and 24% of gunshot wounds were appropriately managed non-operatively.

Overall, as a general guideline regarding penetrating trauma, surgical decision-making should be guided by clinical stability, the grade of injury and the presence of associated injuries. All haemodynamically unstable patients with intra-abdominal injuries should be explored. Stable patients with Grades I or II renal injuries may be managed by observation. The strong association of delayed bleeding with higher grade renal injuries dictates that renal exploration is often required mandatory for this group of patients.

Injury to the Ureter

Since the ureter travels a long distance from the upper flank to the pelvis, it can potentially be injured if external trauma is directed anywhere between the ribs and the bony pelvis. However, in real life, it is very rarely injured (< 1% of urinary trauma), owing both to its protected location in the retroperitoneum, and to its small cross-sectional area. As opposed to renal and bladder injuries, penetrating injuries are more common, especially in places where gunshot wounds are more frequent than stab wounds.

Although not entirely fitting in the acute surgical management context, it is interesting to note that iatrogenic injuries to the ureter does occur. In fact, iatrogenic injuries are more often encountered than external traumatic injuries in routine urological practice. Ureteral injuries largely occur after major surgical procedures in the pelvis and retroperitoneum. In a review by St. Lezin and Stoller,[18] hysterectomy accounted for 54%, followed by colorectal surgery (14%). Since the development of minimal access surgery, laparoscopic injury to the ureter has also been reported. A large percentage of laparoscopic injuries occur during electrosurgical or laser-assisted adhesiolysis in endometriotic disease.[19] Of particular importance, while at least one-third of ureteral injuries are noted intra-operatively in open surgery, the percentage of its being recognised intraoperatively tends to be much lower in laparoscopic surgery. Thus, a high index of suspicion is required when persistent fever, peritoneal signs, and leucocytosis are the only clues, since haematuria and urine leakage leading to pelvic mass formation occur infrequently. Ureteric injuries can also occur during ureteroscopy, especially during rigid ureteroscopy. With the improvement of fibre-optics for semi-rigid scopes, availability of flexible ureteroscopes, as well as with improved intra-corporeal stone fragmentation mechanisms, ureteral perforation are less common in contemporary urological practice.[20]

Imaging

After external injuries, trauma to the ureter — unlike renal injuries — are difficult to detect with the usual array of urine analysis, CT and intravenous urography. The findings of urography are usually subtle and non-specific, including delayed function and ureteral dilatation or deviation. Where CT is used primarily, delayed images must be obtained five to ten minutes after contrast injection, to allow contrast material to extravasate from the injured collecting system, renal pelvis or ureter.[21] It was estimated that insensitivity of the usual diagnostic tools accounts for up to 20% of delayed diagnosis.[22]

Management

External injury

The management obviously depends on the extent of the external injury. Of note is that ureteral contusion may heal with stricture

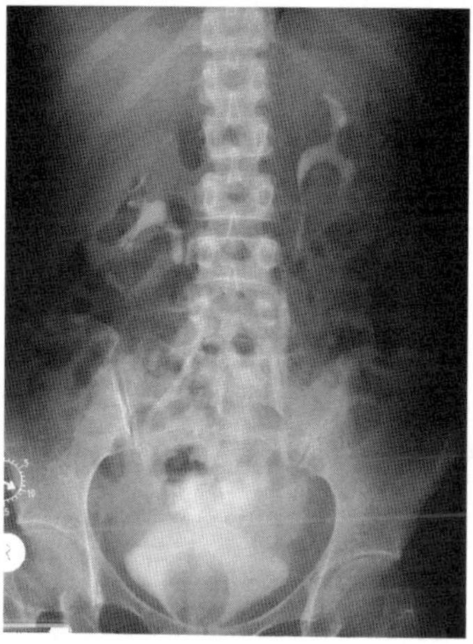

(a)

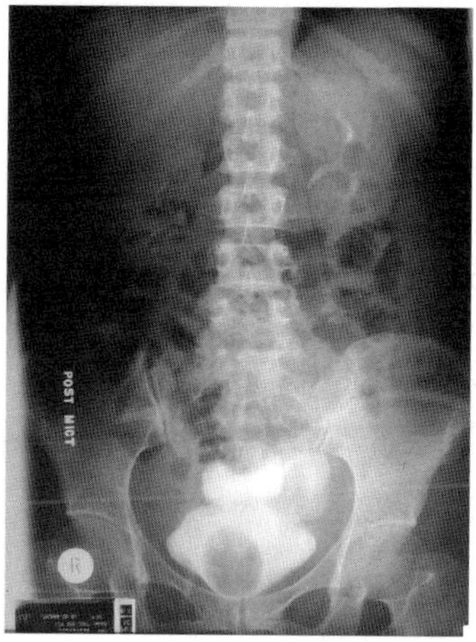

(b)

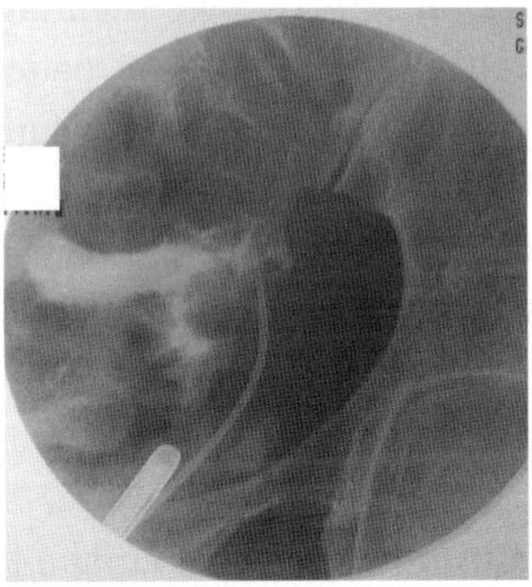

(c)

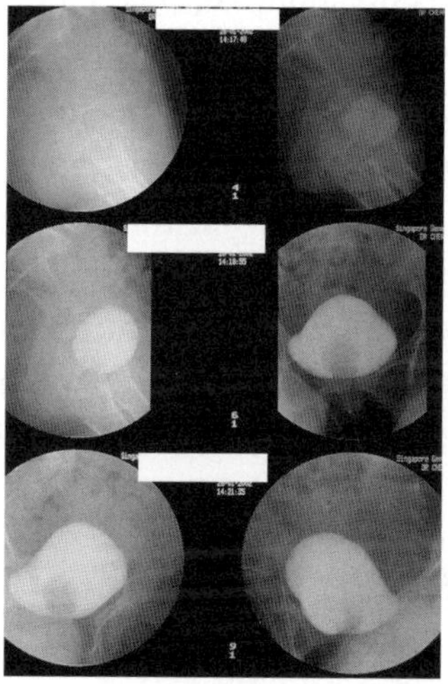

(d)

Figs. 4(a)–(d) A middle-aged lady who underwent elective hysterectomy noted some vaginal discharge early post-operatively. Intravenous urography [Figs. 4(a) and (b)] showed leakage of contrast (urine) to the vagina. However, the exact origin could not be defined. She subsequently underwent exploratory laparotomy. On-table retrograde pyelogram [Fig. 4(c)] demonstrated contrast leakage from the left lower ureter, while on-table cystogram [Fig. 4(d)] demonstrated an intact bladder. The proximal segment of the ureter was then anastomosed to the bladder by way of a raised Boari flap. The lower ureter was subsequently ligated off.

formation. Extensive contusion as well as transection should therefore be treated by excision and primary anastomosis. Direct uretero-ureterostomy would be appropriate for injury of the upper and middle ureter. Lower ureteric injury is often repaired by uretero-neocystostomy, with or without the additional use of a psoas hitch or Boari flap to bridge the gap caused by loss of ureteral length. Minor injuries, especially those recognised during the procedure, can be managed by placement of indwelling ureteral stents.

Surgical injury

Immediate recognition and repair can make a vast difference in the magnitude of repair and the recovery period required (Figs. 4(a)–(d)). Repair of ureteral injury that is recognised during open surgery carries universally high success rates. Similarly, laparoscopic or ureteroscopic injuries, if recognised intra-operatively, can be managed by endoscopic stenting without major complications. Management of delayed diagnosis of ureteral injury is more controversial. Endoscopic stenting has been advocated, but this is possible in only 20% to 50% of patients.[23] In fact, in a series of delayed recognition of laparoscopic ureteral injuries, all the patients ultimately required direct repair.[24]

In many instances, proper pre-operative assessment and pre-operative ureteral stenting could prevent ureteral injuries.

References

1. American College of Surgeons Committee on Trauma (1997). *Advanced Trauma Life Support for Doctors*. Chicago: American College of Surgeons.
2. Cass AS (1989). Renovascular injuries from external trauma. Diagnosis, treatment, and outcome. *Urol Clin North Am* **16**, 213–220.
3. Mee SL, McAninch JW, Robinson AL, Auerbach PS, Carroll PR (1989). Radiographic assessment of renal trauma: a 10-year prospective study of patient selection. *J Urol* **141**, 1095–1098.

4. Moore EE, Shackford SR, Pachter HL, McAninch JW, Browner BD, Champion HR, Flint LM, Gennarelli TA, Malangoni MA, Ramenofsky ML (1989). Organ injury scaling: spleen, liver, and kidney. *J Trauma* **29**, 1664–1667.
5. Miller KS, McAninch JW (1995). Radiographic assessment of renal trauma: our 15-year experience. *J Urol* **154**, 352–355.
6. Goldman SM, Sandler CM (1998). Upper urinary tract trauma — current concepts. *World J Urol* **16**, 62–68.
7. Morey AF, Bruce JE, McAninch JW (1996). Efficacy of radiographic imaging in pediatric blunt renal trauma. *J Urol* **156**, 2014–2018.
8. Morey AL, McAninch JW, Tiller BK, Duckett CP, Carroll PR (1999). Single shot intra-operative excretory urography for the immediate evaluation of renal trauma. *J Urol* **161**, 1088–1092.
9. Santucci RA, McAninch JW (2000). Diagnosis and management of renal trauma: past, present and future. *J Am Coll Surg* **191**, 443–451.
10. Matthews LA, Smith EM, Spirnak JP (1997). Non-operative treatment of major blunt renal lacerations with urinary extravasation. *J Urol* **157**, 2056–2058.
11. Husmann DA, Gilling PJ, Perry MO, Morris JS, Boone TB (1993). Major renal lacerations with devitalized fragments following blunt abdominal trauma: a comparison between non-operative (expectant) versus surgical management. *J Urol* **150**, 1774–1777.
12. Nash PA, Bruce JE, McAninch JW (1995). Nephrectomy for traumatic renal injuries. *World J Urol* **153**, 609–611.
13. McAninch JW Carroll PR, Klosterman PW, Dixon CM, Greenblatt MN (1991). Renal reconstruction after injury. *J Urol* **145**, 932–937.
14. Haas CA, Dinchman KH, Nasrallah PF, Spirnak JP (1998). Traumatic renal artery occlusion: a 15-year review. *J Trauma* **45**, 557–561.
15. Cass AS, Luxenberg M, Gleich, Smith C (1987). Long-term results of conservative and surgical management of blunt renal lacerations. *Br J Urol* **59**, 17–20.

16. Monstrey SJM, Beerthuizen GIJM, Werken CV, Debrune FMJ, Goris RJA (1989). Renal trauma and hypertension. *J Trauma* **29**, 65–70.
17. Wessels H, Deirmenjian J, McAninch JW (1997). Preservation of renal function after reconstruction for trauma: quantitative assessment with radionuclide scintigraphy. *J Urol* **157**, 1583–1586.
18. St. Lezin MA, Stoller ML (1991). Surgical ureteral injuries. *Urology* **38**, 497–506.
19. Grainger DA, Soderstrom RM, Schiff SF, Glickman MG, Decherney AH, Diamond MP (1990). Ureteral injuries at laparoscopy: insights into diagnosis, management and prevention. *Obstet Gynecol* **75**, 839–843.
20. Yip KH, Lee CW, Tam PC (1998). Holmium laser lithotripsy for ureteral calculi: an outpatient procedure. *J Endourol* **12**, 241–246.
21. Kawashima A, Sandler CM, Corriere JN Jr, Rodgers BM, Goldman SM (1997). Ureteropelvic junction injuries secondary to blunt abdominal trauma. *Radiology* **205**, 487–492.
22. Palmer LS, Rosenbaum RR, Gershbaum MD, Kreutzer ER (1999). Penetrating ureteral trauma at an urban trauma centre: 10-year experience. *Urology* **54**, 34–36.
23. Ghali AM, El-Malik EM, Ibrahim AI, Ismail G, Rashid M (1999). Ureteric injuries: diagnosis, management and outcome. *J Trauma* **46**, 150–158.
24. Oh BR, Kwon DD, Park KS, RyuSB, Park YI, Presti Jc Jr (2000). Late presentation of ureteral injury after laparoscopic surgery. *Obstet Gynecol* **95**, 337–379.

26

Trauma to the Bladder and Urethra

Lay-Guat Ng
Chris Cheng

Introduction

Injury to the lower urinary tract can be divided broadly into traumatic or iatrogenic. The latter usually occurs during difficult urological, gynaecological, obstetric or colorectal surgery. This is usually noted at the time of injury, and can be repaired straight away. This chapter will focus mainly on traumatic injuries to the lower urinary tract.

Bladder Injury

Aetiology

In the adult, the bladder is an extraperitoneal organ that is protected by the pelvic bones. Injury to the bladder usually happens when an external force is applied with the bladder distended and has arisen out of the pelvis. Penetrating injuries to the bladder, such as gun shot wounds, are rare in Singapore, but knife wounds and all penetrating injuries need to be explored surgically, debrided and repaired.

Blunt injuries are more common. In Singapore, the most common cause of traumatic bladder injury is that arising from road traffic accidents. The other causes include falls from height or falls with a distended bladder, and abdominal blows.

Classification

Blunt injury to the bladder can be classified according to the extent of injury.

Bladder contusion occurs when there is damage to the mucosa or muscles without loss of continuity to the bladder wall. The cystogram should not show any extravasation, but the bladder may be distorted by the presence of pelvic haematoma.

Intraperitoneal rupture occurs when there is sudden pressure on a distended bladder. The bladder gives way at the weakest and most mobile part of the bladder, that is the dome.

Extraperitoneal rupture occurs in the presence of pelvic fracture. Classical extravasation patterns are described. The site of perforation may be near the fracture, or at a contra-coup site opposite the area of impact.

Diagnosis

History of bladder injuries is not usually specific. The classical history of a drunken man falling onto a pole over his lower abdomen is uncommon. There may be a history of attempts to pass urine, or a strong urge to pass urine, but with the patient being unable to do so. The presence of other injuries in the road traffic accident usually overshadow the symptoms of bladder injury.

Clinically, there may be tenderness at the supra-pubic area. Gross haematuria is usually present. Bowel sounds may be absent in the event of an intraperitoneal perforation.

Diagnosis of bladder injury is usually clinched with a cystogram.[1] This can be done with fluoroscopy or as a CT cystogram.[2] In a patient with pelvic fracture who has not voided spontaneously, urethral catheterisation is contraindicated. Retrograde injection of dilute contrast, with a small catheter at the fossa navicularis of the urethra, will delineate the urethra well. After a normal urethrogram, advancement of the catheter into the bladder, and further contrast studies, should delineate any extravasation of contrast. This may be extraperitoneal or intraperitoneal. Extravasation of contrast in the peritoneal cavity will delineate the cul-de-sac, the loops of the bowel and paracolic gutter. For an extraperitoneal rupture of the bladder, the latter is usually sheared on the anterior and lateral wall. On cystogram, a flame-shaped extravasation of contrast at the perivesical tissues can be seen. Occasionally, the bladder may be lacerated by bony spikes, or lifted up by a large pelvic haematoma. Major extravasation may extend through the obturator foramen in the pelvis into the thigh.

Treatment

All penetrating injuries will require formal exploration and surgical repair. A midline abdominal incision is usually used, and all intra-abdominal viscera and vascular structures should be examined for injuries. Devitalised tissues or bony spikes should be removed. The bladder may be entered intraperitoneally. If the injury is around the ureteric orifices, the ureters should be examined by inserting a small ureteric catheter and injecting a small amount of methylene blue to identify any ureteric injuries. The bladder may be repaired in two layers with an indwelling catheter *in situ*.

Bladder contusions can be treated with an indwelling urethral catheter, as the bladder neck is frequently distorted by the pelvic haematoma, making voiding difficult. For patients with major sacral injuries who are unable to void spontaneously, a delayed urodynamic study may be done to detect any damage to the sacral nerve roots. If no detrusor contractions are seen, the patient may be treated with intermittent self-catheterisation until spontaneous contractions are re-established.

Intraperitoneal rupture of the bladder caused by blunt trauma should undergo formal repair.[3] The bladder should be debrided, and the blood and urine in the peritoneal cavity evacuated. All abdominal organs must be inspected, and any concomitant injuries dealt with. The bladder should be closed in two layers with a urethral catheter left in place and the urethral catheter can be removed after ten days.

Extraperitoneal bladder ruptures may be treated with an indwelling catheter alone.[3] The bladder drainage may be achieved with a urethral catheter or supra-pubic catheter, or both. Good drainage is needed and maintained for about ten days. A cystogram may be done before allowing the patient to attempt voiding spontaneously. If the catheter

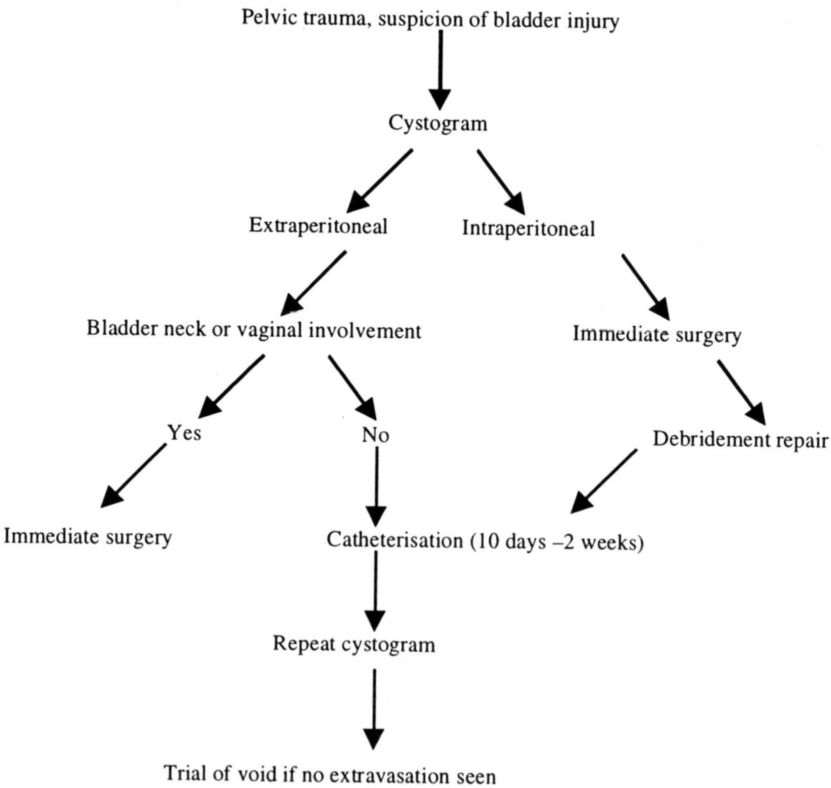

Fig. 1 Bladder trauma.

is unable to drain well, it is probably better to repair the bladder formally.

In cases where the bladder neck or the vagina in females is injured, prompt reconstruction is necessary (Fig. 1).

Complications

The most serious complication of bladder injuries is delayed diagnosis. A high degree of suspicion is important. Infected urine in the peritoneal cavity will result in serious septicaemia. The abscesses need to be drained surgically, and the bladder debrided and closed. Good drainage is of the utmost importance.

Injuries to the bladder neck and vagina may result in problems of incontinence, fistulae or strictures.

Urethral Injuries

Injuries to the male urethra are generally addressed according to the location of the damage. In general, the urethra is divided into the anterior and posterior urethra at the level of the urogenital diaphragm, with the penile and bulbous urethra in the anterior, and membranous and prostatic urethra in the posterior.

Aetiology

Besides iatrogenic injuries such as traumatic catheterisation, trauma to the posterior urethra is generally related to pelvic fractures. This may occur in road traffic accidents, falls or other crush injuries. This classically occurs when the prostate and the puboprostatic ligament is being sheared in one direction, and the membranous urethra, attached to the urogenital diaphragm, in another.

Damage to the anterior urethra occurs mainly with straddle injuries such as falling astride, bicycle injuries or a kick at the groin during contact sports. Another possible cause of anterior urethral injury occurs with penile fracture from sexual intercourse.

Iatrogenic injuries are also common. Penetrating injuries can occur at the anterior as well as the posterior urethra.

Classification

As for bladder injuries, classification of urethral injuries is also according to the extent of damage. Urethral contusion is described when there is blood at the meatus but the urethrogram is normal. *A stretch injury* is an elongated urethra seen on the urethrogram but with no visible extravasation. *Partial rupture* refers to visualisation of the bladder as well as extravasation of contrast. *Complete rupture* occurs when there is extravasation of contrast and no contrast is seen outlining the bladder when instilled retrogradely.

Diagnosis

All patients with pelvic fractures or with injuries to the perineum should be suspected of having urethral injury. Most patients with such injuries will have blood at the meatus. There may be an unsuccessful attempt to pass urine. For an anterior urethral injury, there may be swelling and ecchymosis around the penis, scrotum and perineum. The pattern of the ecchymosis gives an indication as to the extent of injury. If the swelling is limited to the penis, it is probably contained within the Buck's fascia. If it extends to the scrotum, perineum and anterior abdominal wall, it is contained in the Colles' fascia.

Examination rectally may reveal a "high-riding" prostate, in the case of posterior urethral injury. In the position where the prostate is usually felt, a boggy haematoma may be felt.

Imaging

An ascending urethrogram is the definitive imaging done to delineate the urethral injury. This allows classification of the injury depending on the site, and allows planning for subsequent surgery, depending on the distance of separation.

Treatment

Acute management

In the acute situation after the injury has been sustained, the usual trauma management protocol involving the Airway, Breathing and Circulation (ABC) is followed. If urethral injury is suspected, no attempt at urethral catheterisation should be done prior to a normal urethrogram. In this hospital, we prefer to perform the urethrogram on an elective date, after all the acute trauma management has been completed. This may be the next day, or a week later. In the meantime, the patient's urine is drained with a supra-pubic catheter.

In patients whose bladders are easily palpable, insertion of the supra-pubic catheter is very simple. In patients with a substantial amount of pelvic haematoma, the bladder cannot be palpable and the supra-public catheter is best inserted under ultra-sound guidance.

Management of urethral injury

Urethral contusion and stretch injury

The former is characterised by the presence of blood at the meatus, but the urethrogram is normal, while the latter will reveal an elongated urethra. The mechanism of injury for the former is most likely from blunt trauma on the urethra. The latter is caused by stretching of the urethra by a pelvic haematoma. In both situations, a trial of voiding may be allowed by clamping the supra-pubic catheter. The patient may be unable to void urine due to distortion of the bladder neck by external compression. The patient should then be left on the supra-pubic catheter, for trial of voiding at a later date.

Partial urethral rupture

The patient should be left on the supra-pubic catheter for two to three weeks, and the urethrogram repeated. If the extravasation is no longer present, and the calibre of the urethra is normal, the supra-pubic

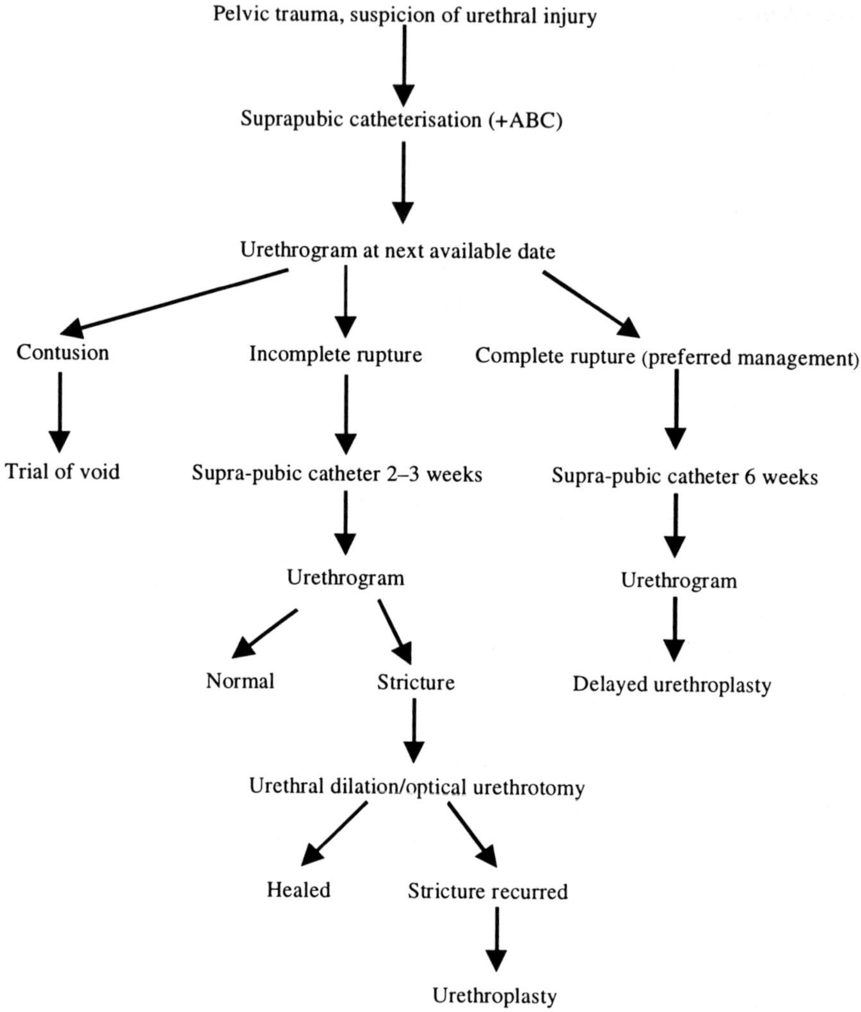

Fig. 2 Urethral trauma.

catheter is removed, and the patient allowed to void urine normally. If healing occurs with a stricture, this may be dilated, or an optical urethrotomy may be done. If the stricture persists or recurs, reconstruction may be done as a delayed procedure (Fig. 2).

Complete urethral rupture

This may be managed by three different approaches: immediate surgical re-alignment, supra-pubic cytostomy, and delayed surgical repair or endoscopic realignment.

Indications for immediate surgical re-alignment are when a stable patient is brought to the operating theatre for pelvic exploration for colorectal or vascular injuries; when there is major displacement of the prostate and bladder; or when there is major bladder neck and prostatic fragmentation. Immediate re-suturing is not done. The patient must be stable, and surgical expertise must be present.

If the above prerequisites are not present, the patient is best left on supra-pubic drainage and the pelvic haematoma allowed to settle. Delayed repair is usually done in after six weeks to three months. A delayed repair may be in the form of an excision and direct anastomosis if the disruption is short. The fibrosis is excised by sharp dissection. Various manoeuvres such as separation of the corporal bodies or excision of part of the pubic bone, are designed to achieve direct anastomosis. Transpubic urethroprostatic anastomosis may be done without excision of scars. Substitution with skin flaps or grafts using buccal mucosa may be done for bulbous injury if the disruption distance is too long for direct anastomosis.

Endoscopic re-alignment has been described but it is not favoured locally. Guided by another cystoscope inserted supra-pubically, directed towards the proximal urethra, the basic principle is "to cut to the light".

Complications

Complications of urethral injuries may be a result of the injury, or from subsequent surgery. Common complications include impotence, incontinence and strictures.

The most common approach, yielding the best results, is the delayed repair. This approach yields the lowest incontinence rate (1–4%) and erectile dysfunction rate (17.6–62%).[4–6] Restricturing after delayed urethroplasty is also rare.[7] The first approach using immediate realignment has a higher restricture (38–53%) and incontinence rate (4–21%). The erectile dysfunction rate is similar (20–50%) as the injury is most likely sustained during the initial trauma.[4, 6] The incontinence rate after endoscopic re-alignment is higher than delayed repair (up to 12.5%) and the erectile dysfunction rate is similar.

The endoscopic approach has the highest restricture rate of 25–100%, and the patient may be subjected to the fate of lifelong repeated dilatation.[8]

Conclusions

Management of injuries of the lower urinary tract depends on a high index of suspicion, early diagnosis and good imaging. Expert care is needed to give good long-term results. Besides possibilities of strictures, incontinence, neurogenic bladders and impotence, there may be other concomitant non-urological problems such as depression, skin problems and social problems. The urologist should thus adopt the holistic approach and treat the patient as a whole.

References

1. Carroll PR, McAninch JW (1983). Major bladder trauma: the accuracy of cystography. *J Urol* **130**, 887–888.
2. Peng MY, Parisky YR, Cornwell EE 3rd, *et al.* (1999). CT cystography versus conventional cystography in evaluation of bladder injury. *AJR Am J Roentgenol* **173**, 1269–1272.
3. McAninch JW, Kahn RI, Jeffrey RB (1984). Major traumatic and septic genital injuries. *J Trauma* **24**, 291–298.
4. Corriere JN Jr, Rudy DC, Benson GS (1994). Voiding and erectile function after delayed one-stage repair of posterior urethral disruption in 50 men with a fractured pelvis. *J Trauma* **37**, 587–589.
5. Elliot DS, Barret DM (1997). Long term follow-up and evaluation of primary realignment of posterior urethral disruptions. *J Urol* **153**, 587–589.

6. Dhabuwala CB, Hamid S, Katsikas DM, Pierce JM Jr (1990). Impotence following delayed repair of prostatomembranous urethral disruption. *J Urol* **144**, 677–678.
7. Morey AF, McAninch JW (1997). Reconstruction of traumatic posterior urethral strictures. *Tech Urol* **3**, 103–107.
8. Chiou RK, Gonzalez R, Ortlips S, Fraley EE (1988). Endoscopic treatment of posterior urethral obliteration: long term follow-up and comparison with traspubic urethroplasty. *J Urol* **140**, 508–511.

Section VII

Perianal Emergencies

27

Genitoperineal (Fournier's) Gangrene

Yik-Hong Ho

Introduction

This uncommon but potentially rapidly fatal condition is characterised by an abrupt onset of infective necrotising fasciitis, affecting the perineal, genital and perianal regions.

Demographics

An average of 97 cases have been reported annually, and the mean age of the patients is about 50 years. It has been reported to be more prevalent among the Nigerian *Igbos* race. Men are much more commonly affected than women (in a ratio of 10:1), but genitoperineal gangrene in women is particularly virulent. In such cases, it has been associated with infected episiotomy wounds and Bartholin's abscesses.

Aetiology and Pathology

The source of infection is usually an anorectal abscess, but urological and dermal causes are also possible. The main predisposing factors are alchoholism and diabetes mellitus. Other factors include leukaemia and human immunodeficiency virus (HIV) infection. Common to these factors is reduced host cellular immunity allowing invasion of the subcutaneous tissue by normal commensal organisms. There may be associated local trauma or surgery such as hernia repair, haemorrhoidal banding, vasectomy, prostate biopsy, and anorectal fish bone impaction. Mixed flora of aerobes and anaerobes have been isolated from most cases; synergism of such bacteria is believed to be the underlying pathogenesis. In this process, one bacterium produces a nutrient for the other, which in turn produces a toxin to protect both of them against phagocystosis. The activity of the aerobes also reduces tissue oxygenation and allows the anaerobes to thrive. The resulting soft tissue suppurative infection leads to thrombosis of subcutaneous vessels and rapid development of gangrene.

Clinical Features

The diagnosis of genitoperineal gangrene is basically clinical, often made with a high index of suspicion. Most patients present with anorectal complaints but insidious presentation at times may be misleading. However, progression of painful erythema, skin necrosis, bullae around an abscess or crepitus, and the lack of frank suppuration, should raise suspicion. The infection can extend from the scrotum to reach the abdominal wall, thigh, chest wall and axilla. The testes are usually spared because the testicular artery is a direct branch or the aorta. When the testes are involved, a retroperitoneal or intra-abdominal source of sepsis should be suspected. Diabetics with drained anorectal abscesses should be given antibiotics, and their progress carefully monitored as progression to genitoperineal gangrene is relatively common in this group.

Investigations

While these go hand-in-hand with urgent resuscitation, investigations would be aimed at possibly identifying the source of the infection.

Where present, foci of sepsis such as ruptured appendicitis, colonic cancer and diverticulitis must be identified and treated. Hence, investigations of the urinary or intestinal tract may be indicated, depending upon the clinical circumstances of the individual patient. However, such tests must often follow after emergency surgical debridement. The best method of culturing anaerobes is to aspirate the tissue pus with a syringe, and to expel any residual air. Where the disease is extensive, CT scans of the abdomen and pelvis may be required. However, the latter does not preclude further debridement, or laparotomy if clinically indicated.

Treatment

Management starts with aggressive fluid resuscitation of the seriously ill patient; blood transfusions may often be required. The aim is to prepare and optimise the patient for surgery. Antibiotics with broad-spectrum aerobic and anaerobic coverage are administered intravenously. Penicillin is recommended for streptococci, metronidazole for anaerobic organisms, and a third generation cephalosporin (with or without gentamicin) is best for coliform organisms and staphylococci. Tetanus prophylaxis is suggested because *C. tetani* is often suspected in fetid, offensive and discharging gangrene. It is very rare that *C. tetani* are actually cultured, but this may be due to technical difficulties in culturing this organism.

The real fundamentals of effective treatment are prompt and adequate surgical debridement. All non-viable tissue has to be removed in order to halt the progression of the infection, and to alleviate systemic toxicity. The wounds are laid open to drain. Debridement must be repeated if necessary, because residual infection is often due to the infiltrative nature of the disease. Faecal diversion is indicated where the anal sphincter is grossly contaminated, but is seldom required to facilitate wound management. Orchidectomy is rarely necessary as the testes have a separate blood supply and are usually spared. Occasionally, this has been reportedly carried out owing to lack of space to house the testes after extensive skin removal. Bladder catheterisation provides initially for monitoring of fluid resuscitation efforts, and later for diversion of urine from the wounds. The effectiveness of hyperbaric oxygenation remains to be proven.

Mortality and Morbidity

The mortality of Fournier's gangrene varies from 3–45%, the better results being due to modern aggressive surgical treatment. Mortality is highest when the origin of the infection is from the anorectal region, and when the involved area is extensive. The usual causes of death include severe sepsis, coagulopathy, acute renal failure, diabetic ketoacidosis and multiple organ failure. Patients who survive may require hospitalisation for several months. The debrided wounds usually heal well by granulation, and seldom require cosmetic reconstruction. Recurrence of genitoperineal gangrene is rare, but not unknown.

References

1. Ong HS, Ho Y-H (1996). Genitoperineal gangrene: experience in Singapore. *Aust NZJ Surg* **66**, 291–293.
2. Eke N (2000). Fournier's gangrene: a review of 1726 cases. *Br J Surg* **87**, 718–728.

28

Acute Management of Haemorrhoids

Sieu-Min Heah

Introduction

Haemorrhoids are vascular cushions in the anal canal that are present from birth. They form a spongy bolster and prevent damage to the anal sphincters during defaecation. This compressible lining permits complete closure of the anal canal and contributes to 10% of the overall continence. The three main cushions lie in the "4, 7 and 11 o'clock" positions when viewed from the lithotomy position. Smaller "secondary" haemorrhoids may occasionally lie between these main bundles. Contrary to what had been previously thought, haemorrhoids are not related to portal hypertension. Increased portal venous hypertension may develop into portosystemic communications between the superior and middle haemorrhoidal veins, resulting in rectal varices. Haemorrhoidal bleeding occurs from presinusoidal arterioles, and is seen to be bright red spurting in nature.

The pain from acutely prolapsed and thrombosed haemorrhoids is mediated through the pudendal and sacral plexus.

Aetiology

Pathological enlargement of the haemorrhoidal tissue results from constipation, prolonged straining, pregnancy and internal sphincter dysfunction. The typical low fibre diet of modern society predisposes the population to constipation and straining. Sitting over the toilet seat for prolonged periods (to read books or newspapers) is an important aggravating problem. This results in congestion and enlargement in the haemorrhoidal tissue. It is important to break this habit, otherwise recurrence is virtually inevitable after treatment.

With time and aging, chronic straining weakens the supporting ligaments, resulting in prolapsation of the haemorrhoids. An abnormally tight internal sphincter leads to venous outflow obstruction and engorgement of the haemorrhoids, which stretches the overlying skin, leading to oedema, prolapse and bleeding.

Classification

External haemorrhoids are located distal to the dentate line, and are covered by anoderm which is innervated by somatic nerves and therefore sensitive to pain. The former are caused by thrombosis of the haemorrhoidal plexus of veins, and appear as a tender bluish mass under the the perianal skin.

Internal haemorrhoids are proximal to the dentate line and covered by columnar mucosa.

Grade 1 haemorrhoids protrude into but do not prolapse outside the anal canal. Grade 2 haemorrhoids prolapse out of the anal canal during straining but spontaneously reduce. Grade 3 haemorrhoids prolapse outside the anal canal and must be reduced manually. Grade 4 haemorrhoids are permanently prolapsed outside the anal canal and cannot be reduced. Haemorrhoids that prolapse outside the canal may develop ischaemia, thrombosis or gangrene in addition to bleeding and oedema.

Symptoms and Signs

Patients with an acute attack of haemorrhoids may complain of severe pain and/or profuse fresh bleeding due to either a prolapsed oedematous, or inflamed haemorrhoids. The thrombosed haemorrhoid is especially tender and tends not to bleed much. Severe anaemia is rare and accounts for 0.5 patients per 100,000. Physical examination reveals a tender, swollen, and often circumferentially prolapsed haemorrhoid which may contain blood clots within.

Differential Diagnosis

Even if haemorrhoids are obvious, one must consider the possibility of anorectal malignancy; a rigid sigmoidoscopy during anaesthesia before the commencement of surgery is mandatory. A malignant melanoma mimicks the appearance of a thrombosed haemorrhoid; suspicious lesions should be sent for histology.

Other conditions which may be mistaken for haemorrhoids include anorectal abscess, fistula-in-ano, anal fissures, foreign bodies such as a fish bone, full thickness rectal prolapse, anal warts and anal cancer.

Management

General

The patient with an acute case of haemorrhoids is in distress; therefore pain control is essential. The prolapsed haemorrhoid may first be reduced manually after generous local application of lignocaine gel (2%) while awaiting surgery. For the irreducible haemorrhoids, warm hypertonic saline baths reduce the oedema and bring relief. This option is appropriate in the medically unfit or pregnant patient in whom surgery may preferably be avoided or deferred. The patient may also be started orally on stool bulking agents (Ispaghula) or stool softeners (Lactulose) and a micronised flavonidic fraction (Daflon). Recommended Daflon dosage is 1 g thrice daily for four days followed by

500 mg thrice daily for the next ten days. It is also given after surgery.[1] NSAIDs are used for analgesia. The acutely bleeding haemorrhoid is managed with neat adrenalin (1:1000) packs and manual pressure. Haemorrhoidectomy should be undertaken in all but the severely ill.

Proctoscopy and sigmoidoscopy

Proctoscopy is unnecessary with painfully prolapsed grade 4 haemorrhoids. A beveled proctoscope provides better views of bleeding internal haemorrhoids, thereby aiding therapy. Immediately prior to surgery, a rigid sigmoidoscopy with the patient under anaesthesia is always performed. A fleet enema should be given before the procedure in order to clear the rectum and sigmoid colon of faeces. A clear view can then be obtained to 25 cm proximal to the anal verge where up to one-third of colorectal cancers occur.

Sclerotherapy

Sclerotherapy aims to cause scarring, thereby causing fixation and eventual shrinkage of the haemorrhoidal tissue. It works by obliterating the vascularity of the haemorrhoids, fixing them to the adjacent anorectal muscularis propia and preventing prolapse. Grade 1 haemorrhoids with acute bleeding are ideally suited to sclerotherapy. The sclerosing agent recommended is phenol 5% in almond oil. After gentle introduction of the proctoscope, 3–5 ml of sclerosant is injected into the submucosa of each haemorrhoidal bundle, 1 cm above the dentate line using a specialised haemorrhoid (Gabriel, Allen & Homburys Ltd., London) needle. Injection is aimed into the tissue just above the haemorrhoidal plexus, and should be deep enough not to blanch the mucosa but not too deep as to injure the internal sphincter. The procedure should be painless if done correctly. Pain occurs if the injection is too deep (causing internal sphincter spasm), or placed below the dentate line where sensitive somatic nerves are irritated.

Contraindications to sclerotherapy include inflammatory bowel disease, immunocompromised states, and anorectal sepsis.

Complications of sclerotherapy occurs from misplaced injections. Most common is the superficial sloughing of the haemorrhoidal mucosa, which heals without treatment. Scarring and stricture formation are rare but may be potentially caused by repeated injections with are best avoided. Thrombosis of an adjacent haemorrhoid may occasionally require surgical evacuation, but mostly can resolve with a protocol of sitz bath, analgesia and stool softeners. The most serious complication is prostatitis caused by deep sclerosant injection into the prostate. The patient complains of dysuria, haematospermia and fever. A week's course of antibiotics (Ciprofloxacin) is recommended. Other rare complications include abscess formation and a granulomatous reaction to the sclerosant.

Rubber band ligation

The procedure first involves introducing a well lubricated bevelled proctoscope into the anus. The haemorrhoidal bundle is seen as falling into view, and a band is placed using a ligator after gentle drawing the apex of the bundle through the loop of the ligator with a pair of atraumatic forceps. The procedure is repeated, and up to three haemorrhoids can be ligated in the same sitting. After successful ligation, the banded haemorrhoids will appear as three red "cherries" at their corresponding positions.

The placement of a tight rubber band around excess haemorrhoidal tissue constricts the blood supply, thereby causing the haemorrhoidal tissue to slough off over five to seven days and forming a small ulcer. This ulcer then heals and fixes the tissue to the underlying muscle. Although best suited for treating bleeding grade 2 haemorrhoids, it can also be used for grade 3 haemorrhoids.

The band should only be placed over the anal mucosa overlying the haemorrhoidal pedicle, well above the the dentate line. Excruciating pain will be experienced if the band is placed over somatically innervated skin distal to the dentate line. If pain is experienced when tissue is grasped by the atraumatic forceps, then it should be released, and more proximally located tissue, not producing pain, should be banded instead. A band that causes pain is immediately removed using specially designed hooked scissors.

After the procedure, the patient is prescribed with stool bulking agents and Daflon. The patient is advised to avoid defaecation if possible, for about six hours. He or she should be warned of the temporary sensation of incomplete evacuation. There may be bleeding at five to seven days when the necrotic tissue sloughs off and exposes a vessel. Other infrequent complications include vasovagal response on placement of the band; anal pain and anal sepsis.

Surgery

Surgery is recommended for complicated grades 3 and 4 prolapsed haemorrhoids or failure of the aforementioned measures. The post haemorrhoidectomy wound has a well deserved reputation of intense postoperative pain, especially upon defaecation. However, patients with prolapsed thrombosed or oedematous haemorrhoids are in so much distress that they cannot wait to have the tissue excised. Surgery will be seen as a procedure bringing relief rather than agony. Although local anaesthesia (LA) is possible,[2] surgery for painful prolapsed haemorrhoids should be done under general or regional anaesthesia. After surgery, recurrence will be minimised if the patient avoids straining or being seated on the toilet seat for prolonged periods. Currently, procedures are categorised as being either "conventional" or "stapled" haemorrhoidectomy techniques.

Conventional haemorrhoidectomy

(1) The Milligan-Morgan (open) technique

This was popularised from St. Mark's Hospital (United Kingdom) in 1937, where the wound is left open to granulate after excision of the haemorrhoidal tissues. The patient is positioned in the lithotomy position, and the surgeon is seated between the patient's legs. Each haemorrhoidal plexus to be excised is infiltrated in the submucosal plane with a diluted adrenalin/marcaine mixture of up to 1 ml. This effectively raises a plane between the haemorrhoidal tissue and the underlying internal sphincter. A well lubricated anal retractor (Eisenhammer) is inserted into the anus and positioned to allow the plexus to be removed, to "drop in". With the assistant holding the retractor, the haemorrhoidal bundle is firmly grasped by a tooth forcep and pulled towards the centre of the anal orifice, thereby providing traction. Dissection begins with the use of diathermy (level 7) cutting the skin and finding the plane between the haemorrhoid tissue and the internal sphincter fibres, identified as white circular fibres going around the anal margin. Once this plane is found and followed, dissection is quite bloodless. One may see "sparks" when dissecting the "oedematous" plane formed by correct infiltration which lifts up the haemorrhoidal tissue from the internal sphincter fibres. Any bleeding point is diathermised. The dissection aims to taper off at the pedicle of the plexus which lies 1 cm above the dentate line. When the pedicle is reached, the surgeon can either transfix it with absorbable sutures (vicryl 3-0) or diathermise the entire pedicle before transecting it, leaving a stump of 2 mm behind. It is easier to see and stop all bleeding points by pulling down the pedicle before transecting it. After haemostasis, the pedicle is transected and the tissue retracts upwards. In this way, each of the three haemorrhoidal bundles are excised in turn. The bundle that is the biggest or bleeding most (i.e. causing the most problems), should be excised first. This provides a clearer view which facilitates the excision of the other bundles.

(2) Ferguson (closed) technique

The dissection stage proceeds as in the "open" procedure. After the pedicle is ligated, the mucosa edges of each excised bundle are approximated with a running suture, including the underlying internal sphincter muscle for additional strength. The suture is then tied close at the most caudal extent of the wound.

Special Points:

(i) Dissection can proceed with either scissors, diathermy[3] or a harmonic scalpel.[4] No individual method has been shown to be superior in terms of post-operative pain, bleeding and strictures. Diathermy dissection is preferred as it is effective and provides good haemostasis.

(ii) The open and closed techniques produce similar results in post-operative pain and bleeding.[5] Occasionally, the closed technique predisposes the patient to small abscess formation (by not allowing the wound to discharge) and delays wound healing.

(iii) There is no difference in postoperative bleeding rate whether the pedicle is ligated or diathermised first before transection. The novice surgeon should start off by ligating the pedicle.

(iv) Only primary haemorrhoids at the 4, 7 and 11 o'clock positions should be excised, even if there is circumferential prolapse. Even if present, secondary haemorrhoids should be left behind in order to preserve mucocutaneous bridges to avoid anal stricture formation. The excess tissue will shrink down when the oedema resolves. Remember that it is easier to treat residual haemorrhoids by banding or ligation subsequently than strictures which often requires skin advancement flaps.[6] Whitehead haemorrhoidectomy involving the circumferential excision of haemorrhoid tissue, gives rise to a high stricture rate and ectropion, and should not be practised.

Post-operative care:

Post-operative care after haemorrhoidectomy focuses on two areas: prevention of complications and relief of pain. A realistic description of post-operative recovery should be given, and the patient should be told that pain will occur but medication can largely reduce the intensity. He is also given assurance that small amounts of bleeding may occur with each bowel movement for approximately ten days. However, should there be torrential bleeding with clots, he should seek medical help immediately. The patient is prescribed with oral analgesia (NSAIDS), stool bulking and softening agents. Daflon has been shown to significantly reduce post-haemorrhoidectomy bleeding.[1] Twice daily shower washes should be performed for at least two weeks. The patient is advised against straining at stools, and to minimise wound pain by squirting Lignocaine gel 2% into the wound, beyond the anal orifice, before and after defaecation. He is discharged and given an appointment to be seen as an outpatient in four weeks.

Complications and treatment:

(i) Haemorrhage

To the patient, this is the most frightening ordeal. Bleeding that occurs within 24 hours (reactionary) is related to inadequate haemostasis at surgery, and may be due to a slipped ligature at the pedicle. Haemostasis under anaesthesia is usually required. Secondary haemorrhage may occur in 4% of cases at seven to 14 days after surgery. The patient experiences several bouts of passing fresh blood and clots per rectum. It is caused by low grade sepsis resulting in friable granulation tissue which sloughs off, exposing a vessel at or near the vascular pedicle. Management begins with an assessment of the haemodynamic status and haemoglobin level, immediate intravenous crystalline infusion and if necessary, blood transfusion.

When haemodynamically stable, the patient is examined with a proctoscope. Often due to intense pain, intravenous pethidine (50 mg) and/or midazolam (5 mg) is given prior to examination. A generous amount of 2% lignocaine gel is squirted into the wound and functions both as a lubricant and analgesia. The smallest size proctoscope with a bevel tip is used to visualise the anal wound in quadrants. Often, the rectum needs to be emptied of clots and stale blood before one can visualise the bleeding point. A powerful light source, with forceps and gauze to clean off blood, are also essential. If no bleeding points are seen, then insertion of a gauze pack for 24 hours, soaked in 1:1000 adrenaline, is appropriate. A bleeding point is identified either as oozing from the wound edge or a spurting vessel, and is effectively treated by injecting the submucosal edges of the wound with a mixture of 1:10000 adrenaline[7] and lignocaine 1%. One to two millilitres is injected via a 23-gauge needle, into the bleeding point. After injection, mild finger pressure is applied onto the wound for two minutes followed by gauze packing. Commonly, one encounters continual wound oozing but the precise point is obscured by blood and cannot be precisely identified. In such instances, 2 ml of the adrenaline and lignocaine mixture can be injected into each quadrant of the wound in a "blind" fashion and then packed with gauze, achieving success in the majority of cases. In the 1% of cases when conservative measures fail, surgical haemostasis by underrunning the wound under anaesthesia is necessary. A Bardia Foley balloon tamponade by gentle traction and strapping the end to the thigh, may minimise blood loss on the way to the OT.

(ii) Urinary retention

The majority affected are males. Post-operative pain and sympathetic "overdrive" are implicated. To reduce its incidence, fluids (less than 250 ml) are minimised and the patient is asked to void soon after surgery. Adequate pain relief is essential. However, about 3% of patients require the catheterisation for 12 hours, after which they are able to void spontaneously once the catheter is removed.

(iii) Rectovaginal fistula

This rare but serious complication occurs when diathermy is used in burning too deeply for haemostasis, or during excision of the 11 o'clock haemorrhoid, especially in older females where the rectovaginal septum may be thinned out. This can be avoided if suture ligation is used for haemostasis when difficulty is encountered.

(iv) Anal stricture

This occurs when insufficient mucocutaneous bridge remains between the quadrants after haemorrhoid excision. Secondary haemorrhoids need not be excised after primary haemorrhoidectomy, and should spontaneously reduce with time. Anal dilatation with metal bougies, lateral internal sphincterotomy or anoplasty with anal advancement flap, may be required.[6]

(v) External thrombosis

This is due to the clotting of a bleeding subcutaneous vessel, and instant relief can be obtained by incision and evacuation of the clot.

(vi) Faecal impaction:

This may predispose the patient to bleeding as the patient is forced to strain to evacuate the stools. It is best prevented by giving stool bulking agents and softeners, but once it has occurred, a gentle olive oil enema may be given. Rarely will the patient require anaesthesia for stool disimpaction.

Stapled haemorrhoidectomy

Since its introduction, stapled haemorrhoidectomy has been enthusiastically received as a novel technique in the management of prolapsed haemorrhoids. Longo[8] refined and popularised the technique, working on the basis that stapling interruption of the feeding superior haemorrhoidal arteries above the base of the haemorrhoids was adequate in treating symptomatic haemorrhoids. The prolapsed anorectal mucosa is drawn upwards and fixed in place by the stapled anastomosis, and the loose redundant mucosa is then conveniently excised in the stapler doughnut. Any residual skin tags not entirely withdrawn upwards are expected to shrivel off to become asymptomatic. The outstanding feature of this technique is the considerable reduction in pain compared to the conventional technique, as the stapled wound overlies the less sensitive mucosa proximal to the dentate line. It is particularly effective in managing circumferential prolapsed haemorrhoids — including thrombosed haemorrhoids. When done properly, it produces a relatively painfree cosmetic result with reduced analgesia usage and earlier return to work compared to conventional surgery.[9]

Technique

The patient is placed in lithotomy under general anaesthesia. Stapled haemorrhoidectomy is performed using PPH™ set (procedure for prolapsed haemorrhoids; Ethicon Endosurgery®, Cincinnati, OH). After the insertion of the anal dilator, any prolapsed haemorrhoid should first be reduced back into the anal canal. The purse string anoscope is then used for the application of a 2-0 Prolene® (Polypropylene, Ethicon, Inc., Somerville, NJ) purse string suture, taking submucosal bites at least 2 cm above the dentate line. The anoscope is removed, and the circular stapler is inserted till the anvil is beyond the level of the purse string. It is then opened completely and the purse string is tied securely around the anvil. The loose end of the tightened purse string is pulled through one of the side holes using the suture threader. Traction is applied on this suture at the same time as the stapler is closed. This serves to hitch up loose anorectal mucosa. Before firing the stapler in female patients, the vagina is examined to ensure that it has not been incorporated into the stapler to avoid rectovaginal injuries. After firing, the jaws are partially opened and removed together with the circular dilator. The purse string anoscope is then used to inspect for bleeding points along the staple line, which can either be diathermised or sutured.

Problems with stapled haemorrhoidectomy

(1) The most serious but infrequent complication is full thickness rectal tear. This arises from improper surgical technique or stapler failure, and results in pelvic sepsis.[10] This may occur when full thickness bites are incorporated into the purse string and the stapler misfires, causing a full thickness defect in the rectum. If the patient has significant pelvic floor descent, the defect may even be intraperitoneal

resulting in peritonitis. The patient complains of pelvic pain and blood stained discharge per rectum. An erect abdominal X-ray shows retropneumoperitoneum. When sepsis persists despite antibiotics and bowel rest, then surgical debridement and defunctioning colostomy are required.

(2) The incidence of secondary haemorrhage is lower than the conventional method, and it can be managed with adrenalin injections as in conventional haemorrhoidectomy.

(3) Stricture formation has an incidence of up to 9% but is usually mild and can be easily dilated by the index finger in the clinic at three weeks following surgery. Some patients may require dilatation by metal bougies under anaesthesia.

(4) Pain is usually mild compared to conventional surgery. However it may be increased in the following instances:

- anal tears upon insertion of a dilator or the stapling instrument; therefore, generous lubrication and gentle insertion of instruments should minimise this
- firing the staplers too low, i.e. near or below the dentate line; one should ensure that the purse string is placed at least 2 cm proximal to the dentate line
- thrombosis of the external haemorrhoidal plexus which resolves with conservative treatment.

(5) Incontinence may result from fragmentation of the internal sphincter upon introduction of the dilator or stapling device.[11] However, this is transient and will invariably resolve in six to eight weeks.

(6) The incidence, management and resolution of urinary retention is similar to that in conventional surgery.

(7) The difference in cost is US$500 more than using the conventional method. However, this should be weighed against earlier return to work and patients improved sense of well-being due to less pain.

Contraindication:

(1) A scarred perianal region from previous surgery may not permit introduction of the stapler.

(2) If there is significant external skin tag components associated with the haemorrhoids, this may not be removed by the stapler. The patient may benefit cosmetically from conventional surgery instead.

The External Thrombosed Haemorrhoid

The patient presents with acute pain which typically lasts for three to five days. The clot underlying the perianal skin is seen as a lump with a bluish tinge, and is exquisitely painful to the touch. Instant relief is obtained by incising into the lump and squeezing out the clot under local anaesthesia. The incision should be wide enough and packed with a small ribbon gauze to avoid reaccumulation of blood and recurrent thrombosis. Stool bulking agents should then be prescribed. Haemorrhoidectomy is rarely required.

Haemorrhoids in Pregnancy

Approximately one-third of pregnant women suffer from haemorrhoids. Constipation is common, and may be due to smooth muscle inhibition by circulating high levels of progesterone, iron supplementation or by mechanical obstruction by the gravid uterus. Venous dilatation and engorgement results from 25–40% increase in circulating blood volume. Hormonal changes result in laxity of connective tissue, especially in the pelvis. A combination of these factors therefore predisposes one to haemorrhoids.

Symptoms vary from mild bloody discharges to severe perianal pain. Since anaesthesia and surgery may pose increased risks to the developing foetus, conservative local therapy should be attempted first. For those with painful prolapsed piles, pain control may be effected by local application of lignocaine 2% gel, manual reduction and oral paracetamol. For haemorrhoids that cannot be reduced, warm hypertonic saline baths can dramatically reduce the oedema and pain over a few days. Daflon and bulk laxatives can safely be prescribed in all stages of pregnancy.

For non-prolapsing (grades 1 and 2) haemorrhoids with acute bleeding, sclerotherapy with phenol is safe and effective, rendering over 80% of patients asymptomatic. For grade 2 or 3 haemorrhoids, rubber band ligation should be undertaken.

Evacuation of thrombus by means of a incision and drainage can be easily performed under local anaesthesia, usually providing immediate relief. Surgery is reserved for painful grade 4 haemorrhoids not resolved with conservative measures. Haemorrhoidectomy under local anaesthesia is preferable to regional or general anaesthesia. Postpartum haemorrhoids is similarly managed conservatively, as delivery results in resolution for most patients. Those with persistent symptoms are advised to elect surgery, especially if further pregnancies are expected.

References

1. Ho YH, Foo CL, Seow-Choen F, Goh HS (1995). Prospective randomized controlled trial of micronized flavonidic fraction to reduce bleeding after haemorrhoidectomy. *Br J Surg* **82**, 1034–1035.
2. Ho KS, Eu KW, Heah SM, Seow-Choen F, Chan YW (2000). Randomised clinical trial of haemorrhoidectomy under a mixture of local anaesthesia versus general anaesthesia. *Br J Surg* **87**, 410–413.
3. Seow-Choen F, Ho YH, Ang GH, Goh HS (1992). Prospective, randomized trial comparing pain and clinical function after conventional scissors excision/ligation versus diathermy excision without ligation of symptomatic haemorrhoids. *Dis Colon Rectum* **35**, 1165–1169.
4. Tan JJ, Seow-Choen F (2001). Prospective, randomized trial comparing diathermy and harmonic scalpel haemorrhoidectomy. *Dis Colon Rectum* **44**, 677–679.

5. Ho YH, Seow-Choen F, Tan M, Leong AFPK (1997). Randomised controlled trial of open and closed haemorrhoidectomy. *Br J Surg* **84**, 1729–1730.
6. Eu KW, Teoh TA, Seow-Choen F, Goh HS (1995). Anal stricture following haemorrhoidectomy: early diagnosis and treatment. *Aust NZ J Surg* **65**(2), 101–103.
7. Nyam DCNK, Seow-Choen F, Ho YH (1995). Submucosal adrenalin injection for posthaemorrhoidectomy haemorrhage. *Dis Colon Rectum* **38**, 776–777.
8. Longo A (1998). Treatment of haemorrhoidal disease by reduction of mucosa and haemorrhoidal prolapse with a circular suturing device: a new procedure. In *Proceedings of the 6th World Congress of Endoscopic Surgery.* Bologna: Monduzzi Editore, pp. 777–784.
9. Ho YH, Cheong WK, Tsang C, Ho J, Eu KW, Tang CL, Seow-Choen F (2000). Stapled haemorrhoidectomy-cost and effectiveness. Randomised controlled trial including incontinence scoring, anorectal manometry, and endoanal ultrasound assessments at up to three months. *Dis Colon Rectum* **43**, 1666–1675.
10. Ripetti V, Caricato M, Arullani A (2002). Rectal perforation, retropneumoperitoneum, and pneumomediastinum after stapling procedure for prolapsed haemorrhoids: report of a case and subsequent considerations. *Dis Colon Rectum* **45**, 268–270.
11. Ho YH, Seow-Choen F, Tsang C, Eu KW (2001). Randomised trial assessing anal sphincter injuries after stapled haemorrhoidectomy. *Br J Surg* **88**, 1449–1455.

Section VIII

Orthopaedic Emergencies

29

Treatment of Multiple Fractures

Tet-Sen Howe

Introduction

The management of multiple fracture made a dramatic improvement in the 1970s when studies showed that early aggressive fracture stabilisation was associated with significant improvements in almost every measurable parameter. In particular, ICU stays, length of stay, sepsis rates, pulmonary complications and patient outcomes were dramatically improved.[1–4] As a direct result of these improvements, cost was also contained.

Pape *et al.* in the early 1990s challenged this dictum.[5] Proposing that early intra-medullary nailing may add additional insult to the lungs, further endangering patients in extremis. Similar concerns regarding "tipping over" of severe head injuries and severely injured patients was also expressed at the same time. The premise was that a severely injured patient could not tolerate the additional surgical insult, and that operating on this subgroup of patients would increase mortality rates. This caused some concern and in some cases encouraged a less aggressive approach.

Most recent studies, however, support the view that early fracture stabilisation with an intra-medullary nail is beneficial even in patients with significant chest injuries, and head injuries.[6,7]

Early Management of the Trauma Patient

Immediate resuscitation is the key to improving survival rates. The ABC's taught on airway, breathing and circulation remain cornerstones of early resuscitation. The cervical spine must be assessed simultaneously to prevent further injury in occult injuries. If there is any doubt, the spine should be immobilised and treated as unstable.

Accurate diagnosis has always been a problem in the busy emergency room. Injuries missed because of incomplete physical examination are common in any situation, and even more so when one severe injury distracts attention from other injuries. The advent of imaging in the emergency room must be coupled with an accurate history and clinical examination.

The timing of investigations and surgical procedures should be made by a team leader. This person should be an experienced member of the trauma team. No particular system has priority over another system: the only factor in deciding the importance of a particular investigation/procedure is that the injury most likely to kill or disable the patient should have priority. No one particular organ system is more important than another.

Systemic Effects of Trauma

Trauma constitutes an insult to the organism that must be coped with, and homeostasis must be restored if the organism is to survive. The wound is an inflammatory site with devitalised necrotic tissue.[8] Additional surgery constitutes an additional insult with an aim to restore homeostasis to the severely injured patient. If the patient is already in severe extremis, this surgical insult will cause death. If, however, the patient can tolerate this insult in the early phase, the long-term probability of survival is improved.

As always, the decision to operate on a severely injured patient is a calculated risk aimed at improving a patient's chances of survival. The trick is to identify the patients that do not benefit from surgical intervention, and treat them with alternative strategies. This is an extremely complex decision process that must be guided with a combination of objective data, experience and intuition.

The response to trauma is characterised by two distinct phases:

(1) The Ebb phase — short period of hypometabolism immediately following an insult. This phase is characterised by extreme instability in blood pressure, fluid volumes and oxygen delivery. The body attempts to preserve blood flow to essential organs. Resuscitative measures during this phase are critical to an improved outcome.

(2) The Flow phase — variable period of hypermetabolism following an insult resulting in potentially severe state of protein and energy malnutrition. These are secondary responses with marked hyperdynamic states, glucose intolerance, fever, and negative nitrogen balance. This phase constitutes a mobilisation of the body's repair mechanisms. Multiple fractures have been shown to increase resting energy expenditure up to 30%. This hypermetabolic state drains the body's reserves and accentuates any pre-existing malnutrition state and may compromise the recovery from the initial insult.

Immune effects of trauma

Sepsis is a common problem in trauma patients. Patients become septic either as a result of direct inoculation of pathogenic organisms, or enteric microbial translocation. This resulting sepsis is thought to play a large role in end-organ failure seen in multiple trauma patients. A severe hyperdynamic state causes starvation with protein malnutrition

Table 1 Mortality Rates with Acute and Delayed Fracture Stabilisation

	ISS 18–34 Delayed Stabilisation	ISS 18–34 Acute Stabilisation	ISS 35–45 Delayed Stabilisation	ISS 35–45 Acute Stabilisation
Less than 50 years of age	11.8	5.1	25.8	11.5
More than 50 years of age	26.4	8.0	42.3	18.4

Source: Bone *et al.* (1994). *J Trauma* **37**.

leading to immunosupression. The intestinal barrier also becomes more permeable to bacteria as a result of hypoxia. This results in not only sepsis but in the release of further inflammatory substances, resulting in a vicious cycle of increased hypermetabolism. This converts a negative feedback system into a positive feedback one. Unchecked, this will result in death.

Concept of Early Stabilisation

The largest benefit from early fracture fixation is the markedly decreased rate of pulmonary complications. Additional benefits are: immediate patient mobilisation, reduction in fat embolism syndrome, and a decreased tissue necrotic load.

This was shown first by Bone *et al.* in a prospective randomised study on early versus late stabilisation of femoral fractures.[3]

Patients and medical staff are also less taxed, and general morale is significantly higher. Even greater in significance was the fact that early surgical stabilisation reduced mortality in young and old patients with significant Injury Severity Scores (ISS) (Table 1).

Immobilisation of a traumatised patient encourages sepsis, decubitus ulcers, muscle wasting, joint stiffness, a negative nitrogen balance and a general poor emotional state.

Methods of Stabilisation

Lower limb

The intra-medullary nail remains the standard of care in the stabilisation of lower-limb fractures. It has proven over time to be effective, safe and efficacious in the treatment of both femur and tibial fractures. Advances such as locked nails, unreamed nails, solid nails and retrograde insertion of the nails, have greatly extended their use.

The intra-medullary nail is an excellent load-sharing device and allows early mobilisation and weight bearing. Infection rates are also extremely low — well under 1%. Union rates are also extremely high — in excess of 95%.

The use of intra-medullary nails in open fractures is now widely accepted in mild to moderately contaminated wounds. In severe contamination an external fixator remains the gold standard.

The intra-medullary nail is also an excellent choice for segmental fractures, as well as fractures involving the metaphyseal region of

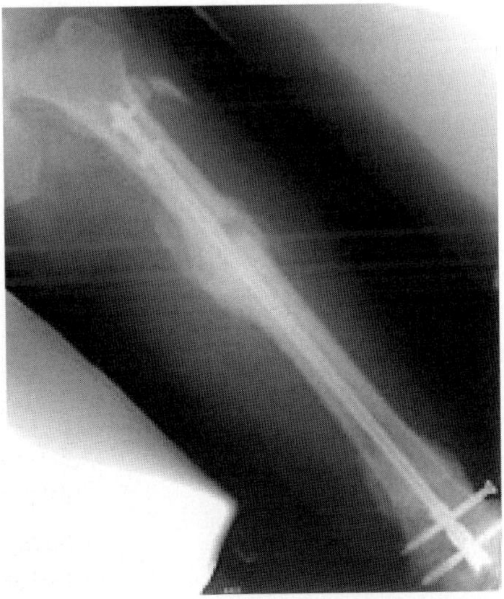

Fig. 1 Retrograde nail used to stabilise a segmental open femur fracture.

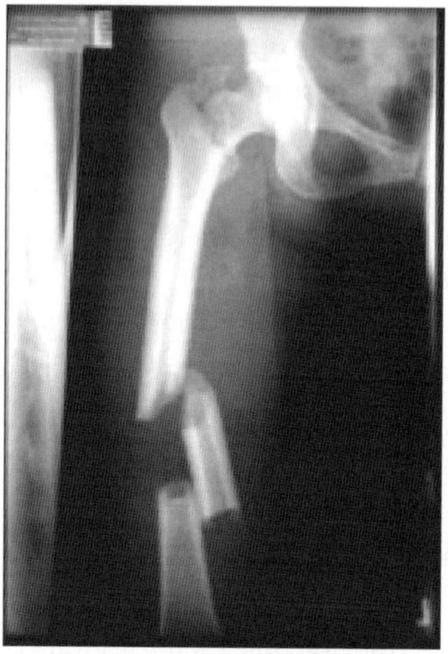

Fig. 2 Segmental fermur fracture with associated inter-trochanteric fracture.

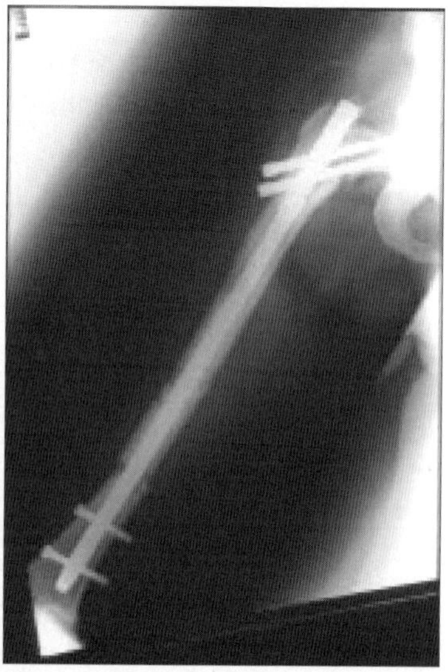

Fig. 3 Stabilisation with reconstruction nail.

the femur, because a single implant will bridge both fractures and also restore load bearing functions. The advent of locked nails and retrograde nails (Fig. 1) has extended the role of nails to most of the femur and tibia except for the extreme ends of the bone.[9]

The use of plates still has a role in some circumstances. Plates are still a fast, reliable method of fracture stabilisation, and have a good track record provided they are used in appropriate circumstances. The recent introduction of minimally invasive plate osteosynthesis — where the plate is introduced — through two small incisions away from the fracture site — may confer some of the benefits similar to that of the intra-medullary nail. Plates with locking screws may also be advantageous in some situations (Figs. 2 and 3).

Upper limb

The use of plates remains the mainstay of treatment in the upper limb. The use of intra-medullary nails has not proven to be as advantageous in the upper limb as in the lower limb. Plates give reliable fracture stabilisation and satisfactory union rates. Infection rates in open fractures remain low even in open fractures. In vascular injuries, the use of plates allows rapid and rigid fracture stabilisation, allowing vascular anastamosis to be performed with a minimum delay.

Intra-medullary nailing in the upper limb is advantageous in segmental and extremely comminuted fractures. There is, however, a small risk of injury to the radial nerve in the humerus.

Pelvis

Most pelvic fractures cause significant haemodynamic instability by large volume losses into the retroperitoneal cavity. This is most often due to venous bleeding. As such, stabilisation reduces pelvic volume and allows the haematoma to tamponade. Pelvic volumes rise exponentially with pelvic incongruity. Early pelvic stabilisation has a marked effect on reducing bleeding. Pelvic stabilisation is initially achieved with either an external fixator or a pelvic C-clamp. These devices are useful, and may be configured so that they do not interfere with subsequent abdominal surgery.

An arterial bleeder may be the cause of persistent haemodynamic instability after pelvic stabilisation, and an angiogram should be ordered if hypotension persists. If found, embolisation should be performed at the same time.

Open surgery is rarely needed in the early phase of treatment. Surgery is more often used in pelvic fractures, but its role is to prevent secondary disability from pain, leg length inequality or deformity. It should be performed after acute resuscitative measures are completed, and adequate assessments of other injuries has been performed. Often, this will require extensive imaging to assess the pelvic injury, and extensive fluid and clotting factor replacement. The ideal window for pelvic surgery should be within two weeks of the fracture.

Anaesthesia

Anaesthesia is a necessary overhead in dealing with the traumatised patient. However, most of this overhead occurs on induction and reversal, where the risk are the greatest. Within large limits, time spent under anaesthesia does not significantly affect morbidity or mortality. This holds true only if homeostasis is maintained, and hypothermia is avoided. Most operating theatres are too cold for prolonged anaesthesia and a conscious effort must be made to warm the patient to at least 22°C.

It should be remembered that most anaesthetic agents are myocardial depressants, and cardiac output diminishes with their use.

Transport of the critically ill patient from the ICU to the operating room may also compromise the haemodynamic stability of the patient. It has been estimated that as many as 10% of these patients will have significant disturbances in their cardiovascular or respiratory systems.[10]

Coagulopathy

Coagulopathy is a problem that must be anticipated early in the management of a trauma patient, if it is to be prevented. Trauma rapidly depletes the host's clotting factors and platelets. Replacement blood products and fluids are generally deficient in factors V, VIII and platelets.

Use of prothrombin time (PT), partial thromboplastin time (PTT), platelets and serum fibrinogen levels to monitor the patient will warn of early coagulopathy. Fresh frozen plasma early in the resuscitative process is essential to prevent problems.

Hypothermia results in platelet segregation, and impairs release of platelet factor. The trauma patient should be warmed, as the OT is an inhospitable environment for the trauma patient. If possible the patient should be warmed to at least 22°C. If there is sufficient time the fluids should also be warmed. Severe head injuries also cause coagulopathy, probably by releasing tissue thromboplastin.

Special Cases

Head injury

Head injury is responsible for almost 50% of deaths in the severely traumatised patient. Fracture fixation in the presence of head injuries is controversial. There is, however, increasing data to show that this is a safe procedure. With adequate monitoring of intra-cranial pressures, most orthopaedic procedures can proceed with minimal problems. One exception to this may be in the first one to two hours after trauma, where fluid shifts are still in progress, and the severity of the head injury may not have fully declared itself.

Orthopaedic procedures may often proceed simultaneously with neurosurgical procedures.

Lung injury

Lung injury is not a contra-indication to orthopaedic stabilisation of fractures. Indeed, one of the greatest benefits of fracture stabilisation is better pulmonary function from lesser fat embolism. Mortality rates from fat embolism approach zero with fracture stabilisation and good monitoring and supportive therapy. The early mobilisation and upright posture after skeletal stabilisation also helps to improve lung function.

Open fractures

Open Fractures can often be treated with intra-medullary devices except in severe contamination or extensive tissue damage. In severe contamination an external fixator is still preferred.

Table 2 Classification of Open Fractures

Fracture Type	Description
Type I	Skin opening of 1 cm or less; quite clean. Most likely from inside to outside. Minimal muscle contusion. Simple transverse or short oblique fractures.
Type II	Laceration more than 1 cm long, with extensive soft tissue damage, flaps, or avulsion. Minimal to moderate crushing component. Simple transverse or short oblique fractures with minimal comminution.
Type III	Extensive soft tissue damage including muscles, skin, and neurovascular structures. Often a high-velocity injury with severe crushing component.
Type IIIa	Extensive soft tissue laceration, adequate bone coverage. Segmental fractures, gunshot injuries.
Type IIIb	Extensive soft tissue injury with periosteal stripping and bone exposure. Usually associated with massive contamination.
Type IIIc	Vascular injury requiring repair.

Source: Gustilo RB *et al.* (1984). *J Trauma* **24**, 742–746.

The most commonly used is the classification of Gustilo and Anderson (Table 2).

The mangled extremity: Often the orthopaedic surgeon must decide if limb preservation is in the best interest of the patient. Severely ischaemic or crushed limb exerts a significant necrotic load on the body. Necrotic tissue must be removed before it causes coagulopathy or renal dysfunction. In general, a limb that is insensate is better sacrificed in the lower limb as the lack of protective propioception results in a poor long term outcome. A quick decision regarding limb salvage or amputation by a senior surgeon can avoid numerous complications in the early postoperative patient. Modern orthopaedic procedures including micro-vascular reconstruction, bone lengthening procedures and free tissue transfers allow solutions to most problems except nerve injury.

The geriatric patient: This is often the most difficult patient to deal with. Often done in an emergency theatre by a junior staff. These patients constitute a neglected group with many medical problems and inadequate reserves. Minor trauma, easily survivable by a younger, fitter patient may have disastrous results in this population.

These patients are often admitted with hip fractures. Many studies show that early operation has better results but this is only true if medical problems are resolved first. Many of these patients are admitted with cardiac failure, anaemia, uncontrolled hypertension and fluid and electrolyte disturbances. These need to be fully corrected before surgery. These patients also rapidly develop chest infections, urinary tract infections and decubitus ulcers if surgery is prolonged. Often, it is better to start on antibiotics and proceed with surgery in cases of minor sepsis.

There is increasing data from meta-analysis showing that regional anaesthesia is better than a general anaesthesia in this group of patients. Patients with a regional anaesthesia have less chest infection, deep vein thrombosis, better pain control and better mental function. There is often a drop in mental function in this group of patients after surgery and anaesthesia.

The aim in this group of patients is to return them to as active a lifestyle as possible, as soon as possible. Sadly, mortality rates may exceed 20% at one year, and high proportions never attain pre-operative levels of activity or cognitive function.[11]

Decision Making

The management of the multiply injured patient is centred on patient survival with normal brain and major organ system function. Thus in the early phase the sole aim is to "improve the physiology". The principle doctor must rapidly decide which organ systems are most severely affected and where the patient is most at risk. These organ systems are tackled first and lesser injuries temporised and treated when the patient is more stable.

This differs significantly from the management of a multiply fractured patient where an optimum orthopaedic result is the desired outcome.

This difference exists because modern orthopaedics has acceptable means with dealing secondarily with complications that include massive bone loss, significant joint incongruity, malunions and to some extent severe infections.

As such the surgeon may trade lesser procedures that "wound" the patient less, and choose to deal with the problems that result at a later date. Thus many simple procedures such as wound toilet and debridement, splinting, external fixation and application of pelvic clamps may be done in the ICU without shifting the patient. Even fasciotomies may be performed at the bedside with only minimal sedation and/or anaesthesia.

Only after relative homeostasis is secured will a concerted plan be made to transport the patient to the operating theatre and definitively treat his fractures. If fracture fixation is planned then the optimum procedure should be performed, as operating time has little effect on outcome. Despite this, it is still preferable to work in multiple teams to keep operating time to a minimum.

Bad Prognostic Factors

In certain cases, it may be prudent to postpone all except life saving procedures. When the patient has severe injuries and is metabolically decompensating, further surgery may kill him. Certain parameters warn the surgeon of this.

These include: massive transfusions of more then 10–15 units of blood
Significant coagulopathy
Metabolic acidosis
Hypoxia
Mixed venous-oxygen saturation
Decreased core temperature

Rehabilitation

This begins the moment the patient is admitted. Chest and limb and physiotherapy begin as soon as the patient is stable. An advantage of intra-medullary fixation is that patients can begin weight bearing almost immediately. This has significant benefits for muscle strength and joint range of motion. For the same reason, upper limb fractures should be fixed to allow the patient to perform activities of daily living. External fixators may be safely exchanged to a nail within ten days of the initial surgery providing there is no pin tract infection. Early bone grafting should be considered at 4 to 8 weeks for bone defects.

Summary

Management of the multiply fractured patient is a difficult but satisfying task.

The surgeon must distinguish between the multiply fractured patient and the multiply injured patient. The orthopaedic surgeon must then consider how his surgical treatment affects patient physiology and alter his strategies accordingly.

Advances in our approach to this group of patients have become more aggressive with a better understanding of the pathophysiology of the traumatised patient. We have seen marked improvements in chest complications, sepsis, fat and pulmonary embolism.

References

1. Behrman SW, Fabian TC, Kudsk KA, Taylor JC (1990). Improved outcome with femur fractures: early versus delayed fixation. *J Trauma* **30**, 792–798.
2. Bone L, Bucholz R (1986). Current concepts review. The management of fractures in the patient with multiple trauma. *J Bone Joint Surg* **68A**, 945–949.
3. Bone LB, Johnson KD, Weigelt J, Scheinberg R (1989). Early versus delayed stabilisation of femoral fractures. *J Bone Joint Surg* **71A**, 336–340.
4. Bone LB, McNamara K, Shine B, Border J (1994). Mortality in multiple trauma patients with fractures. *J Trauma* **37**, 262–264.
5. Pape H-C, Auf'mKolk M, Paffrath T, *et al.* (1993). Primary intramedullary femur fixation in multiple trauma patients with associated lung contusion — A cause of post-traumatic ARDS? *J Trauma* **34**, 540–548.
6. McKee MD, Schemitsch EH, Vincent LO, Sullivan I, Yoo D (1997). The effect of a femoral fracture on concomitant closed head injury in patients with multiple injuries. *J Trauma* **42**(6), 1041–1045.
7. Reynolds MA, Richardson JD, Spain DA, Seligson D, Wilson MA, Miller FB (1995). Is the timing of fracture fixation important for the patient with multiple trauma? *Ann Surg* **222**(4), 470–478; discussion 478–481.
8. Bessey PQ (1995). Metabolic response to critical illness. In *American College of Surgeons: Care of the Surgical Patient.* Wilmore DW, Cheung LY, Harken AH, *et al.* (eds.) New York: Scientific American, p. 3.

9. Howe TS (1998). Double level fractures of the femur treated with closed intramedullary nailing. *Ann Acad Med Singapore* **27**(2), 188–191.
10. Insel J, Weissman C, Kemper M, *et al.* (1986). Cardiovascular changes during transport of critically ill and postoperative patients. *Crit Care Med* **14**, 539.
11. Wong MK, Arjandas, Ching LK, Lim SL, Lo NN (2002). Osteoporotic hip fractures in Singapore — costs and patient's outcome. *Ann Acad Med Singapore* **31**(1), 3–7.

30

Acute Management of Pathological Fractures

Mann-Hong Tan

Introduction

The definition of a pathological fracture includes a break in the continuity or integrity of any bony structure as a result of an underlying loss in its ability to withstand a normal physiological load.

Therefore a pathological fracture, in the complete sense, would encompass any fracture resulting from the following aetiologies:

- primary bone disease
- metastatic bone disease
- metabolic bone disease including osteoporosis
- iatrogenic bone disease including post irradiation therapy.

Much of this chapter will focus on the management of pathological fractures resulting from metastatic bone disease.

Most series of metastatic bone disease rates range from 30 to 85% of cancer patients.[1] Autopsy series reported actual incidences of up to 70%.[2,3]

With improved cancer therapy, patient survival have improved with increased disease-free periods. However, distressingly, the "long arm of cancer" can stretch to as long as 10 to 15 years after the original tumour, and manifest as metastatic disease. Long-term survivors will imply that follow-up care is needed, and will require orthopaedists to detect and provide treatment of bone metastases for some cases.

Both benign primary bone tumours such as simple bone cysts, giant cell tumours and the much rarer bone sarcomas (forming only 0.4% of all cancers) can have the first presentation as pathological fractures. However, these tumours are beyond the scope of this chapter. Metabolic bone disease such as hyper-parathyroidism and osteoporosis are also not the subject of this review.

Clinical Features and Diagnosis

History

Metastatic bone diseases and pathological fractures may present with or without a history of a known primary malignancy. With a known history of a primary malignancy, any subsequent fracture must arouse a high index of suspicion of an underlying pathological nature. This is especially so if the degree of trauma is not likely to cause fractures in normal circumstances.

Likewise, even when there is no known malignancy history, any fracture that had resulted from a degree of trauma that is out of proportion to the inciting force should raise the possibility of a pathological fracture as well. The presence of rest pain, especially relentless night pain, swelling or both, can precede metastatic bone disease or pathological fracture.

Spinal metastases can present as backpain, with or without neurological features such as paraparesis, paraplegia and bladder and bowel symptoms.

Constitutional complaints of weight and/or appetite loss, risk factors such as family history, social history (like cigarette smoking) or exposure to radiation, should be noted.

Radiological features

Metastatic bone disease can present radiologically with two main features, namely, osteolytic and osteoblastic.

Osteolytic lesions are more common in most metastatic cancers (such as lung, colorectal and breast carcinomas), myelomas and leukaemias. These result from bone destruction and osteoclastic and lytic enyzymatic activities.[4]

Osteoblastic lesions can result from stromal new bone formation as a result of blastic activities or reactive bone formation from stress response to weakened bone.[4] Common examples include breast and prostate cancers.

Standard radiographs of the fracture may not be obvious in showing the underlying pathological fracture. This is especially so when malignancy was not previously suspected or noted (see Fig. 1).

Certain sites pose notorious difficulty for the picking up of pathological fractures: the spinal vertebral body compression fracture masquerading as a mere "post traumatic" or osteoporotic fracture in the elderly, and pelvic, iliac and sacral sites are some examples. Also, beware the adolescent patient with a pathological fracture of a bone sarcoma presenting as a "healing fracture" with "reactive bone formation".

For long-bone related metastases, more than 50% cortical involvement is needed to be radiologically obvious. Needless to say, careful scrutiny of any "suspicious" fracture should be done, especially if the patient has had a history of malignancy.

Evaluation and Work-up

Once the pathological fracture has been suspected or established, the patient should be admitted and properly evaluated with a complete history, including obtaining prior medical records, past biopsy and histo-pathological reports. Patients above 40 years of age are at risk.

Complete physical examination will include simple screening physical examinations of the "paired central organs" such as the thyroid, breasts, kidneys, prostate and lungs. The neck and groin lymph nodes should be palpated.

If the patient does not have an obvious primary malignancy, then a series of simple screening examinations could be done to provide a reasonable yield of the primary tumour:

- chest X-ray — anterior-posterior and lateral views
- mammogram (in women)
- urinalysis
- neck examination of thyroid and nodes
- digital rectal examination of prostate and rectum.

Blood work-up is needed to help perioperative preparation and assessment, diagnose malignancy possibilities with tumour markers and allow optimisation for treatment.

- full blood count and erythrocyte sedimentation rate
- urea/electrolytes
- serum electrophoresis (to look for myeloma)
- tumour markers — PSA, CEA, CA125, alpha foeto-protein, etc.
- liver function test and alkaline phosphatase
- coagulation profile
- serum calcium, phosphate (to exclude hyper-parathyroidism and hyper-calcemia).

Specialised imaging studies

Radionuclide imaging is more relevant in its use in the surveillance of the patient with known malignancy. Technetium 99 m scans are the most sensitive modalities (95% sensitivity) especially for most carcinomas.[5] However, beware the occasional "cold" spot in myeloma and certain renal cell carcinomas.

Computer Tomography (CT) scan is useful in at least three situations:

(1) To define certain metastatic sites and extent of bony destruction where the osseous architecture is not obvious from plain radiographs, such as the pelvis, sacrum and spine.
(2) To detect the occult primary in a first presentation of metastatic bone disease (CT scans of the abdomen and chest usually provide the best yield).
(3) To detect lung metastases or define associated intra-thoracic pathologies in primary lung cancers.

Magnetic Resonance Imaging (MRI) scans are useful in spinal metastases in defining possible cord compression, epidural metastases and for evaluating the number of spinal segmental involvement.

Biopsy

The diagnosis would have been obvious in some cases where there is a previous history of primary malignancy and radiological features of the pathological fracture are evident.

If surgical stabilisation of the fracture is intended or already planned, then some specimen from the fracture site could be sent for histology during the surgery itself.

If no prior history of malignancy is available, or the diagnosis is in any doubt, then a biopsy should be planned. This may be done through a fine needle or core needle biopsy, with or without image guidance. If the pathologist is not comfortable with needle biopsy specimens, or if they are insufficient for making a clear diagnosis, then an open biopsy may be needed.

In special situations such as spinal metastases, image guided needle biopsies are desired so as to minimise the need for many separate spinal procedures, and reduce their attendant risks in an already ill and compromised patient.

Options in Surgical Management

The initial management of the patient with a pathological fracture consists of recognition of the pathological nature of the fracture, pain management, and stabilisation of the fracture with external splints or immobilisation devices.

Patients with metastatic bone disease will need variations and combinations of radiation therapy, chemotherapy and surgical stabilisation.

A consult with the oncologist is helpful in getting an idea of the tumour progression, prognosis and need for adjuvant or hormonal therapy.

The life expectancy of the patient must at least be two to three months, and be able to withstand the anaesthesia.

Other than spinal metastases with impending or obvious cord compression that constitute surgical emergencies, there should be a deliberate and well thought-out strategy in approaching the pathological fracture.

For bone metastases with or without fractures, the approach may be divided into two broad categories: wear-bearing versus non-weight bearing bones. This is at best an arbituary division, because the upper extremity may be called into bearing some weight whilst holding walking aids for the lower extremity.

Surgical devices in stabilisation of fractures may be divided into:

- fixation devices — such as plates, screws, intramedullary nails, plate-screw devices, rods, cages
- bone substitutes/fillers — bone grafts (autografts, allografts) polymethylmethacrylate (PMMA)
- joint arthroplasty prostheses — hip, shoulder, knee
- mega-endoprosthesis — that allow both segmental bone replacements with joint arthroplasties.

Combinations of the above devices are required to surgically stabilise the various permutations of fracture and tumour involvement.

In general, the fixation devices will have to span the entire length of the bone, as well as the fracture, to forestall any impending fracture proximal or distal to the site of fracture. For example, a midshaft femoral fracture is best fixed with an intramedullary nail.

In addition, certain devices allow a more "weight bearing" mechanical advantage after implantation. Again, intramedullary nails for the femur, tibia and humerus have this special advantage, and may allow a "speedier" rehabilitation and recovery.

In relationship to intramedullary devices, there is also another advantage in their use in metastatic bone disease and pathological fractures — the need for added protection after radiotherapy. Radiotherapy is often given both to retard further tumour progression and to provide pain relief, but can weaken the bone considerably as well.

Location of the fracture

Upper extremity fractures are mainly in the humerus (50%) and are managed with shoulder hemiarthroplasties for the proximal head and neck region.[6]

The humeral shaft can be resected and shortened, plated or nailed. The distal humeral metaphyseal region can be double plated. Bone cement can be used to augment the fixations.

Lower extremity fractures involving the head and neck region of long bones can be treated with hemiarthroplasties, preferably cemented. If an impending fracture is encountered in the head and neck region, either a hemiarthroplasty or an augmented nail-plate device can be used. However, it is sobering to note that 44% of fixation devices failed at 5 years.[7]

Inter-trochanteric region fractures can be fixed with angled plate-screw devices, or gamma nail devices, with or without PMMA augmentation. Similarly, sub-trochanteric region fractures can be fixed with angled plate-screws, or by calcar replacing hemiarthroplasty or proximal modular endoprosthesis.

Femoral shaft fractures are best dealt with using locked intramedullary nail devices (see Fig. 2), and tibial shaft fractures can likewise be nailed. Distal femoral metaphyseal fractures can be fixed with retrograde nails or a distal femoral modular prosthesis.

Tibial condylar or metaphyseal metastases can be augmented with PMMA. Tibial shaft fractures can also be nailed.

Spinal metastases

Spinal metastases are believed to be the most frequent site for bone metastases.[8]

These present special challenges not only to bony stability and pain, but can also give rise to possible and distressing neurological compromise.

Thoracic spine involvement is commonest (70%), followed by lumbar (20%) and cervical spine (10%).[9]

Treatment of spinal metastases remained controversial due to historical and biased interpretation of older literature. This was due to the then dogmatic approach to using radiation therapy, versus the simple posterior surgical approach of laminectomy.

Then, no significant difference between radiation was demonstrated over simple laminectomy plus radiation in terms of neurological outcome.[10,11]

Presently, the anterior, anterolateral and posterior approaches to spinal tumours and fractures take into account the underlying pathology and the relationship to segmental stability. If the tumour is located anteriorly in the vertebral body, then an anterior approach with a view to resection, partial or complete corpectomy or decompression of the epidural metastases, makes a rational solution.

Better understanding of tumour biology, and better instrumentation with spinal fixation devices and prosthetic replacements, have led to better salvage of spinal cord compression and instability from spinal metastases.

Pelvic metastases

The presence of pelvic metastases presents great problems, especially in the weight bearing peri-acetabular regions. Harrington has classified these periacetabular lesions and recommended treatments.[7]

These lesions tend to be challenging and will require the use of hip arthroplasties, reinforcement cups, methylmethacrylate augmentation and protrusio cups.

Options in Medical Management

Most cancer patients are now treated in a multi-modality setting, involving all three modalities of radiation, chemotherapy and surgery.

Radiation therapy is the commonest follow-on treatment for bone metastases and pathological fractures.

Radiation retards tumour growth and progression, provides medium to long term control of the tumour in the location, and also provides long term pain relief.

Pain relief is a serious issue in advanced cancer patients. These would encompass pharmacologic approaches using opiod therapy, non-opiod and adjuvant analgesics. Neural blockade using neurolytics, neurosurgical techniques like cordotomy and neurostimulation, are now available in achieving relief for patients.

Biphosphonates can also help in reducing the pain and morbidity of bone metastases. These are effective in addressing cancer-induced hypercalcemia through inhibition of osteoclastic activities.

Conclusion

The increasingly longer surviving cancer patient in some groups will translate into higher likelihood of metastatic bone disease manifestations.

Current managements are adequate in handling pathological fractures, but the challenge is in preventing the fractures before they occur.

This may mean a greater need for skeletal surveillance, and heightened awareness in detecting bone metastases, prophylactic fixation and stabilisation of impending fractures.

Appendix

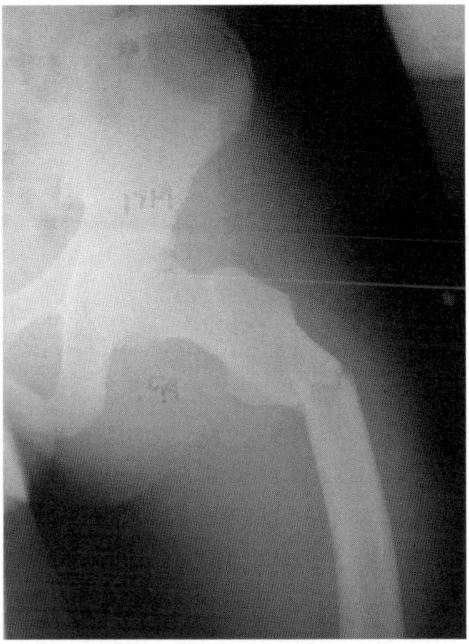

Fig. 1 X-rays of a patient with left proximal femoral pathological fracture. Note the irregular lytic area at the fracture site.

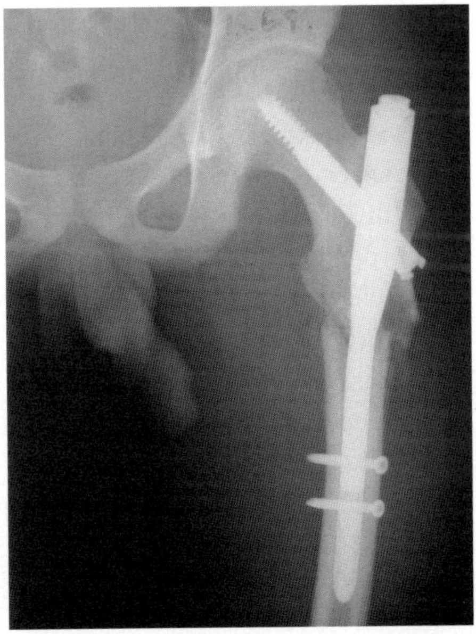

Fig. 2 Post-operative X-rays of a patient with left femoral pathological fracture after a proximal femoral nail fixation.

References

1. Cadman E, Bertino JR (1976). Chemotherapy of skeletal metastases. *Int J Radiat Oncol Biol Physiol* **1**, 1211–1215.
2. Jaffe HL (1967). Palliation of metastatic bone disease. In *Palliative Care of the Cancer Patient.* Hickey RD (ed.) Boston: Little Brown, pp. 313–340.
3. Sherry HS, Levy RN, Siffert RS (1982). Metastatic disease of bone in orthopaedic surgery. *Clin Orthop* **169**, 44–52.
4. Levine AM (1992). Pathologic fractures. In *Skeletal Trauma.* Browner BD, Jupiter JB, Levine AM, Trafton PG (eds.) Philadelphia: W.B. Saunders, p. 403.
5. Citrin DL, Greig WR (1977). A comparison of the sensitivity and accuracy of technetium 99 phosphate bone scan and skeletal radiograph in the diagnosis of bone metastases. *Clin Radiol* **28**, 107.
6. O' Connor MI (2000). Symposium: metastastic bone disease. In *Program and Abstracts of the 67th Annual Meeting of the Americam Academy of Orthopaedic Surgeons, 15–19 March 2000, Orlando, Florida.*
7. Harrington KD (1981). The management of acetabular insufficiency secondary to metastatic malignant disease. *J Bone Joint Surg* **63(A)**, 653–664.
8. Malawer MM, Delaney TF (1993). Treatment of metastatic cancer to bone. In *Cancer: Principles and Practice of Oncology*, 4th Ed. Devita VT, Hellman S, Rosenberg SA (eds.) Philadelphia: Lippincott-Raven, p. 2225.
9. Gokasian ZL, York JE, Walsh GL (1988). Transthoracic vertebrectomy for metastatic spinal tumours. *J Neurosurg* **89**, 599–609.
10. Black P (1979). Spinal metastasis: current status and recommended guidelines for management. *Neurosurgery* **5**, 726–746.
11. Gilbert RW, Kim JH, Posner JB (1978). Epidural spinal cord compression from metastatic tumour: diagnosis and treatment. *Ann Neurol* **3**, 40–51.

Section IX

Hand Surgical Emergencies

31

Open Injuries of the Hand — Assessment and Treatment

Lam-Chuan Teoh

Introduction

The hand is made up of five different tissue components: the skin and subcutaneous tissues; nerves; blood vessels; tendons and muscles; bones and joints. In the hand, these five tissues are closely related. A small penetrating injury can easily transect the tendons, nerves or arteries. In injury of a severe magnitude, the five tissue structures can be damaged in any combination.

The hand can be injured while at work, during recreational activities or during the tasks of daily living. It is the open injuries with bleeding and pain that prompt the patient to seek treatment with urgency. Open injuries of the hand can range from a small laceration to severe mutilation, crushing and amputation. Any of the five tissue components can be injured. Therefore, the surgeon treating the patient should be aware that seemingly minor open injuries could have an associated injury of deeper vital structures. The attending surgeon should have good knowledge of hand anatomy and be trained to conduct a proper assessment. Hand injuries have a tremendous negative economic impact to the patient and the society.[1,2] The injury should be treated promptly, aiming at an early recovery of function and the patient's return to gainful employment.[3]

Assessment

This process is performed to establish comprehensively and precisely, the extent and severity, of the injury to the five-tissue components of the hand. The injury is then categorised.

Surgical anatomy

The palmar skin, has ample sweat glands, is hairless, glabrous and ideal for contact functions. Hence, the loss of palmar skin should ideally be replaced with a sensate like-for-like skin. The dorsal skin is loose on digital extension, but tightly stretched with digital flexion. Therefore, dorsal skin loss should not be underestimated.

The flexor tendon is covered by a fibrous flexor sheath called flexor pulleys, which extends from the head of the metacarpal, to the base of the distal phalanx. The integrity of the flexor pulleys is necessary for proper mechanical function of the flexor tendons. The synovial lining of the flexor tendons extends as the bursae proximally into the palm, across the carpal tunnel, and into the distal forearm. In injection injury, the injected substance can spread through the synovial bursae to reach the forearm.[4]

History

The history taking is to ascertain the nature of the offending objects and mechanism of the injury, the time of occurrence, and any other associated injuries. The patient's previous medical history should also be recorded.

The environment that the injury was sustained in could be in farm, sewerage or construction sites. Injuries occurring in soiled environment with heavy contamination have a higher risk of developing wound infection.[5] Human bites are associated with the risk of *Eikenella corrodens* infection while animal bites are associated with *Pasteurella multocida* infection.[6,7] Infection with *Mycobacterium marinum* has being reported in fishermen and fish-handlers.[8,9] Injuries in contact with river water may run the risk of *Aeromonas hydrophila* infection.[10]

The type of machinery causing the injury should be noted down in detail, and the nature of the injury understood by the surgeon. Sharp penetrating injury, although small in dimension, often lacerates the tendons. A rotating saw causes sharp injury with the zone of tissue loss corresponding to the width of the saw blade. A punch press injury causes a broad segment of multiple tissue damage. A roller injury causes tissue degloving and skin flap ischaemia.

High-pressure industrial equipment can cause injection injury to the hand. These equipments could be waterguns, grease guns, paint guns, fuel injection apparatus or machinery with hydraulic systems. The severity of the injury is dependent on the volume and nature of the injectant.[11–13]

The duration of contact is important in hot press and chemical injuries. In amputations, the warm and cold ischaemic time influence the success of the replantation surgery.

The treatment plan has to be modified in patients with associated cardiovascular, endocrine, haematological and renal diseases. Complex microvascular procedures with prolonged anaesthesia may not be advisable for medically unfit patients.

Physical Examination

The surgeon usually encounters the injured hand covered up in a bulky dressing with blood soaking through the dressing from active bleeding. The necessary preparation for the examination should be in place before the dressing is removed. The examination should be carried out in a well-lit room. A pressure-regulated tourniquet should be placed over the arm and inflated, and the examination should be done under a bloodless field. The necessary dressing implements should be available to redress the hand upon conclusion of the examination.

The physical examination is to assess and document the extent of injury to the five-tissue components of the hand. The order of

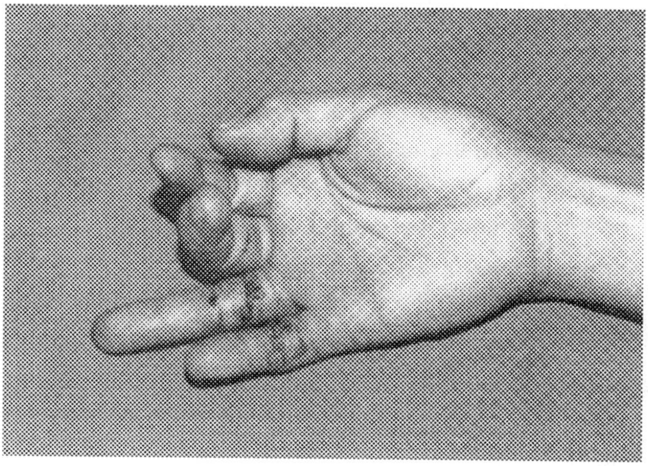

Fig. 1(A) A factory packer had his right ring and little finger cut by a blade. This is a "single tissue transection". The sharp injury over the palmar aspect of the fingers lacerated the flexor tendons. The natural cascade of the fingers was disrupted and he lost the ability to actively flex the finger.

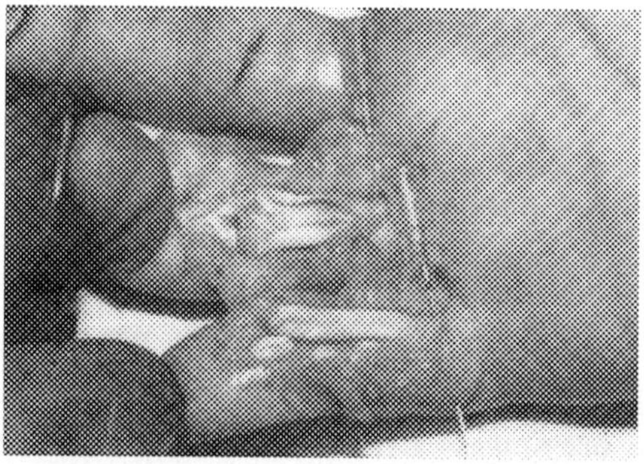

Fig. 1(B) He had a zone II flexor tendon injury. The flexor tendons were exposed through a palmar Brunner's incision and repaired.

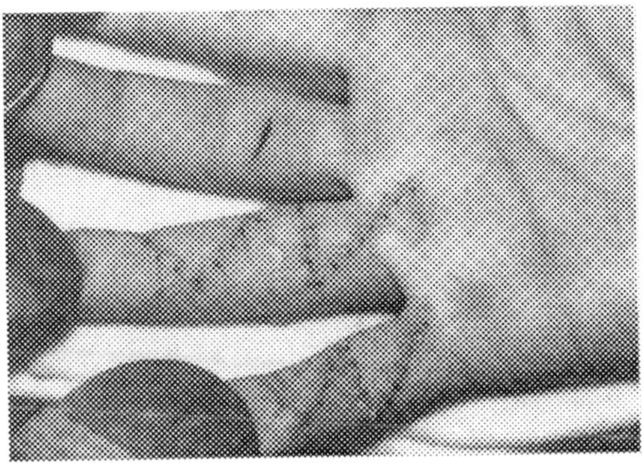

Fig. 1(C) The original wound was incorporated into the design of the Brunner's incision.

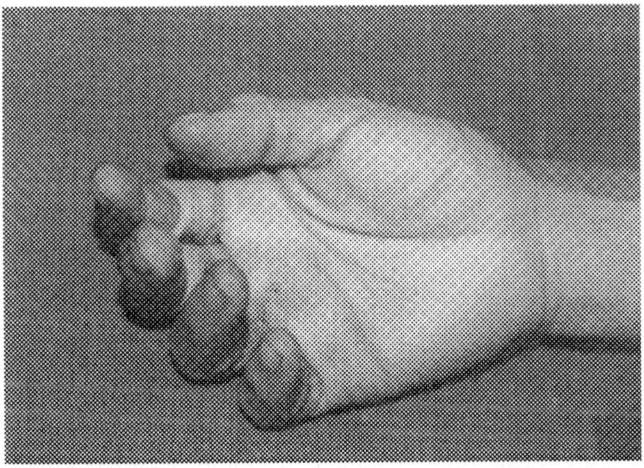

Fig. 1(D) The natural cascade of the fingers was restored after repair of the tendons.

examination is that of inspection, testing of functions and assessment of perfusion.

Inspect the posture of the hand. A loss of the natural palmar cascade of the fingers indicates transected flexor tendons (Figs. 1(A) and (B)), and drop fingers indicate transected extensor tendons. Swellings and

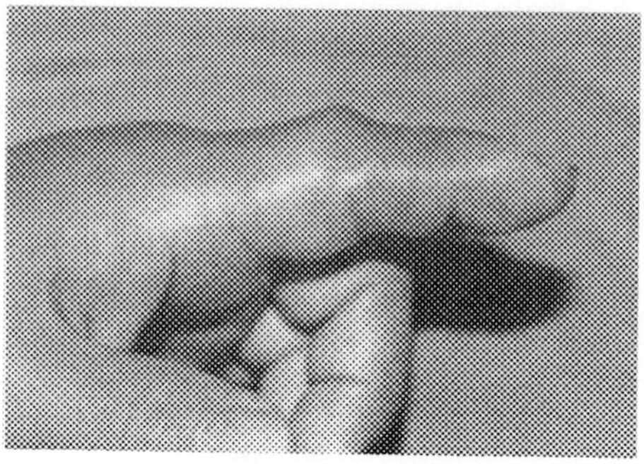

Fig. 2 A mechanic sustained a grease gun injury. The injection was over the index fingertip. There was a tiny entry wound over the pulp, but there was swelling, emphysema and tenderness extending to the forearm.

deformities are from bony fractures and joint dislocations. Inspect the nature of the wound. It can be a small, clean, tidy wound, or a macerated large wound from a crush or avulsion injury. Assess the width of the zone of crushing and segmental damage.

In injection injury, the entry wound can be very small, ranging from one to several millimeters in diameter (Fig. 2). However, there is associated subcutaneous emphysema from the air accompanying the injection. The foreign material that is introduced follows the least resistant tissue planes and may reach the forearm.

Test the functions of the nerves and tendons. Test for touch sensation by running a blunt paper clip over the tip of the fingers. The patient can easily appreciate the difference of touch sensation of an injured digital nerve. A proper two-point discrimination test is difficult to do in a patient who is in pain.[14,15] Active flexion or extension of the finger is performed on the suspected fingers. Loss of active flexion indicates a transected flexor tendon, and inability to extend a finger indicates a transected extensor tendon.

Assess perfusion. Perfusion is assessed with the tourniquet deflated. Colour, refill, turgidity and temperature are the four clinical parameters for assessing perfusion. An adequately perfused finger is

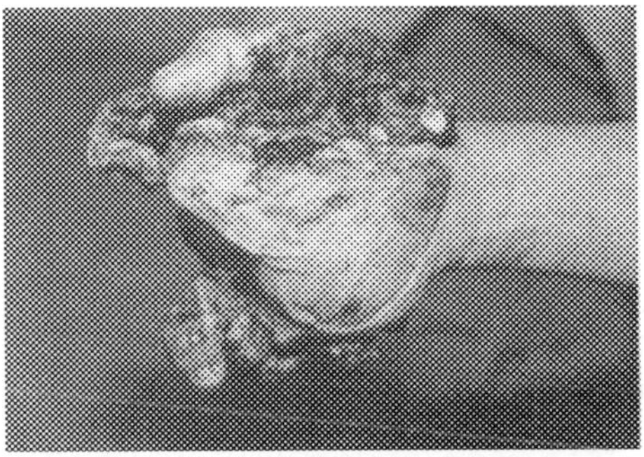

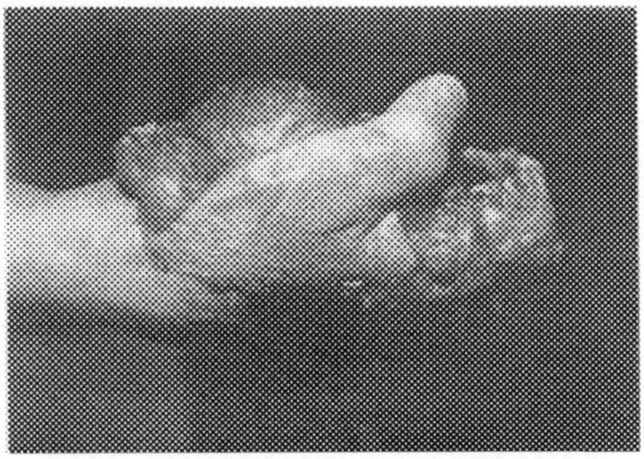

Figs. 3(A) and (B) A mould maker had his right hand crushed by a punch press machine. This is a mutilating injury with "all tissues loss". The ulnar four digits and the palm were completely pulverised. The thumb had both neurovascular bundles damaged and was not viable. In the assessment, the only possible part that can be saved was the thumb.

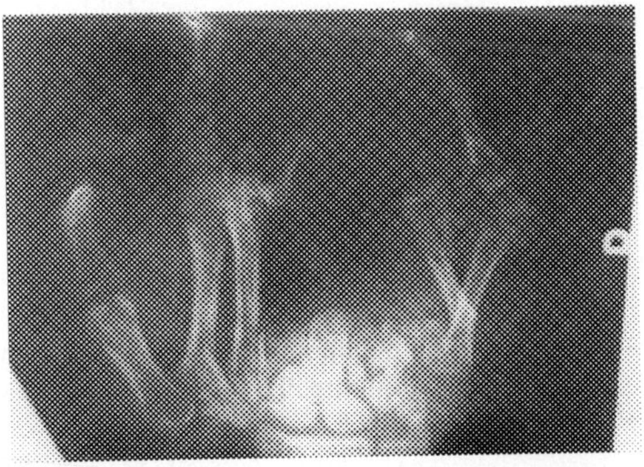

Fig. 3(C) X-ray showing a severely damaged hand, the thumb was dislocated with the trapezial bone from the scaphoid bone.

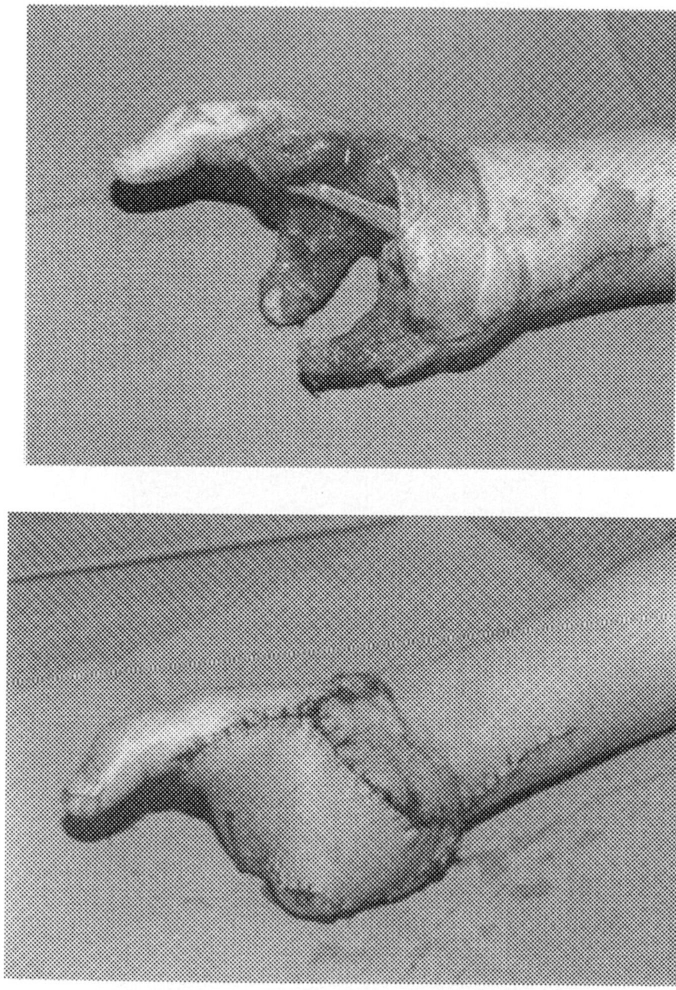

Figs. 3(D) and (E) A meticulous debridement was performed to his hand, removing all the non-viable and contaminated tissues. The thumb was salvaged and it was revascularised with vein grafts. The digital nerves were repaired with grafts harvested from the crushed digits. The large metacarpal defect was immediately resurfaced with a 30 × 5 cm free lateral arm flap.

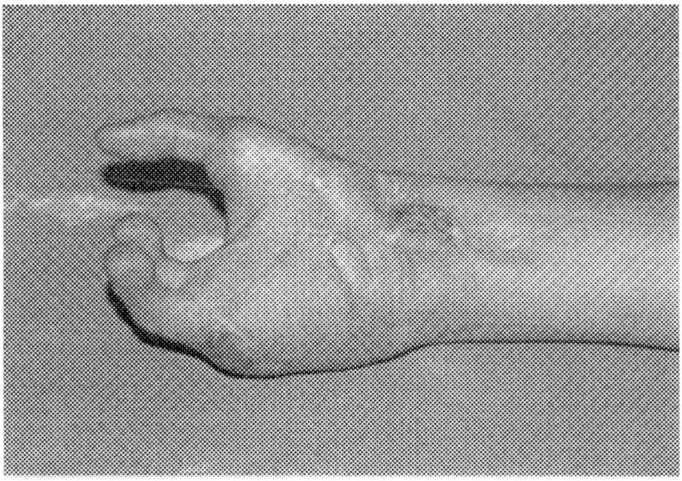

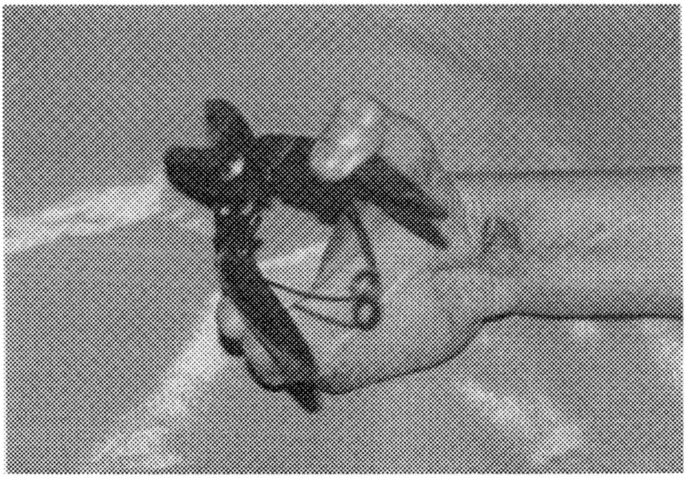

Figs. 3(F) and (G) A staged combined second and third toe transfer was done for him at four months after the initial injury. He recovered sufficient function and dex terity after ten months, and he returned to his original occupation.

pink in colour, comparable to the uninvolved finger, has a refill within one second, and feels full and warm.

In mutilating injuries, the severe crushing injury results in complete loss of a large part of the hand, leaving some functional parts intact. In these cases the examination is to evaluate the intact parts that can still be salvaged and reconstructed (Figs. 3(A) and (B)).

Investigations

Plain radiographs of the hand are the most useful investigation for open injuries of the hand. X-rays of the hand and fingers including the amputated parts in postero-anterior, lateral and oblique views are routinely done for all the cases (Figs. 3(B), 4(B), 8(B) and 9(B)).

Complex imaging is seldom indicated in open injuries of the hand. However, computed tomography is useful for evaluating difficult intraarticular fractures.

Examination under anaesthesia

Thc final examination is completed under anaesthesia. Intra-operative exploration under anaesthesia and a bloodless field further delineate the nature of the injury.

Classification of Open Injuries of the Hand

Open injuries of the hand are very diverse, and therefore classification is necessary to guide treatment.[16,17] Open injuries of the hand are classified based on the five-tissue components of the hand. The injury can be a transection or actual loss of a single tissue component, or multiple tissue components of the hand.

(1) *Single tissue transection*

It is a laceration of the skin, tendon, nerve, artery or a bone fracture (Figs. 1(A) and (B)).

(2) *Single tissue loss*

Loss of skin is the commonest injury under this category (Fig. 4(A)), followed by fracture with bone loss, nerve and vascular injury with a damaged segment.

(3) *Multiple tissues transection*

Dorsal injury of cut extensor tendon and fracture, and volar injury of cut flexor tendon, nerves and arteries are the commonest injuries under this category (Figs. 5(A) and (B)).

(4) *Multiple tissues loss*

Classified under this category are dorsal combined loss of skin and extensor tendon associated with fracture (Fig. 6(A)), and volar combined loss of skin, flexor tendon, nerves and arteries. Severe fingertip injury with loss nail matrix, bone and pulp tissue is included in this category (Figs. 7(A) and (B)). Ulnar and radial combined injury are less common. Loss of skin can be associated with partial loss of extensor tendon, one neurovascular bundle and bone.

(5) *All tissues transection (amputation)*

All amputations comes under this category (Fig. 8(A)).

(6) *All tissues loss (mutilating injury)*

Mutilating injuries are classified under this category (Figs. 3(A) and (B)). Multiple digits or the whole hand are completely crushed and pulverised beyond salvage.[18,19]

Treatment

There is no role for conservative treatment. All open injuries of the hand should be expeditiously and surgically treated. Tetanus immunisations, both active and passive, are necessary in all open injuries. Prophylactic antibiotics are not indicated in minor clean open injuries.[20,21] However, prophylactic antibiotics are indicated in complex open injuries with wound contamination.[22,23] The use of prophylactic antibiotics is also well justified in human and animal bites.[6,7,24]

Surgical debridement

All open injuries of the hand are possibly contaminated. Surgical debridement has to be properly carried out in all the injuries. Under anaesthesia, a sterile scrub of the hand before final cleansing should be done in injuries that are heavily soiled or contaminated. The damaged skin is excised until it reaches a healthy and clean margin. In a heavily soiled wound, to remove the contamination effectively, a thin layer of tissue over the entire wound surface should be excised (Fig. 3(D)).

In injection injuries, it should be recognised that under the small and innocuous puncture wound is an extensive lesion proximally (Fig. 2). All injection injuries should be treated urgently with surgical decompression and debridement.[25,26]

The wound is then irrigated with copious amount of saline solution to further dilute the residual contamination. In heavily soiled and contaminated wounds, the use of pulse irrigation lavage that delivers a large volume of irrigation fluid over a short time, is recommended.[27] In these severe cases, the addition of an antibiotic to the irrigation solution can be beneficial.[28]

Repair of single tissue transection

In this category it is a direct repair: all transected tissues should be promptly repaired. There is no loss of skin, and direct skin closure following the repair is always possible. However, skin incisions should be carefully planned for the exposure to repair the cut structures. The palmar incision should be a zig-zag Brunner's incision, and the dorsal incision should be a gentle curve incision to avoid crossing the joint directly. The original wound, often transverse or oblique, should be incorporated into the design of the incision (Fig. 1(C)). The mid-lateral incision gives limited exposure and is seldom useful.

The flexor tendon injury is divided into five zones. Zone II injury is the most difficult to repair. In this zone both flexor digitorium superficialis and flexor digitorium profundus tendons pass through a tight fibro-osseous tunnel of flexor sheath pulleys. These important flexor sheath pulleys are preserved; the cut tendon ends are delivered through a small perforation for the repair, and then return into the sheath. Both the tendons are repaired with an inner core suture and an outer epitendon running suture (Figs. 1(A)–(D)). The six-strain core suture technique is recommended for the flexor tendon repair, as it offers a better repair strength.[29]

The extensor tendon injury is divided into eight zones. The extensor tendons are small in diameter, and flat. Zone I to IV repairs are done with external interrupted or running sutures and no inner core suture. The repairs are tenuous and require a K-wire pinning of the joints to protect the repair. For Zone 1 and II repair the distal interphalangeal joint is pinned, and for Zone III and IV the proximal interphalangeal joint is pinned.

Cut nerves and arteries are repaired with microsurgical techniques. The repair is performed under a microscope with micro instruments and sutures.

Fractures of the hand that are unstable and displaced are considered for open reduction and internal fixation. The fixation should be of good stability to allow early mobilisation. The approach is dependent on location of the fracture. The method of fixation is dependent on the configuration of the fracture and size of the fracture fragment. Plate-and-screw fixation offers the best mechanical strength and is the fixation of choice.[30–33]

Replacement of single tissue loss

Direct repair is not possible, the missing tissues has to be replaced. Skin loss is the commonest problem, and it is usually due to shaving injury. Except for treatment of some minor fingertip injuries, secondary intention healing with the simple dressing method is not recommended.[34] The method of resurfacing depends on the size and depth of the defect. Skin grafting is indicated for superficial defects. A full thickness grafting is preferred for the hand resurfacing as it gives better padding, durability and less scarring.[35,36] Resurfacing

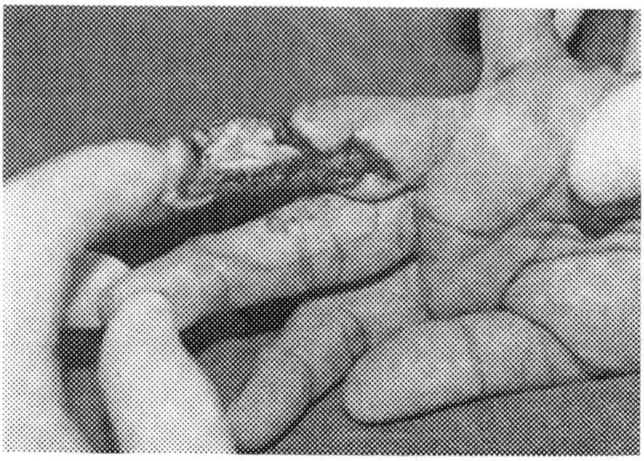

Fig. 4(A) A cook sustained a deep shaving injury to his left ring finger. There were exposed radial neurovascular bundle and flexor tendon. Delay in seeking appropriate treatment resulted in infection. The infection was treated and the wound redebrided. The final defect was 4 × 5 cm. This is a "single tissue loss".

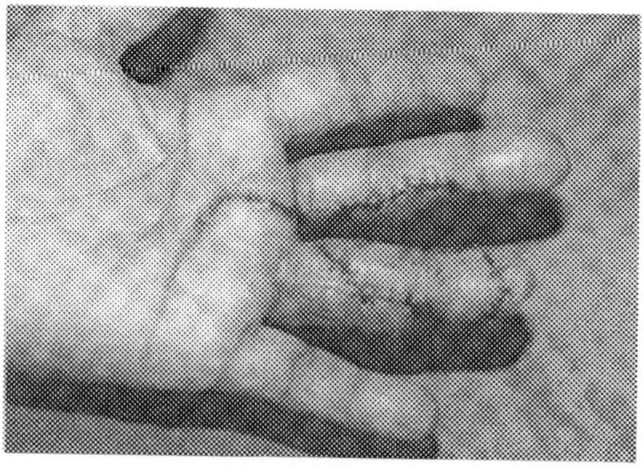

Figs. 4(B)–(D) The skin defect was re-surfaced with a heterodigital arterialised flap harvested from the ulnar aspect of the middle finger. The flap was based on the ulnar digital artery and a dorsal vein of the finger. The wound healed very quickly and he recovered excellent function in two months.

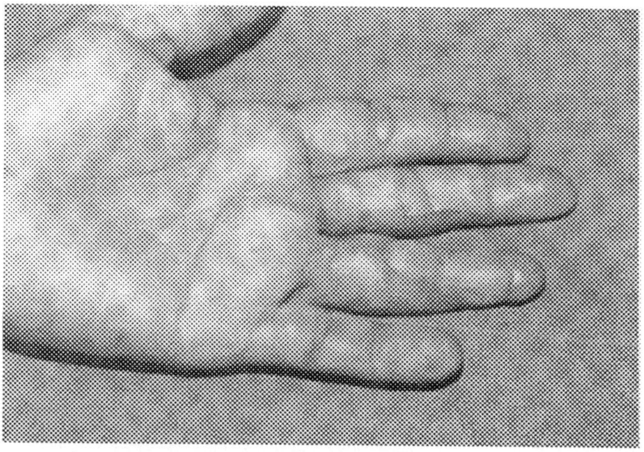

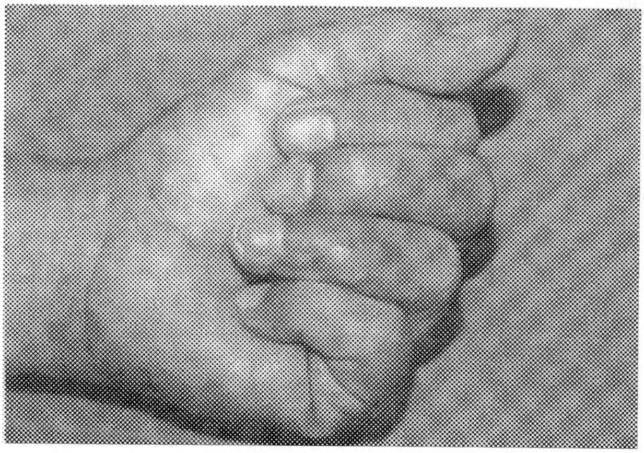

Figs. 4(B)–(D) (*Continued*)

with a skin flap is indicated when there is exposed bare bone, joint and tendon (Figs. 4(A)–(D)). For smaller skin defects of 5–15 cm^2, local advancement flaps and regional flaps are adequate.[37–42] In a larger defect of more than 15 cm^2, the injury is more complex. These defects may need to be resurfaced with distant flaps or free tissue transfers.[43–46]

Bone loss occurs in comminuted phalangeal fractures. Bone loss can result in failure of the fixation construct, leading to a delayed union or non-union of the fracture. Bone grafting is indicated when there is insufficient contact between the bone ends from excessive bone loss. If the soft tissue injury is not severe, conventional bone grafting is sufficient.[47,48]

Flexor and extensor tendon loss can be replaced with a tendon graft. The palmaris tendon, plantaris tendon and long extensor tendons of the second and third toes are the possible sources of tendon grafts.

Loss of nerves can be repaired with a nerve graft. The medial cutaneous nerves of the forearm and sural nerve are possible sources of nerve grafts. Nerve repair should be done without tension with the fingers and wrist in the neutral position. A digital nerve gap of more than 5 mm, and medial nerve gap of more than 1 cm, is indicated for nerve grafting.

Loss of a segment of artery from direct damage or excision of thrombosis should be repaired with a vein graft. Veins over the dorsum of the hand or the palmar aspect of the distal forearm are a good source of grafts.

Repair of multiple tissues transection

The repair technique of each tissue individually, is as described in the single tissue transection category. The approach to repair of combined injuries is in the order of deeper tissue first, and superficial tissue last.

In dorsal combined injury, fracture stabilisation is mandatory and precedes repair of extensor tendons. Extensor tendon rehabilitation is ineffective without a stable fracture fixation (Figs. 5(A)–(E)).

In volar combined injuries, the flexor tendon is first to be repaired. Repair of the flexor tendons may require many manipulative steps and may damage the fine microsurgical repair of nerve and artery. Therefore, microsurgical repair of nerve and artery is last in the order of the repairs.

Replacement of multiple tissues loss

The replacement technique of individual tissue components is similar to that of replacing a single tissue loss. However, the reconstruction

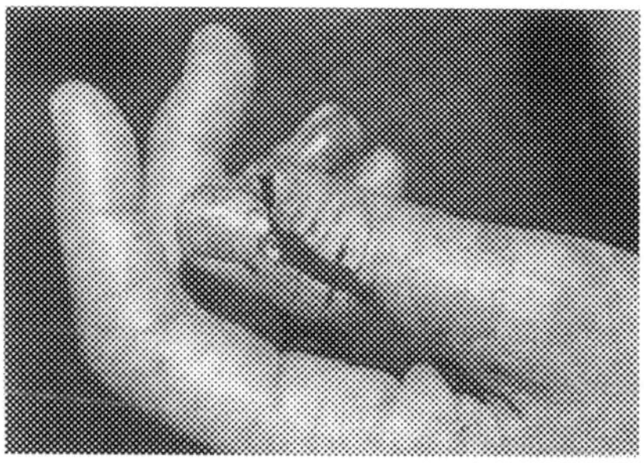

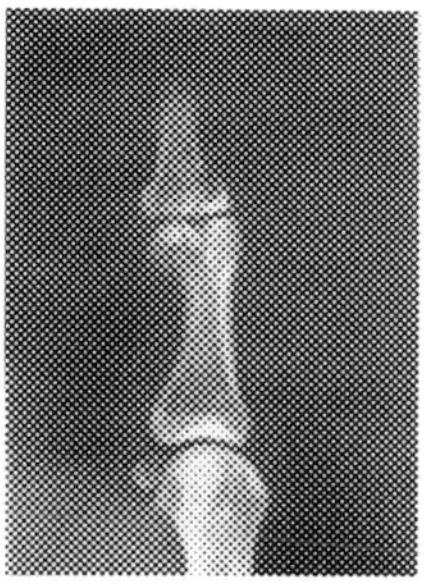

Figs. 5(A) and (B) A metal worker had her left thumb sliced by a metal cutter. She sustained radial oblique transection through the IP joint with laceration of extensor tendon and radial neurovascular bundle. X-rays showing fracture of proximal phalanx condylar and base of distal phalanx. This is a "multiple tissues transection". Rigid internal fixation of the fracture was accomplished with 1.5 mm interfragmentary screws and K-wires. Direct repair of radial neurovascular bundle was done under magnification. Direct repair of extensor tendon and wound closure were possible.

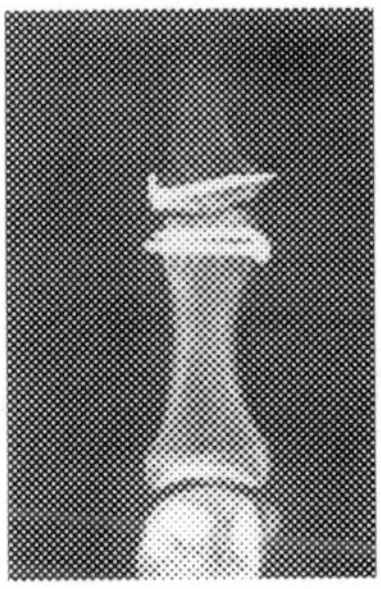

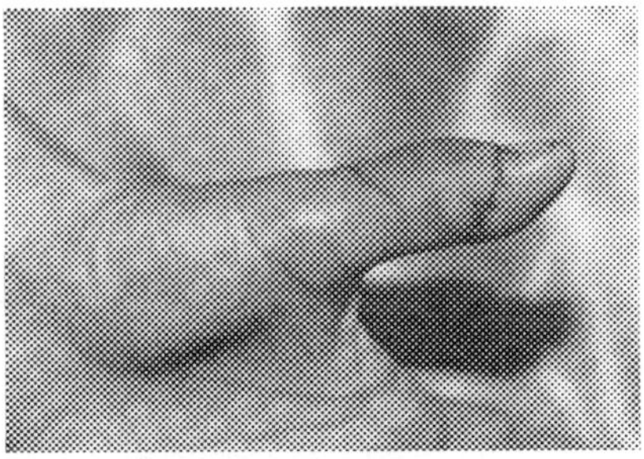

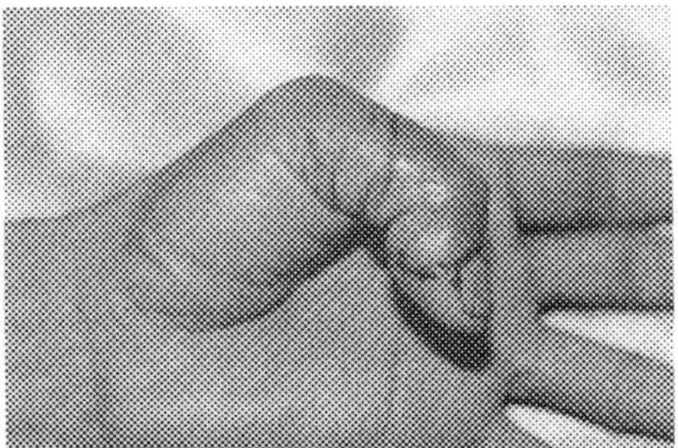

Figs. 5(C)–(E) X-rays showing rigid internal fixation of the fractures. She had uncomplicated wound healing and recovered normal motion of her thumb in six weeks.

of a combined injury needs careful planning.[49] The reconstruction can be in a multi-staged, or in a combined single stage approach. The reconstruction usually involves fracture stabilisation and bone grafting, tendon grafting and skin flap cover. Microvascular free flaps and composite tissue transfers may be necessary for reconstruction of these defects.[50–57] Emergency free tissue transfer may also be indicated for the reconstruction.[58,59]

In dorsal combined loss of skin and extensor tendon associated with fracture bone loss. The tendon, nerve and bone loss can be replaced with non-vascularised grafts. However, the skin coverage has to be a flap that carries its own blood supply (Figs. 6(A)–(D)). If the bone loss is extensive, a vascularised bone graft that gives a rapid bone healing should be considered.[56,60]

In volar combined loss of skin, flexor tendon and neurovascular bundle, similarly the loss of tendon and nerves can be grafted with non-vascularised grafts. The finger is revascularised with a vein graft

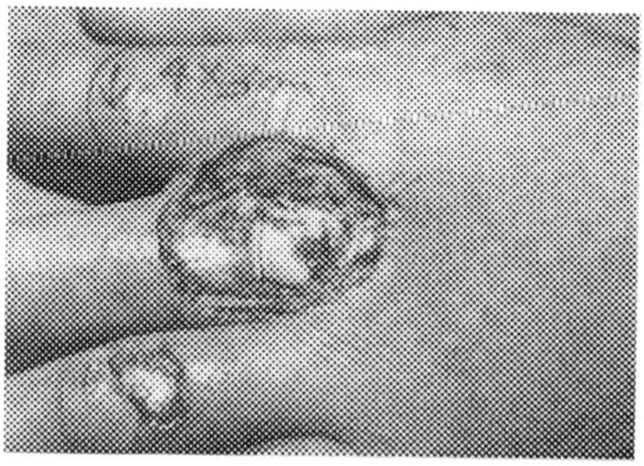

Fig. 6(A) A carpenter had a deep shaving injury to the dorsum of his left hand. He sustained a "multiple tissues loss" over the dorsal MCP joint of middle finger. There was a 4 × 3 cm skin defect with a 4 cm extensor tendon loss.

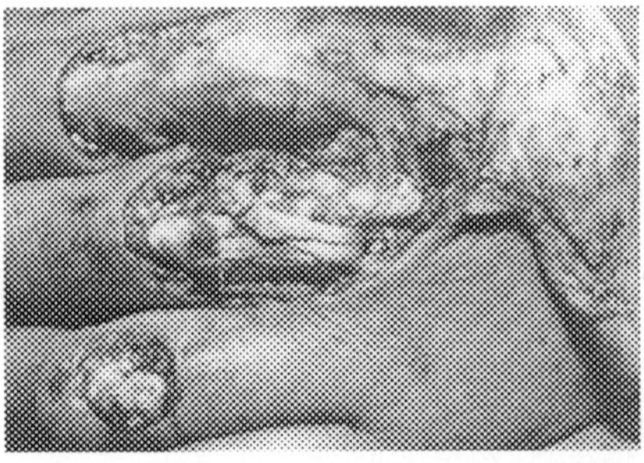

Fig. 6(B) The extensor tendon defect was reconstructed with a palmaris longus tendon graft. The skin defect was resurfaced with transposition flap from the dorsum of index finger.

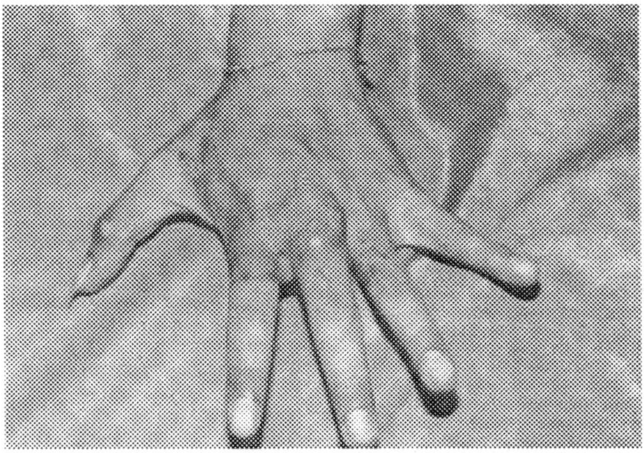

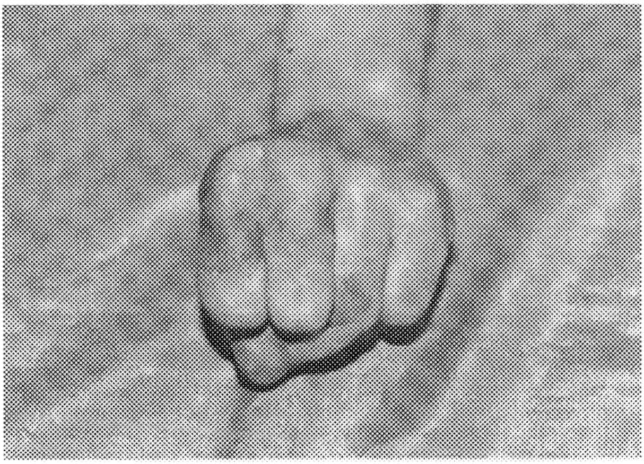

Figs. 6(C) and (D) He had uncomplicated wound healing and a successful reconstruction. The extension of the middle finger had fully recovered in six weeks.

to the artery. The skin defect must be covered with a flap. A regional flap from the same hand is preferred. Otherwise the coverage is with a distant flap or free flap. The loss of artery and skin can be reconstructed with a flow-through flap. The distal end of the flap artery is used to revascularise the finger and hand distally.

Reconstruction of ulnar and radial loss follows the approach of replacing the tendon, nerve and bone loss with non-vascularised grafts. The skin coverage is again with a skin flap.

Severe fingertip injury with loss nail matrix, bone and pulp tissue can be successfully reconstructed if sufficient nail germinal matrix in still intact. Sufficient nail growth will occur with an intact germinal matrix, and the fingertip does regain acceptable aestheticism (Figs. 7(A)–(D)). The pulp loss is resurfaced with a local and regional flap such as V-Y plasty[38] or cross-finger flap.[37] Bone grafting is not required for the distal phalanx bone loss. The residual bone length is usually sufficient to restore the fingertip. A sterile nail matrix can be successfully grafted during the acute surgery.

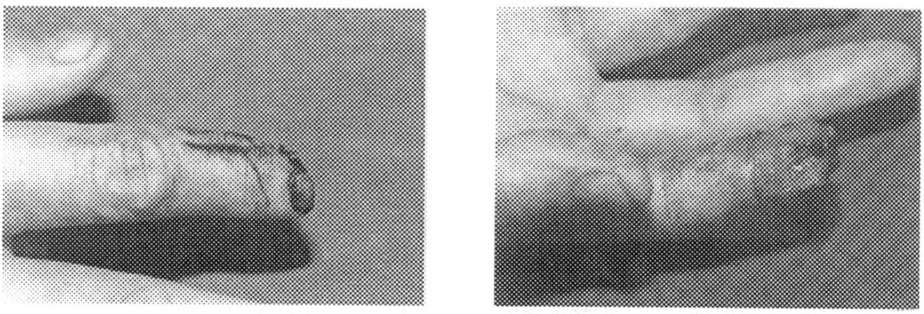

Figs. 7(A) and (B) A production worker had her right index finger crushed by a punching machine. There was extensive loss of pulp tissue, however sufficient amount of nail matrix was still intact. This is an example of "multiple tissues loss".

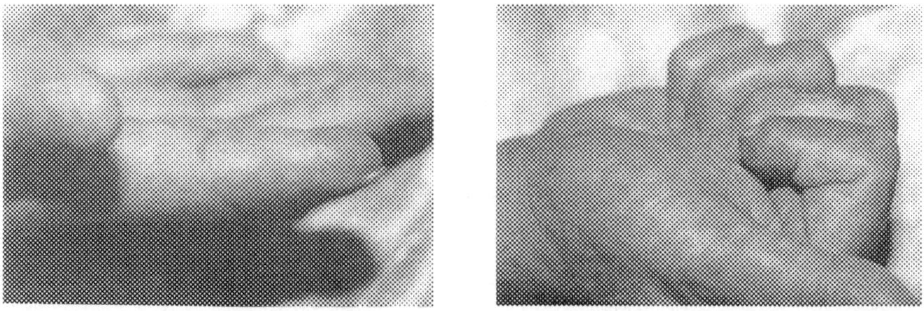

Figs. 7(C) and (D) Her index finger was reconstructed with a cross finger flap harvested from the adjacent middle finger. No bone grafting or nail bed grafting were necessary. Her index fingertip was successfully salvaged. She recovered good function with acceptable aestheticism.

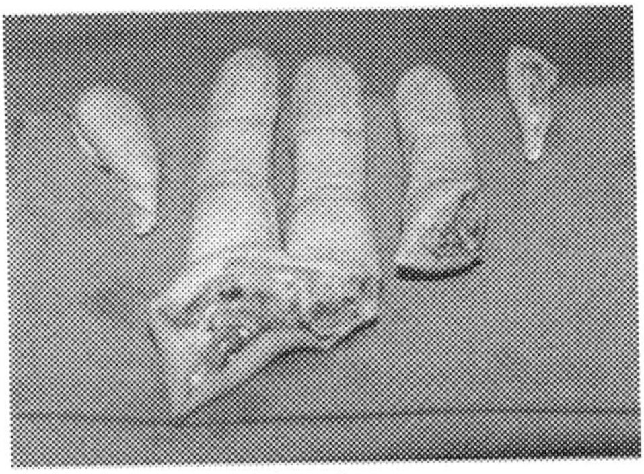

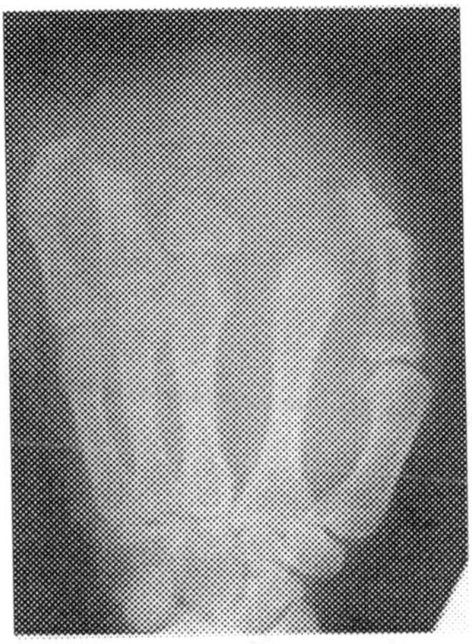

Figs. 8(A) and (B) A printer had a guillotine injury to his left hand by a paper-cutting machine. All the five digits were amputated but at varying levels. This is an amputation injury of "all tissues transection". The index amputation had damaged the MP joint and the ring finger was damaged at the PIP joint. The thumb and little finger were amputated at a distal level.

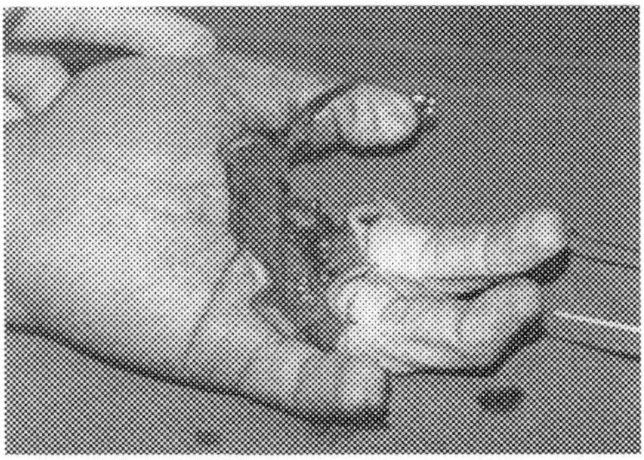

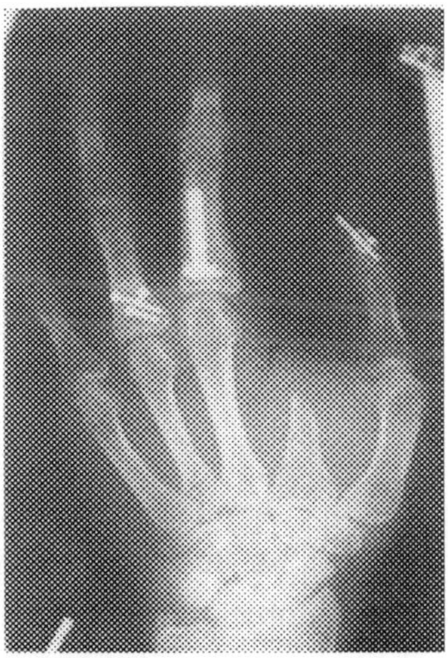

Figs. 8(C) and (D) To restore all the joints to the replanted fingers, the index and middle fingers were replanted onto the middle and ring fingers. The ring finger was salvaged and replanted to the thumb as an augmentation. Bone stabilisation was achieved with plating, interfragmentary screws and interosseous wire fixations. Comprehensive quality repair of all the tendons, nerves and vessels was performed.

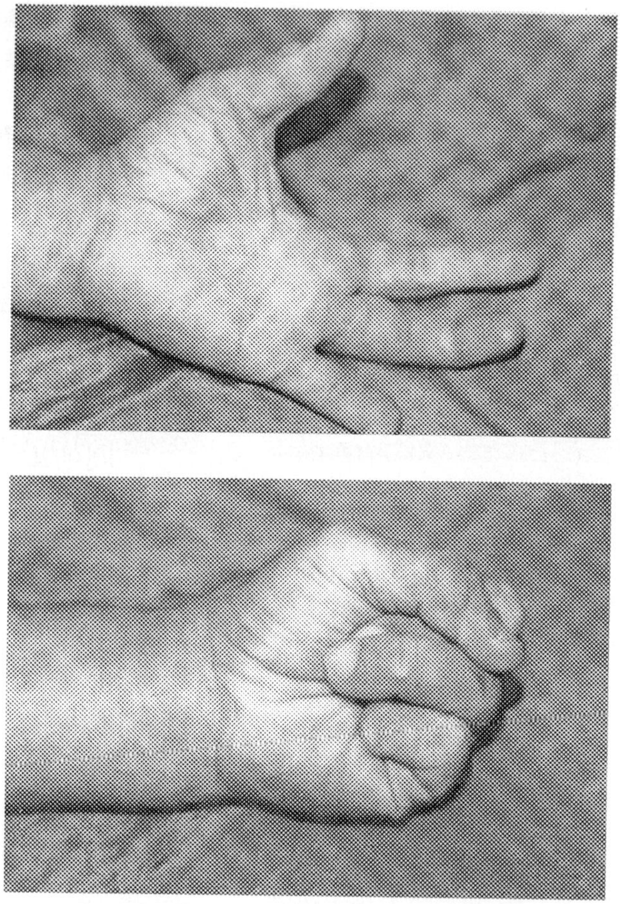

Figs. 8(E) and (F) He recovered excellent function by the sixth month and returned to his original job as a printer.

In a severe combined injury, if three of the five tissue components are lost and need to be replaced, the functional outcome is unfavourable. However, it takes experience and judgment in deciding when a severely damaged digit becomes non-reconstructable. If it is decided to amputate a non-reconstructable digit, salvage for spare grafts to reconstruct the remaining digits should always be considered (Figs. 9(A)–(D)).[61,62]

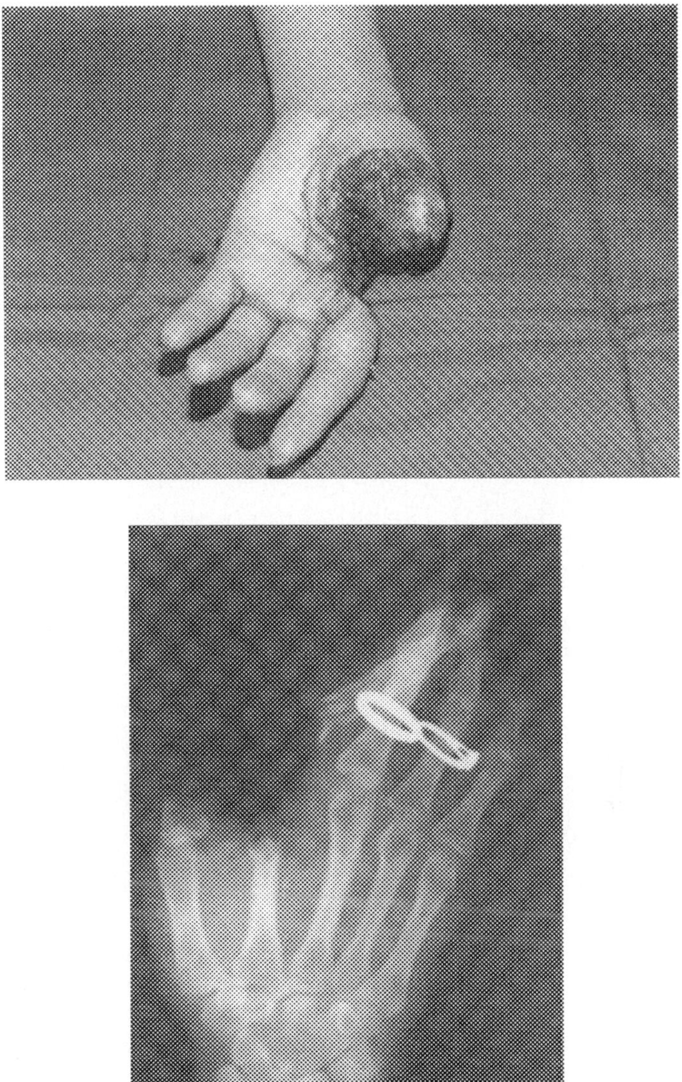

Figs. 9(A) and (B) A young female working on a metal punching machine had a punched-out injury to her left hand. The thumb was completely crushed. The index finger sustained a 5 cm missing segment over the MP joint and was devascularised. The index finger had three out of five tissue components missing and was deemed not reconstructable.

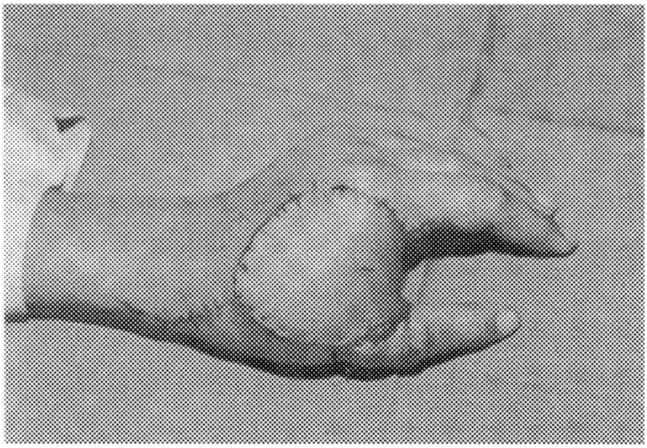

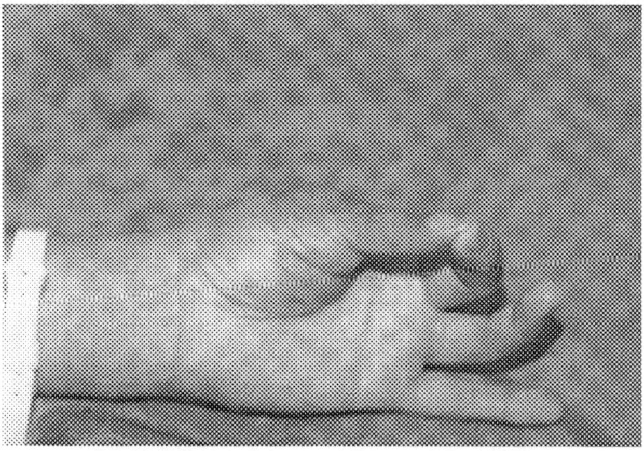

Figs. 9(C) and (D) Double microsurgical procedures were performed to her left hand in an emergency setting. The index finger was excised and transplanted to the thumb. A free lateral arm flap was used to cover the large defect over the web space. She recovered excellent function and aestheticism, and returned to work in six months.

Repair of all tissues transection (Amputation)

The treatment of amputation injury is replantation surgery. Replantation surgery is an extension of repair of multiple tissue transection. It is the repair and reconstruction of all tissues in a complete total transection (Figs. 8(A)–(F)).

Replantation is most indicated for the thumb, multiple digits, and proximal level amputations.[63] Amputation in children should always be considered for replantation.[64,65] Replantation of a single digit is less indicated, but the surgery should be considered for the individual who demands it.

Replantation should be done under a tourniquet to minimise unnecessary blood loss. However, after debridement the tourniquet should be deflated to ascertain the quality of blood flow from the proximal recipient artery. Longitudinal lateral incisions over the digit and hand provide excellent exposure for identification and repair of the tissues.

Bone shortening is always necessary, and this effectively obliterates the segmental tissue loss from the injury.

The order of the repair is from the deepest tissue to the most superficial tissue. Stable fixation of the bone is the first to be done, followed by repair of the tendons and muscles. The nerve and vascular repairs are done with microsurgical techniques. There is no preference in the order of the vein and artery repair. "Passive patency" is a reliable technique of checking the success of a vascular repair when the tourniquet is inflated. The transversely opposing skin edges should be closed to protect the vascular repair. However the lateral incision should be left open to accommodate the post-operative swelling.[66,67]

Reconstruction of all tissues loss (Mutilating injury)

Mutilating injuries require complex microsurgical reconstruction.[68] A comprehensive reconstruction plan should be formulated for every case. Full reconstitution of the hand is not possible. Therefore the functional goal must be realistic. In most severe injuries, it is only possible to reconstruct a "basic hand" or "opposable hand". This is a two-digit hand that is capable of a simple pinch function.[69–72] In less severe cases, it is possible to reconstruct a more functional three-digit hand. There is a thumb opposable to two other digits, and the hand is capable of a more stable chuck pinch, and some grasping function (Figs. 3(A)–(G)).

The reconstruction may require multi-stage microvascular free tissue transfer. In a typical reconstruction, the first stage is to resurface the huge defect over the hand with a large skin flap, and the second stage involves two toes to hand transfer a few months later.[73–76]

Post-operative Rehabilitation

All cases should go through a post-operative rehabilitation programme. In an injured hand adhesion quickly developes between the tissues, and a delay in rehabilitation leads to irreversible stiffness and loss of function.

Rehabilitation should be started early, while the tissues are still in the healing phase. Therefore, mobilisation during the initial six weeks post-operatively is most effective in restoring the tissue gliding planes. This "window of opportunity" must not be missed.

References

1. Kelsey JL, Pastides H, Kreiger N, Harris C, Chernow RA (1980). *Upper Extremity Disorders. A Survey of Their Frequency and Cost in United States*. St. Louis: CV Mosby.
2. O'Sullivan ME, Colville J (1993). The economic impact of hand injuries. *J Hand Surg* **18B**, 395–398.
3. Pulvertaft RG (1973). Twenty five years of hand surgery. Personal reflections. *J Bone Joint Surg* **55B**, 32–55.
4. Kaplan EB (1968). *Functional and Surgical Anatomy of the Hand.* Philadelphia: Lippincott.
5. Cooney WP 3rd, Fitzgerald RH Jr, Dobyns JH, Washington JA 2nd (1982). Quantitative wound cultures in upper extremity trauma. *J Trauma* **22**, 112–117.
6. Arons MS, Fernando L, Polayes IM (1982). *Pasteurella multocida* — The major cause of hand infections following domestic animal bites. *J Hand Surg* **7A**, 47–52.
7. Mann RJ, Hoffeld TA, Farmer CB (1977). Human bites of the hand: twenty years of experience. *J Hand Surg* **2A**, 97–104.

8. Kullavanijaya P, Sirimachan S, Bhuddhavudhikrai P (1993). *Mycobacterium marinum* cutaneous infections acquired from occupations and hobbies. *Int J Derm* **32**, 504–507.
9. Phillips SA, Marya KS, Dryden MS, Samuel AW (1995). *Mycobacterium marinum* infection of the finger. *J Hand Surg* **20B**, 801–802.
10. Liseki EJ, Curl WW, Markey KL (1980). Hand and forearm infections caused by *Aeromonas hydrophila*. *J Hand Surg* **5A**, 605.
11. Gelberman R, Posch JL, Jurist JM (1975). High-pressure injection injuries of the hand. *J Bone Joint Surg* **57A**, 935–937.
12. Couzens G, Burke FD (1995). Veterinary high pressure injection injuries with inoculations for large animals. *J Hand Surg* **20B**, 497–499.
13. Sena T, Brewer BW (1999). Natural gas inflation injury of the upper extremity: a case report. *J Hand Surg* **24A**, 850–852.
14. Dellon AL (1978). The moving two-point discrimination test: clinical evaluation of the quickly adapting fiber/receptor system. *J Hand Surg* **3A**, 474–481.
15. Moberg E (1964). Evaluation and management of nerve injuries in the hand. *Surg Clin North Am* **44**, 10–19.
16. Tonkin M (1992). Hand surgery: the skin and its contents. *J Hand Surg* **17B**, 381–382.
17. Campbell DA, Kay SPJ (1996). The hand injury severity scoring system. *J Hand Surg* **21B**, 295–298.
18. Midgley RD, Entin M (1976). Management of mutilating injuries of the hand. *Clin Plast Surg* **3**, 99–109.
19. Wei FC, Epstein MD, Chen HC, Chuang CC, Chen HT (1993). Microsurgical reconstruction of distal digits following mutilating hand injuries: results in 121 patients. *Br J Plast Surg* **46**, 181–186.
20. Grossman JA, Adams JP, Kunec J (1981). Prophylactic antibiotics in simple hand lacerations. *JAMA* **245**, 1055–1056.
21. Peacock KC, Hanna DP, Kirkpatrick K, Breidenbach WC, Lister GD, Firrell J (1988). Efficacy of perioperative cefamandole with postoperative cephalexin in the primary outpatient treatment of open wounds of the hand. *J Hand Surg* **13A**, 960–964.

22. Madsen MS, Neumann L, Andersen JA (1996). Penicillin prophylaxis in complicated wounds of hands and feet: a randomized, double-blind trial. *Injury* **27**(4), 275–278.
23. Hoffman RD, Adams BD (1998). The role of antibiotics in the management of elective and post-traumatic hand surgery. *Hand Clin* **14**, 657–666.
24. Chadaev AP, Jukhtin VI, Butkevich Ats, Emkuzhev VM (1996). Treatment of infected clench-fist human bite wounds in the area of metacarpophalangeal joints. *J Hand Surg* **21A**, 299–303.
25. Stark HH, Ashworth CR, Boyles JH (1961). Grease gun injuries of the hand. *J Bone Joint Surg* **43A**, 485–491.
26. Scher C, Schun FD, Harvin JS (1973). High pressure paint gun injuries of the hand. *Br J Plast Surg* **26**, 167–171.
27. Gross A, Cutright DE, Bhaskar SN (1972). Effectiveness of pulsating water jet lavage in treatment of contaminated crushed wounds. *Am J Surg* **124**, 373–377.
28. Scherr DD, Dodd TA (1976). *In vitro* bacteriological evaluation of the effectiveness of antimicrobial irrigating solution. *J Bone Joint Surg* **58A**, 119–122.
29. Gill RS, Lim BH, Shatford RA, Toth E, Voor MJ, Tsai TM (1999). A comparative analysis of the six-strand double-loop flexor tendon repair and three other techniques: a human cadaveric study. *J Hand Surg [Am]* **24**(6), 1315–1322.
30. O'Sullivan ST, Limantzakis G, Kay SP (1999). The role of low-profile titanium miniplates in emergency and elective hand surgery. *J Hand Surg [Br]* **24**(3), 347–349.
31. Ouellette EA, Freeland AE (1996). Use of the minicondylar plate in metacarpal and phalangeal fractures. *Clin Orthop* **327**, 38–46.
32. Bischoff R, Buechler U, De Roche R, Jupiter J (1994). Clinical results of tension band fixation of avulsion fractures of the hand. *J Hand Surg [Am]* **19**(6), 1019–1026.
33. Dabezies EJ, Schutte JP (1986). Fixation of metacarpal and phalangeal fractures with miniature plates and screws. *J Hand Surg [Am]* **11**(2), 283–288.
34. Allen MJ (1980). Conservative management of fingertip injuries in adults. *The Hand* **12**, 257–265.

35. Holevich J (1965). Early skin grafting in the treatment of traumatic avulsion injuries of the hand and fingers. *J Bone Joint Surg* **47A**, 944–957.
36. Ross R (1979). Inhibition of myofibroblasts by skin grafts. *Plast Reconstr Surg* **63**, 473–481.
37. Cronin TD (1951). The cross finger flap — A new method of repair. *Ann Surg* **17**, 419–425.
38. Atasoy E, Ioakimidis E, Kasdan M, Kutz JE, Kleinert HE (1970). Reconstruction of the amputated fingertip with a triangular volar flap. *J Bone Joint Surg* **52A**, 921–926.
39. Foucher G, Braun JB (1979). A new island flap transfer from the dorsum of the index to the thumb. *Plast Reconstr Surg* **63**, 344–349.
40. Teoh LC, Tay SC, Yong FC, Tan SH, Khoo DB (2003). Heterodigital arterialized flaps for large finger wounds: results and indications. *Plast Reconstr Surg* **111**, 1905–1913.
41. Bertille JA (1997). Neurocutaneous island flaps in upper limb coverage: experience with 44 clinical cases. *J Hand Surg* **22A**, 515–526.
42. Brunelli F, Vigasio A, Valenti P, Brunelli GR (1999). Arterial anatomy and clinical application of the dorsoulnar flap of the thumb. *J Hand Surg* **24A**, 803–811.
43. Lister GD, McGregor IA, Jackson IT (1973). Groin flap in hand injuries. *Br J Accident Surg* **4**, 229–239.
44. Upton J, Havlik RJ, Khouri RK (1992). Refinements in hand coverage with microvascular free flaps. *Clin Plast Surg* **19**, 841–857.
45. Braun RM, Rechnic M, Neil-Cage DJ, Schorr RT (1995). The retrograde radial fascial forearm flap: surgical rationale, technique, and clinical application. *J Hand Surg* **20A**, 915–922.
46. Woo SH, Jeong JH, Seul JH (1996). Resurfacing relatively large defects of the hand using arterialized venous flaps. *J Hand Surg* **21B**, 222–229.
47. Freeland AE, Jabaley ME, Burkhalter WE, Chaves MV (1984). Delayed primary bone grafting in the hand and wrist after traumatic bone loss. *J Hand Surg* **9A**, 22–28.

48. Stahl S, Lerner A, Kaufman T (1999). Immediate autografting of bone in open fractures with bone loss of the hand: a preliminary report. Case reports. *Scand J Plast Reconstr Surg Hand Surg* **33**, 117–122.
49. Beasley RW (1983). Principles of soft tissue replacement for the hand. *J Hand Surg* **8A**, 781–784.
50. Ohmori K, Harii K (1976). Free dorsalis pedis sensory flap to the hand, with microneurovascular anastomoses. *Plast Reconstr Surg* **58**, 546–554.
51. Katsaros J, Schusterman M, Beppu M, Bannis JC, Acland RD (1984). The lateral upper arm flap: anatomy and clinical applications. *Ann Plast Surg* **12**, 489–500.
52. Upton J, Rogers C, Durham-Smith G, Swartz WM (1986). Clinical applications of free temporoparietal flaps in hand reconstruction. *J Hand Surg* **11A**, 475–483.
53. Yoshimura M, Shimada T, Matsuda M, Hosokawa M, Imura S (1989). Double peroneal free flap for multiple skin defects of the hand. *Br J Plast Surg* **42**, 715–718.
54. Kuek LB, Teoh LC (1991). The extended lateral arm flap: a new modification. *J Reconstr Microsurg* **7**, 167–173.
55. Tropet Y, Brientini JM, Garbuio P, Ridoux PE, Vichard P (1995). Reconstruction of a complex defect of the dorsum of the hand. *J Hand Surg* **20B**, 591–595.
56. Teoh LC, Khoo DB, Lim BH, Yong FC (1995). Osteocutaneous lateral arm flap in hand reconstruction. *Ann Acad* **24**, 15–20.
57. Ninkovic MM, Schwabegger AH, Wechselberger G, Anderl H (1997). Reconstruction of large palmar defects of the hand using free flaps. *J Hand Surg* **22B**, 623–630.
58. Godina M (1986). Early microsurgical reconstruction of complex trauma of the extremities. *Plast Reconstr Surg* **78**, 285–292.
59. Ninković M, Deetjen H, Öhler K, Anderl H (1995). Emergency free tissue transfer for severe upper extremity injuries. *J Hand Surg* **20B**, 53–58.
60. Bengoechea-Beeby MP, Pellicer-Artigot JL, Abascal-Zuloaga A (1998). Vascularised bone graft from the second metacarpal to the thumb: a case report. *J Hand Surg* **23A**, 541–544.

61. Gainor BJ (1985). Osteocutaneous digital fillet flap. A technical modification. *J Hand Surg* **10B**, 79–82.
62. Libermanis O, Krauklis G, Kapickis M, Krustins J, Tihonovs A (1999). Use of the microvascular finger fillet flap. *J Reconstr Microsurg* **15**, 577–580.
63. Graham B, Adkins P, Tsai TM, Firrell J, Breidenbach WC (1998). Major replantation versus revision amputation and prosthetic fitting in the upper extremity: a late functional outcome study. *J Hand Surg* **23A**, 783–791.
64. Tan AB, Teoh LC (1995). Upper limb digital replantation and revascularisation in children. *Ann Acad* **24**, 32–36.
65. Cheng GL, Pan DD, Zhang NP, Fang GR (1998). Digital replant in children: a long-term follow-up study. *J Hand Surg* **23A**, 635–646.
66. Morrison W, O'Brien B, MacLeod A (1978). Digital replantation and revascularisation. A long term review of one hundred cases. *The Hand* **10**, 125–134.
67. Kleinert HE, Jablon M, Tsia TM (1980). An overview of replantation and results of 347 replants in 245 patients. *J Trauma* **20**, 390–398.
68. Brown HC, Williams HB, Woolhouse FM (1968). Principles of salvage in mutilating hand injuries. *J Trauma* **8**, 319–332.
69. Burkhalter WE (1986). Complex injuries of the hand. In *The Hand and Wrist: Current Management of Complications in Orthopaedics*. Sandzen SC Jr (ed.) Baltimore: Williams & Wilkins.
70. Vilkki SK (1985). Free toe transfer to the forearm stump following wrist amputation — a current alternative to the Krukenberg operation. *Handchir Mikrochir Palst Chir* **17**, 92–97.
71. Wei FC, Coessens B, Ganos D (1992). Multiple microsurgical toe-to-hand transfer in the reconstruction of the mutilated hand. A series of fifty-nine cases. *Ann Chir Main Memb Super* **11**, 177–187.
72. Yu ZJ, Huang YC, Yu S, Sui SP (1999). Thumb reconstruction in a bilateral upper extremity amputee: an alternative to the Krukenburg procedure. *J Hand Surg* **24A**, 194–197.
73. Koshima I, Etoh H, Moriguchi T, Soeda S (1993). Sixty cases of partial or total toe transfer for repair of finger losses. *Plast Reconstr Surg* **92**, 1331–1338.

74. Wei FC, el-Gammal TA, Lin CH, *et al.* (1997). Metacarpal hand: classification and guidelines for microsurgical reconstruction with toe transfers. *Plast Reconstr Surg* **99**, 122–128.
75. Wei FC, Chen HC, Chuang CC, Noordhoff MS (1998). Simultaneous multiple toe transfers in hand reconstruction. *Plast Reconstr Surg* **81**, 366–377.
76. Yu Z, Huang Y (2000). Sixty-four cases of thumb and finger reconstruction using transplantation of the big toe skin-nail flap combined with the second toe or the second and third toes. *Plast Reconstr Surg* **106**, 335–341.

32

Infection of the Hand

Fok-Chuan Yong
Lam-Chuan Teoh

Introduction

Infections in the hand seem small and trivial, but the severity of onset may be unexpected, as the tissue planes are thin and in close proximity to each other. Thus, any surgical indication should be prompt and adequate to avoid severe disability. Infection of the hand may be acute or chronic depending on the infective organism.

Concepts of Surgical Treatment

Surgery in infection of the hand is based on these five principles:

(1) Diagnosis.
(2) Antibiotics treatment.
(3) Incision and Debridement.
(4) Repair or Reconstruction.
(5) Rehabilitation.

Diagnosis

One should come to a diagnosis as to: (1) the stage of the infection, i.e. cellulitis, abscess, abscess-associated gross tissue necrosis; (2) the extent of the infection, i.e. level of involvement of the tissue planes in depth and in proximal extension, as in any involvement of tendon, bone or joint; and (3) the type of infection, e.g. necrotising soft tissue infection. This will indicate any surgical intervention needed, and the extent of the surgical procedure. Patients often present with a multiple tissue plane involvement. The six tissues in the hand are: (1) skin and subcutaneous tissue, (2) tendon, (3) bone, (4) joint, (5) blood vessels and lymphatics, (6) nerves. Thus, these tissues need to be assessed in the clinical examination.

History

A history of skin abrasion or penetration may or may not be apparent. However, the environment of "infective organism inoculation" is important, and will indicate the probable organism and local tissue condition. Infection arising from a "prick", "stab", or "laceration" is commonly due to *Staphalococcus aureus*, the common resident bacterial flora on the skin. A history of biological material contamination is relevant as one would suspect organisms like *Escherichia coli* or *Enterobacter* species causing the infection. Animal bites will alert the surgeon to "deep" penetrating contamination, thus causing multi-tissue plane infection. The common organism in human bites is *Eikenella corrodens*; in dog bites it is *Pasteurella multocida*. If the patient had been working in an aquatic environment or on a fish-tank, a chronic infection from atypical *Mycobacterium marinum* is likely. A rare infection from *Mycobacterium avium* occurs in patients handling birds.

A crushing injury compromises the local blood supply, injures the skin and subcutaneous tissue and makes it more prone to infection. This has to be considered during the surgical procedure where ischaemic tissues may need to be excised.

In cases of fungal or viral infections, the environment of contact may be the predisposing cause of the infection, and will be of help in post-treatment advice, e.g. contact with tree trunk and wood associated with herpes virus infection.

Medical history is important, especially in note of the age of the patient, presence of any diabetes mellitus or peripheral vascular disease, pre-existing chemotherapy or immuno-suppression therapy, etc.

Clinical examination

One should be aware of the tissue planes in the hand during clinical examination. Local signs of an infection include swelling, redness, warmth, tenderness, painful motion. Suppurative tenosynovitis typically presents with the four Kanavel's signs, i.e. redness, fusiform swelling, flexed posture of the finger, and tenderness along the synovial sheath. Tenosynovitis in the thumb or little finger may extend proximally along the radial or ulnar bursa, and communicate at the wrist (space of Parona) with each other, resulting in a "horse-shoe" infection. The clinical signs are manifested over a U-shape area in the hand like a horseshoe. This will alert the surgeon to achieve an effective surgical intervention. One should note the site of any penetrating injury. A nidus of abscess at the web usually presents with gross swelling and redness over the dorsum of the hand. This is due to the anatomy of lymphatic drainage which drains dorsally and proximally. Thus, one should not mistakenly diagnose a dorsal hand infection but a palmar infection that is associated with gross lymphangitis and cellulitis on the dorsum of the hand. Moreover, the palmar skin is thick and held firmly via septae to the palmar fascia, which is in turn held firmly to the deep tissues. Any abscess or swelling in the palm will not be obvious to the unsuspecting.

At the fingertip, one should determine whether there is subungual involvement or pulp tissue extension from an obvious paronychia or eponychia. This will help in deciding the extent of operative procedure. In the palm, clinical signs are not grossly apparent especially in infection of the deep tissues. Palmaris fascia or sub-cuticular infection presents as a triangular shaped redness and swelling similar to the surface anatomy of the fascia.

Investigations

In addition to haematological studies, X-ray radiographs of the digit or hand are done to exclude osteomyelitis or septic arthritis. Any bone or joint erosion (and the extent of it) will influence the pre-operative planning of the surgical procedure. Features of air in the soft tissue indicate a severe infection by gas-forming organisms like *Clostridia* or *Streptococcus* species. In patients with peripheral vascular disease, "vascular" calcifications seen in the radiographs indicate significant ischaemia to the tissues in the hand.

Antibiotics Treatment

Prescription of antibiotics may be divided into two phases, namely: (1) commencement phase, and (2) definitive phase. A history of any allergy to drugs, especially penicillin, should be determined. The patient's age and expected renal function, etc. are also considered when prescribing antibiotics.

Commencement phase

Antibiotics treatment is commenced on diagnosis of an infection. The choice of antibiotics is expectant as in assessing the most likely organism causing the infection, and prescribing the antibiotics that it is sensitive to. The mode of delivery should be intravenous initially, and later continued or converted to oral as indicated by the type of antibiotic and the status of the infection. Assessment of the most likely organism is described above in diagnosis of the infection. In hand surgery, the most common organism is the resident skin flora of *Staphalococcus aureus*. Other organisms that may be expected will be indicated by the history of the "environment" of contamination or injury. We also prefer a dual antibiotic commencement phase. Thus our initial choice of antibiotics is cloxacillin for the common *Staphalococcus aureus* organism, and gentamicin for likely gram-negative organisms. In our experience, this combination covers about 85% of the aerobic organisms cultured in infections of the hand. Additional specific antibiotics like penicillin are prescribed in a diagnosis of dermal infection or cellulitis where *Streptococcus* is the most likely organism, or suspected anaerobic organism, causing the infection. Nevertheless, in suspected atypical mycobacterium infection the specific antibiotic may be withheld until culture and sensitivity confirmation. However, initial prescription of doxycycline may be indicated following the physician's assessment and diagnosis.

This choice and dosage of the antibiotics should be adjusted according to age factor, renal status, severity of the infection, or associated septicaemia.

Definitive phase

The antibiotics treatment is reviewed and changed appropriately as the definitive diagnosis unfolds, or as the culture and sensitivity of the causative organism is determined. The duration of treatment is influenced by the progress of various clinical parameters, the plane of tissue involvement and the type of organisms. Further reference may be made in other relevant texts.

Incision and Debridement

The concept of surgical treatment is to convert the "infective wound" to a "clean surgical wound". Therefore the abscess and necrotic and ischaemic tissues need to be excised rather than drained or curetted. The use of a surgical blade to excise the necrotic tissues is tedious and difficult, and the use of a curette does not "completely" excise them. We find that the use of a bone rongeur is the best for this. The technique is to gently grasp the tissues and pull away. Any necrotic tissue will be easily pulled off, and firm tissues that cannot be pulled off (presumed to be still vascularised and not dead) is left behind. This procedure is done to preserve the neurovascular structures. The technique is to place the jaws of the rongeur perpendicular to the neurovascular bundle so that the rongeur will not grasp it, but push it away and thus not avulse it.

The procedure is followed by copious irrigation to further reduce the local bacterial and necrotic tissue load. The wound is left open for daily irrigation and antibiotic dressing. It is also "plugged" with tulle-grasse or a piece of gauze to prevent the skin edges from apposing together and "sealing up" the wound, preventing drainage and irrigation.

Incisions

Sub-cuticular and dermal abscess/cellulitis: This should be tangentially excised beyond the margin of the erythema.

Paronychia and felon at the fingertip: A lateral incision is made from the tip to the level of the eponychium. Thereafter it may be extended obliquely dorsally or volarly as needed. The lateral incision should not be extended distally to cross over to the other side like a "fish-mouth" incision. If the felon is associated with cutaneous necrosis, the incision should be volar oblique, incorporating excision of the necrotic tissue and extended in a zig-zag manner if needed.

Suppurative tenosynovitis and infections in the digit: In the early tenosynovitis, a surgical option of limited distal and proximal incision to expose the synovial sheath for "closed" drainage and irrigation has been described. However, the author prefers the "open" concept of exposure of the whole extent of the infection, as is clinically and per-operatively apparent for the objective of drainage and debridement in addition to irrigation. Various incisions have been described for the volar aspect of the digit, mainly the zig-zag incision. Nevertheless, the principle is that it should be zig-zag in manner, the incision angle is about 60° to the transverse line, and the apex is at the antero-lateral line (surface marking of the neurovascular bundle) to avoid accidental laceration of the digital artery or nerve. Dorsal digital incisions are made longitudinally so that blood supply to the skin is not compromised. The main arterial blood supply to the dorsal skin comes from dorsal communicating branches of the digital artery laterally towards the midline. Zig-zag incisions may lead to apical necrosis of the skin.

Web abscess: Surgical incisions should not cross the webs of the digits. The wounds may heal with resultant scar contractures of the webs. It is not necessary to add a dorsal incision if a palmar incision has been made. The dorsal web area is easily accessed through the palmar exposure. The palmar incision may be transverse or oblique, and extended in a zig-zag manner to follow the thenar crease to the carpal tunnel as needed. If the abscess had extended distally to one digit, the incision may be easily extended distally to it in a zig-zag manner. However if it had extended to two adjacent digits, the incision had to be well planned. This is to avoid a resultant necrosis of the web skin in the middle. The distal web skin will be similar to a distal-based flap laceration with risk of proximal edge necrosis. Thus, the planned incision places the web skin as wide as possible, and the proximal confluence of the incision as obtuse as possible.

Septic arthritis: A dorsal longitudinal exposure is direct and simple. The extensor tendon is incised longitudinally in the midline. In an early infection, the joint capsule may be incised transversely. In the advanced infection, the volar recess of the head of the metacarpal or condyle of the proximal phalanx may be involved. This is a "blind spot" and is difficult to be accessed dorsally. Thus an additional volar incision and approach may be necessary to excise the affected tissues.

Necrotising soft tissue infection: In addition to excision of the whole extent of the necrotic tissue, incision should be made along the whole extent of the erythema and cellulitis. In the necrotising fasciitis, the normal looking skin may be harvested as a split thickness skin graft and stored for later use. This area of skin will invariably result in necrosis because of devascularisation by the underlying fascia necrosis.

Irrigation

Copious, pulsed irrigation is done after satisfactory debridement. A mechanical pulse-lavage device may be used in the large wound. Topical antibiotic is applied with the dressing of the wound.

Indication for amputation

The concept is that if three or more tissues are affected that needed grafting or replacement reconstruction, amputation of the part is indicated and must be seriously considered. The hand is an organ of prehension function. Our experience is that the above damage situation results in a useless and functionless part in the hand. It obstructs the function of the unaffected parts in the hand and is a "nuisance". The appearance of the hand is not improved.

In the fingertip (a three-tissue complex), reconstruction to a cosmetic and functional unit is possible if the nail bed tissue and the dorsal cortex of the distal phalanx are spared in the infection. Thus, in a case of a felon with necrosis of the pulp tissue and osteomyelitis affecting both the cortices of the distal phalanx (involvement of two tissues), amputation of the distal phalanx of the finger is indicated. Amputation of the infected part is also indicated in a case of an infection over a gangrenous part ("wet" gangrene) of the hand.

The objective in amputation surgery in infection is to achieve wound closure and primary healing. Thus the concept of a "clean surgical wound" is observed, and the blood supply to the skin edge is ensured to achieve a primary wound healing. The wound closure may be done as a delayed procedure if there is residual oedema or underlying peripheral vascular or small vessel disease. It should be done without tension (e.g. bone can be shortened, ligamentous tissue can be excised) and interrupted sutures placed a reasonable distance apart without tension, to ensure minimal compromise to the skin edge circulation.

Repair/Reconstruction

Following debridement is daily cleansing, irrigation and antibiotic dressing of the wound. The infection is reviewed daily. Reversal of the infection will be apparent by the third day in the majority of patients who do not have significant associated medical problems affecting the recovery. Signs of reversal of the infection include: (1) minimal discharge as observed in the removed dressing and the wound itself, (2) a "squeeze" test may be done to note whether there is residual purulent discharge, and (3) surrounding oedema and redness subsiding as indicated by the "wrinkling" of the skin and the colour. Thus a surgical decision is made at this time for (1) a re-debridement and irrigation under anaesthesia when there is no sign of reversal of the infection, (2) a repair and/or secondary suture of the wound, or (3) a reconstruction surgical procedure.

The need for a simple repair or a reconstruction procedure is best assessed and planned during the first surgical procedure. Wound healing is associated with skin edge contraction, and it is difficult to assess at three to four days later the possibility of a simple wound repair. If there is minimal soft tissue or skin loss, repair or closure of the wound is possible. At surgery, a debridement of the fibrinous and early granulation tissue is done before skin suture.

Reconstruction procedures in treatment of hand infections are mainly for skin defect re-surfacing. These include a split-thickness skin grafting, pedicled cutaneous flap, and free cutaneous flap.

Rehabilitation

Rehabilitation therapy commences early on the first post-operative day. The therapy includes ensuring a correct resting posture of the hand,

and joint mobility. Pain and swelling results in a tendency to a bad posture of the hand i.e. with the wrist flexed, metacarpo-phalangeal joints extended, and inter-phalangeal joints flexed. The function of the hand is severely affected if stiffness occurs in this posture. Thus a volar intrinsic-plus splint may be required in-between dressing and exercises. Pain and swelling also discourages mobilisation of the joints in the hand. Therapy addresses this, and aims to regain normal mobilisation of the hand. Mobilisation of the hand in a fluid media is less painful and has a soothing effect. An antiseptic solution or silicon oil has been used for this, especially when there is a large wound. The granulation tissue formation and myofibroblast cells differentiation in wound healing result in fibrotic scar formation and contracture. Thus, early mobilisation therapy is important to prevent formation of a contracted scar. Following reconstruction surgery, functional reintegration therapy is also commenced early.

Infection in the hand often presents as a multiple tissue plane involvement. Surgical indication should be prompt and definitive to ensure a functional outcome. One may occasionally meet the painful task of advising amputation of the part when too many tissues are necrotic and lost in the infection. Surgical management based on the five principles described here has proved to be effective.

Section X

Skin and Soft Tissue Injuries

33

Acute Burn Care

Erik SW Ang
Colin Song
Kok-Chai Tan

Introduction

Paradigm shifts in burn management

Considerable strides were made in burn care in the 20th century,[1] and these continue into the 21st century. The "great awakening" occurred in the 1940s, and this was due to (1) the availability of plasma, sulphanilamide and penicillin to treat shock and sepsis; (2) the experience gained from treating casualties in World War II; and (3) the introduction of the scientific method to clinical medicine and surgery. The first specialised burn care facilities in the world were established in the U.K. and the U.S. in the 1960s.

Milestones in burn care include the introduction of various fluid resuscitation regimes, the practice of early excision of burn eschar in the 1970s, the use of artificial skin substitutes in the 1980s and 1990s, and the use of cultured epithelial autografts and anti-inflammatory mediators. These advances in the science of burn care resulted in considerable improvements in mortality rates.[2]

In Singapore, a burns centre was set up in 1982. Lee[3] documents the history and growth of the unit from the 1960s to the 1980s. In line with current practice, the management of major burn patients in Singapore is characterised by early surgery and wound coverage, increased use of allograft and synthetic wound coverage material, reliance on a multi-disciplinary approach, and a better understanding of critical care management.[4]

Scope of the problem

The Department of Plastic Surgery in the Singapore General Hospital treats two to eight new patients with burn injuries daily. This figure excludes patients with minor burns that are treated in other hospitals and by primary health physicians. Annually, about 300 patients are admitted to the Burns Centre, out of which about 10–20% of patients have major and severe burns requiring intensive care. Scalds (40%) and flame burns (40%) make up the majority of cases for all surface areas; the rest are due to chemicals (10%) and others like electrical, hot exhaust and hot metals.[5,6]

The impact of burn injuries

Patients with burn injuries are affected in many different ways. The course of the injury, the impact on the patient as a whole, and the eventual appearance of the burn wound depends mainly on the *extent* of the burn injury as a percentage of the body surface area (BSA), the *depth* of each burn wound, *associated injuries* (especially respiratory burns), and the patient's age, *pre-existing medical condition* and nutritional status. In general, the deeper and the more extensive the burn, the more severe the physiological derangements are.[4,7]

Patients with more extensive injuries by surface area fare worse than those with smaller areas of involvement. A burn injury results in loss of integrity of the epidermal-dermal barrier, predisposing the patient to the risk of infection.[8] In addition, plasma fluids and proteins are lost through the raw surface. The body is able to compensate for fluid losses that arise from a burn area of less than 15% BSA in adults, and less than 10% BSA in children. Patients with burn wounds in excess of these areas require fluid replacement therapy to prevent the development of burn shock and hypovolaemic renal failure.[9] Beyond 30% BSA, burn patients may also develop systemic complications like renal failure, systemic inflammatory response syndrome,[4] and gastrointestinal haemorrhage.[10] Release of inflammatory mediators as a response to the trauma, together with loss of the normal protective integument, threaten the survival of the victim.

The deeper the burn wounds, the longer it takes to heal spontaneously, and the greater its impact on the overall condition. In general, superficial burns heal within ten to 14 days with minimal scarring and long-term morbidity, and are usually treated conservatively. Deeper wounds that take longer than 14 days to heal and will eventually produce significant wound contraction and scarring. Morphological and functional morbidity may result if these wounds are not excised and skin-grafted.[11]

The presence of *respiratory burns* adds to the morbidity, and causes the risk of mortality to be increased by up to 50%.[12] Patients in the extremes of ages are less able to tolerate trauma and stress, as are patients with significant predisposing medical illnesses. Illnesses like diabetes mellitus and hypoproteinaemic conditions compromise recovery by impairing wound healing.

The First Contact

Burn injuries may range from a minor burn to a major catastrophe. Whatever the area and severity, every patient requires a careful assessment obtained from the history taking and clinical examination.

History of the injury

Accurate and complete information about the incident is essential, either from the patient, or from eyewitnesses if the patient has impaired consciousness. This includes the time, the location and the mechanism of the incident, what the burn agent was, and the duration in which the victim was in contact with the burn agent.

Associated injuries may be sustained while the victim attempted to escape a fire. For example, a person trapped in a burning room for a few minutes may sustain respiratory burns as opposed to one who has been scalded by hot water. Water heater, propane gas, and other explosions may throw the patient some distance and may result in internal injuries or fractures, resulting in involvement of the intracranial, myocardial, pulmonary, or abdominal systems.

The history from the patient or relative should include a brief survey of pre-existing illnesses like diabetes, hypertension, cardiac, pulmonary and/or renal disease, and drug therapy. Allergies and sensitivities are also important. The patient's tetanus immunisation status should be ascertained.

Clinical examination

General assessment

The patient's airway, breathing and circulation (ABC) status is checked. Every body system of the patient is then examined to ensure that all injuries are noted.

Assessment of the burn wound

(1) Extent of injury (in terms of body surface area)

This is very important as it helps to determine the fluid requirements and condition of the patient. Special charts are available to help assess the extent accurately. Our unit currently uses an adapted Lund Browder chart. As a rough guide, the size of the patient's palm is equivalent to 1% BSA. Body proportions vary considerably in children. For example, the young child's head represents a larger proportion of the surface area, and the lower extremities a lesser proportion, than the adult's. The percentage of total body surface of the infant's head is twice that of the normal adult. When Lund

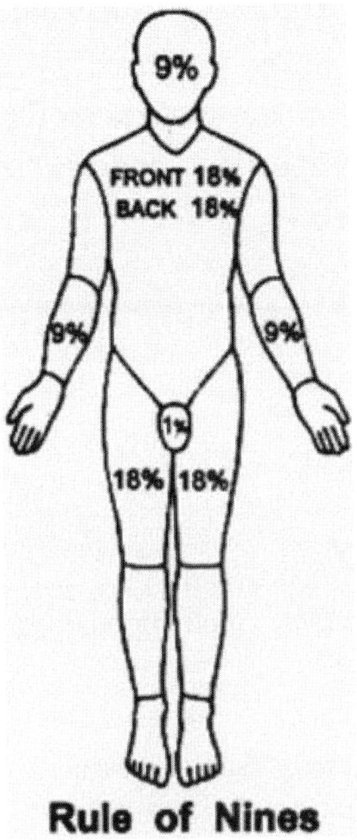

Fig. 1 "Rule of Nines" Chart. The surface area of each body region is estimated in multiples of nine. Thus, the head-scalp is 9%, each upper limb is 9%, each surface of the trunk is 18%, each lower limb is 18%, and the perineum is assigned 1% body surface area. When added up, the total is 100%.

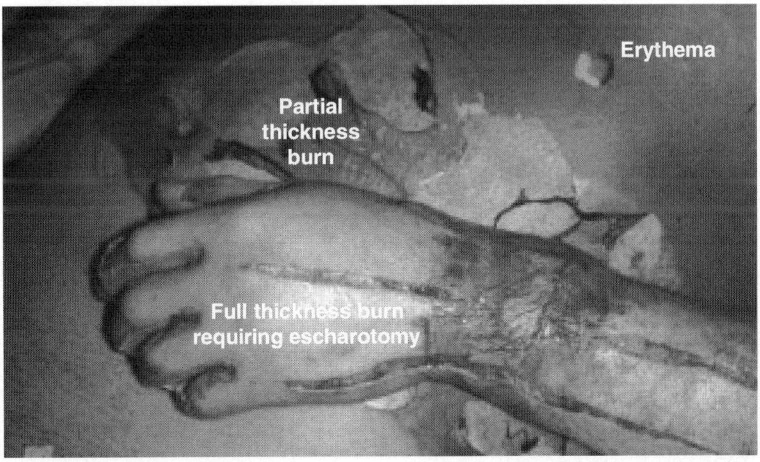

Fig. 2 Different burn depths demonstrated in one patient with flame burns. The trunk has areas of erythema and partial thickness burns, whereas the left hand and forearm has full-thickness areas. Escharotomy incisions have been made to relieve the compressive effects. Note the relatively unburnt area where the patient's watch strap had been.

Browder charts are unavailable, a simple way of estimating the extent is according to the "Rule of Nines" (Fig. 1).

The larger the extent of burn involvement, the more serious the condition will be.[4] Patients with burns involving 30% BSA and above are considered to have major burn injuries, and can be quite ill. Burns involving more than 80% BSA are usually fatal.

(2) Depth of injury (Fig. 2)

Burn depth is graded in the following manner:[13]

Name	Depth	Appearance	Characteristic	Treatment
Erythema (1st degree)	Superficial	Reddish, like a sunburn; epidermis intact	Painful to touch; heals without scarring	Soothing ointment
Partial thickness (2nd degree)	Part of thickness of skin; varying thickness	Reddish to whitish if deeper; epidermis not intact	Painful to touch; more superficial ones heal without scarring; deeper areas heal with scarring if not operated	Sterile dressing changed daily to once in two days; deeper areas may need operation to prevent scarring and deformity
Full thickness (3rd degree)	Both epidermis and dermis	Whitish, greyish, "leather-like"	No sensation; will not heal	Operation

Initial Management

At the site of injury, the burn should be covered with a clean dressing. The application of soap or toothpaste is probably not harmful if only a limited and superficial area is involved, but may introduce wound infection if larger areas are involved.

The initial management depends on the severity of the injury. For convenience, burns injury is divided into minor burns, intermediate and major burns.

Minor burns

Adults with small (less than 1% BSA) erythema or superficial burns in non-functional areas are considered to have minor burns. The wounds of these patients are dressed with paraffin gauze or Opsite® and the patients may be discharged to be followed up at outpatient clinics (Fig. 3).

Patients with burns more than >1% but do not fulfil admission criteria should be given adequate analgesics (Avoid NSAIDS in those above 35 years old to minimise risks of gastro-intestinal tract bleeding, antibiotics not required), referral for outpatient change of dressings, a follow-up date at the Specialist Outpatient Clinic (Plastic Surgery) and medical leave to cover till the follow-up date.

Intermediate burns

Patients who fulfil the admission criteria should be admitted to the Burn Centre. Our Burn Centre admission criteria include the following:

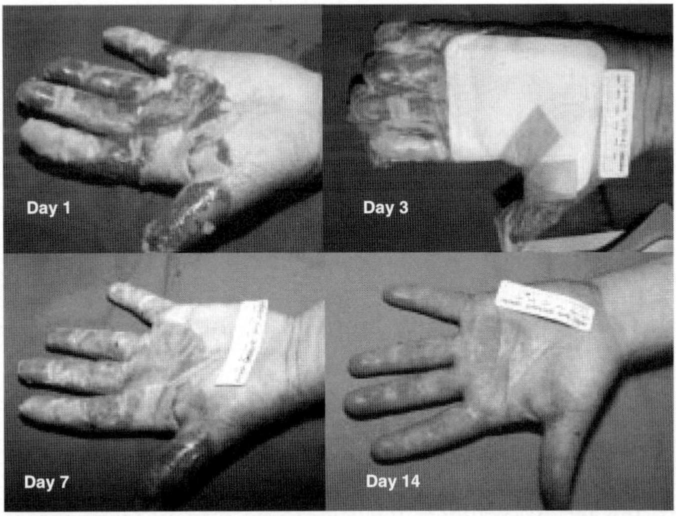

Fig. 3 Conservative treatment of superficial burns of the palmar surface of the hands with Opsite® dressing results in complete wound healing in two weeks.

- burns in adults > 15% Total Body Surface Area (TBSA) or in children > 10% TBSA who require special fluid replacement (fluid replacement)
- burns involving special areas like the face, hands and perineum
- deep burns requiring early surgery
- burns due to smoke inhalation
- burns resulting from contact with electricity, chemicals or hot metals
- infected burns.

Minimal investigations required for these patients upon admission include:

- Full Blood Count (FBC), urea/electrolytes, liver function test
- Calcium/Phosphate if TBSA > 15% in adults and > 10% in children
- Chest X-Ray (CXR) if > 35 years old or if inhalation burns suspected
- Electrocardiogram (ECG) if > 35 years old, if inhalation burns suspected or if electrical burns
- Group and Match (GXM) and Prothrombin Time/Partial Thromboplastin Time (PT/PTT) if TBSA > 15 % in adults and > 10% in children
- Arterial Blood Gas (ABG) if chemical burn, if inhalation burns suspected, or if > 65 years old.

Major burns

A patient who has sustained a burn injury in excess of 30% TBSA is generally regarded to have major burns.[4]

Airway

Although the larynx protects the subglottic airway from direct thermal injury, the supraglottic airway is extremely susceptible to obstruction due to oedema as a result of exposure to heat. Signs of airway obstruction may not be immediately obvious, but if present, they may warn the examiner of potential airway obstruction. When a patient is admitted to the hospital after sustaining a burn injury, the physician should be alert to the possibility of airway involvement, and should identify signs of respiratory distress, and initiate supportive measures. Clinical indications of inhalation injury include:

- facial burns
- singeing of the eyebrows and nasal vibrissae
- carbon deposits and acute inflammatory changes in the oropharynx
- carbonaceous sputum
- history of impaired mentation and/or confinement in a burning environment
- history of explosion.

The presence of any of these findings suggests acute inhalation injury. Such injury requires immediate and definitive care, including airway support, which may involve endotracheal intubation and early admission (Fig. 4).

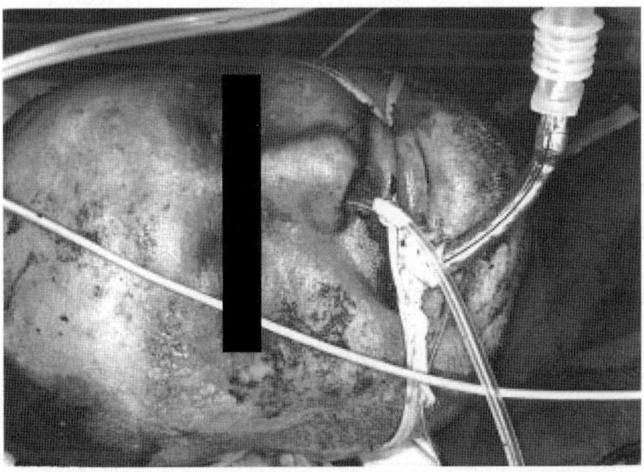

Fig. 4 Patient with facial burn and inhalation injury requiring emergent endotracheal intubation for airway protection.

Intravenous lines

After establishing airway patency and identifying and immediately treating life-threatening injuries, intravenous access must be established. Any patient with burns over more than 20% of the BSA needs circulatory volume support. Large calibre intravenous cannulas must be established in the peripheral vein. If the extent of burns precludes placement of the venous cannula through unburned skin, overlying burned skin should not deter placement of the catheter in an accessible vein. The upper extremities are preferable to the lower extremities for venous access because of the high incidence of phlebitis and septic phlebitis in the saphenous veins. Begin fluid therapy with Hartmann's solution.

Wound care

The aim of burn wound care in the major burns patient is to minimise wound infection, limit the extension of burn injury depth, reduce the burden of devitalised tissue, and to promote wound healing.

In general, superficial burns can be treated conservatively with dressing changes and these will heal spontaneously within two weeks. Deeper burns require excision and grafting.[11,14] These operations should be carried out on the next available Burn Theatre elective operating list.[a] Split skin autografts, cadaveric allografts, and semi-synthetic/synthetic material are employed in wound coverage.

Pre-operative Preparation of the Patient for Emergency Surgery

Candidates for emergency surgery

There are a few instances where burn patients require emergency surgery. These include, but are not limited to, the following situations:

---

[a]In this centre, the Burn Operating Theatre is located within the Burn Unit, and operates every Monday, Wednesday and Friday.

- Circulation to the limbs is threatened
- Major severe burns requiring skin biopsy for autogenous cell culture, and/or early debridement of eschar
- Other associated trauma like intra-abdominal trauma, neurosurgical trauma, and extremity skeletal trauma injuries
- Severe upper airway inhalation injury requiring emergency tracheostomy.

Pre-operative investigations

For major procedures like escharotomy and excision and grafting, the routine pre-operative investigations for surgery include: a full blood count, urea and electrolytes, blood clotting profile, blood gases, chest radiograph, and electrocardiogram. In addition, serum is cross-matched for blood transfusion for two to six units of blood. As the coagulation profile of these patients is often deranged, serum is also cross-matched for fresh frozen plasma and platelet transfusion.

Intra-operative Procedures

Skin biopsy for cell culture

This procedure is performed under local anaesthesia, and requires harvesting an ellipse of skin measuring 1×2 cm under sterile conditions for cell culture. The piece of skin is placed in sterile saline and sent to the Skin Laboratory for further processing. Preferred sites for harvesting include the groin crease, the posterior auricular region, and the scalp. This procedure should be performed within 24 hours of the burn injury.

Escharotomy and fasciotomy

Circumferential deep and full thickness burns are constrictive and compromise circulation to the peripheries. When such burns occur on the chest, these restrict respiratory function. In such circumstances, it is essential to release the constrictive tissue.

This procedure is performed under local anaesthesia under sedation. Longitudinal incisions along the axial lines are made in the skin, and the pressure in the underlying tissue can be seen to be immediately released. The incisions should extend a short way into normal skin in order to achieve a proper release. It is not necessary to deepen the cut to include the fascia layer.

In patients with full thickness burns caused by electricity, there is usually a compartment syndrome caused by oedema of the underlying muscles. In such cases, the incisions should include a fasciotomy.

Debridement of burn wounds

From time to time, patients present to our Burn Centre a few days after the burn injury, either because of personal choice, or because there is a delay in the transfer from a treatment facility or country that does not offer specialised burn care. These patients may have burn wounds that are infected and necrotic. Some limbs may be gangrenous, like diabetics with neglected foot burns and patients with neglected electrical injuries. Emergency surgery including debridement and amputation in some cases, is necessary to reduce the bacterial load and necrotic burden.

Surgery of other anatomical sites

A burn patient may suffer trauma to the other organs. These can be seen in victims of road traffic accidents, where the vehicles had caught fire, and the patient had suffered blast injuries. Occasionally, patients with burn injuries have gastrointestinal bleeding requiring emergency surgery for surgical haemostasis.

In these cases the burnt skin overlying the intended surgical access routes need to be excised, and following completion of surgery of underlying structures, these areas have priority for the limited autogenous skin grafts that should have been harvested at the same time.

Early Post-operative Care of the Patient

Monitoring

Close monitoring of the patient in the immediate post-operative period is essential. This includes the monitoring of the vital parameters (blood pressure, pulse rate, oxygen saturation, and respiratory rate) and fluid balance (central venous pressures, fluid intake and urine output) on an hourly basis.

Operated sites

Attention needs to be paid to the operated sites with regard to haemostasis and general wound care. The circulation to the extremities is monitored hourly for colour and capillary refill.

Pain control

Burn wounds and skin graft sites are often painful, and patients require adequate analgesia in the form of intravenous opiates.

Conclusion

Over the past few decades, there have been significant improvements in home and industrial safety standards, leading to a steadily declining incidence of patients with burn injuries. This has recently been offset, however, by the growing threat and reality of terrorist action employing explosives. The participation of our Burn Centre in the management of victims from the Bali (2002) and Jakarta Marriott Hotel (2003) terror attacks emphasises the strategic importance and relevance of appreciating and understanding the treatment of acute burn injuries.

References

1. Ang SW (1999). Burns Care in the 21st Century. SGH Proceedings. **8**, 100–105.
2. Jackson DM (1991). The evolution of burn treatment in the last 50 years. *Burns* **17**, 329–334.
3. Lee ST (1982). Two decades of specialised burns care in Singapore, 1961–1982. *Ann Acad Med Singapore* **11**, 358–365.
4. Nguyen TT, Gilpin DA, Meyer NA, Herndon DA (1996). Current treatment of severely burned patients. *Ann Surg* **223**(1), 14–24.
5. Ang SW, Lee ST, Gan CSG, See PGJ, Chan YH, Ng LH, Machin D (2001). Evaluating the role of alternative therapy in burn wound management: randomized trial comparing moist exposed burn ointment with conventional methods in the management of patients with second degree burns. *Medscape Gen Med*, 6 April.
6. Ang SW, Lee ST (1992). Emergence of a multiply resistant strain of acinetobacter in a burns unit. *Ann Acad Med Singapore* **21**, 660–663.
7. Allgower M, Schoenenberger GA, Sparkes BG (1995). Burning the largest immune organ. *Burns* **21**(Suppl. 1), S7–S47.
8. Ang SW, Lee ST (1997). The pattern of burn infection in the Singapore National Burns Centre. *Ann Acad Med Singapore* **26**(5), 599–603.
9. Muir IFK, Barclay TL, Settle JAD (1987). Treatment of burns shock. In *Burns and Their Treatment*, 3rd Ed. Butterworths: Somerset, p. 1454.
10. Nathan S, Ang SW, Chia KH, Huang MH, Lee ST (1999). Severe gastrointestinal bleeding resulting in total gastrectomy in a patient with major burns — a case report. *Burns* **25**(6), 531–536.
11. Engrav KH, Heimbach DM, Reus JL, Harnar TJ, Marvin JA (1983). Early excision and grafting versus non-operative treatment of burns of indeterminate depth: a randomized prospective study. *J Trauma* **23**, 1001–1004.

12. Lee ST, Leung CM (1992). Epidemiology and management of respiratory burns in National Burns Centre, Singapore. *Ann Acad Med Singapore* **21**, 612–618.
13. Lawrence JC (1996). Burns and scalds: aetiology and prevention. In *Principles and Practice of Burns Management*. Settle JAD (ed.). Edinburgh: Churchill Livingstone, pp. 3–25.
14. Janzekovic Z (1970). A new concept of skin grafting in burns. *J Trauma* **10**, 1103.

34

Soft Tissue Injuries

Colin HJ Tham
Ying-Chien Tan
Karen WE Sng
Vincent KL Yeow

Introduction

Soft tissue injuries deserve special attention because in addition to their functional significance, the aesthetic result is often at least as important in the patient's eyes.

Initial Care

Soft tissue injuries may occur in isolation as a result of minor trauma. However, they may also occur as a component of the complex pattern of injuries encountered in polytrauma victims. In these cases, treatment should be instituted in accordance with Advanced Trauma Life Support® (ATLS®) guidelines giving priority to patient stabilisation.

Diagnosis

Comprehensive diagnosis and assessment of the injuries must be completed before initiating definitive treatment. Detection of soft tissue injuries logically begins with inspection for surface indications.

The range of possible soft tissue injuries is varied, and may include contusion with or without haematoma, abrasion, traumatic tattoo, foreign body retention, puncture, laceration, avulsion flap or avulsion injury resulting in a soft tissue defect. These soft tissue injuries may occur either in isolation or in combination with deeper injuries.

Following the resolution of life- or limb-threatening problems, the soft tissue injuries are addressed under local, regional or general anaesthesia, depending on the severity of the injury. When definitive treatment has to be postponed, simple accurate approximation of the wound initially will aid in achieving a better eventual end result. If this is not possible, the wounds should be properly cleaned and dressed, and systemic antibiotics prescribed while awaiting the opportunity for secondary wound closure.

Photographic records taken before initiating treatment may aid in the understanding and prediction of the final result, as well as that of any secondary complications. These may also prove invaluable in the event of legal or even, medicolegal proceedings.

Anaesthesia

Minor soft tissue injuries in a reasonably cooperative patient may be repaired under local anaesthesia. This is safer and more expedient, bearing in mind that acute trauma victims have often just ingested food, alcohol or blood. If not contraindicated, sedation delivered via oral, intramuscular or intravenous routes may make the experience more bearable for the patient.

When dealing with young children who are unable to cooperate despite authoritative assurance, the use of gentle physical restraint may become necessary. This may be in the form of a skillful assistant or a calm parent, if the operation can be swiftly concluded. For more lengthy procedures, the child's torso and limbs may be effectively restrained by "mummying" the patient in an ordinary blanket or draw-sheet. If the former method limits exposure of the injury, or if the head requires restraining, an infant restraining board with Velcro straps would be more suitable. Oral sedation in the form of Chloral Hydrate (maximum dose 50 mg/kg up to 1 g total dose) may aid in reducing the child's agitation.

Treatment

Contusion (with or without haematoma)

A contusion is a bruising injury caused by blunt forms of trauma. Rarely does it result in any permanent damage to the skin, and observation of the injury will usually suffice. An exception is if the contusion is associated with an underlying haematoma.

Small haematomas frequently resorb spontaneously. Larger ones may form an inflammatory pseudocapsule and require surgical evacuation. Left untreated, the latter would lead to permanent disfiguring subcutaneous scar contracture.

When the haematoma is in a fluid state, aspiration with a large-bore needle (18-gauge or larger) may be possible. If, however, the haematoma is in a solid or semi-solid "currant jelly" state, formal incision and evacuation is the most appropriate treatment. Aspiration of haematomas using liposuction cannulae has also been described and may be appropriate in certain circumstances. Systemic proteolytic enzyme preparations may be helpful in the treatment of small haematomas.

Abrasion

Superficial abrasions should be cleaned with a mild, non-irritating antiseptic solution. Epithelialisation of the wound should be encouraged by keeping it moist via application of a topical hydrocolloid and/or covering it with an occlusive dressing depending on the depth of skin loss.

Traumatic tattoo

Traumatic tattoos are caused when small foreign body particles become embedded in the dermis as a result of trauma. Prompt efforts should be made to remove the particles from the wound before they become fixed in the tissues. Tissue fixation usually occurs approximately 12 hours post-injury.

If performed early, scrubbing the affected area with a stiff sterile scrub brush and a soap solution will usually succeed in removing most embedded foreign particles. When grease or oil is present in the wound, solvents such as ether or acetone may be required. Once the particles become tissue-fixed, formal surgical abrasion is the best solution. Occasionally, when there are only a few, isolated yet deeply embedded particles, a needle or scalpel blade may be used to tease them out individually.

When scrubbing or abrading the wound, care must be taken not to violate the deep dermis, as this may result in permanent scarring. For treatment of extensive areas, the techniques described above are best performed under regional or general anaesthesia.

Left untreated, traumatic tattoos will result in permanent, disfiguring discolouration in the skin.

Foreign bodies

Retained foreign bodies are larger than the particles that cause traumatic tattoos, and should be routinely removed if these are large and located in the superficial soft tissue. If the object is totally embedded, removal can be difficult, and may require extension of the entrance wound and/or radiologic localisation.

Bullets or missile fragments are an exception. These are sterile and penetrate deeply. If these only elicit minimal reaction, attempting to remove the fragments usually results in more damage than leaving them *in situ*.

Failure to remove foreign bodies can lead to cellulitis, abscess or pyogenic granuloma formation.

Puncture

When faced with a puncture wound, one must always be aware of the possibility of injury to deeper structures. If in doubt, formal exploration of the wound is mandatory.

Foreign bodies such as graphite from lead pencils, wooden splinters, rust particles and paint chips, are commonly implanted in puncture wounds. These must be thoroughly removed to prevent infection, pigmentation or scar formation. It is sometimes necessary to excise the puncture tract itself to achieve optimal scarless healing. Arteriovenous fistula formation may occur as a late complication of puncture wounds.

Laceration

Lacerations are the most common form of soft tissue injury, and may be subdivided into simple, beveled, tearing, burst or stellate types. Repair of lacerations should only be undertaken after associated injury to underlying structures has been addressed. The time interval between injury and definitive treatment is proportional to the risk of subsequent wound infection. This, in turn, influences management decisions with regards to the timing of surgical repair and choice of repair technique. With the exception of animal or human bites and traumatic tattoos, as a general rule, most properly cleaned and dressed soft tissue wounds can be repaired primarily, up to 24 hours after time of injury. If more than a day has lapsed, the risk of infection increases substantially, and delayed wound closure may be advisable.

Meticulous wound toilet consisting of cleaning, irrigation and thorough debridement should be performed. Devitalised tissue must be removed lest it forms a nidus for bacterial contamination. Jagged, beveled or severely contused wound edges are best conservatively excised to ensure perpendicular skin edges which will heal with minimal scar deformity. Closely parallel lacerations should be converted to a single wound by excising the thin intervening skin bridge, reducing the risk of tissue ischaemia and scar formation. Displaced viable tissue should be replaced in its original anatomical position.

Suturing

Muscular and subcutaneous tissues are best apposed with interrupted absorbable sutures to minimise dead space, and to prevent the formation of a haematoma or seroma. Placement of key interrupted absorbable dermal stitches serves to minimise skin tension. External skin closure with interrupted nylon stitches is the method of choice. This method of closure allows the removal of one or two sutures to permit drainage of blood, pus or serum, should the need arise. The use of absorbable sutures for external wound closure is advocated in lacerations involving mucosa-lined surfaces such as the oral or nasal cavity.

Timing of the removal of sutures is dependent on the site of the wound. As a general guide, sutures on the face are left for four to six days; ears, ten to 14 days; scalp, seven to ten days; trunk, eight to ten days; and extremities, 12 to 14 days. Delay in removal will lead to epithelialisation of the suture tracks, which may then be more obvious than the scar itself.

Avulsion flap

Also known as a flap laceration, the avulsion flap is an undermined laceration which can lead to extremely disfiguring scars. Broad bands of tangentially-oriented scar within the dermis and subcutaneous tissue interfere with free drainage of venous blood and lymph from the avulsion flap to the surrounding skin. Consequently, there is venous engorgement and lymphoedema, which swells the flap leading to spreading and depression of the peripheral scar. As the scar contracts, the swollen flap bordered by the depressed scar results in the formation of a "pin-cushion" or "trap-door" scar.

If the flap is small and in an amenable location, it can be totally excised, and the resulting wound closed primarily. If the flap is too large to be excised, efforts must be made to cut away the thin, beveled peripheral portions of the flap, thus creating perpendicular skin edges for accurate closure. Pressure dressings are often applied for weeks to months following an injury of this type. These dressings help to minimise dead space, restrict venous and lymphatic engorgement, thus reducing fibrin deposition and subsequent scar formation.

Soft tissue defects

Soft tissue defects, if left to heal spontaneously, may result in excessive scar formation. Direct primary closure should be performed when possible. If the defect is too large and there is undue tension in the skin on attempted primary closure, coverage of the defect with a skin graft or an appropriate flap may be in order.

Special Considerations in Facial Soft Tissue Injury

Forehead and brow

The eyebrow must be carefully repaired to preserve its shape and borders, as it is an important anatomical feature. If the muscle underneath the brow is breached, it must be repaired to prevent spreading and depression of the scar. One must always make sure that there are no fractures of the supraorbital ridge or frontal sinuses, as these fractures are often missed in routine facial X-rays.

Eyelids

When treating patients with injuries to the eyelids it is important to first determine whether there is associated injury to the globe.

A search should be conducted for foreign bodies. However, when removing the foreign body, one must be careful not to cause further damage. When encountering a wound that penetrates deeply into the orbit through the upper eyelid or globe, one must exclude intracranial injury as the superior orbital plate is thin and fragile.

Eyelid infection is rare because the blood supply is abundant; nevertheless, eyelid lacerations should be cleaned by irrigation with saline. Avulsed eyelid tissue should be gently cleaned in saline and replaced as an autograft whenever possible.

Eyelid lacerations can be divided into two groups: superficial and deep. Superficial lacerations can be further divided into those that are parallel to the lid margin, and those that are perpendicular to it. Superficial lacerations that run parallel to the lid margin would require only simple closure of the skin, and smaller ones may even be left alone. Perpendicular lacerations cross normal skin lines and tend to gape. Hence, these require absorbable sutures in the underlying muscle and subcutaneous tissue prior to skin closure. If conjunctival lacerations are small, these tend to heal well without suture repair; but when suturing is necessary, 6/O catgut on a swaged ophthalmologic needle should be used. Burying of the suture should be ensured to prevent the development of corneal abrasions.

Deep lacerations should be thoroughly explored to exclude any injury to underlying muscles. Lacerations extending through the lid margin should be promptly repaired or contracture of the orbicularis muscle may cause the wound to gape. If repair is delayed for more than seven days, the muscle fibres will undergo fibrosis, the tarsal plate will thicken and retract, and the wound edges will no longer be apposable.

The simplest type of anatomically accurate approximation with sutures is generally the best way to repair eyelid lacerations, even though one is often tempted to perform complicated procedures such as Z-plasties to realign the scar. Care must also be taken to preserve the integrity of the lacrimal apparatus and the canthal ligaments. Should the lacrimal system be found to be divided and grossly displaced, one would need to cannulate it with a 3/O nylon suture, and repair it with fine sutures. However, in instances of incomplete division, the lacrimal system may simply be approximated with the expectation of good functional return, often without direct suture.

Ears

It is important to attempt to repair the ear primarily, since secondary reconstruction is not only more difficult — the outcome is often less than satisfactory. When debriding a wound over the ear, one must always be conservative. This is because the tissues that make up the ear are unique and are not easily replaceable. As the ear has an excellent cutaneous blood supply, narrow-based avulsion flaps or even completely avulsed skin can often survive just by accurate replacement of the tissue.

The cartilage should be accurately repaired with absorbable stitches. The placement of perichondrial-cutaneous sutures will provide additional support. Injuries involving the cartilage should be covered with systemic antibiotics.

Nose

The soft tissue components of the nose consist mainly of the skin, cartilage and mucous membrane. Its muscular layer is thin and adherent to the overlying skin. Management of soft tissue injuries of the nose is generally straightforward. Most of the time, once the bony architecture of the nose is accurately restored, the soft tissue just has to be approximated with anatomical accuracy to ensure a good aesthetic outcome.

Should the injury be full thickness, it is easier to repair the deepest layers first (the mucous layer) using an absorbable suture. Similar to injuries of the ear, lacerations in the cartilage should be repaired with interrupted absorbable stitches. A non-absorbable suture is used for skin closure.

It is important not to miss the diagnosis of a septal haematoma, since it may result in chondromalacia if left untreated. This condition can result in either loss or thickening of the septal cartilage, and may eventually cause obstruction of the nasal airway.

Lips

The vermilion border is an important landmark in the repair of the lip. Lip repair is always performed with respect to this. An absorbable suture (3 or 4/O) is used to appose the muscles of the lip first. This is followed by external closure commencing at the vermilion border; a fine (6 or 7/O) non-absorbable suture is used. Mucosa is closed last with an absorbable suture.

Cheeks

Management of cheek lacerations is fairly straightforward. However, special attention needs to be paid to the branches of the facial nerve, the parotid gland and its duct. This applies particularly when the injury is located in the posterior and inferior aspects of the cheek.

Branches of the facial nerve

Major branches of the facial nerve lie deep to the muscles of facial expression. Unless there are signs of paralysis of any of these muscles, exploration to determine injury to the nerve is unnecessary. Since the superficial facial muscles are innervated in the posterior portions, division of nerve branches anterior to the mid-pupillary line usually does not cause any permanent loss of muscle function.

Should any injury of the nerve require repair, the use of magnifying loupes or an operating microscope is necessary. If the nerve has been cleanly divided (for example, with a knife), the neural sheaths can be approximated with fine sutures. However, if it is a blunt injury, each end would require some debridement before commencement of the repair. It is important to note that although some recovery of nerve function is expected, complete recovery is rare.

Parotid gland and Stensen's Duct

The parotid gland is superficial to the branches of the facial nerve and hence, is easily damaged. The buccal branch of the facial nerve usually runs parallel to, and sometimes crosses, the parotid duct. As a result, it is often damaged at the same time.

The gland need not be repaired. However, the patency of the duct has to be ensured before closure of the wound. The surface marking of the parotid duct follows a line drawn from the tragus of the ear to the midportion of the upper lip. If the wound overlies the point of division of the duct, a fine prolene suture can be used to cannulate the duct. Alternatively, the cannulation may be performed in a retrograde fashion through the ostium which lies opposite the second upper molar tooth. Once this is done, the divided ends are anastomosed with a fine suture. If there is only partial division of the duct, the suture used for cannulation may be removed. However, if there is relatively severe injury in the region, or if the duct has been completely divided, the suture should be left as a stent. The suture is looped out of the corner of the mouth, and taped to the cheek. If repair is not possible, the proximal portion of the duct may be brought out to the oral mucosa separately, creating a new ostium. If this too is not feasible, the duct may be ligated. Following ligation, the gland becomes atrophic and will stop functioning.

References

1. McGregor AD, McGregor IA (2000). *Fundamental Techniques of Plastic Surgery and Their Surgical Applications*. London, New York: Churchill Livingstone.
2. Schultz RC (1988). *Facial Injuries*. Chicago: Year Book Medical Publishers.

PART II

SUPPORT SERVICES

Section XI

Radiology

35

Computed Tomography Imaging of Blunt Abdominal Trauma

Siew-Kune Wong

Introduction

Computed tomography (CT) has become the primary modality in the evaluation of abdominal trauma, because it is a relatively quick and non-invasive procedure. CT is as accurate as diagnostic peritoneal lavage (DPL) and more sensitive than a focused ultrasound examination in the evaluation of abdominal trauma.[1] Due to its cross-sectional imaging ability and superior soft tissue resolution, CT can give a detailed anatomic assessment of injuries, quantification of haemorrhage and detection of active arterial extravasation. CT is also able to detect retroperitoneal injuries which are usually not detected by DPL or ultrasound.

Imaging Technique

Helical CT is the preferred technique compared to conventional CT, as it is a faster procedure with fewer respiratory motion artefacts and better intravenous contrast enhancement. Administration of intravenous contrast is essential as parenchymal organ injuries may not be demonstrated without intravenous contrast. Active bleeding also requires the presence of contrast extravasation before a definitive diagnosis can be made. Optimal assessment of the gastrointestinal tract requires the use of oral contrast.[2] It helps to identify bowel rupture and abnormal bowel wall thickening, and to differentiate fluid-filled bowel loops from free fluid.

The exact protocol may vary in different imaging centres but in our department, a helical scan is done at 7 mm collimation with a pitch of 1.0 to 1.5 about 90 seconds after initiating an injection of 100 ml of 300 mg/ml low osmolar intravenous contrast medium at 2 ml per second. Oral contrast (300 ml of 2–3% iodinated water-soluble oral contrast medium) should be given orally or via a nasogastric tube as soon as a decision to perform the CT is made. This will allow the contrast to travel as far as possible through the gastrointestinal tract. A second drink can be given if more than 30 minutes have elapsed between the initial drink and the scan. In patients with possible colon injuries, an additional 400 ml and 1000 ml of colon contrast can be administered rectally for left- and right-sided colonic injuries respectively. CT cystography can also be performed to detect any urinary bladder rupture. This is done by instilling 300–400 ml of water-soluble contrast via an existing Foleys catheter inserted by the emergency physician.

Solid Organ Injury

Spleen

This is the most commonly injured abdominal organ following blunt trauma. Contrast enhanced CT is approximately 95% sensitive and specific for the detection of splenic injury. This may be classified as contusions, lacerations, fractures, intraparenchymal haematomas, subcapsular haemorrhages and vascular pedicle injuries.[3]

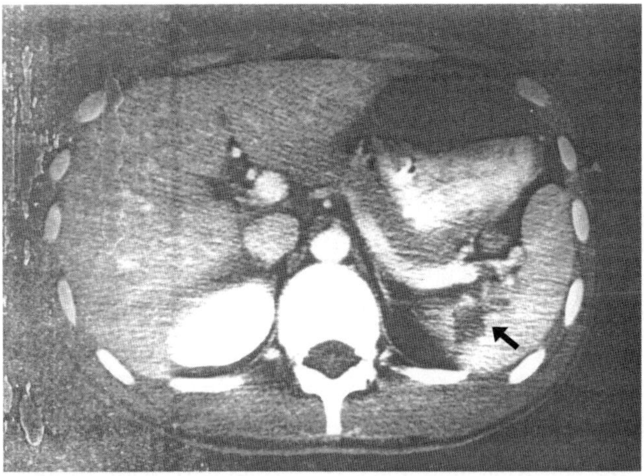

Fig. 1 Splenic laceration seen along the medial aspect of the spleen (arrow).

Contusions appear as focal, poorly-defined areas of low attenuation. Lacerations are focal, linear or branching areas of low attenuation within the normal enhancing splenic parenchyma (Fig. 1). If the laceration extending to the surface results in complete separation of the splenic fragments, this is defined as a fracture.

An intraparenchymal haematoma is due to parenchymal disruption filled with blood products, appearing as rounded areas of low attenuation. Subcapsular haematomas are peripheral lentiform collections, and may compress the contour of the spleen. Vascular pedicle injuries may result from intimal dissection or avulsion of the artery.

While CT can accurately stage splenic injuries, it cannot predict which patients can be managed conservatively, because delayed splenic haemorrhage (defined as active haemorrhage that occurs more than 48 hours following the initial injury) may occur from mild splenic injuries. Another complication is the formation of a pseudoaneurysm. This appears as a focal, well-defined area of increased attenuation within the spleen, and is frequently accompanied by a halo of low density haematoma.

Liver

The liver is the second most frequently injured organ in blunt trauma. The right lobe is more commonly injured than the left[4,5] — particularly the posterior segment. Right lobe injuries may be associated with rib fractures, and lung, renal and adrenal injuries, while the left lobe may be associated with pancreatic, duodenal and colonic injuries. As with injuries to the spleen, the classification of liver injuries can be divided into contusion, laceration, fracture, intraparenchymal haematoma and subcapsular haemorrhage. Lacerations are the most common liver injury[4] and can be linear or stellate in appearance (Fig. 2). The lacerations frequently parallel branches of the hepatic and portal veins and the fissures, and may be associated with biliary tract injuries. A fracture implies that the laceration had extended to involve two visceral surfaces, and a part of the liver may have been avulsed (Fig. 3). Contusions appear as poorly-defined low-attenuation areas, with no mass effect or any obvious laceration noted. Haematomas are collections of blood due to parenchymal laceration or disruption, and

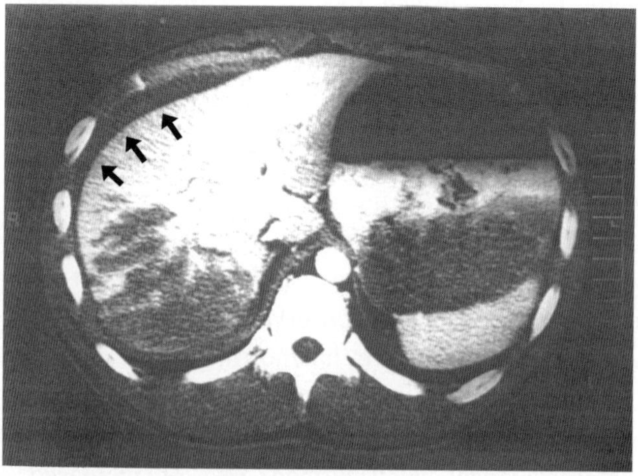

Fig. 2 Liver laceration. Liver laceration appearing as low attenuation areas in the right lobe of the liver. There is haemoperitoneum noted in the perihepatic space (arrows).

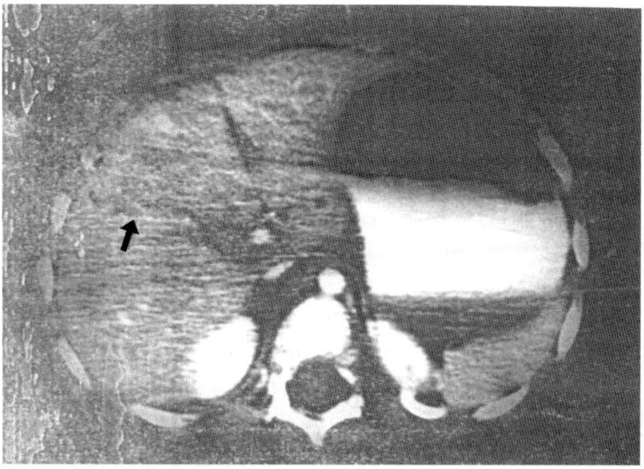

Fig. 3 Fracture of the liver (arrow) is seen extending from the porta hepatis to the liver capsule at the lateral aspect of the right lobe of the liver.

can be intraparenchymal or subcapsular. In the latter, the capsule is intact and the liver contour may be deformed due to the mass effect.

In a study by Shanmuganathan and colleagues, about one-third of liver injuries may not result in haemoperitoneum.[6] Therefore a negative DPL or focused abdominal sonography for trauma (FAST) should be interpreted with caution in light of a suspected liver injury. Haemoperitoneum is usually resorbed significantly by one week. The presence of an unchanged or increased volume of intraperitoneal fluid on follow up scans should suggest continuous haemorrhage or bile leakage.

Anatomically, a sheath of connective tissue surrounds the portal veins, hepatic artery branches, bile ducts and lymphatics creating the portal triads. In trauma, there is likely disruption of the small trigonal vessels and the adjoining hepatic parenchymal, resulting in bleeding. This appears as a region of low attenuation, and parallels the portal vein and and its branches (Fig. 4). This may be the only sign in liver injury.[7] Another reason for the cause of the periportal low density in trauma is the development of periportal lymphatic dilatation. This could be due to obstruction of hepatic lymphatic drainage, volume

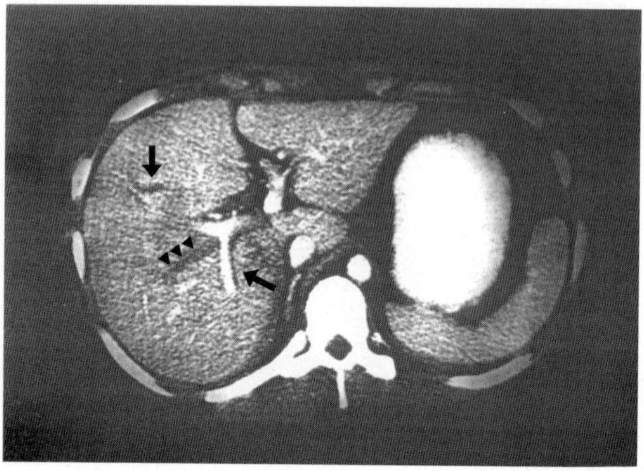

Fig. 4 Periportal tracking of fluid. Periportal zones of low attenuation (arrows) in the periportal region due to liver laceration (arrowheads).

overload secondary to vigorous fluid resuscitation, or elevated central venous pressure from cardiac tamponade, tension pneumothorax or pericardial effusion.[8,9]

Biliary injury

Gallbladder injuries are rare. These may be contused, disrupted or avulsed. CT may showed an ill-defined contour of the gallbladder wall, a contracted or non-visualised gallbladder, pericholecystic fluid and intraperitoneal low attenuation bile.

Both the intrahepatic and extrahepatic bile ducts may be injured in abdominal trauma. Intrahepatic biliary injury usually occurs as a result of liver laceration disrupting the ducts, while extrahepatic biliary injury usually occurs at where the hepatic duct exits the liver or where the common bile duct enters the pancreas.[10] Biliary injuries are often found incidentally at surgery or on follow up. Complications include the formation of a biloma (which may be intrahepatic or within the peritoneum), haemobilia, and bilehaemia or jaundice due to a large subcapsular haematoma compressing on the biliary ducts.

Pancreas

As the pancreas is a deep retroperitoneal organ, it is more commonly injured secondary to a penetrating rather than a blunt injury. A direct blow to the epigastrium is usually due to a steering wheel or handlebar, and there may be associated viseral injuries in up to 90% of cases. The pancreatic injuries may be classified as a contusion, laceration or transection. On CT, contusion can result in focal or diffuse swelling of the pancreas. Lacerations appear as a linear low attenuation area while a transection extends through the entire pancreas (Fig. 5). The most common site of laceration is at the neck of the pancreas. The pancreatic duct is usually injured if the laceration involves more than 50% of the thickness of the pancreas.[11] Endoscopic retrograde cholangiopancreatography (ERCP) or intraoperative pancreatography may be required to establish pancreatic duct integrity.[12] Other CT scan findings include peripancreatic fat stranding or fluid, fluid in the lesser sac, fluid between the pancreas and splenic vein,[13] and thickening of the left anterior renal fascia.[14]

Complications of pancreatic trauma include pancreatitis, pseudocyst and fistula formation.

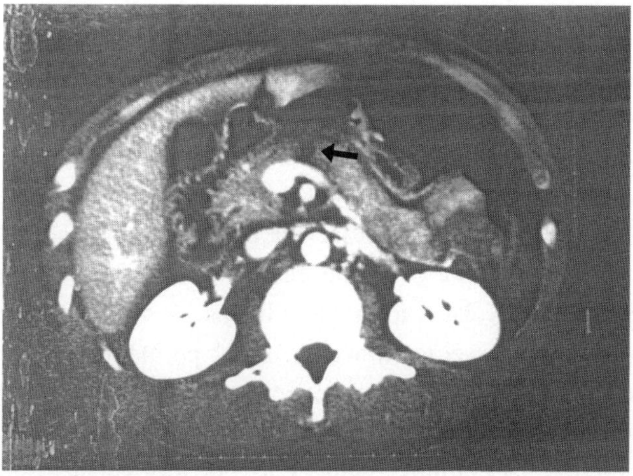

Fig. 5 Pancreatic transection. Linear area of decreased attenuation extending through the entire pancreas at the pancreatic neck (arrow) from a direct blow to the epigastrium.

Adrenal gland

Adrenal injuries result in the formation of a haematoma, diffuse irregular haemorrhage or uniform swelling of the adrenal gland.[15] It is usually unilateral, occurring more on the right. This is because the right adrenal is easily compressed by the liver, and the raised venous pressure from the inferior vena cava may elevate the intra-adrenal venous pressure, resulting in haemorrhage. As with the pancreas, adrenal injury is associated with ipsilateral thoracic, abdominal or retroperitoneal injuries in up to 95% of cases. Unilateral haemorrhage is of little clinical significance but bilateral haemorrhages can result in adrenal insufficiency.

Adrenal injury may appear as a discrete round or oval haematoma expanding the gland, diffuse irregular haemorrhage obliterating the gland or a uniformly enlarged adrenal gland with indistinct margins. Periadrenal findings include stranding of the periadrenal fat, and haemorrhage in the posterior pararenal space mimicking a thickened diaphragmatic crus.[15]

Urinary Tract Injuries

Kidneys

Blunt renal injury is the third most common injury after those of the spleen and liver. The types of injury may be classified as contusion, laceration, fracture, subcapsular haematoma, and vascular pedicle injuries. Contusion appears as focal areas of decreased parenchymal enhancement, while a subcapsular haematoma appears as a crescenteric collection of blood over the renal surface that may flatten the renal parenchyma. A laceration is a linear or wedge-shaped cortical defect, and may be associated with a focal perinephric or subcapsular haematoma (Fig. 6). It may be superficial or deep, and may involve the collecting system, resulting in extravasation of contrast. Renal fracture occurs when the lacerations connect to cortical surfaces through the hilum. A shattered kidney results from multiple deep lacerations, with the renal fragments held together by the vascular scaffolding.

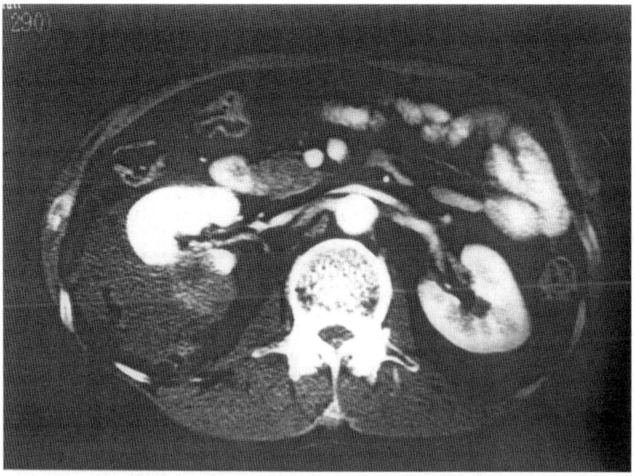

Fig. 6 Laceration of the right kidney associated with a large perinephric haematoma. The kidney is displaced anteriorly by the haematoma.

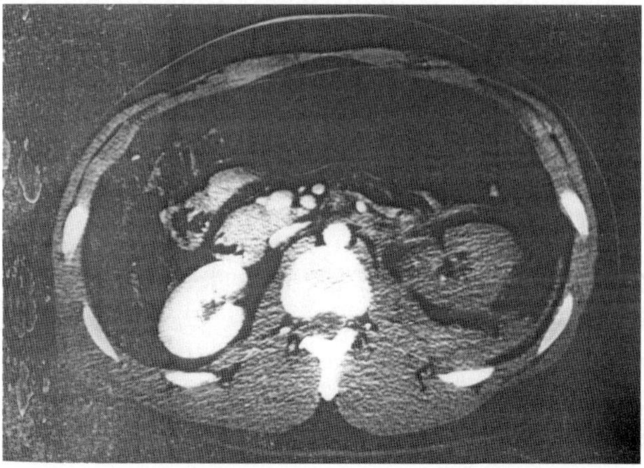

Fig. 7 Total renal infarct. There is non-enhancement of the left kidney which could be due to renal artery thrombosis or avulsion.

There is usually a large perinephric haematoma, and some of the renal fragments may be infarcted. Renal infarct can be segmental, due to injury to the segmental division of the renal artery, or total, due to dissection, thrombosis or avulsion of the main renal artery (Fig. 7).

Collateral supply from capsular arteries may result in peripheral renal cortical enhancement ("cortical rim sign").

Computed tomography is more sensitive and specific than urography in the evaluation of suspected blunt genitourinary trauma.[16] As the ureter is fixed in the retroperitoneum (while the kidney is relatively mobile), the most common site of injury due to blunt trauma is at the ureteropelvic junction (UPJ) followed by the mid and distal ureter. The UPJ avulsion may be a complete transection or laceration when contrast material is seen in the ipsilateral ureter distal to the point of injury. Ureteropelvic junction injuries are usually seen in children, and the presence of perinephric extravasation of contrast material at the medial aspect is highly suggestive of UPJ injury.[17] A distinctive pattern of contrast extravasation at CT termed "circumrenal urinoma" was found to be specific for UPJ injury.[17] As contrast-laden urine may not be visualised in the early vascular phase CT, delayed scanning may be needed to show contrast extravasation. Potential complications of non-operative management would include the formation of a urinoma which may become infected if the patient is immunocompromised, or when there is associated bowel injury or sepsis.

Bladder injuries

Extraperitoneal bladder rupture accounts for 70–80% of all bladder ruptures from blunt trauma, while intraperitoneal bladder injuries are more common in penetrating injuries. The diagnosis can be made by either radiographic or CT cystography. In the latter, the CT should be done at the same time when the abdomen is being evaluated.

The CT signs of extraperitoneal bladder injuries include the flame-shaped perivesical extravasation of contrast, and the spreading of the contrast along fascial planes of the anterior abdominal wall, scrotum or the thigh (Fig. 8). Intraperitoneal bladder injuries result in contrast media collecting in the vesicorectal or vesicouterine peritoneal recess, along paracolic gutters, between bowel loops and under the surface of the liver (Fig. 9).

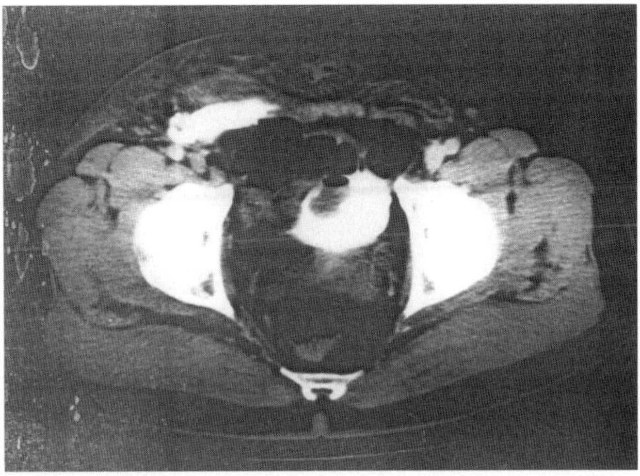

(A)

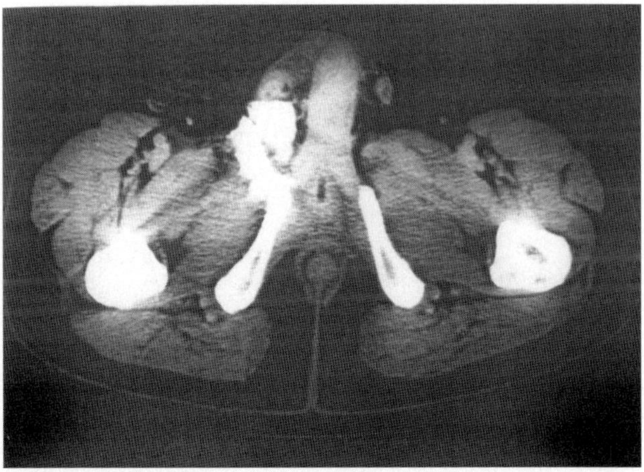

(B)

Fig. 8 Extraperitoneal bladder rupture. **(A)** Contrast material extravasates extraperitoneally into the paravesical spaces and the anterior abdominal wall fascial planes. **(B)** CT scan caudad to that in (A) shows extension of contrast material into the scrotum.

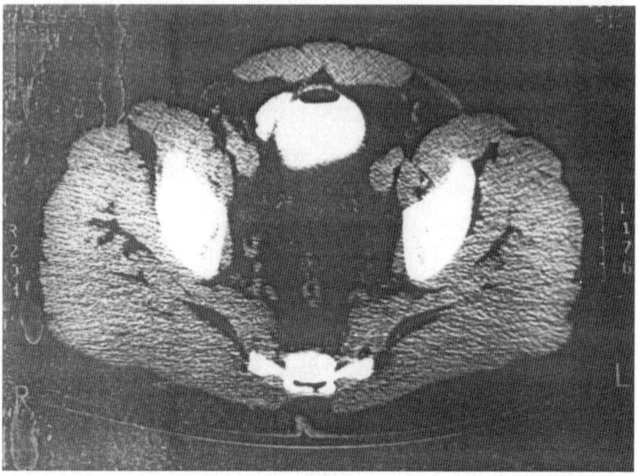

(A)

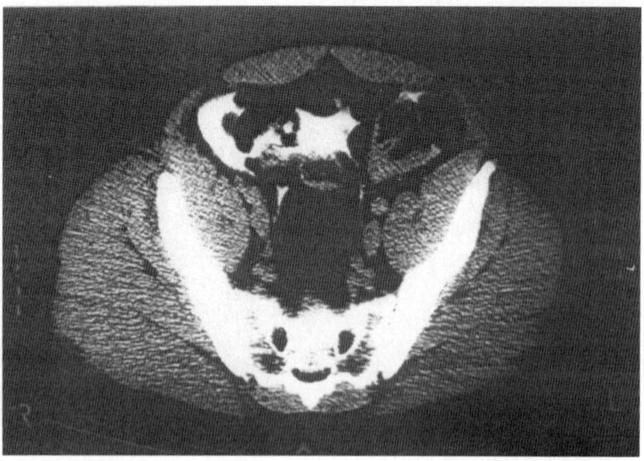

(B)

Fig. 9 Intraperitoneal bladder rupture. **(A)** CT near the bladder dome shows laceration of the right side of the bladder. **(B)** CT scan cephalad to that in (A) shows intraperitoneal extravasated contrast between bowel loops.

Gastrointestinal Injuries

Bowel injuries

Bowel and mesenteric injuries are found in approximately 5% of all patients undergoing laparotomy after blunt abdominal trauma, and are most often associated with motor vehicles accident.[18] Computed tomography is 88% to 93% sensitive in detecting blunt abdominal injuries.[19–21] Blunt trauma to the bowel may cause contusions resulting in paralytic ileus, intramural haematomas, which can cause obstruction or perforation. Hollow viscus injuries occur less commonly in blunt trauma as compared to penetrating trauma, and usually involve the small bowel. This is commonly seen near the points of attachment (ligament of Treitz and the ileocaecal valve) but can occur anywhere along the length of the small bowel.[22] Blunt injuries to the stomach and jejunum are less common and usually occur in children.[23] The anterior wall of the stomach and the second and third part of the duodenum are the most common sites respectively. Blunt colonic injuries are rare and usually involves the transverse colon.[24]

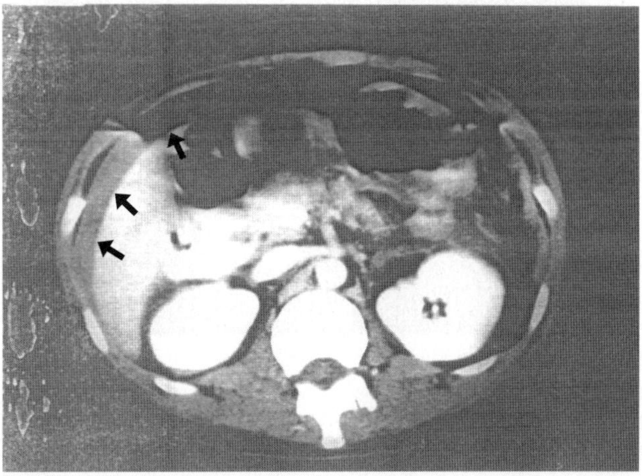

Fig. 10 Bowel perforation. CT shows the presence of pneumoperitoneum and extravasation of bowel luminal contents (arrows).

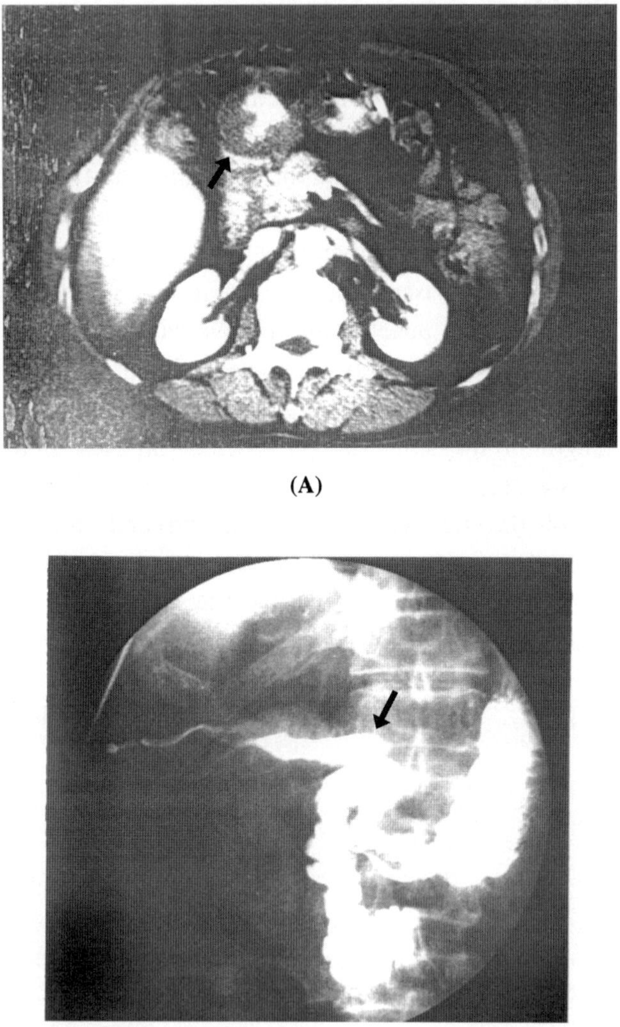

Fig. 11 Duodenal perforation. **(A)** Abnormal thickening of the duodenal wall (arrow) is noted. Extravasation of contrast material is seen in the perihepatic space, resulting in a fluid-fluid level. **(B)** A gastrograffin meal confirms the perforation with leakage of contrast material (arrow) seen at the level of the duodenum.

Computed tomography signs that are diagnostic of bowel perforation include: pneumoperitoneum, mesenteric, intramural or retroperitoneal free gas, visualisation of discontinuity of the bowel wall, or extravasation of luminal contents or contrast media (Figs. 10 and 11).[19] Computed tomography signs suggestive of bowel rupture include thickening of bowel wall, intense enhancement of the bowel wall, free fluid in the anterior pararenal space, and intraperitoneal fluid or blood without an obvious source or fluid or blood between bowel loops.

Mesenteric injuries

Computed tomography signs of mesenteric injury include the detection of mesenteric haematoma or fluid.[25] These appear as a triangular fluid collection between the leaves of the mesentry, between bowel loops, or as mesenteric streaking. Moderate to large amounts of intraperitoneal fluid may also be present. While a large mesenteric tear can result in intestinal hernia, vascular injuries can cause life-threatening haemorrhage, bowel ischaemia or infarction with delayed rupture or delayed ischaemic stricture due to segmental ischaemia.

Vascular Injuries

Intraperitoneal fluid in blunt trauma may be due to blood, intestinal fluid, urine, bile, lymphatic fluid or ascites. With the exception of blood, the attenuation of the above fluids as measured on CT in Hounsfield units (HU) is less than 20. Unclotted blood measures between 30–45 HU; clotted blood, between 40–70; while 85–370 HU would indicate active haemorrhage due to extravasation of contrast material.[26,27] However, due to volume averaging, underlying anaemia and lysis of red blood cells, the measurement of blood may be less than 20 HU.[28]

When multiple sites of haematoma are seen in the peritoneal cavity after blunt trauma, the site of the highest attenuation represents the most likely source of haemorrhage (Fig. 12). This is known as the

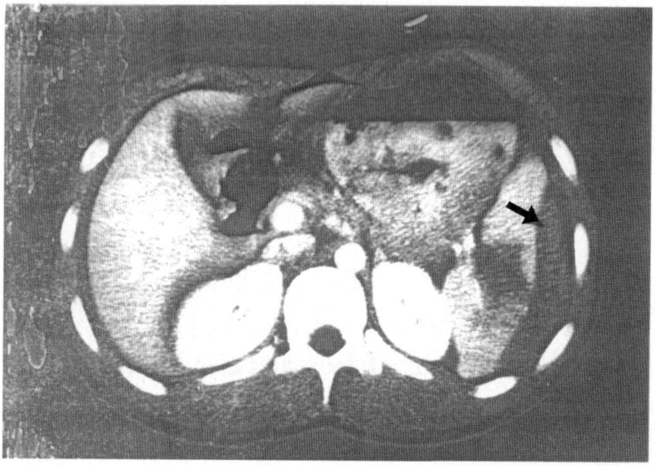

Fig. 12 Sentinel clot sign. Laceration of the spleen with haemoperitonuem noted in the perihepatic and perisplenic spaces. The dense haematoma adjacent to the spleen (arrow) indicates the spleen as the likely source of the haemorrhage.

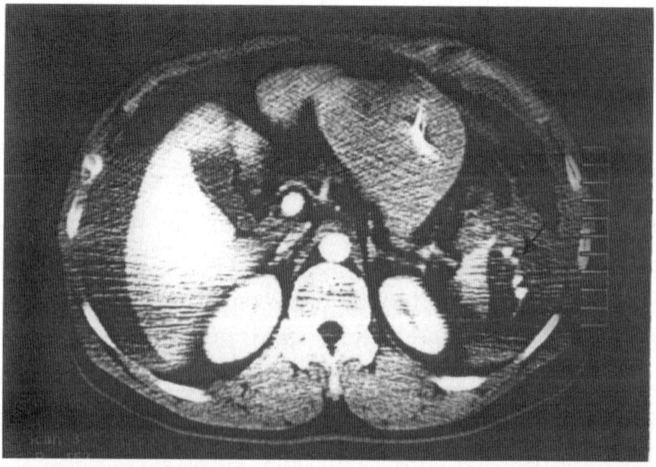

Fig. 13 Laceration of the spleen is noted. There is extravasation of contrast from the spleen indicating active haemorrhage (arrow).

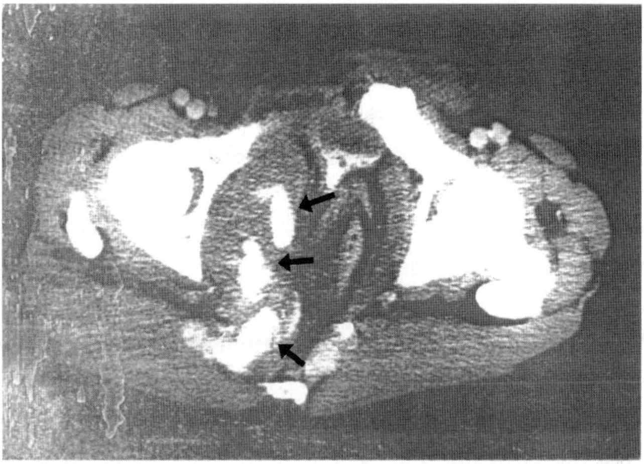

Fig. 14 CT shows active arterial extravasation (arrows) due to bleeding from the right obturator artery.

"sentinel clot sign".[29] Among the abdominal viscera, the spleen is the most common site of active haemorrhage observed on CT (Fig. 13). The liver and kidneys are also common sites. Life-threatening retroperitoneal haemorrhage can arise from injury to a number of vessels like the lumbar arteries, inferior vena cava, abdominal aorta and the iliac vessels (Fig. 14). Computed tomography can aid in the detection and localisation of the acute haemorrhage before surgery or angiography. The primary finding on CT is a focal dense collection of contrast enhanced blood with a surrounding haematoma.

Conclusion

Helical CT is now the principal diagnostic modality to evaluate blunt abdominal trauma in major trauma centres. It is quick, well tolerated and accurate for the assessment of any solid organ, urinary tract or bowel injuries. Immediate surgery or angiographic embolisation can be planned if any potential life-threatening haemorrhage is detected on CT. Computed tomography is also an essential imaging tool with which to follow up on patients who have been treated conservatively.

References

1. Liu M, Lee CH, P'Eng FK (1993). Prospective comparison of diagnostic peritoneal lavage, computed tomographic scanning, and ultrasonography for the diagnosis of blunt abdominal trauma. *J Trauma* **35**(2), 267–270.
2. Federle MP (1998). Diagnosis of intestinal injuries by computed tomography and the use of oral contrast medium. *Ann Emerg Med* **31**(6), 51–53.
3. Roberts JL (1996). CT of abdominal and pelvic trauma. *Semin Ultrasound CT MR* **17**(2), 142–169.
4. Foley WD, Cates JD, Kellman GM, Langdon, T, Aprahamian C, Lawson TL, Middleton WD (1987). Treatment of blunt hepatic injuries: role of CT. *Radiology* **164**(3), 635–638.
5. Moon KL, Ferderle MP (1983). Computed tomography in hepatic trauma. *Am J Radiol* **141**(2), 309–314.
6. Shanmuganathan K, Mirvis SE, Sherbourne CD, Chiu WC, Rodriguez A (1999). Hemoperitoneum as the sole indicator of abdominal visceral injuries: a potential limitation of screening abdominal US for trauma. *Radiology* **212**(2), 423–430.
7. Macrander SJ, Lawson TL, Foley WD, Dodds WJ, Erickson SJ, Quiroz FA (1989). Periportal tracking in hepatic trauma: CT features. *J Comput Assist Tomogr* **13**(6), 952–957.
8. Shanmuganathan K, Mirvis SE, Amoroso M (1993). Periportal low density on CT in patients with blunt abdominal trauma: association with elevated venous pressure. *Am J Radiol* **160**(2), 279–283.
9. Patrick LE, Ball TI, Atkinson GO, Winn KJ (1992). Pediatric blunt abdominal trauma: periportal tracking at CT. *Radiology* **183**(3), 689–691.
10. Parks RW, Diamond T (1995). Non-surgical trauma to the extra-hepatic biliary tract. *Br J Surg* **82**(10), 1303–1310.
11. Wong YC, Wang LJ, Lin BC, Chen CJ, Lim KE, Chen RJ (1997). CT grading of blunt pancreatic injuries: prediction of ductal disruption and surgical correlation. *J Comput Assist Tomogr* **21**(2), 246–250.

12. Lane MJ, Mindelzun RE, Jeffrey RB (1996). Diagnosis of pancreatic injury after blunt abdominal trauma. *Semin Ultrasound CT MR* **17**(2), 177–182.
13. Lane MJ, Mindelzun RE, Sandhu JS, McCormick VD, Jeffrey RB (1994). CT diagnosis of blunt pancreatic trauma: importance of detecting fluid between the pancreas and the splenic vein. *Am J Radiol* **163**(4), 833–835.
14. Sivit CJ, Eichelberger MR, Taylor GA, Bulas DI, Gotschall CS, Kushner DC (1992). Blunt pancreatic trauma in children; CT diagnosis. *Am J Radiol* **158**(5), 1097–1100.
15. Burks DW, Mirvis SE, Shanmuganathan K (1992). Acute adrenal injury after blunt abdominal trauma.: CT findings. *Am J Radiol* **158**(3), 503–507.
16. Sandler CM, Toombs BD (1981). Computed tomographic evaluation of blunt renal injuries. *Radiology* **141**(2), 461–466.
17. Kawashima A, Sandler CM, Corriere JN, Rodgers BM, Goldman SM (1997). Ureteropelvic junction injuries secondary to blunt abdominal trauma. *Radiology* **205**(2), 487–492.
18. Rizzo MJ, Federle MP, Griffiths BG (1989). Bowel and mesenteric injury following blunt abdominal trauma: evaluation with CT. *Radiology* **173**(1), 143–148.
19. Mirvis SE, Gens DR, Shanmuganathan K (1992). Rupture of the bowel after blunt abdominal trauma: diagnosis with CT. *Am J Radiol* **159**(6), 1217–1221.
20. Sherck J, Shatney C (1996). Significance of intraabdominal extraluminal air detected by CT scan in blunt abdominal trauma. *J Trauma* **40**(4), 674–675.
21. Janzen DL, Zwirewich CV, Breen DJ, Nagy A (1998). Diagnostic accuracy of helical CT for detection of blunt bowel and mesenteric injuries. *Clin Radiol* **53**(3), 193–197.
22. Hagiwara A, Yukioka T, Satou M, Yoshii H, Yamamoto S, Matsuda H, Shimazaki S (1995). Early diagnosis of small intestine rupture from blunt abdominal trauma using computed tomography: significance of the streaky density within the mesentry. *J Trauma* **38**(4), 630–633.

23. Allen GS, Moore FA, Cox CS Jr, Wilson JT, Cohn JM, Duke JH (1998). Hollow visceral injury and blunt trauma. *J Trauma* **45**(1), 69–75.
24. Nghiem HV, Jeffrey RB Jr, Mindelzun RE (1993). CT of blunt trauma to the bowel and mesentry. *Am J Radiol* **160**(1), 53–58.
25. Dowe MF, Shanmuganathan K, Mirvis SE, Steiner RC, Cooper C (1997). CT findings of mesenteric injury after blunt trauma: implications for surgical intervention. *Am J Radiol* **168**(2), 425–428.
26. Shanmuganathan K, Mirvis SE, Sover ER (1993). Value of contrast-enhanced CT in detecting active hemorrhage in patients with blunt abdominal or pelvic trauma. *Am J Radiol* **161**(1), 65–69.
27. Jeffrey RB Jr, Cardoza JD, Olcott EW (1991). Detection of active intraabdominal arterial hemorrhage: value of dynamic contract-enhanced CT. *Am J Radiol* **156**(4), 725–729.
28. Levine CD, Patel UJ, Silverman PM, Wachsberg RH (1996). Low attenuation of acute traumatic hemoperitoneum on CT scans. *Am J Radiol* **166**(5), 1089–1093.
29. Orwig D, Federle MP (1989). Localised clotted blood as evidence of visceral trauma on CT: the sentinel clot sign. *Am J Radiol* **153**(4), 747–749.

36

The Role of Interventional Radiology in Acute Haemorrhage

Kiang-Hiong Tay
Winston Eng-Hoe Lim
Bien-Soo Tan

Introduction

The role of radiologists in the management of patients with acute haemorrhage has traditionally been to perform diagnostic procedures. Catheter angiography is a time-honoured tool for the diagnosis and localisation of acute haemorrhage. However, advances in ultrasound, computed tomography (CT) and magnetic resonance imaging (MRI) as well as endoscopy, have led to decreased indications for diagnostic angiography. At the same time, remarkable technological innovations in imaging equipment, catheters, guidewires and intra-vascular prostheses have enabled the adaptation of percutaneous approaches, evolved originally for purely diagnostic imaging purposes, to a variety of therapeutic applications. Therapeutic transcatheter manipulations have expanded the role of radiologists, moving the radiologist to the front line of patient management.

Angiographic techniques have proven themselves to be life-saving in patients with acute haemorrhage. Such techniques may be used as an adjunct to surgery but increasingly, control of haemorrhage can be achieved by percutaneous techniques alone, without recourse to further operative intervention. In some instances, transcatheter therapy may be the only option available when surgical access or vascular control is difficult, or when the patient cannot tolerate surgery due to severe co-morbidities.

Embolisation is the principal angiographic technique for control of haemorrhage. The technique involves the deliberate occlusion of a vessel by intravascular delivery of an occluding agent via percutaneous means. Vessels treated by embolisation are typically expendable. These vessels are likely to be ligated if treated surgically. Bleeding vital vessels that cannot be sacrificed without dire effects usually require surgical repair or reconstruction with surgical grafts. Stent grafts or covered stents are recent additions to the percutaneous armamentarium that allow treatment of these vessels. They exclude the site of haemorrhage from the circulation without causing vessel occlusion. Other transcatheter techniques available for control of acute haemorrhage include: catheter directed infusion of vasopressin for treatment of gastrointestinal haemorrhage, and transjugular intrahepatic porto-systemic shunt (TIPS) creation for the management of acute variceal bleeding.

Percutaneous management of acute haemorrhage in the head and neck regions falls within the realm of interventional neuroradiology and will be discussed at the end of this chapter.

General Principles of Embolisation

Although transcatheter embolisation was first described in the early 1970s, the principle of vascular embolisation is not new, and dates back to 1904, when Dawbarn described the pre-operative injection of melted paraffin into the external carotid arteries of patients suffering from head and neck tumours to reduce operative blood loss.[1] Since the early attempts at transcatheter embolisation in the 1970s, there have been tremendous advances in catheter technology and embolic materials. Development of highly sophisticated catheterisation methods, including co-axial microcatheter systems, has allowed super-selective catheter placement, making possible highly selective delivery of embolic agents. Vascular occlusion can now be accomplished with greater precision than is possible with surgery, minimising hazards to non-target tissues.[2,3]

Many different materials have been used to embolise vessels (Table 1).[4,5] Embolic agents can broadly be classified into particulate agents (such as gel foam, polyvinyl alcohol), mechanical agents (such as metallic coils, detachable balloons) and liquid agents (such as alcohol, glue). Embolic agents function by causing direct mechanical obstruction of the vessel as well as providing a framework for

Table 1 Embolic Agents

Category	Duration of Occlusion
Particulate Agents	
Autologous blood clots	Hours
Gelatin sponge (Gelfoam®)	Days to weeks
Oxidised cellulose (Oxycel®)	Days to weeks
Microfibrillar collage (Avitene®)	Days to weeks
Polyvinyl alcohol (PVA)	Permanent
Mechanical Agents	
Gianturco steel coils	Permanent
Platinum microcoils	Permanent
Gugliemi detachable coils (GDC®)	Permanent
Detachable balloons	Permanent
Liquid Agents	
Polymerising fluids	
N-butyl-2-cyanoacrylate (Histocryl®)	Permanent
Ethylene vinyl alcohol (Onyx®)	Permanent
Sclerosing fluids	
Absolute alcohol	Permanent
Sodium tetradecyl sulfate (Sotradecol®)	Permanent
Sodium morrhuate (Variocid®)	Permanent
Boiling contrast medium	Permanent
Hypertonic glucose solution	Permanent

thrombus formation. Sclerosing agents such as alcohol cause direct destruction of the vascular endothelium and denaturation of proteins, resulting in thrombotic occlusion of the vessel. Certain agents also incite an inflammatory reaction in and around the vessel wall, which further accentuates vessel occlusion.

The size of the embolic agents determines the level of vascular occlusion, and this can be anywhere from a large vessel to a distal arteriolar or capillary level. Liquid and particulate agents tend to produce distal occlusion. Mechanical agents, because of their larger size, result in proximal vessel occlusion, which in effect simulate surgical ligation. Depending on the agents used, vascular occlusion may be permanent or temporary. In general, non-absorbable agents give rise to permanent vascular occlusion, while absorbable agents allow temporary occlusion lasting from days to weeks.

Although a wide variety of embolic agents have been described and utilised, the vast majority of embolisations are performed with one of three agents: gel foam, polyvinyl alcohol (PVA) and metallic coils. Gelfoam is the most commonly used embolic agent. It is non-toxic, resorbable and is available in both powder and sheet forms. The sheets can be divided into various sized pledgets and strips, or made into a slurry by mixing gel foam shavings with contrast and saline. Gelfoam provides a temporary occlusion lasting approximately three to six weeks, after which the vessel will completely recanalise. Gelfoam is widely used in situations where temporary occlusions are desired, such as with pelvic trauma, priapism and peripartum haemorrhage. Polyvinyl alcohol is an inert plastic polymer available as particles ranging in size from 50 microns to 2000 microns. It causes mechanical occlusion of the vessel lumen and induces a foreign body type reaction with permeation of the particles by granulation tissue. Polyvinyl alcohol is a permanent agent and is widely utilised for tumour embolisation as well as pre-operative devascularisation of other lesions. It is also the preferred agent for bronchial artery embolisation.

Metallic coils are constructed of stainless steel or platinum, and Dacron fibers are attached to the coils to enhance thrombogenicity. These are available in sizes from 2 mm to 30 mm diameters, and can be delivered through microcatheters. Coils produce a permanent focal occlusion leaving the vessel distal to the coils patent. The use of coils is analogous to a focal surgical ligature of the vessel.

The choice of embolic agent depends on the permanency and desired level of the vascular occlusion required to achieve the therapeutic goal. For example, in traumatic haemorrhage, a temporary agent like gelfoam is preferable as the aim of embolisation is not to cause tissue infarction, but rather, to decrease perfusion to the point that endogenous haemostatic mechanisms stop the bleeding. The vessel is occluded long enough to allow healing. Eventually it will recanalise, restoring optimal tissue perfusion for the long term. On the other hand, for unresectable tumours, permanent occluders like PVA are agents of choice, as complete tissue ablation is usually the goal. The desired level of vascular occlusion is the other critical factor in selecting an appropriate embolic agent. Very small particulate and liquid agents can reach the capillary level, resulting in significant ischaemia and infarction, especially in non-target tissues. They should be avoided unless permanent tissue or tumour ablation is the aim. Proximal vessel occlusion carries less risk of tissue necrosis because of the potential for development of collateral vessels with the distal circulation. In the treatment of arteriovenous fistulas and malformations, embolic agents may shunt through the site of the fistula or malformation with subsequent embolisation to the pulmonary circulation. The size of the embolisation particles should be adjusted to minimise this possibility. The choice of embolic agents will also be influenced by its availability at a particular institution, as well as the operator's experience and comfort level with the agent.

A thorough knowledge of the relevant vascular anatomy, its normal variation and anastomotic communications is essential to ensure success of embolisation and to prevent complications. Because of pre-existing collateral networks, and the potential for formation of collaterals secondary to an occlusion, one should always attempt to embolise on both sides of the bleeding site to prevent reconstitution of the bleeding via collateral supply (Fig. 1). A complete proximal coil embolisation of a feeding vessel should be avoided as this could

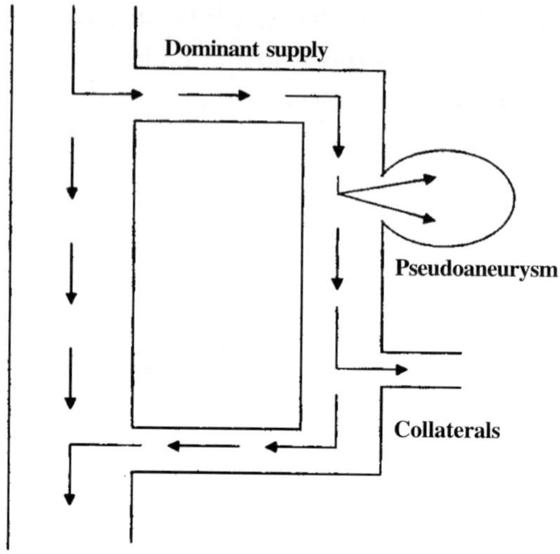

(A)

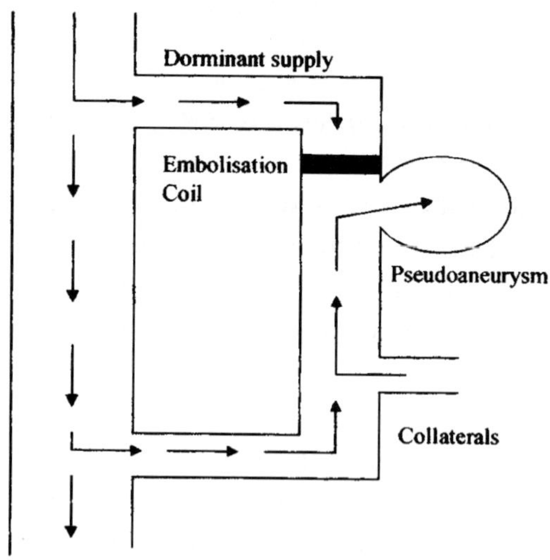

(B)

Fig. 1 Principles of pseudoaneurysm embolisation. **(A)** A pseudoaneurysm fills from its dominant supply. **(B)** Embolisation proximal to the pseudoaneurysm neck prevents filling from the dominant supply (closing the front door). However, flow in the collateral vessels reverses and reconstitute the pseudoaneurysm (filling via the back door). **(C)** Embolisation across the pseudoaneurysm neck prevents filling by both the dominant and collateral supplies (closing both the front and back doors).

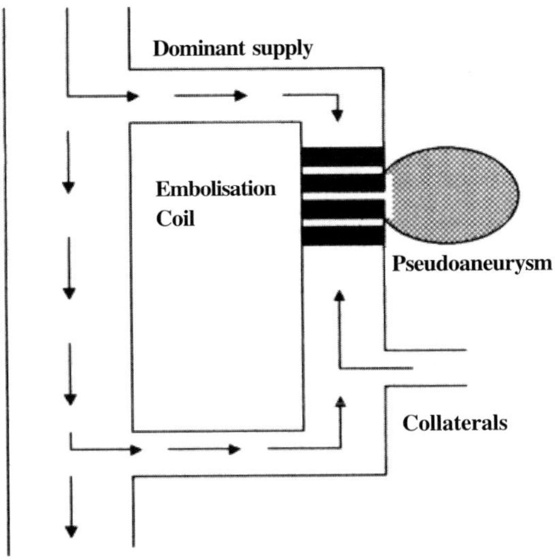

(c)

Fig. 1 (*Continued*)

hamper subsequent efforts to recannulate the vessel to access the bleeding site if haemorrhage recurs.

The most significant untoward complication of embolisation is non-target embolisation with unintentional occlusion of other vessels. This can be prevented with meticulous technique. Embolisation should always be preceded by high quality angiography to define precisely the vascular territory under consideration. Embolisation catheters should be sited as selectively as possible to prevent reflux of embolic agents into adjacent vascular territories. Co-axial microcatheters are often required to achieve the necessary degree of selectivity. Common to all angiographic procedures, contrast nephropathy and reactions, puncture site haematoma, thrombosis and pseudoaneurysms as well as catheter-induced complications like dissection, perforation or rupture of vessels, are other complications that may be encountered during embolisation.[6]

Post-embolisation syndrome comprises a constellation of symptoms including fever, pain, nausea, vomiting and leucocytosis. The symptoms arise shortly after embolisation and usually resolve within three days, but may persist up to a week. These symptoms are due to tissue ischaemia or infarction. The syndrome is more common with solid organ embolisation than embolisation at other sites, and it can be difficult to differentiate the syndrome from infection. Prophylactic antibiotics are often instituted to prevent super infection of ischaemic tissues, especially in embolisation of large solid organs like the liver.

Patient Preparation

Embolisation is a major procedure, and preparation of the patient should be no different than preparing the patient for surgery. Informed consent should be obtained after a frank discussion of the benefits and risks of the procedure, including the possibility of non-target embolisation. Details of any previous surgery should be obtained, as vascular anatomy may be altered; in particular, collateral vessels may be compromised, increasing the risk of ischaemic complications following embolisation. The clotting profile should be checked and corrected if possible prior to the procedure, otherwise fresh frozen plasma and/or platelet coverage during the procedure needs to be arranged. The patient should be well hydrated to minimise the risk of contrast nephropathy. If renal function is impaired, the interventional radiologist should be informed so that alternative contrast media like carbon dioxide or gadolinium (which are non-nephrotoxic) can be used during the procedure. Prophylactic antibiotics are generally recommended, especially for solid organ embolisation.

Clinical Scenarios

Haemoptysis and bronchial artery embolisation

Massive haemoptysis defined as 300–600 ml per 24-hour period carries a 50–85% mortality with conservative treatment. Severe haemoptysis most commonly presents in patients with chronic inflammatory lung disease, of which pulmonary tuberculosis is the most

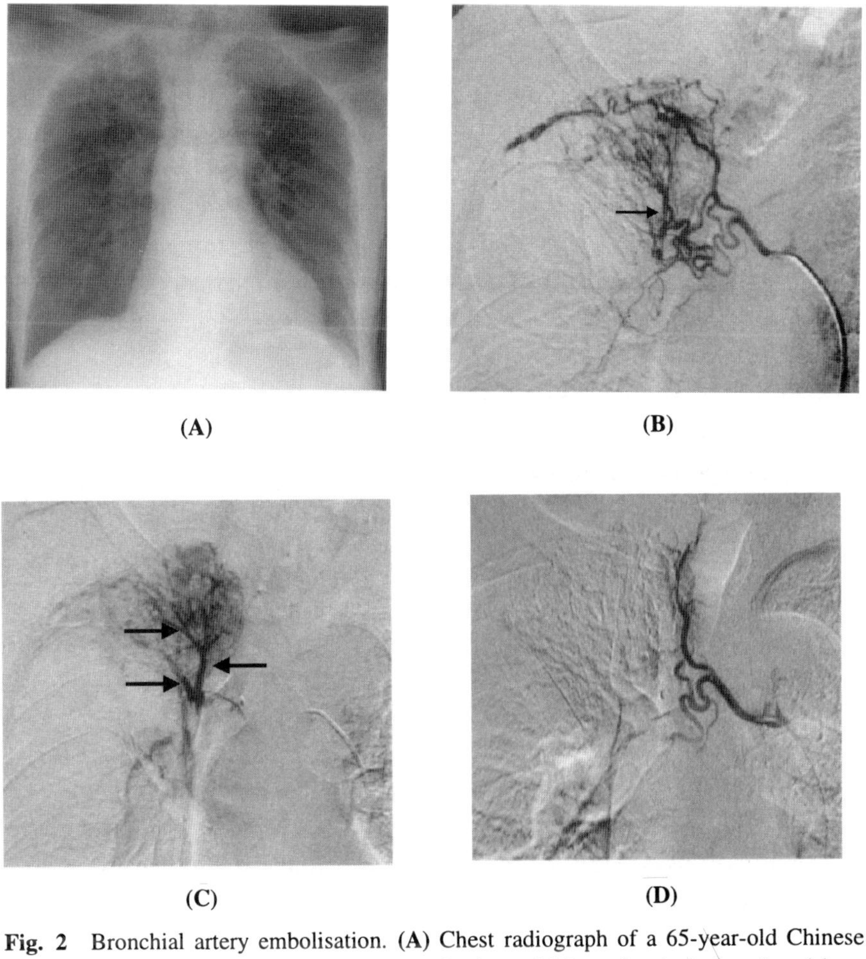

Fig. 2 Bronchial artery embolisation. **(A)** Chest radiograph of a 65-year-old Chinese man who presented with massive haemoptysis showed bilateral apical pleural and lung scarring in keeping with chronic pulmonary tuberculosis. The hyperinflated lungs suggest underlying chronic obstructive airway disease. The chest radiograph often provides valuable clues to the probable sites of bleeding. **(B)** and **(C)** Selective injection of the right intercostobronchial trunk (B: arterial phase image, and C capillary phase image) revealed hypertrophy and marked tortuosity of the bronchial vessels. The area of pleural scarring showed intense hypervascularity as well as shunting into the pulmonary veins (arrows). **(D)** Post-embolisation angiography revealed eradication of lung hypervascularity and shunting indicating successful embolisation. In this patient, embolisation was performed with PVA particles delivered via a co-axial microcatheter.

common aetiology worldwide. In most cases, severe haemoptysis results from a systemic arterial source rather than the pulmonary circulation, and tends to be episodic. Patients with chronic lung disease often have unacceptable surgical risks due to limited pulmonary reserve. Bronchial artery embolisation is now the treatment of choice for haemoptysis of inflammatory origin. The technique is well established and has been shown to effectively and rapidly control massive haemoptysis with minimal complications. Immediate success rates range from 86–91%. Long-term control of haemoptysis can be achieved in 70–80% of patients and is largely determined by the natural progression of the underlying disease.[7–12]

Bronchial arteries most commonly arise from the thoracic aorta at the T5 to T6 levels, and a single right intercostobronchial trunk with a single left bronchial artery is the most frequent angiographic variation described.[9] In cases of chronic inflammation, the bronchial arteries are hypertrophied and tortuous. Other signs include hypervascularity, systemic to pulmonary artery or venous shunting and bronchial artery aneurysms. Frank contrast extravasation into a bronchus during angiography is rare. With haemoptysis, hypervascularity or enlargement of the bronchial arteries is enough evidence to proceed with embolisation.

Prior to embolisation, a review of previous chest radiographs or CTs should be made, as probable sites of bleeding can often be identified. Bronchoscopy is also useful as it may localise the source of bleeding to a particular lobe or lung. This will help the interventional radiologist to concentrate on the affected region.

Currently, PVA is the agent of choice for bronchial artery embolisation, although the use of gelfoam has been described in a few large series. Distal embolisation should be performed whenever possible. Proximal coil embolisation of the bronchial arteries should be avoided as collateral vessels will develop to reconstitute supply to hypervascular areas. Further, future access to the main bronchial artery may be lost. Liquids such as absolute alcohol and fine particles should be avoided as they can occlude the capillary bed, leading to tissue infarction.

Patients who have undergone previous bronchial artery embolisation should not be excluded from repeat embolisation procedures. Recurrent haemorrhages may be due to recanalisation of embolised vessels, but more frequently, other systemic arterial sources such as the internal mammary, intercostal, lateral thoracic and inferior phrenic arteries contribute to the abnormal hypervascularity and bleeding. These vessels should be embolised if they are hypertrophied.

The most feared complication of bronchial artery embolisation is inadvertent embolisation of the spinal artery leading to spinal cord infarction and paraplegia. A spinal artery may arise from the intercostobronchial trunk or bronchial artery, and can certainly branch off from an intercostal artery. The spinal artery should be actively sought out before embolisation. Acquisition of high quality diagnostic angiography prior to embolisation is mandatory. The complication, is fortunately, uncommon and is less than 1% in reported series.[7–12]

Gastrointestinal bleeding

In 1963 Nausbaum and Baum, in a landmark paper, demonstrated that bleeding at rates as low as 0.5 ml/minute could be detected angiographically.[13] This report set the stage for transcatheter management of haemorrhage. This was first achieved with selective intra-arterial infusions of vasopressin[14] and in 1972, Rosch, Dotter and Brown reported controlling acute gastric haemorrhage by embolisation of the gastroepiploic artery with autologous blood clots.[15]

Endoscopy is a well established first line diagnostic and therapeutic modality for acute gastrointestinal (GI) haemorrhage. The role of angiography in GI bleeding is complementary to that of endoscopic techniques. When endoscopy fails to detect or precisely localise a source of bleeding, angiography can be utilised. This is true if the haemorrhage is from endoscopically inaccessible regions like the small bowel, liver and pancreas, or when massive bleeding impairs endoscopic visualisation. Angiography may also be performed in anticipation of transcatheter therapy of GI bleeding, particularly in patients with poor surgical risks, and in patients where there is continued haemorrhage after an exploratory laparotomy for unidentified source(s) of bleeding from the GI tract, or optimal endoscopic therapy. Selective intra-arterial injection of methylene blue to guide surgical resection is another application of angiography. Bleeding sites in the small bowel, or lesions of angiodysplasia and other small arterio-venous malformations can be difficult to identify at surgery. The pathologic bowel segment can be demonstrated by selectively catheterising the specific mesenteric branch involved prior to laparotomy. After the bowel is surgically exposed, methylene blue is injected into the catheter, resulting in a transient staining of the abnormal bowel. The technique precisely localises the pathologic segment of bowel and helps to limit the extent of bowel resection.

The typical angiographic appearance of GI bleeding is a localised puddle of extravasated contrast material within the bowel lumen. The extravasated contrast may even outline an ulcer crater or a colonic diverticulum. When contrast extravasation is not detected, indirect evidence of haemorrhage such as the presence of aneurysm, pseudoaneurysm, aorto-enteric fistula, arterio-venous malformation, angiodysplasia and tumour staining, should be sought.

In acute GI bleeding, angiography is most likely to be positive if blood loss exceeds four to six units within 24 hours (1.5 to 2 ml/minute) or if continued intravenous fluids and blood transfusions are required to keep the patient stable. Less rapid bleeding is difficult to detect, although it has been reported that bleeding rate as low as 0.5 ml/minute can be detected angiographically.[13] Carbon dioxide angiography has been shown to improve the diagnostic efficacy in GI haemorrhage.[16] Due to its buoyancy and lower viscosity (1/400 that of iodinated contrast), carbon dioxide has a greater propensity to extravasate through a small tear in an artery.

Another limitation of angiography relates to the intermittent nature of GI bleeding, which can result in a negative study if the bleeding had temporarily stopped at the time of contrast injection. Some angiographers have attempted to provoke bleeding in these cases using heparin, tolazoline, urokinase and tissue plasmingogen activator (tPA), but the technique is not widely accepted or practised.[17–19] Radionuclide scanning using tagged red blood cells (RBC) can address the problem of intermittent bleeding. The technique can detect bleeding at rates as low as 0.1 ml/minute and does not require bleeding to be occurring at the time of injection. If the scans are negative, the patient can be sent back to the ward and the scans repeated as and when clinically indicated. If bleeding occurs in the interim, the extravasated tagged RBC can be detected on the repeat scans.[20,21] Tagged RBC scan is very useful for selecting patients who are actively bleeding for angiography, and its use has reduced the incidence of negative angiography.

The main transcatheter options for emergency control of GI bleeding include catheter directed infusion of vasopressin and transcatheter embolisation.[22–26] Vasopressin infusion has been shown to be effective in controlling GI haemorrhage, but it has fallen out of favour due to several disadvantages associated with the technique. Vasopressin therapy requires a prolonged infusion, typically 24–48 hours, during which careful observation in an intensive care unit is required. Catheter-related complications such as infection and pericatheter thrombosis are more likely to occur because of the length of time the catheter is required to stay in place. A potent vasoconstricter, vasopressin can cause coronary ischaemia, particularly in patients with ischaemic heart disease. Other adverse consequences of vasopressin infusion include volume overload and hyponatraemia (from the antidiuretic effect of the drug), arrhythmias and hypertension. There is also a high rate (up to 50% of cases) of recurrent bleeding following vasopressin infusion.

Transcatheter embolisation does not incur the systemic risks associated with vasopressin infusion, and the effect of embolisation is prolonged since the embolic agent remains in place after the procedure is terminated. However, embolisation is technically more difficult as it demands safe, super-selective catheter positioning and deposition of embolic agents. The advent of steerable, atraumatic guidewires and microcatheters has made this possible.

Upper gastrointestinal bleeding

Upper GI bleeding is defined as bleeding proximal to the ligament of Treitz. Transcatheter embolisation is the treatment of choice for haemorrhage in the gastroduodenal region where collateral supply is generally rich enough to prevent ischaemic complications. Bleeding ulcers unresponsive to endoscopic therapy are the most common aetiology for angiographic intervention of upper GI bleeding. Embolisation of the left gastric and gastroduodenal arteries (GDA) is often required, and gelfoam is the embolic agent of choice in this setting.[27] In patients with massive upper GI bleeding from documented (endoscopy or barium studies) lesions in the left gastric territory and normal angiographic findings, prophylactic embolisation of the left gastric artery has been shown to decrease the risk of rebleeding.[28]

In patients with a history of prior gastric or duodenal surgery, potential collateral vessels could have been ligated. Embolisation in this setting can result in ischaemic complications. In such patients, careful diagnostic angiography to evaluate collateral supply and highly selective embolisation is necessary if ischaemic complications are to be avoided.

Lower gastrointestinal bleeding

Beyond the ligament of Treitz, the potential for collateral perfusion is not as great, and the bowel is more susceptible to ischaemia and infarction. Early experience with colonic embolisation resulted in significant bowel infarction rates of up to 20%.[29–32] As such, lower GI bleeds have been traditionally treated with vasopressin infusion. However, in the last decade, improvements in equipment allowing easier and safer super-selective catheterisation and embolisation of the GI vasculature, have prompted a renewed interest in lower GI tract embolisation. At this point, over 80 colonic embolisations have been reported since 1990.[33–37] Technical success rates have ranged from 62–100%, immediate haemostasis was achieved in 54–100%, and most of which has translated to long-term definitive control of

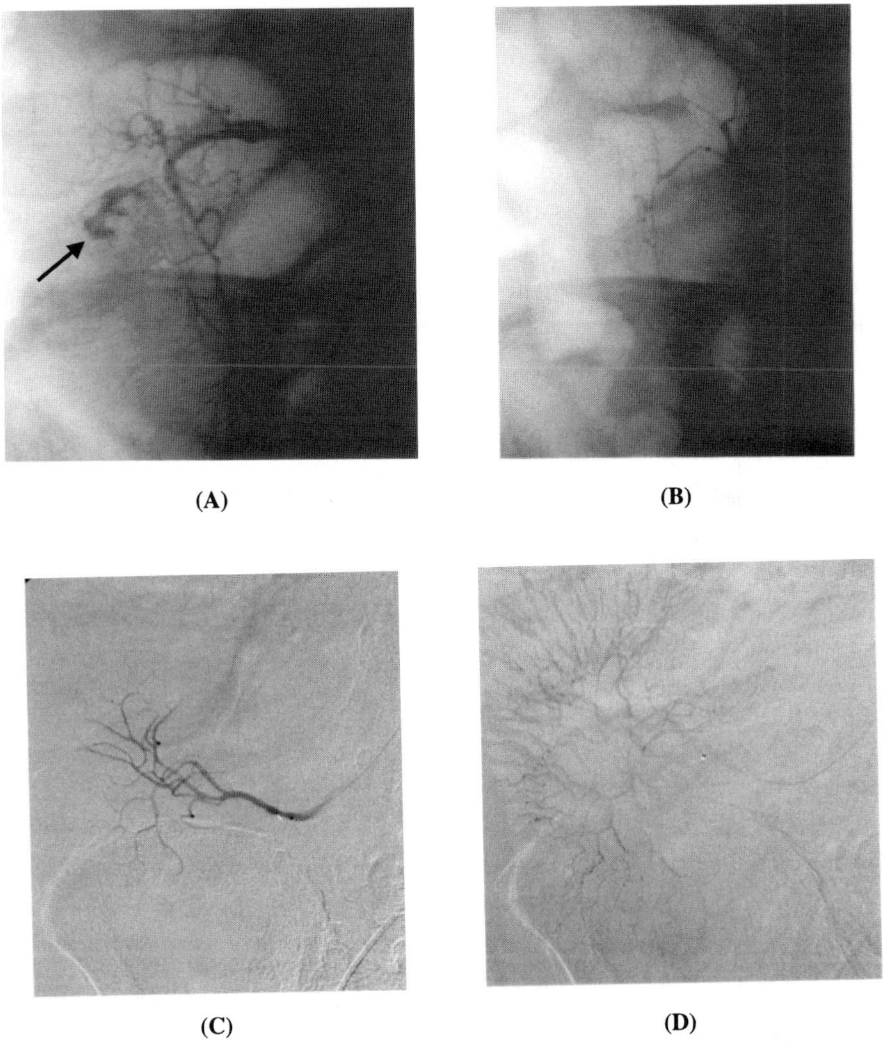

Fig. 3 Catheter directed vasopressin infusion for lower gastrointestinal haemorrhage. **(A)** Selective injection of the ileo-colic artery revealed contrast extravasation into the bowel lumen (arrow) indicating active bleeding. **(B)** Repeat angiography after 20 minutes of vasopressin infusion showed that the bleeding was successfully arrested. Embolisation was not performed in this patient, as it was not possible to manipulate the microcatheter into the bleeding branch vessel. Embolisation in a proximal location may lead to significant bowel ischaemia and infarction. **(C)** and **(D)** check angiography the next day showed no evidence of bleeding. Catheter directed vasopressin infusion therapy typically span over 24 to 48 hours.

haemorrhage. Significantly, there has not been any case of colonic infarction in these reports. Although ischaemic sequelae have occurred which included symptoms of abdominal pain and fever, as well as mucosal changes and ischaemic strictures on endoscopy, the majority of these have been self-limited or asymptomatic.

For lower GI embolisation, it is important to deposit the embolic material as close to the bleeding site as possible without compromising adjacent branches. This usually entails embolisation at the vasa recta or distal vascular arcade level via flexible microcatheters. If such a position cannot be reached, vasopressin infusion or surgical therapy should be considered. Although these cause permanent occlusion, the metallic microcoil is the favoured embolic agent as it is easily visible on fluoroscopy, and can be placed with extreme precision into very distal locations.

Acute variceal haemorrhage

Variceal haemorrhage remains the most feared and lethal complication of portal hypertension. Endoscopic sclerotherapy or variceal band ligation are usually the first line treatment for bleeding oesophageal varices. Percutaneous transhepatic embolisation of varices was popular in the 1970s but is no longer performed due to the high complication and rebleeding rate.[38,39] An innovative treatment of patients with complications of portal hypertension has been the non-surgical creation of decompressive shunts. Transjugular intrahepatic porto-systemic shunt (TIPS) creation was first described in 1969 by Rosch and colleagues in animals.[40] Colapinto and colleagues reported the first human application in 1982 but the shunt tract did not remain consistently patent.[41] In 1990, Richter and colleagues reported the first creation of TIPS with stents in humans.[42] The vascular stents prevent the collapse of the shunt tract which greatly improve the efficacy of the shunt. In this technique, a curved needle is introduced via a long sheath through the right internal jugular vein into the right hepatic vein. Under fluoroscopic guidance, the needle is advanced through the liver parenchyma into the right portal vein to create the shunt. A stent is then deployed along the shunt tract to keep it patent. Embolisation of varices can also be performed from the jugular approach via the TIPS shunt. Transjugular intrahepatic porto-systemic shunt is now indicated for acute or recurrent variceal bleeding that cannot be controlled by medical or endoscopic therapy, as well as for refractory cirrhotic ascites and hydrothorax. Technical success rates for TIPS range from 93–100%. Acute bleeding is controlled in 96–100% and ascites improves in approximately 85% of patients. Thirty-day mortality after TIPS is in the range of 5–20% but most who died had pre-morbid conditions (with poor Child-Pugh's or Apache II scores). The main limitation of the technique is the poor primary patency (25–65% at six months) of the shunt due to tissue growth within the stent, or outflow veins leading to shunt stenosis and recurrence of variceal bleeding or ascites. Although shunt stenosis is easily treatable with repeat angioplasty or stent insertion such that secondary shunt patency approaches 100%, re-stenosis requiring multiple repeat interventions frequently occurs.[43–50] The use of covered stents has been shown to improve primary shunt patency.[51,52] Clinical trials are currently underway in both Europe and the U.S.

Trauma

Angiography was the primary tool in the diagnosis of trauma prior to the 1980s. Advances in cross-sectional imaging, in particular duplex ultrasound and spiral CT, have enabled non-invasive, rapid and accurate diagnosis in trauma patients. Increasingly, angiography is performed in anticipation of transcatheter therapy to control haemorrhage and occlude or repair vessels rather than for purely diagnostic purposes.

The classical angiographic appearance of haemorrhage is contrast media extravasation from a vessel. Other angiographic findings in vascular trauma include pseudoaneurysm, complete disruption of the vessel, spasm, thrombosis, intimal flaps, vessel displacement and

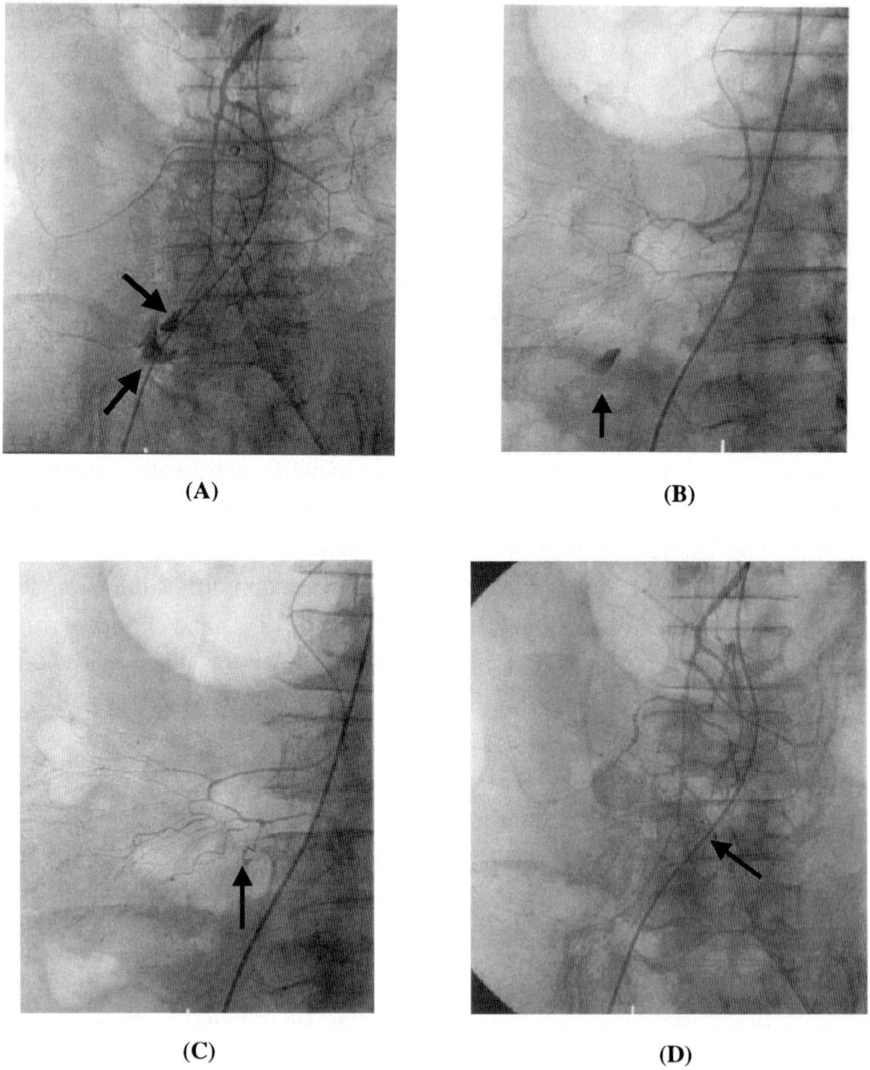

Fig. 4 Coil embolisation in lower gastrointestinal haemorrhage. (**A**) Superior mesenteric angiography of a 75-year-old Malay lady who was hypotensive from bleeding per rectum revealed contrast extravasation (arrow) over the right lower quadrant of the abdomen indicating active bleeding. (**B**) Super-selective injection of the jejunal artery confirmed active haemorrhage (arrow). (**C**) Post-embolisation angiography showed cessation of haemorrhage. Embolisation was performed with a platinum microcoil (arrow). (**D**) Completion superior mesenteric angiography confirmed successful haemorrhage control.

compression by extrinsic haematoma as well as arterio-venous fistula. As in GI haemorrhage, carbon dioxide angiography has been shown to be more sensitive than iodinated contrast for detection of traumatic haemorrhage due to the buoyancy and low viscosity of carbon dioxide.[53]

Embolisation is the main transcatheter therapeutic option in traumatic haemorrhage. Active haemorrhage, pseudoaneurysms and AV fistulas are all amenable to treatment by embolisation. The principal considerations in selecting an embolic agent in the trauma setting are speed and reliability of delivery, permanency of occlusion and preservation of normal tissues. Coils and gelfoam are the two most frequently used agents. Coils provide controlled delivery with rapid occlusion, and are available in a wide range of sizes. They are therefore ideal for single vessel injuries, larger vessels, and where the site of occlusion must be precise. Where injuries are multiple, distal in location, or where numerous collateral pathways are present, the use of particulate agents is indicated. Gelfoam is the ideal agent in this setting as it provides temporary occlusion, and the gelfoam pledgets can be tailored to sizes appropriate to the clinical situation at hand. If the bleeding vessel is vital and cannot be sacrificed, placement of an occlusion balloon across the injury site for a short period of time may sometimes arrest haemorrhage. If bleeding recurs after deflation of the balloon, the balloon should be re-inflated to tamponade bleeding while the patient is being transferred to the operating room for definitive surgical repair.

Abdominal trauma

With a growing trend towards more conservative management to achieve greater organ preservation, an increasing number of patients with hepatic, splenic and renal trauma are managed expectantly.[54–59] Superselective transcatheter embolisation that can effectively control haemorrhage and at the same time minimise damage to normal tissues, is increasingly being applied to this enlarging group of patients. The liver is well suited for transcatheter embolisation because of its dual blood supply (30% hepatic artery, 70% portal vein). Arterial embolisation is unlikely to result in tissue infarction unless there is concomitant injury to the portal system. Splenic artery embolisation is also relatively safe as collateralisation via pancreatic and short gastric branches allows splenic preservation. The kidney, on the other hand, is an end-artery organ. Occlusion of renal branch vessels will cause parenchymal infarction congruent to the size of the vessel embolised. Super-selective embolisation is therefore highly desirable. Arterial injuries that can be treated percutaneously include extravasation, pseudoaneurysm, arteriovenous fistula and arterio-biliary fistula. Gelfoam, PVA and microcoils are commonly used. Successful control of haemorrhage in the order of 84–100% has been reported for transcatheter embolisation of hepatic, splenic and renal arterial injuries.[60–69]

Pelvic trauma

Uncontrolled pelvic haemorrhage arising from blunt or penetrating pelvic trauma is associated with high mortality despite aggressive transfusion. The confined pelvic space and presence of extensive haematoma makes surgical localisation of bleeding sites extremely difficult. Proximal ligation of the internal iliac arteries is frequently unsuccessful because of rich collateral supply within the pelvis. In addition, surgical incision into the retroperitoneum will release any tamponading effect of the haematoma, further worsening bleeding. Even without incision into the retroperitoneum, haemorrhage may not be adequately tamponaded as the injured bony and ligamentous structures no longer prevent expansion of the pelvis. Application of a pelvic fixator to stabilise pelvic fractures helps to address this issue, but this may not be sufficient to arrest haemorrhage.

Angiographic techniques, on the other hand, are well suited for management of traumatic pelvic haemorrhage. Angiography reliably and rapidly identifies sites of haemorrhage. Transcatheter therapy does

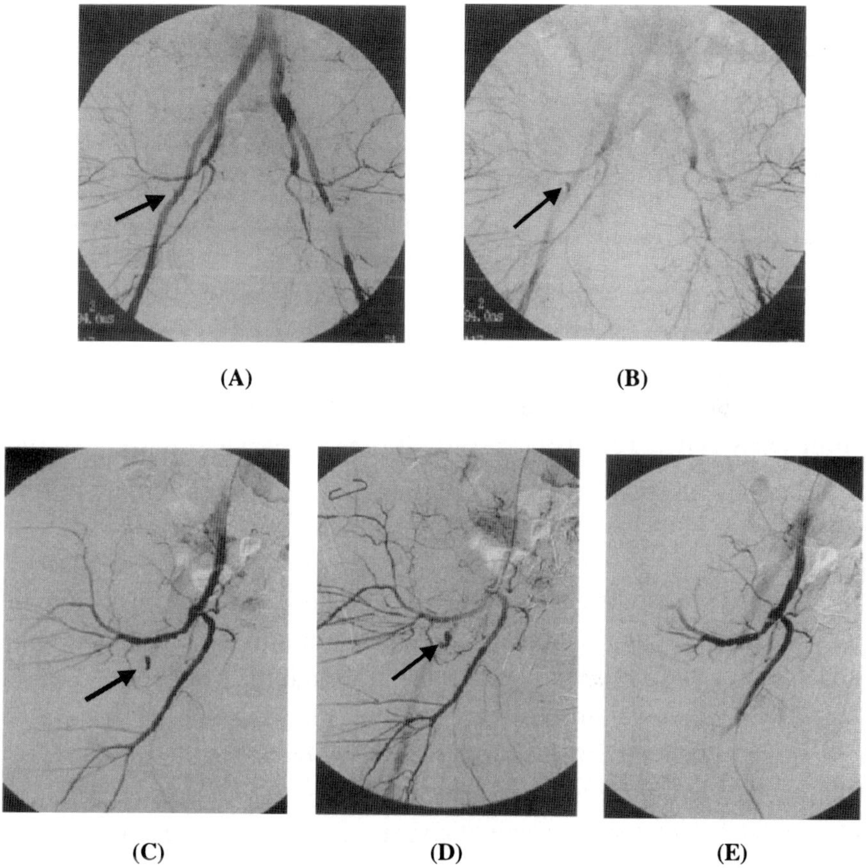

Fig. 5 Pelvic embolisation in acute haemorrhage secondary to pelvic fracture. **(A)** and **(B)** Flush pelvic angiography revealed contrast extravasation in the region of the right hemipelvis (arrows). The extravasated contrast was better seen on the late arterial phase image (Fig. 4(B)). **(C)** and **(D)** Selective right internal iliac angiography confirmed active bleeding where contrast extravasation was clearly demonstrated (arrows). **(E)** Post-embolisation angiography showed that the bleeding was successfully arrested. In this patient, embolisation of the entire right internal iliac territory was performed with gel foam slurries. Selective cannulation and embolisation of the bleeding branch vessel, a tedious and time consuming process, was not attempted as the patient was haemodynamically unstable and may not tolerate a prolonged procedure.

not disrupt the peritoneal covering and its tamponade effect. It can precede or follow application of a pelvic fixator or surgical abdominal exploration, and may be performed in stable or unstable patients. Transcatheter control of arterial haemorrhage related to pelvic trauma can be expected in approximately 90% of cases.[70–74]

With pelvic trauma, the goal is to temporarily reduce the pressure head so that endogenous haemostatic mechanisms can stop the bleeding. As such, gelfoam is the embolic agent of choice. Because of the extensive collateral network within the pelvis, proximal vessel occlusion with coils, like proximal surgical ligation of the internal iliac arteries, is usually ineffective and is to be avoided. Distal embolisation with gelfoam slurry is preferred, and it is often necessary to embolise the internal iliac arteries on both sides to prevent bleeding from cross-pelvic collateral vessels. If a focal bleeding point could be selectively cannulated, coil embolisation may be performed. However, prolonged attempts at superselective catheterisation of bleeding sites are not advisable as these patients are often unstable, and embolisation should be performed expeditiously. There should be no hesitation in embolising the entire internal iliac artery to shorten procedure time and contrast load, especially when there are multiple punctate bleeding sites from various branches of the internal iliac artery.

The principles of management for post-partum haemorrhage secondary to childbirth injuries are similar to pelvic trauma, and are best treated with gelfoam embolisation. If a single bleeding vessel is identified and is accessible, coil embolisation can be performed.[75,76] Occasionally, patients may have conditions (for example, placenta accreta) that predispose them to significant risk of bleeding during childbirth or obstetric intervention. These patients may benefit from placement of occlusion balloon catheters into both internal iliac arteries prior to delivery, to allow proximal vascular control.

The Future

While bleeding vessels that are expendable are eminently treatable with transcatheter embolisation, vital vessels that cannot be sacrificed

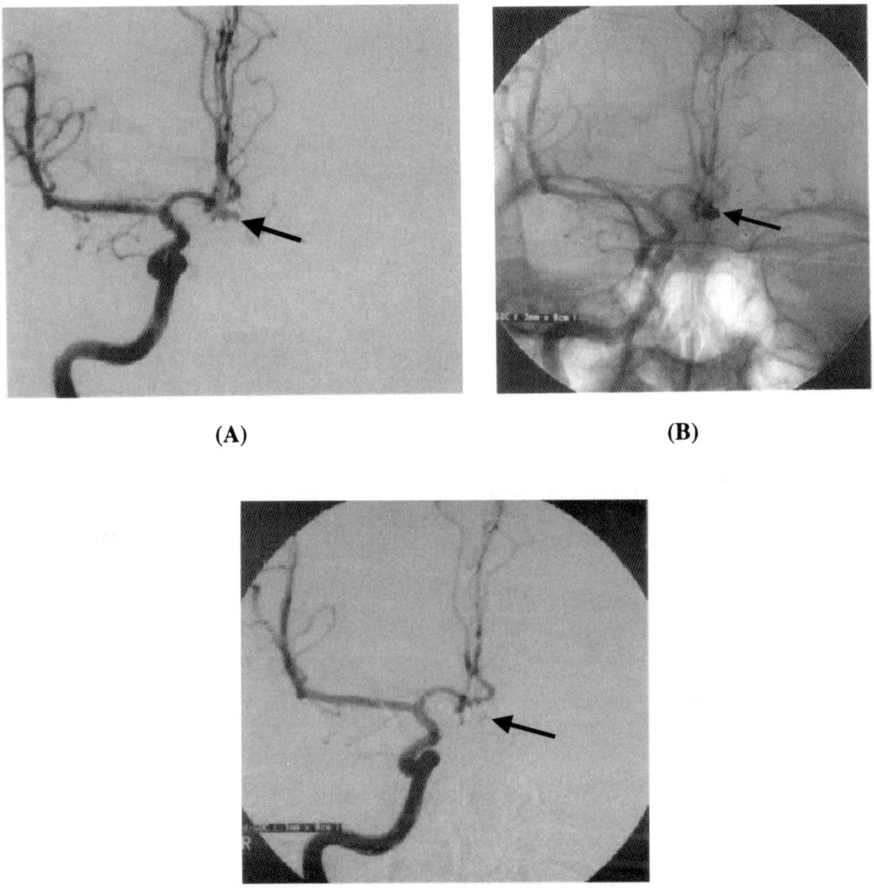

(A) (B) (C)

Fig. 6 Embolisation of anterior communicating artery aneurysm with Guglielmi Detachable Coils (GDC). **(A)** Right internal carotid angiogram of a 45-year-old Japanese tourist who presented with acute subarachnoid haemorrhage showed an anterior communicating artery aneurysm (arrow). **(B)** and **(C)** Post-GDC (arrows) embolisation right internal carotid angiography (B: unsubtracted image, and C: subtracted image) showed successful aneurysm occlusion without compromising parent artery patency.

without dire effects are traditionally treated with surgical repair or reconstruction with surgical grafts. Two recent developments in transcatheter therapies have allowed repair of such vessels without vessel occlusion. Guglielmi detachable coils (GDCs), developed primarily for embolisation of cerebral aneurysms, have been used to pack pseudoaneurysms to induce pseudoaneurysm thrombosis and occlusion, and yet preserving the patency of the parent vessel. These coils are very soft and are attached to the pushing wire. They are detached from the wire electrically once the desired coil position or configuration is achieved. If there is mal-positioning, the coil can be retrieved and repositioned or removed from the body.

Of even greater significance has been the introduction of stent grafts and covered stents in the 1990s. These are vascular stents that are covered by Dacron or polytetrafluoroethylene (PTFE). These exclude the underlying lesion from the circulation without causing vessel occlusion, which in effect, is akin to insertion of surgical interposition grafts. Successful treatment of traumatic thoracic aortic injuries with stent grafts has been described.[77] As covered stents require relatively large delivery catheters, their use is presently restricted to fairly large vessels like the iliac, femoral, subclavian, proximal renal and carotid arteries.[78,79] Covered coronary stents are now available, and may be adapted for use in the smaller peripheral vasculature.[80] While the minimally invasive nature of these devices makes them attractive, their long-term durability remains unknown.

Interventional Neuroradiology for Acute Haemorrhage in the Head and Neck Region

Acute intracranial haemorrhage

Cerebral aneurysms

Rupture of an intracranial aneurysm is the most common cause for spontaneous subarachnoid haemorrhage (SAH), with an incidence of 11 per 100,000 population in the West. Locally the reported incidence appears to be lower (one per 100,000). However, this figure probably reflects under-reporting and under-diagnosis of the condition in an earlier era. The true incidence is probably higher, as would be expected, with an ageing population and better diagnostic techniques. The consequences of aneurysmal SAH are severe, with mortality rates of 20–40% and a rebleeding rate of up to 29%.

While computed tomography is the best initial modality to detect the presence of SAH, catheter-based cerebral angiography remains the gold standard for the diagnosis of cerebral aneurysms. With newer three-dimensional angiography techniques, detailed assessment of the angio-architecture of the lesion is now possible prior to endovascular therapy or neurosurgical intervention.[81]

One of the more exciting developments over the last decade has been the use of soft, controlled detachable coils in the treatment of intracranial aneurysms (Guglielmi Detachable Coils — GDC Target Therapeutics, Boston Scientific).[82] The ability to precisely deposit the coil within the aneurysm and reposition it, if necessary, prior to detachment, has revolutionised the endovascular management of cranial aneurysms. Morbidity rates of about 6–8% and mortality rates of about 2–3% are quoted for this mode of therapy, figures that are comparable to those of surgical clipping.

Occasionally SAH may be secondary to trauma, or from rupture of a mycotic aneurysm with a resultant pseudoaneurysm formation. These aneurysms are best treated with occlusion of the parent vessels, with a variety of occlusion devices including tissue glue (cyanoacrylate), detachable balloons and embolisation coils.

Arteriovenous malformations

Arteriovenous malformation associated intracerebral haemorrhage is usually intraparenchymal or intraventricular in location. Urgent CT may be followed by an angiogram to confirm the diagnosis and to delineate the lesion, the feeding and draining vessels, should urgent evacuation of the haematoma be required. Definitive treatment is usually delayed until the patient and the brain recover from the effects of the haematoma. Embolisation alone can achieve total cure in only

10% of arteriovenous malformations. These are usually small lesions with finite and favourable feeding vessels. More commonly, embolisation is used to decrease the size of the arteriovenous malformation prior to surgery or radiosurgery.[83,84]

Dural arteriovenous fistulas

These lesions are either single-hole (traumatic) or multiple-hole (spontaneous) connections between arteries and veins or dural sinuses of the cranium. Single-hole lesions are due to tears in the carotid vessels, or may be related to rupture of skull base aneurysms. Single-hole lesions can be treated either with detachable balloons or coils placed within the proximal venous component of the lesion to seal up the rent in the arterial wall. If this defect is too large, the parent vessel may have to be occluded. Multiple-hole fistulae usually do not present acutely, and are often difficult to diagnose. However, in a subgroup where there is involvement of the cortical cerebral veins, there is an associated mortality of 10–20% when there is a rupture of the draining vein. Multiple-hole lesions can be approached from the arterial side with either tissue glue (cyanoacrylate) or PVA particle embolisation, and retrogradely from the venous side with embolisation coils.[84,85]

Head and neck haemorrhage

Carotid blow-out pseudoaneurysms

Injury of the carotid vessels can result from either blunt trauma or penetrating injury (such as gun-shot or stab wounds). Blunt trauma injuries are rare (under 1%) and are not usually associated with acute haemorrhage. However, the estimated mortality rates from such injuries can be as high as 20–40%.

Direct injury of the vessel wall initially results in vessel dissection. About 30% of these develop pseudoaneurysms which have a natural history of progression to either haemorrhage or becoming an embolic source to the cranial vasculature. Traditionally, pseudoaneurysms have been treated with either trapping or proximal parent vessel occlusion.[86] More recently Dacron® covered stents have been utilised to seal off these areas of weakness.

Epistaxis

Epistaxis is a common problem, with up to 60% of the population experiencing this symptom. Fortunately only a tenth of these require medical consultation. The aetiology of epistaxis is varied and includes tumour (angioneurofibromas, nasopharyngeal carcinoma), congenital (hereditary haemorrhagic telangiectasia) and last but not least idiopathic. Initial treatment in epistaxis is nasal packing or cautery. If this fails, the bleeding point may then be occluded with a variety of embolic agents alluded to above.[87]

Conclusion

The management of acute haemorrhage remains challenging. Transcatheter techniques have proven to be safe and highly effective in arresting haemorrhage throughout the body. These are more tissue sparing than surgery, and increasingly can be the definitive treatment in appropriate lesions. Interventional radiology has gone beyond a solely diagnostic role and has become a valuable adjunct in the management of patients with acute haemorrhage. The role of interventional radiology will continue to grow as better techniques for minimally invasive and non-operative management develop.

References

1. Dawbarn G (1904). The starvation operation for malignancy in the external carotid area. *J Am Med Assoc* **43**, 792–795.
2. Seppanen SK, Leppanen MJ, Pimenoff G, Seppanen JM (1997). Microcatheter embolisation of hemorrhages. *Cardiovasc Intervent Radiol* **20**, 174–179.

3. Teitelbaum GP, Reed RA, Larsen D, Lee RK, Pentecost MJ, Finck EJ, Katz MD (1993). Microcatheter embolisation of non-neurologic traumatic vascular lesions. *JVIR* **4**, 149–154.
4. Coldwell DM, Stokes KR, Yakes WF (1994). Embolotherapy: agents, clinical applications and techniques. *Radiographics* **14**, 623–643.
5. Pentecost MJ, Teitelbaum GP (eds.) (1992). Embolotherapy. *Semin Intervent Radiol* **9**, 1–71.
6. Hemingway AP, Allison DJ (1988). Complications of embolisation: analysis of 410 procedures. *Radiology* **166**, 669–672.
7. Remy J, Arnaud A, Fardou H, Giraud R, Voisin C (1977). Treatment of hemoptysis by embolisation of bronchial arteries. *Radiology* **122**, 33–37.
8. Hayakawa K, Tanaka F, Torizuka T, Mitsumori M, Okuno Y, Matsui A, Satoh Y, Fujiwara K, Misaki T (1992). Bronchial artery embolisation for hemoptysis: immediate and long term results. *Cardiovasc Intervent Radiol* **15**, 154–158.
9. Uflacker R, Kaemmerer A, Picon PD, Rizzon CF, Neves CM, Oliveira ES, Oliveira ME, Azevedo SN, Ossanai R (1985). Bronchial artery embolisation in the management of hemoptysis: technical aspects and long term results. *Radiology* **157**, 637–644.
10. Rabkin JE, Astafjev V, Gothman LN, Gringorjev YG (1987). Transcatheter embolisation in the management of pulmonary hemorrhage. *Radiology* **163**, 361–365.
11. Mal H, Rullon I, Mellot F, Brugiere O, Sleiman C, Menu Y, Fournier M (1999). Immediate and long term results of bronchial artery embolisation for life threatening hemoptysis. *Chest* **115**, 996–1001.
12. Goh PYT, Lin M, Teo N, Wong DES (2002). Embolisation for hemoptysis: a six year review. *Cardiovasc Intervent Radiol* **25**, 17–25.
13. Nusbaum M, Baum S (1963). Radiographic demonstration of unknown sites of gastrointestinal bleeding. *Surg Forum* **13**, 374.

14. Baum S, Nusbaum M (1971). The control of gastrointestinal hemorrhage by selective mesenteric arterial infusion of vasopressin. *Radiology* **98**, 497.
15. Rosch J, Dotter CT, Brown MJ (1972). Selective arterial embolisation. A new method for control of acute gastrointestinal bleeding. *Radiology* **102**, 303–306.
16. Hawkins IF, Caridi JG (1998). Carbon dioxide (CO2) digital subtraction angiography: 26-year experience at the University of Florida. *Eur Radiol* **8**, 391–402.
17. Bloomfeld RS, Smith TP, Schneider AM, Rockey DC (2000). Provocative angiography in patients with gastrointestinal hemorrhage of obscure origins. *Am J Gastroenterol* **95**, 2807–2812.
18. Malden ES, Hicks ME, Royal HD, Aliperti G, Allen BT, Picus D (1998). Recurrent gastrointestinal bleeding: use of thrombolysis with anticoagulation in diagnosis. *Radiology* **207**, 147–151.
19. Ryan JM, Key SM, Dumbleton SA, Smith TP (2001). Non localised lower gastrointestinal bleeding: provocative bleeding studies with intra arterial tPA, heparin and tolazoline. *JVIR* **12**, 1273–1277.
20. Bentley DE, Richardson JD (1991). The role of tagged red blood cell imaging in the localisation of gastrointestinal bleeding. *Arch Surg* **126**, 821–824.
21. Orecchia PM, Hensley EK, McDonald PT, Lull RJ (1985). Localisation of gastrointestinal hemorrhage: experience with red blood cells labelled *in vitro* with technetium Tc-99m. *Arch Surg* **120**, 621–624.
22. Conn HO, Ramsby GR, Storer EH, Mutchnick MG, Joshi PH, Phillips MM, Cohen GA, Fields GN, Petroski D (1975). Intra arterial vasopressin in the treatment of upper gastrointestinal hemorrhage: a prospective, controlled clinical trial. *Gastroenterology* **68**, 211–221.
23. Athanasoulis CA, Baum S, Rosch J, Waltman AC, Ring EJ, Smith JC Jr, Sugarbaker E, Wood W (1975). Mesenteric arterial infusions of vasopressin for hemorrhage from colonic diverticulosis. *Am J Surg* **129**, 212–216.

24. Encarnacion CE, Kadir S, Beam CA, Payne CS (1992). Gastrointestinal bleeding: treatment with embolisation. *Radiology* **183**, 505–508.
25. Keller FS, Rosch J (1988). Embolisation for acute gastric haemorrhage. *Semin Intervent Radiol* **5**, 25–31.
26. Rossen RJ, Sanchez G (1994). Angiographic diagnosis and management of gastrointestinal hemorrhage: current concepts. *Radiol Clin North Am* **32**, 951–967.
27. Lang EK (1992). Transcatheter embolisation in the management of hemorrhage from duodenal ulcer: long term results and complications. *Radiology* **182**, 703–707.
28. Lang EV, Picus D, Marx MV, Hicks ME, Friedland GW (1992). Massive upper gastrointestinal hemorrhage with normal findings on arteriography: value of prophylactic embolisation of the left gastric artery. *AJR* **158**, 547–549.
29. Shenoy SS, Satchidanand S Wesp EH (1981). Colonic ischemic necrosis following therapeutic embolisation. *Gastrointest Radiol* **6**, 235–237.
30. Walker WJ, Goldin AR, Shaff MI, Allibone GW (1980). Per catheter control of hemorrhage from the superior and inferior mesenteric arteries. *Clin Radiol* **31**, 71–80.
31. Rosenkrantz H, Bookstein JJ, Rosen RJ, Goff WB, Healy JF (1982). Post embolic colonic infarction. *Radiology* **142**, 47–51.
32. Uflacker R (1987). Transcatheter embolisation for treatment of acute lower gastrointestinal bleeding. *Acta Radiol* **28**, 425–430.
33. Guy GE, Shetty PC, Sharma RP, Burke MW, Burke TH (1992). Acute lower gastrointestinal hemorrhage: treatment by superselective embolisation with polyvinyl alcohol particles. *AJR* **159**, 521–526.
34. Peck DJ, Mcloughlin RF, Hughson MN, Rankin RN (1998). Percutaneous embolotherapy of lower gastrointestinal hemorrhage. *JVIR* **9**, 747–751.
35. Evangelista PT, Hallisey MJ (2000). Transcather embolisation for acute lower gastrointestinal hemorrhage. *JVIR* **11**, 601–606.

36. Gordon RL, Ahl KL, Kerlan RK, Wilson MW, LaBerge JM, Sandhu JS, Ring EJ, Welton ML (1997). Selective arterial embolisation for control of lower gastrointestinal bleeding. *Am J Surg* **174**, 24–28.
37. Bandi R, Shetty PC, Sharma RP, Burke TH, Burke MW, Kastan D (2001). Superselective arterial embolisation for the treatment of lower gastrointestinal hemorrhage. *JVIR* **12**, 1399–1405.
38. Benner KG, Keefe EB, Keller FS, Rosch J (1983). Clinical outcome after percutaneous transhepatic obliteration of esophageal varices. *Gastroenterology* **85**, 146–153.
39. L'Hermine C, Chastanet P, Delemazure O, Bonniere PL, Durieu JP, Paris JC (1989). Percutaneous transhepatic embolisation of gastroesophageal varices: results in 400 patients. *AJR* **152**, 755–760.
40. Rosch J, Hanafee WN, Snow H (1969). Transjugular portal venography and radiologic portacaval shunt: an experimental study. *Radiology* **92**, 1112–1114.
41. Colapinto RF, Stronell RD, Gildiner M, Ritchie AC, Langer B, Taylor BR, Blendis LM (1983). Formation of intrahepatic portosystemic shunts using balloon dilatation catheter: preliminary clinical experience. *AJR* **140**, 709–714.
42. Richter GM, Noeldge G, Palmaz JC, Roessle M, Slegerstetter V, Franke M, Gerok W, Wenz W, Farthman E (1990). Transjugular intra hepatic portosystemic stent shunt: preliminary clinical results. *Radiology* **174**, 1027–1030.
43. LaBerge JM, Ring EJ, Gordon RL, Lake JR, Doherty MM, Somberg KA, Roberts JP, Ascher NL (1993). Creation of transjugular intrahepatic portosystemic shunt (TIPS) with the Wallstent endoprosthesis: results in 100 patients. *Radiology* **187**, 413–420.
44. Rossle M, Haag K, Ochs A, Sellinger M, Noldge G, Peramau JM, Berger E, Blum U, Gabelmann A, Hauenstein K, *et al.* (1994). Using transjugular intrahepatic portosystemic stent shunt procedure for variceal bleeding. *N Engl J Med* **330**, 165–171.
45. Haskal ZJ, Cope C, Shlansky-Goldberg RD, Baum RA, Pentecost MJ, Soulen MC (1994). Transjugular intrahepatic portosystemic

shunts: early and midterm efficacy into 100 patients. *Radiology* **193**, 130–137.

46. Hausegger KA, Sternthal HM, Klein GE, Karaic R, Stauber R, Zenker G (1994). Transjugular intrahepatic portosystemic shunt: angiographic follow-up and secondary interventions. *Radiology* **191**, 177–181.
47. Haskal ZJ, Pentecost MJ, Soulen MC, Shlansky-Goldberg RD, Baum RA, Cope C (1994). Transjugular intrahepatic portosystemic shunt stenosis and revision: early and midterm results. *AJR* **163**, 439–444.
48. Jalan R, Elton R, Redhead DN (1995). Analysis of prognostic variables in the prediction of mortality, shunt failure, variceal rebleeding and encephalopathy following transjugular intrahepatic portosystemic stent shunt for variceal hemorrhage. *J Hepatol* **23**, 123–128.
49. Martin M, Zajko AB, Orons PD, Dodd G, Wright H, Colangelo J, Tartar R (1993). Transjugular intrahepatic portosystemic shunt in the management of variceal bleeding: indications and clinical results. *Surgery* **114**, 719–727.
50. Stanley AJ, Jalan R, Forrest EH, Redhead DN, Hayes PC (1996). Long term follow-up of transjugular intrahepatic portosystemic shunt for the treatment of portal hypertension: results in 130 patients. *Gut* **39**, 479–485.
51. Andrews RT, Saxon RR, Bloch RD, Petersen BD, Uchida BT, Rabkin JM, Loriaux MM, Keller FS, Rosch J (1999). Stent grafts for de novo TIPS: technique and early results. *JVIR* **10**, 1371–1378.
52. Otal P, Smayra T, Bureau C, Peron JM, Chabbert V, Chemla P, Joffre F, Vinel JP, Rousseau H (2002). Preliminary results of a new expanded-polytetrafluoroethylene-covered stent-graft for transjugular intrahepatic portosystemic shunt procedures. *AJR* **178**, 141–147.
53. Hashimoto S, Hiramatsu K, Sato M. CO_2 as an intra-arterial digital subtraction angiography agent in the management of trauma. *Semin Intervent Radiol* **2**, 163–173.

54. Pachter HL, Knudson MM, Esrig B, Ross S, Hoyt D, Cogbill T, Sherman H, Scalea T, Harrison P, Shackford S, *et al.* (1996). Status of non-operative management of blunt hepatic injuries in 1995: a multicenter experience with 404 patients. *J Trauma* **40**, 31–38.
55. Croce MA, Fabian TC, Menke PG, Waddle-Smith L, Minard G, Kudsk KA, Patton JH Jr, Schurr MJ, Pritchard FE (1995). Non-operative management of blunt hepatic trauma is the treatment of choice in hemodynamically stable patients. Results of a prospective trial. *Ann Surg* **221**, 744–753.
56. Demetriades D, Rabinowitz B, Sofianos C (1986). Non-operative management of penetrating liver injuries: a prospective study. *Br J Surg* **73**, 736–737.
57. Cogbill TH, Moore EE, Jurkovich GJ, Morris JA, Mucha P Jr, Shackford SR, Stolee RT, Moore FA, Pilcher S, LoCicero R, *et al.* (1989). Non-operative management of blunt splenic trauma: a multicenter experience. *J Trauma* **29**, 1312–1317.
58. Villalba MR, Howells GA, Lucas RJ, Glover JL, Bendick PJ, Tran O, Jafri SZ (1990). Non-operative management of adult ruptured spleen. *Arch Surg* **125**, 836–839.
59. Mathews LA, Spirnak JP (1995). The non-operative approach to major blunt renal trauma. *Semin Urol* **13**, 77–85.
60. Schwartz RA, Teitelbaum GP, Katz MD, Pentecost MJ (1993). Effectiveness of transcatheter embolisation in the control of hepatic vascular injuries. *JVIR* **4**, 359–365.
61. Sclafani SJ, Shaftan GW, McAuley J, Naryaranaswamy T, Mitchell WG, Gordon DH, Glanz S (1984). Interventional radiology in the management of hepatic trauma. *J Trauma* **24**, 256–262.
62. Hagiwara A, Yukioka T, Ohta S, Tokunaga T, Matsuda H, Shimazaki S (1997). Non-surgical management of patients with blunt hepatic injury: efficacy of transcatheter arterial embolisation. *AJR* **169**, 1151–1156.
63. Hagiwara A, Yukioka T, Ohta S, Nitatori T, Matsuda H, Shimazaki S (1996). Non-surgical management of patients with blunt splenic

injury: efficacy of transcatheter arterial embolisation. *AJR* **167**, 159–166.

64. Sclafani SJ, Weisberg A, Scalea TM, Phillips TF, Duncan AO (1991). Blunt splenic injuries: non-surgical treatment with CT, arteriography and transcatheter arterial embolisation of the splenic artery. *Radiology* **181**, 189–196.
65. Davis KA, Fabian TC, Croce MA, Gavant ML, Flick PA, Minard G, Kudsk KA, Pritchard FE (1998). Improved success in non-operative management of blunt splenic injuries: embolisation of splenic artery pseudoaneurysms. *J Trauma* **44**, 1008–1015.
66. Kantor A, Sclafani SJ, Scalea T, Duncan AO, Atweh N, Glanz S (1989). The role of interventional radiology in the management of genitourinary trauma. *Urol Clin North Am* **16**, 255–265.
67. Corr P, Hacking G. Embolisation in traumatic intrarenal vascular injuries. *Clin Radiol* **43**, 262–264.
68. Heyns CF, Van Vollenhoven P (1992). Increasing role of angiography and segmental artery embolisation in the management of renal stab wounds. *J Urol* **147**, 1231–1234.
69. Eastham JA, Wilson TG, Larsen DW, Ahlering TE (1992). Angiographic embolisation of renal stab wounds. *Urology* **148**, 268–270.
70. Ben-Menachem Y, Coldwell DM, Young JW, Burgess AR (1991). Hemorrhage associated with pelvic fractures: causes, diagnosis and emergent management. *AJR* **157**, 1005–1014.
71. Katz MD, Teitelbaum GP, Pentecost MJ (1992). Diagnostic arteriography and therapeutic transcatheter embolisation for post-traumatic pelvic hemorrhage. *Semin Intervent Radiol* **9**, 4–12.
72. Agolini SF, Shah K, Jaffe J, Newcomb J, Rhodes M, Reed JF 3rd (1997). Arterial embolisation is a rapid and effective technique for controlling pelvic fracture haemorrhage. *J Trauma* **43**, 395–399.
73. Panetta TM, Sclafani SJ, Goldstein AS, Phillips TF, Shaftan GW (1985). Percutaneous transcatheter embolisation for massive bleeding from pelvic fractures. *J Trauma* **25**, 1021–1029.
74. Wells I (1996). Internal iliac artery embolisation in the management of pelvic bleeding. *Clin Radiol* **51**, 825–827.

75. Pelage JP, Le Dref O, Mateo J, Soyer P, Jacob D, Kardache M, Dahan H, Repiquet D, Payen D, Truc JB, Merland JJ, Rymer R (1998). Life-threatening post-partum hemorrhage: treatment with emergency selective arterial embolisation. *Radiology* **208**(2), 359–362.
76. Yamashita Y, Harada M, Yamamoto H, Miyazaki T, Takahashi M, Miyazaki K, Okamura H (1994). Transcatheter arterial embolisation of obstetric and gynaecological bleeding: efficacy and clinical outcome. *Br J Radiol* **67**, 530–534.
77. Rousseau H, Soula P, Perreault P, Bui B, Janne d'Othee B, Massabuau P, Meites G, Concina P, Mazerolles M, Joffre F, Otal P (1999). Delayed treatment of traumatic rupture of the thoracic aorta with endoluminal covered stent. *Circulation* **99**, 498–504.
78. Redekop G, Marotta T, Weill A (2001). Treatment of traumatic aneurysms and arteriovenous fistulas of the skull base by using endovascular stents. *J Neurosurg* **95**, 412–419.
79. Becker GJ, Benenati JF, Zemel G, Sallee DS, Suarez CA, Roeren TK, Katzen BT (1991). Percutaneous placement of a balloon-expandable intraluminal graft for life-threatening subclavian arterial hemorrhage. *JVIR* **2**, 225–229.
80. Venturini M, Angeli E, Salvioni M, De Cobelli F, Trentin C, Carlucci M, Staudacher C, Del Maschio A (2002). Haemorrhage from a right hepatic artery pseudoaneurysm: endovascular treatment with a coronary stent-graft. *J Endovasc Ther* **9**, 221–224.
81. Hurst RW (ed.) (1997). *Cerebral Aneurysms*. Neuroimaging Clinics of North America.
82. Guglielmi G, Vinneula F, Dion J, Duckwiler G (1991). Electrothrombosis of saccular aneurysms via endovascular approach. Part 2: preliminary clinical experience. *J Neurosurg* **75**, 8–14.
83. Wilkins RH (1985). Natural history of intracranial vascular malformations: a review. *Neurosurgery* **16**, 421-430.
84. Russel EJ, Meyer JR (eds.) (1998). *Neurovascular Malformations: Diagnosis and Intervention.* Neuroimaging Clinics of North America.

85. Cognard C, Gobin Y, Pierot L, Bailly AL, Houdart E, Casasco A, Chiras J, Merland JJ (1995). Neurological symptoms of intracranial dural arteriovenous fistulas: clinical and angiographic correlation in 205 cases. A revisited classification of the venous drainage. *Radiology* **194**, 671–680.
86. Serbinenko FA (1974). Balloon catheterisation and occlusion of major cerebral vessels. *J Neurosurg* **41**, 125–145.
87. Elden L, Montanera W, Terbrugge K, Willinsky R, Lasjaunias P, Charles D (1994). Angiographic embolisation for the treatment of epistaxis: a review of 108 cases. *Ortolaryngol Head and Neck Surg* **111**, 44–50.

Further Reading

88. Baum S, Pentecost MJ (eds.) (1996). *Abram's Angiography: Vascular and Interventional Radiology*, 4th Ed. Lippincott Williams & Wilkins.
89. Castaneda-Zuniga WR, Tadavarthy SM (eds.) (1997). *Interventional Radiology*, 3rd Ed. Lippincott Williams and Wilkins.
90. Bulter P (ed.) (2000). *Endovascular Neurosurgery — A Multidisciplinary Approach*, 1st Ed. Springer Verlag Inc.
91. Lasjaunias P (ed.) (1987). *Surgical Neuroangiography Vol. 2: Endovascular Treatment of Craniofacial Lesions*, 1st Ed. Springer Verlag Inc.
92. Berenstein A (ed.) (1992). *Surgical Neuroangiography Vol. 4: Endovascular Treatment of Cerebral Lesions*, 1st Ed. Springer Verlag Inc.
93. Conners and Wojak (eds.) (1999). *Interventional Neuroradiology — Strategies and Practical Techniques*, 1st Ed. Saunders WB Co.
94. Mukherji SK (ed.) (February 2000). Paediatric Head and Neck Imaging. *Neuroimaging Clinics of North America*.
95. Chi SZ, Go JL (eds.) (May 2002). Imaging of Head Trauma. *Neuroimaging Clinics of North America*.

Section XII

Perioperative Anaesthetic Care

37

Optimisation of Patients for Emergency Surgery

Christine JC Cheng
Nian-Chih Hwang

Introduction

Adequate pre-operative preparation is vital in minimising morbidity and mortality from anaesthesia and surgery. Integral in this process is the identification of factors that place individual patients at increased risk, and the optimisation of co-existing medical problems.

Patients presenting for emergency surgery frequently present challenges in pre-operative preparation. They may have medical conditions that are either poorly controlled or previously undiagnosed. There may also be problems specific to the surgical conditions that require special attention, for prevention of unnecessary increases in morbidity and mortality.

The American Society of Anesthesiologists (ASA) has stratified patient risk according to the pre-existing state of health, so producing the ASA classification (Table 1). In general terms, the higher the ASA grade, the more effort will be required to maintain patient stability in the peri-operative period. The critically ill patients have greater potential for developing post-operative complications, particularly if

Table 1 American Society of Anesthesiologists (ASA) Physical Status with Overall Mortality Rate

Category	Description of Patient	Mortality (%)
I	Healthy	0.06–0.08
II	Suffers mild systemic disease with no functional limitation	0.27–0.4
III	Suffers severe systemic disease with definite functional limitation	1.82–4.3
IV	Suffers severe systemic disease that is a constant threat to life	7.76–23.4
V	Is moribund and unlikely to survive 24 hours with or without an operation	9.38–50.7

The suffix "E" is added to the ASA grade if the operation is performed under emergency circumstances.

the surgical procedure is prolonged, and when there is greater surgical trespass. Facilities for increased monitoring and nursing care (high dependency, intermediate care or intensive care) in the post-operative period for such high risk patients may have to be arranged prior to major surgery.

Mandatory Preparation Guidelines

Fasting

All patients due for surgery under general anaesthesia, regional anaesthesia or sedation should undergo a period of fasting. This is to allow time for gastric emptying to occur.[1] Although there has been much controversy about the duration of fasting, most anaesthesiologists accept the omission of all but clear fluids for six hours prior to elective operations.[2] If the patient does not suffer from gastro-intestinal immotility, clear fluid may be allowed up to two hours before surgery. However, acute trauma and abdominal pathology both predispose patients to a reduction in the rate of gastric emptying. Thus there may be residual food in the stomach even after the required period of starvation has been observed. Unless there is risk to life or limb without immediate surgery, the guidelines for starvation should be adhered to in order to minimise the risk of gastro-oesophageal reflux and aspiration pneumonitis. As patients presenting for emergency surgery generally do not have a confirmed operation time, it is usual practice to deny the patient all food and drink from the time the need for operation is decided. In situations where there is a definite delay in operation time, it should be possible to feed patients whenever feasible, should there not be surgical contra-indications to this.

Investigations

Laboratory investigations are an integral part of peri-operative management. These are useful as an assessment of adequacy of control of medical problems; an indication of the severity of the presenting problem, and a useful tool in the detection of unrecognised disease states. The tests are also useful to record baseline parameters for patients undergoing major surgical procedures.

The investigations requested must take the patient's health and proposed surgery into consideration. Extensive investigations in healthy patients presenting for minor surgery are often unnecessary, particularly if the results are unlikely to alter clinical management.

The *haemoglobin concentration* should be checked in all females and in males above the age of 50 years. In addition, it should be checked prior to major surgery, in patients of racial origins with a high incidence of haemoglobinopathies and when clinically indicated, such as, a history of bleeding. For major surgery, the pre-operative haemoglobin concentration should ideally be 10 g/dl or greater. For minor surgery, and in patients with chronic renal failure, a haemoglobin concentration of 8 g/dl should suffice. (Refer to the management of patients with renal disease.)

The *full blood count* is useful when investigating conditions where infections or sepsis have a role, or where aberrations in platelet count are suspected.

Pre-operative serum *urea and electrolyte* concentrations should be determined when there is a history of diarrhoea, vomiting or metabolic disease (like renal disease, hepatic disease or abnormal nutritional states); after dialysis; and when drugs like diuretics, digoxin, anti-hypertensive agents and steroids are used. The use of bowel preparation can result in dehydration and electrolyte imbalance.

Hyponatraemia[3] is one of the most common biochemical abnormalities in hospitalised patients. Often, it is mild and easily reversible with treatment of the underlying condition. However, in severe cases, this can lead to severe life-threatening neurological deficit. Table 2 lists the mechanisms of hyponatraemia.

Table 2 Mechanisms of Hyponatraemia

(1) Decreased free water clearance caused by antidiuretic hormone (ADH)

- Administration of vasopressin or its analogues
- Inappropriate ADH secretion (malignancies, brain lesions, pulmonary tuberculosis, pneumonia, artificial ventilation)
- Appropriate secretion in the presence of extracellular fluid volume contraction
- Congestive cardiac failure, nephrotic syndrome and cirrhosis
- Secretion in response to increased sympathetic nervous system activity
- Baroreceptor stimulation
- "Stress"

(2) Decreased free water clearance caused by other agents, for example: oxytocin, diuretic agents

(3) Water retention secondary to renal disease

(4) Decreased free water clearance caused by local reversible renal causes

- Decreased delivery of solute load to diluting segment as a result of decreased renal blood flow and glomerular filtration rate and increased proximal tubular sodium re-absorption
- Change in water permeability of loop of Henle and collecting ducts not caused by ADH (such as with steroid deficit)

(5) Movement of water from intra- to extra-cellular compartments

- Potassium depletion
- Infusion exerting high osmotic pressure (such as mannitol and dextran)
- Hyperglycaemia

Pseudo-hyponatraemia is an apparent decrease in serum sodium concentration caused by measurement error in the presence of severe hyperlipidaemia and hyperproteinaemia. This condition is identified by the presence of normal serum osmolality (275–295 mosm/l).

There remains much controversy regarding the need for (and speed of) correction of hyponatraemia. There is evidence that rapid correction of hyponatraemia can result in central pontine myelinosis. Chronic hyponatraemia is corrected by treating the underlying condition. Severe acute hyponatraemia carries great neurological risks, so correction should occur to a target of 120–130 mmol/l by means of water restriction and the infusion of calculated amounts of saline. Increments in serum sodium should be limited to 20 mmol/l/day. Avoid infusing sodium concentrations that exceed twice that of normal saline, to avoid major acute changes in serum concentration. Serum electrolytes should be checked every two to three hours. Frusemide should be administered when the hyponatraemia is associated with fluid overload.

Hypokalaemia ($K^+ < 3.5$ mmol/l) is frequently encountered in patients taking loop diuretic agents and after dialysis. Unless the hypokalaemia is severe ($K^+ < 3.0$ mmol/l) or the effects of hypokalaemia (such as cardiac arrhythmias) are evident, aggressive replacement of potassium before surgery is not necessary. Hypokalaemia must be corrected if the patient is on digoxin therapy.

Blood sugar concentrations should be routinely monitored. This will enable the identification of abnormal random blood glucose concentrations, and may lead to the diagnosis of diabetes mellitus. Repeated measurements (twice to four times daily) are mandatory for diabetics and patients receiving corticosteroid therapy. (Refer to the management of the diabetic patient.)

Coagulation profiles (*prothrombin time and activated partial thromboplastin time*) should be investigated for patients scheduled for major surgery, patients taking anticoagulant medication, those with liver disease, and patients with a history of bleeding. Fresh frozen plasma should be made available if excessive intra-operative bleeding is anticipated.

Thyroid function tests must be done on all patients with a history of thyroid dysfunction or with previous thyroid surgery. The peri-operative management of patients with thyroid dysfunction should include the input of an endocrinologist. For urgent surgery, rapid stabilisation of hyperthyroidism with beta blockade and sodium iodide may have to be instituted.

Electrocardiographs (*ECG*) should be routinely obtained in all patients over the age of 50 years. They are also required in patients with hypertension and/or cardiovascular disease. Diabetic patients with autonomic neuropathy may not complain of angina during episodes of ischaemia. Electrocardiographic evidence of ischaemia may be the first hint of the presence of coronary artery disease.

Chest X-rays should be obtained if the history or physical examination suggests cardiac or respiratory disease; for the exclusion of pulmonary metastases; before thoracic surgery; in patients from countries where tuberculosis is endemic; and if comparison between post-operative and pre-operative chest X-rays is intended.

Cervical spine X-rays are required in patients with rheumatoid arthritis, even when they do not complain of neck pain. Both flexion and extension views are required, to exclude atlanto-axial subluxation.

Medical Conditions

This section deals with the management of the more commonly encountered medical conditions.

Ischaemic heart disease

Ischaemic heart disease is one of the leading causes of death in Singapore. It is associated with increased peri-operative morbidity and mortality in terms of congestive cardiac failure (CCF) and myocardial infarction (MI). The incidence of peri-operative myocardial infarction is in the range of 0.1–0.4% in previously healthy patients. This rises to 3.2–7.7% for patients who had suffered a previous MI. The risk is much greater if surgery proceeds within six months of the MI.

Patients can present with angina that is either stable (on exertion) or unstable (not related to exertion) in nature. They may have had myocardial infarctions, and/or had angioplasty or coronary artery bypass grafting performed in the past. The peri-operative risk from surgical procedures has been stratified by Goldman (Table 3).[4]

Assessment of patients with ischaemic heart disease has to include defining the stresses that precipitate angina, establishing the presence of congestive cardiac failure, and determining the degree of exercise tolerance. The New York Heart Association (NYHA) Functional Classification is a useful tool for assessment of the functional disability

Table 3 Goldman's Index of Cardiac Risk in Non-cardiac Procedures (Modified)[4]

Risk Factor	Points
Third heart sound or jugular venous distension	11
Myocardial infarction in preceding 6 months	10
Rhythm other than sinus or premature atrial contractions	7
More than 5 ventricular ectopic beats per minute	7
Abdominal, thoracic or aortic operation	3
Age > 70 years	5
Important aortic stenosis	3
Emergency operation	4
Poor condition as defined by one of the following:	
$PaO_2 < 8$ kPa	
$PaCO_2 < 6.5$ kPa	
$K^+ < 3.0$ $mmol.litre^{-1}$	
$HCO_3^- < 20$ $mmol.litre^{-1}$	
Urea > 7.5 $mmol.litre^{-1}$	
Creatinine > 270 $\mu mol.litre^{-1}$	
SGOT abnormal	
Chronic liver disease	Total: 53

0–5 points: major cardiac complications 0.3–3%.
6–12 points: major cardiac complications 1–10%.
13–25 points: major cardiac complications 3–30%.
26–53 points: major cardiac complications 19–75%.

Table 4 New York Heart Association (NYHA) Functional Classification of Stable Angina

Class	Functional Capability
I	Ordinary physical activity does not cause angina
II	Ordinary physical activity results in angina
III	Comfortable at rest, but angina occurs with mild physical exertion
IV	Angina occurs at rest; inability to carry out any physical activity without discomfort

Table 5 New York Heart Association (NYHA) Functional Classification for Congestive Symptoms

Class	Functional Capability
I	Ordinary physical activity does not cause dyspnoea
II	Ordinary physical activity results in dyspnoea
III	Comfortable at rest, but dyspnoea occurs with mild physical exertion
IV	Dyspnoeic at rest; inability to carry out any physical activity without discomfort

of patients with stable angina (Table 4). There is a second NYHA classification for congestive symptoms secondary to cardiac failure (Table 5).

Patients with significant cardiac disease should be referred to a cardiologist for assessment, investigation and optimisation of their cardiovascular status. Wherever possible, the cardiology records should be made available for anaesthetic assessment.

Hypertension

Chronic hypertension may be associated with cardiac ischaemia and left ventricular dysfunction.[5] Patients with uncontrolled hypertension

Table 6 Definitions and Classification of Blood Pressure Levels for Adults Aged 18 Years and Over[5]

Category	Systolic BP (mmHg)	Diastolic BP (mmHg)
Normal BP	< 130	< 85
High normal BP	130–139	85–89
Grade 1 hypertension (mild)	140–159	90–99
Grade 2 hypertension (moderate)	160–179	100–109
Grade 3 hypertension (severe)	≥ 180	≥ 110
Isolated systolic hypertension*	≥ 140	< 90

*Isolated systolic hypertension is graded according to the same level of systolic BP.

have poor vascular compliance, which may result in marked intra-operative variations in cardiovascular parameters. Ideally, pre-operative control of blood pressure should be for a period of six weeks in order to minimise these problems. As this is not a viable option under emergency circumstances, the patients must be advised of the attendant anaesthetic risks associated with uncontrolled hypertension, particularly with regard to myocardial ischaemia and the risks of per-operative myocardial infarction and strokes.

The severity of hypertension has been classified by the Ministry of Health, Singapore, and is displayed in Table 6.

Pulmonary disease

Patients at risk of developing pulmonary complications include smokers, patients with pre-existing lung disease, the obese, and those undergoing thoracic and abdominal operations. For patients with pre-existing lung disease, blood gas analysis may help predict the need for post-operative ventilation. It should therefore be routinely performed for all patients with severe lung disease, as well as those scheduled for thoracic operations. The peak expiratory flow rate (PEFR) is a useful measure of disease severity for patients with asthma and chronic bronchitis. Medical optimisation will be required if the observed PEFR is 70% or less than the predicted value.

Diabetes mellitus

This common endocrine dysfunction[6] may be due either to insufficient insulin production (Type 1) or to end-organ resistance to insulin (Type 2). Type 1 diabetes usually has a juvenile onset, and requires treatment with insulin. Type 2 diabetes affects older, often obese patients, and is usually treated with oral hypoglycaemic agents. The latter may require insulin therapy as the disease progresses, or during episodes of sepsis.

Diabetes mellitus is a multi-system disorder, with effects on the vascular system and the nervous system. Vascular insults result in coronary artery disease, peripheral vascular disease and nephropathy. Diabetics are prone to autonomic neuropathy and gastroparesis. Patients with autonomic neuropathy lose beat-to-beat heart rate variability (HRV) in response to respiration. They may complain of postural hypotension and be unable to compensate for haemodynamic changes secondary to anaesthetic and surgical causes. Gastroparesis may result in delayed gastric emptying and/or persistent nausea. Its presence increases the risk of regurgitation and aspiration pneumonitis intra-operatively. In addition, such patients may be immuno-compromised and have poor wound healing.

Preparation of a diabetic patient for surgery involves identifying the presence of co-existing medical problems, and ensuring that these, and the control of diabetes, are optimised prior to surgery. A diabetologist may have to be involved in this process. Better glycaemic control in diabetic patients undergoing major surgery has been shown to improve peri-operative mortality and morbidity. Simple avoidance of hypoglycaemia and gross hyperglycaemia are thus no longer acceptable. During anaesthesia, an acceptable range of blood glucose concentration is between 4–11 mmol/l.

When diabetic patients present as surgical emergencies, the presence of acute infection, prolonged fasting and dehydration can lead to major biochemical derangement, including diabetic ketoacidosis. Even in conditions whereby surgery is essential for the removal of the source of sepsis, effort must be made to improve the hydration status and biochemical profile prior to the patient presenting for anaesthesia and surgery. Complete correction of biochemistry may not be possible in diabetic patients with sepsis. In these situations, correction of dehydration with ongoing attempts at correcting the biochemistry should be undertaken, and surgery should then proceed prior to further deterioration of the patient's condition.

Continuous infusions of soluble insulin (administered via a syringe pump) titrated to blood glucose concentration is a convenient method of controlling blood glucose concentration. Compared to the previously used Alberti's regime, there is no wastage of the accompanying infusion solutions. A recommended concentration of insulin in the syringe may be 1 IU/ml if the diluent is a colloidal solution such as gelatin. As the insulin molecules adhere to plastic in the presence of a cystalloid diluent (normal saline), a higher concentration (2 IU/ml) is needed to ensure effective insulin therapy.

Regular assessment of blood sugar concentrations should be performed during the peri-operative period, particularly prior to the resumption of normal feeding.

Renal disease

This may result from a variety of causes (examples include diabetes mellitus, hypertension, auto-immune diseases), and have a spectrum of severity ranging from proteinuria to renal impairment to renal failure. Patients with a history of renal disease must have their serum urea and electrolyte concentrations checked, and any abnormalities such as hyperkalaemia ($K^+ > 5.5$ mmol/l) corrected. Dialysis is required in patients with renal failure, although aggressive haemodialysis just prior to surgery may result in hypovolaemia.

Patients in renal failure are often anaemic. Without erythropoietin therapy, the haemoglobin concentration is usually in the range of 6–8 g/dl. Blood must be available for transfusion. In cases where the starting haemoglobin levels are below 8 g/dl or the proposed operation is likely to result in haemorrhage, it is advisable to transfuse the patient prior to surgery.

Drug History

Many patients take long-term medication for chronic conditions without making the effort to remember the names of these drugs. Although anaesthesia can usually be conducted safely without the identification of concurrent therapy, it is good practice to identify all the prescribed drugs so as not to inadvertently cause adverse drug interactions. Patients should be advised to bring their drugs with them when admitted for surgery, failing which, they should be encouraged to call on their family members to find out the names of the drugs. The prescribed medication can provide clues as to any underlying medical conditions which the patients may have neglected to disclose.

It is important to document all drug allergies in detail. This includes the names of the agents and the types of reaction seen. A history of food intolerance (such as an allergy to egg protein) may also be important, as the patient may develop anaphylactic reactions to anaesthetic agents with egg phosphatide in the formulation (such as propofol).

Latex allergies[7] are becoming a major problem in many developed countries. Contact with latex can result in anaphylactic reactions in susceptible individuals. Theatre staff and anaesthesiologists require advanced warning, as alternative equipment (such as silicone urinary catheters and latex-free gloves) has to be made available for such individuals.

Postponement of Emergency Surgery

The presence of a disease process that necessitates emergency surgery usually negates the usual reasons for postponement of elective surgery. In particular, respiratory tract infections, inadequate fasting and suboptimally controlled medical conditions do not prohibit emergency surgery. Ideally, surgery should be delayed for a short period of time to allow relevant specialists to optimise or stratify risks from co-existing medical problems.

Inadequately resuscitated emergency patients need to be optimised over a limited period of time, usually in terms of hours, prior to surgery. This may be circumvented in the situation of extensive continuous haemorrhage, where early surgery is life-saving. Failure to obtain informed consent may be a problem, but where relatives are not available and if the patient is too ill to give consent, a minimum of two specialists should be able to come to an agreement should immediate surgery make a difference between life and death.

Blood Transfusions

A patient may require the transfusion of blood or blood products because of a chronic insufficiency, as a result of the acute medical problem, or secondary to intra-operative losses.

With a shortage of blood and blood products for transfusion, and the risks of blood-borne infections associated with transfusion, it is essential to recognise which patients require transfusions as part of the operative course.

Blood transfusions may be required pre-operatively, particularly if there are signs of decompensation, like breathlessness, tachycardia, ECG changes or angina. Patients with renal failure may be an exception to this rule, as they are chronically anaemic with adequate physiological compensation. With such patients, the decision for blood transfusion must be balanced, taking haemoglobin concentration, physiological reserves and potential for haemorrhage into consideration. Thought must also be given to transfusing patients presenting for cancer surgery. Research has shown that the recurrence rate is higher after transfusions, so a certain degree of anaemia should be tolerated before embarking upon the transfusion pathway.[8] Anaemic patients should be transfused pre-operatively as opposed to intra-operatively. This is because transfused blood lacks 2,3-diphosphoglycerate (2,3-DPG) and remains poor at oxygen delivery for a few hours after transfusion.

Intra-operative transfusions may be required, depending on the type of surgery and the development of intra-operative complications. In procedures where transfusions are usually required, cross matched blood should be available in the theatre at the start of the procedure. Where the risk of transfusion is moderate, cross matched blood should be available in the hospital blood bank. When the risk of bleeding is low, the patients' blood may be grouped and saved, so that cross matching occurs only if the need for transfusion arises. For minor body surface surgery, transfusion of blood is rarely required.

Blood products may be required in the preparation of patients for surgery. Patients with coagulopathies will require pre-operative transfusion of fresh frozen plasma, and often, fresh frozen plasma should also be available for intra-operative transfusion, particularly if the surgery is associated with a risk of haemorrhage. Platelet transfusions should be arranged for patients who are thrombocytopaenic (platelet count less than $100 \times 10^9/l$) for intraoperative transfusion. Other clotting factors may be needed for specific conditions, for example haemophilia; and these should be given after consultation with the haematologist.

Stabilisation Prior to Emergency Surgery

There is often an interval between the decision for emergency surgery, adequate patient preparation (in terms of investigations and optimisation) and the availability of operating theatre time for the procedure to proceed. It is vital that the patient's condition does not deteriorate during this time. As most patients are kept nil by mouth during this time, adequate hydration by means of an intravenous infusion may be required in dehydrated patients, and in those for whom a prolonged fast is anticipated.

For critically ill patients optimisation of the medical condition is vital prior to surgery. Where aggressive resuscitation is required, transfer to a high dependency ward is justified, particularly if fluid resuscitation with the aid of central venous monitoring is required. Patients with very high peri-operative risk should be considered for optimisation in an intensive care setting. There is evidence that goal-orientated enhancement of oxygen delivery in an intensive care setting prior to surgery can reduce the morbidity and mortality compared to

Table 7 Criteria Suggesting a Patient may Benefit from Admission to an Intensive Care Unit Before Operation for Cardiovascular Augmentation and Pharmacological Enhancement of Physiology, to Achieve a Tissue Oxygen Delivery of at Least 600 ml/min/m^2 Body Surface Area Before Surgery

(1)	Previous severe cardiopulmonary illness with current reduced cardiopulmonary reserve (such as acute myocardial infarction, chronic obstructive airways disease, cerebrovascular accident)
(2)	Respiratory failure requiring mechanical ventilation
(3)	Shock (mean arterial pressure less than 60 mmHg, central venous pressure lower than 15 mmHg, urine output less than 0.5 ml/kg/h, cold and clammy)
(4)	Acute abdominal catastrophe with haemodynamic instability
(5)	Age over 70 years and evidence of reduced physiological reserve in one or more organs
(6)	Acute renal failure (urea > 20 mmol/l, creatinine > 200 μmol/l of sudden onset)
(7)	Planned extensive abdominal surgery for carcinoma (e.g. gastrectomy, oesophagectomy)
(8)	Late-stage vascular disease associated with aortic disease

those admitted into the intensive care unit after surgery.[9,10] Such aggressive management may require the insertion of a pulmonary artery flotation catheter (which has inherent risks); and optimisation of oxygen delivery with hydration, support with inotrope therapy, and supplemental oxygen. The aim is to achieve arterial haemoglobin oxygen saturation of at least 95%, pulmonary artery occlusion pressures of 12–14 mmHg, haemoglobin concentration greater than 12 g/dl, mean arterial pressures of 80–100 mmHg and a urine output of over 0.5 ml/kg/h. Should this not produce an oxygen delivery of at least 600 ml/min/m^2, intravenous inotrope with or without vasodilator therapy is commenced. Patients with two or more of the criteria shown in Table 7 with operations estimated to last longer than 90 minutes, are likely to benefit from optimisation in intensive care prior to surgery.

Conclusion

The risk of surgical and anaesthetic complications may be increased in the presence of ASA physical health status that is higher than 3, and/or severe cardiopulmonary disease and medical conditions with organ dysfunction.

By recognising patients who are at increased risk, and by adequately preparing the patient for surgery, and planning for appropriate post-operative care, the risks of morbidity and mortality can be reduced. A multi-disciplinary approach may be required to optimise high risk patients. When indicated, referrals for consultation by other relevant specialty physicians should be made preferably after the results of all appropriate investigations have been obtained. Anaesthesiologists should be made aware of patients who may pose airway management problems, and informed about critically ill patients, particularly if they are likely to need intensive care in the post-operative period.

References

1. Mendelson CL (1946). The aspiration of stomach contents into the lungs during obstetric anesthesia. *Am J Obstet Gynecol* **52**, 191–205.
2. Strunin L (1993). How long should patients fast before surgery? Time for new guidelines. *Br J Anaes* **70**, 1–3.
3. Swales JD (1991). Management of hyponatraemia. *Br J Anaes* **67**, 146–153.
4. Goldman L, Caldera DL, Nussbaum SR, Southwick FS, Krogstad D, Murray B, Burke DS, O'Malley TA, Goroll AH, Caplan CH, Nolan J, Carabello B, Slater EE (1977). Multifactorial index of cardiac risk in non-cardiac surgical procedures. *New Engl J Med* **297**(16), 845–850.
5. MOH Clinical Practice Guidelines (2000). Hypertension. Singapore: Ministry of Health.
6. McAnulty GR, Robertshaw HJ, Hall GM (2000). Anaesthetic management of patients with diabetes mellitus. *Br J Anaes* **85**, 80–90.
7. Dakin MJ, Yentis SM (1998). Latex allergy: a strategy for management. *Anaesthesia* **53**, 774–781.

8. Blumberg N, Chuang-Stein C, Heal JM (1990). The relationship of blood transfusion, tumour staging and cancer recurrence. *Transfusion* **30**, 291–294.
9. Curran JE, Grounds RM (1998). Ward versus intensive care management of high-risk surgical patients. *Br J Surg* **85**, 956–961.
10. Wilson J, Woods I, Fawcett J, Whall R, Dibb W, Morris C, McManus E (1999). Reducing the risk of major elective surgery: randomised controlled trial of pre-operative optimisation of oxygen delivery. *Br Med J* **318**(7191), 1099–1103.

Further Reading

1. Smith G (1996). Preoperative assessment and premedication. In *Textbook of Anaesthesia*, 3rd Ed. Aitkenhead AR, Smith G (eds.) Edinburgh: Churchill Livingstone, pp. 305–318.
2. Hwang NC (ed.) (1998). *Anaesthesia: A Practical Handbook.* Singapore: Oxford University Press (ISBN 0-19-588422-1).
3. Hwang NC, Sinclair M (1997). *Cardiac Anaesthesia — A Practical Handbook.* Oxford, U.K.: Oxford University Press (ISBN 0-19-262836-4).

38

Anaesthesia for Emergency Surgery

Sook-Muay Tay
Chee-Seng Kong

Introduction

Unlike patients scheduled for elective surgery, patients undergoing emergency surgery may not be optimally prepared. The surgical diagnosis and the severity of the surgical condition may not be apparent. In addition, the patients may be inflicted with known or undiagnosed concomitant medical illnesses that influence the outcome of the surgery.

It is therefore paramount that in considering anaesthesia for patients for emergency surgery, careful preparation and close attention to detail are necessary to:

- ensure a smooth perioperative period
- avoid known potential complications like pulmonary aspiration, hypotension secondary to hypovolaemia and abnormal reactions to drugs in the presence of metabolic and electrolyte derangements
- be prepared to deal with any adverse events.

The perioperative management of these patients can be divided into: (1) preoperative assessment and optimisation, (2) induction of anaesthesia and intraoperative management, and (3) postoperative management.

Preoperative Management

Every patient needing emergency surgery should be in the best possible condition, taking into account the time and means available to evaluate and correct any specific problems like cardiac and respiratory failure, fluid and electrolyte abnormalities, coagulopathies and anaemia.

The topic "preoperative optimisation" will be covered in another chapter, but two important aspects relevant to anaesthesia for emergency surgery will be highlighted here. These are:

- assessment and optimisation of fluid status (Tables 1 and 2)[1,2]
- the problem of the "full stomach".

Assessment and optimisation of fluid status

Induction of general anaesthesia causes vasodilatation that can produce a circulatory collapse in the presence of hypovolaemia. Thus, the circulatory volume must be carefully evaluated and any deficit corrected. Clinical signs like heart rate, blood pressure, pulse pressure and peripheral perfusion are useful. It should be remembered that, in the young and healthy, there may be little change in these parameters until more than 20% blood volume is lost. However, for the elderly with cardiovascular disease, severe signs of hypoperfusion can occur at less than 15% loss.

Assessment of extravascular volume is more difficult because considerable losses have to occur before clinical signs like loss of skin turgour and reduced intraoccular pressure are apparent. Guidance is obtained from the nature of the surgical condition, duration of impaired fluid intake, and the presence of symptoms with abnormal losses. For example, by the time there is radiological evidence of

Table 1 Clinical Indices of Extent of Blood Loss

Grade of Hypovolaemia	1 Minimal	2 Mild	3 Moderate	4 Severe
Percentage of blood lost (%)	10	20	30	Over 40
Volume lost (ml)	500	1000	1500	Over 2000
Heart rate (beats/min)	Normal	100–120	120–140	Over 140
Arterial pressure (mmHg)	Normal	Orthostatic hypotension	Systolic less than 100	Systolic less than 80
Urinary output (ml/hr)	Normal 0.5–1 ml/kg/h	20–30	10–20	Nil
Sensorium	Normal	Normal	Restless	Impaired consciousness
State of peripheral circulation	Normal	Cool and pale	Cool, pale, slow capillary refill	Cold, clammy peripheral cyanosis
CVP (cmH_2O)	Normal	−3	−5	−8

Table 2 Indices of Extent of Loss of Extracellular Fluid

Percentage body weight lost as water	ml of fluid lost per 70 kg	Signs and symptoms
Over 4% (mild)	Over 2500	Thirst, reduced skin elasticity, decreased intraoccular pressure, dry tongue, reduced sweating
Over 6% (moderate)	Over 4200	As above, plus orthostatic hypotension, reduced filling of peripheral veins, oliguria, nausea, dry axillae and groin, low CVP, apathy, haemoconcentration
Over 8% (severe)	Over 5500	As above, plus hypotension, thready pulse with cool peripheries
10–15% (life-threatening)	7000–10,500	Coma, shock, followed by death

intestinal obstruction, there may be 1500 ml of fluid sequestered in the lumen and if there has been vomiting, the deficit may be 3000 ml. The loss is usually expressed as the percentage of the body weight loss.

Laboratory investigations may help to confirm the extent of the deficit; the haematocrit and blood urea concentration are increased, and the urine volume will be decreased with low urinary sodium.

The deficit in extracellular fluid is corrected using normal saline or Hartmann's solution. The ideal time for anaesthesia and surgery is when the intracellular and extracellular fluid deficits are fully corrected but if there are valid surgical reasons to expedite surgery, a compromise is necessary.

The full stomach

Vomiting and regurgitation of gastric contents may result in pulmonary aspiration during induction of anaesthesia, or emergence from anaesthesia. This may cause mild inflammation of the upper and lower respiratory tree but can also result in adult respiratory distress syndrome with or without superimposed lung infection.

Vomiting is an active process occurring in the lighter planes of anaesthesia. Tight adduction of the vocal cords occurs if stimulated by saliva, blood or gastric contents, thus offering some protection to the tracheobronchial tree. The secretions should be cleared by the anaesthesiologist before resumption of ventilation, or paralysis of the vocal cords will occur.

At deeper planes of anaesthesia or muscle paralysis, the laryngeal reflexes are obtunded so that passive regurgitation and aspiration can occur at any time during general anaesthesia. The incidence and degree of gastric regurgitation in this state are affected by function of the lower oesophageal sphincter tone, intragastric pressure and the rate of gastric emptying.

It is recommended that the patients be fasted for six hours or more in the *elective* setting to minimise the risk of vomiting or regurgitation of gastric contents. This risk is clearly higher in the emergency surgical patient undergoing general anaesthesia. They may not be fasted for 6 hours; gastric emptying is reduced due to the pain and stress of the surgical condition, especially if an opioid has been administered, or if the gastrointestinal tract is involved.

During the second and third trimester of pregnancy, the lower oesophageal sphincter tone is relaxed, resulting in gastro-oesophageal reflux.[3] In addition, gastric emptying may be reduced during the third trimester. For patients undergoing caesarean section, they are given ranitidine 50 mg intravenously and 0.3 M sodium citrate 30 ml orally prior to departure to the operating theatre, and metoclopramide 10 mg intravenously prior to induction of anaesthesia, to reduce the acidity and the volume of gastric contents respectively.

Situations in which vomiting or regurgitation may occur:

(1) Full stomach

- peritonitis of any cause
- postoperative ileus
- metabolic ileus: hypokalaemia, uraemia
- drug-induced ileus: anticholinergic agents; those with anticholinergic side effects like phenothiazines and droperidol; opioids, alcohol
- small or large bowel obstruction
- gastric carcinoma
- pyloric stenosis
- hypotension of any cause
- fear, pain or anxiety
- pregnancy (second or third trimester)
- deep sedation
- recent solid or fluid intake
- trauma.

(2) Other causes

- hiatus hernia
- oesophageal strictures
- pharyngeal pouch

- reduced lower oesophageal sphincteric tone (LOS): immaturity of LOS in the infant, anaesthetic agents, pregnancy.

Trauma cases need to be considered as high risk for pulmonary aspiration of gastric contents. This is because gastric emptying virtually ceases at the time of significant trauma as a result of increased sympathetic discharge secondary to pain and anxiety, and as a side-effect of opioid analgesics.[4] In these cases, the time interval between ingestion of food and the accident is taken as the period of fasting. Even if this period is more than six hours, most anaesthesiologists still recommend that full precautions be taken to prevent regurgitation and aspiration.

In the absence of the above factors, and if the patient has been fasted for more than six hours, it may be safe to assume that the stomach is empty and one can conduct general anaesthesia in the normal way.

Intraoperative Management

Techniques of anaesthesia

(1) General anaesthesia

- mask/oral airway with spontaneous ventilation
- laryngeal mask airway (LMA) with spontaneous ventilation
- endotracheal tube intubation with spontaneous or mechanical ventilation

(2) Regional anaesthesia

- spinal or intrathecal anaesthesia
- epidural anaesthesia
- combined spinal epidural technique

(3) Local anaesthesia with monitored anaesthesia care

- wound infiltration of local anaesthetic agents
- plexus or nerve blocks

(4) A combination of the above

The choice of the appropriate anaesthetic technique for a surgical procedure is made after due consideration of factors related to the patient, surgery and anaesthesia in terms of available expertise, equipment and support staff.

Whichever technique is chosen, the principles of preoperative evaluation, optimisation and preparation still hold, and a smooth intraoperative course with adequate monitoring is the objective. Even if a non-general anaesthetic technique is employed, the same operating theatre preparation as for general anaesthetic cases should be carried out so that a "rescue" general anaesthetic can be given in the event of an inadequate regional anaesthetic or nerve block. In addition, if unexpected complications like cardiac events occur, resuscitation can be performed promptly, with a reduced risk of pulmonary aspiration.

As most patients in emergency surgery require general anaesthesia and endotracheal intubation, the next section will describe ways of reducing the risk of pulmonary aspiration and address the management of such a case in the operating theatre.

Preoperatively, besides fasting, a nasogastric tube can be inserted into the stomach to aspirate as much stomach contents as possible, for example, in bowel obstruction. An antacid like the non-particulate 0.3 M sodium citrate 30 ml orally, or histamine (H_2) antagonist like ranitadine 50 mg intravenously, can be administered to neutralise the acidity in the gastric contents so that the risk of pulmonary pneumonitis is diminished if pulmonary aspiration occurs. Lastly, a prokinetic agent like metoclopramide can be administered to increase gastric emptying but its effectiveness may be reduced if opioids have been given.[5]

Preparation of operating theatre

Before the case arrives in the operating theatre (OT) the following equipment need to be available and checked to be functioning:

- anaesthetic machine, including the gas supply, anaesthetic breathing system, ventilator

- suction apparatus
- operating table, including its usability in the head-down or Trendenlenburg position
- airway management equipment, including endotracheal tube (ETT) of estimated size mounted with a stillete and another ETT a size smaller, bougie, LMA, oral airway and mask
- the relevant monitors.

The anaesthetic drugs and drugs for resuscitation, are drawn up and labelled. The presence of a trained anaesthetic nurse or technician is mandatory to perform cricoid pressure on the patient upon induction of general anaesthesia.

If there is any suspicion that the airway is going to be difficult to secure, the anaesthesiologist will have to decide if an awake intubation with the aid of fibre-optic bronchoscopy, or a tracheostomy under local anaesthesia, is warranted.

The topic of "Managing the Difficult Airway in the Emergency Setting" will be discussed more fully in another chapter.

On arrival in the OT, the patient's consent is checked. The patient is then transferred onto the operating table. If there is potential need for blood transfusion, the blood bank will be asked to release the requested units of blood. Emergency major vascular and trauma cases require a minimum of six units of blood. If there is immediate need for blood transfusion, emergency "O" negative blood from the OT suite will be summoned.

An appropriate-size intravenous cannula will be placed in the patient's arm if none has been inserted prior to transfer to the OT. In conditions where continuous blood pressure monitoring is necessary, an arterial cannula will be inserted. A central venous cannula will help to monitor preload or volume status, and this line can be placed before or after induction of general anaesthesia.

Appropriate *monitors* will be applied to the patient prior to induction of anaesthesia. A minimum of basic monitoring like non-invasive blood pressure (NIBP), pulse oximetry (SpO_2), electrocardiograph (ECG) and inspired gas oxygen concentration (FiO_2) is *mandatory* for monitoring the patient, no matter how simple the case. Capnography (end-tidal CO_2) and measurement of inspired and expired volatile anaesthetic concentrations, are useful in assessing adequacy of ventilation, and in setting the depth of anaesthesia. Monitoring of body temperature is useful for minimising the problem of hypothermia, especially in major cases where there are large fluid shifts, and to detect a sharp rise in body temperature seen in malignant hyperthermia. The use of a nerve stimulator can be used to gauge neuromuscular transmission if muscle relaxants are given.[6]

Induction of anaesthesia

The accepted technique employed in the induction of anaesthesia is known as the "*Rapid Sequence Induction*".[7] This technique balances the risk of losing control of the airway against the risk of aspiration. It breaks one of the fundamental rules of airway management in anaesthesia, which is never to give muscle relaxants until it is certain that the airway can be secured. The anaesthesiologist must have a contingency plan should intubation fail.[8]

The patient's head should be in the "sniffing" position, with the head flexed on the shoulder and extended on the neck. The patient is then preoxygenated with 100% oxygen for 3–5 minutes in order to provide a reservoir of oxygen for the patient during laryngoscopy and intubation. A skilled assistant like an anaesthetic nurse is positioned on the patient's right side, ready to perform cricoid pressure (*Sellick's manoeuvre*)[9] (Fig. 1). Correctly applied cricoid pressure presses the cricoid cartilage, the only extrinsic laryngeal cartilage with a complete ring, posteriorly compressing the oesophagus onto the vertebral column (Fig. 2). Incorrectly applied pressure on the thyroid cartilage distorts the laryngeal anatomy, making laryngoscopy and intubation more challenging. The techniques of cricoid pressure application are discussed more fully in chapter 7.

Intravenous induction of anaesthesia is achieved using predetermined doses of thiopentone (2–5 mg/kg) followed by suxamethonium (1–1.5 mg/kg)) without waiting for complete loss of consciousness.

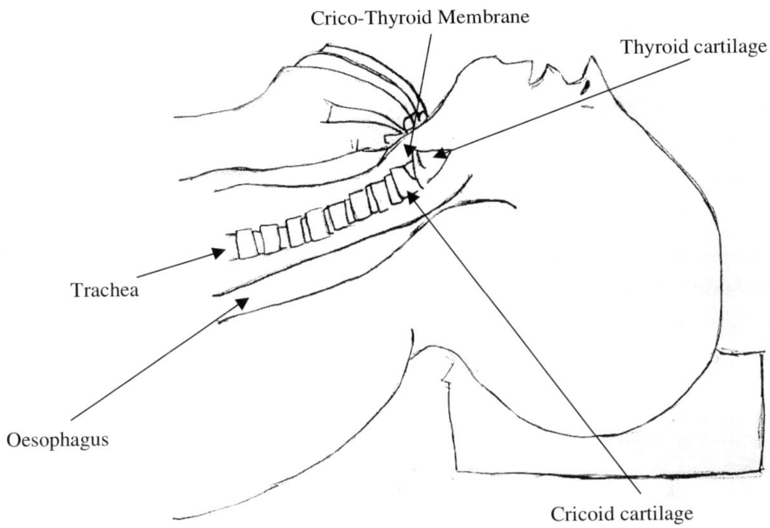

Fig. 1 Sellick's Manoeuvre.

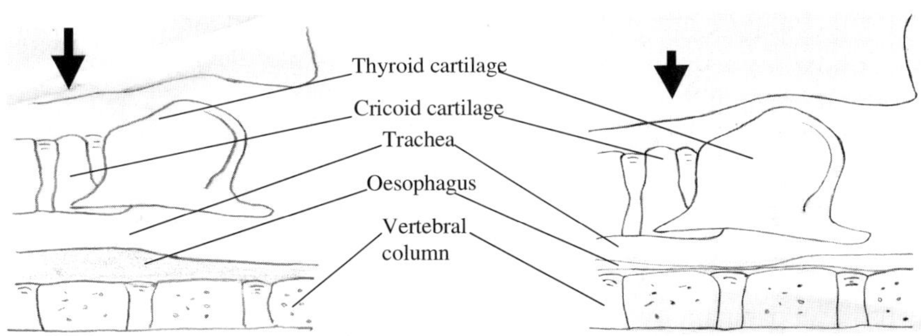

Fig. 2 Direction of cricoid pressure.

Cricoid pressure is applied as consciousness is lost because the laryngeal reflexes are obtunded.

As soon as muscle fasciculations from suxamethonium has occurred, and the jaw relaxes, laryngoscopy and endotracheal intubation are performed. Cricoid pressure is maintained until the endotracheal tube with its cuff inflated, is confirmed to be in the trachea by auscultation and the evidence of carbon dioxide on the capnograph.

A disadvantage of the rapid sequence induction technique is that the predetermined dose of induction agent may be excessive, resulting in hypotension, or inadequate — with consequent tachycardia and hypertension.

Other intravenous induction agents can be used. In young healthy patients, propofol (1–2 mg/kg) can be used, but in older patients with cardiovascular impairment, etomidate (0.1–0.3 mg/kg) may be more appropriate as it may cause less severe drops in blood pressure. It is quite common to add fentanyl (1–2 μg/kg) to obtund the response to laryngoscopy.

Other techniques for endointubation

(1) Awake intubation
(2) Deep inhalational anaesthesia
(3) Tracheostomy under local anaesthesia.

These techniques are useful if the risk of a difficult or failed intubation following a rapid sequence induction is considered too hazardous. During a difficult or failed intubation the patient is subjected to the risks of hypoxia, hypercapnia, light anaesthesia which may result in hypertension, tachycardia, arrhythmias or awareness and pulmonary aspiration. A failed intubation at rapid sequence induction would require the anaesthesiologist to recognise that further attempts would be futile and hazardous. He or she must refrain from further attempts. Cricoid pressure must be maintained until the patient wakes up and regains his laryngeal reflexes. Manual ventilation is possible until then. It is often said that the patient does not die from failure to intubate the trachea, but from failure to ventilate and oxygenate.

If appropriate, the surgery can be performed under local or regional anaesthesia. If not, alternative techniques of securing the airway with the help of more experienced colleagues must be considered.

Inhalation induction is useful in situations like acute epiglottitis, where there is some doubt about the ease to intubate the trachea but confident that an airway can be maintained during anaesthesia.

If there is considerable risk of airway obstruction when loss of consciousness occurs, awake intubation or tracheostomy under local anaesthesia would be the safest option. These situations include angioneurotic oedema, trismus from dental abscesses, large goitre or invading laryngeal tumours.

Maintenance of anaesthesia

As in elective surgery, the patient has to be provided with anaesthesia (loss of consciousness and awareness), analgesia (attenuation of autonomic reflexes in the presence of painful stimuli) and muscle relaxation (obliteration of movement and establishment of mechanical ventilation). A balanced anaesthesia technique allows a much lighter plane of anaesthesia and a quicker emergence from anaesthesia. This is achieved by using different classes of drugs in smaller doses to achieve each of the above effects, thus reducing the side-effects, as compared to using a single drug like isoflurane alone. In other words, this technique allows titration to response and reduces the risk of overdosing, particularly in patients who may be inadequately resuscitated or have multiple organ impairment.

During the maintenance phase the patient is mechanically ventilated and anaesthesia is achieved using nitrous oxide in oxygen and a volatile anaesthetic (isoflurane, desflurane, sevoflurane). Fentanyl in bolus doses of (0.5–1.0 μg/kg) and morphine (0.1–0.2 mg/kg) are suitable analgesic agents, while the choice of muscle relaxants (atracurium, vecuronium or pancuronium) will depend on the length of the operation and the likelihood of postoperative ventilation.

Fluid management

Intravenous fluids are administered in almost all patients for emergency surgery. Administering the correct amount is important particularly in patients with impaired cardiovascular and renal function, so that cardiac output and urine output are adequate, whilst avoiding fluid overload which may lead to postoperative pulmonary oedema.

During emergency intra-abdominal or multiple trauma surgery, a large volume of blood or fluid losses may occur. These include evaporative losses from the exposed intestines and mesentery, haemorrhage and third-space losses into inflamed and traumatised tissues. In these cases, invasive monitoring with intermittent laboratory investigations like arterial blood gases, serum electrolyte concentrations and haemoglobin concentration or haematocrit, are needed to guide fluid management.

Intraoperatively, maintenance fluids are usually electrolyte fluids like Hartmann's or normal saline solution infused at 2 mls/kg/hr, and at 2–10 mls/kg/hr if replacing third-space and evaporative losses, depending on the extent, duration of the surgery and the underlying surgical pathology.

Haemorrhages of more than 10% blood volume in the elderly, neonates and the young, or those with anaemia, ischaemic heart disease or expected large postoperative losses, will generally require blood transfusion. Previously healthy patients may be able to tolerate losses of 15–20% blood volume before necessitating blood transfusion. A haematocrit of 28–32% is a satisfactory balance between ensuring adequate oxygen carrying capacity and preventing hypoperfusion due to hyperviscosity. However, young healthy adults can tolerate haematocrits of 24–28%. They can compensate for the decrease in haemoglobin oxygen-carrying capacity by increasing their cardiac output and thus matching oxygen delivery to metabolic demands.

Emergence from anaesthesia

The majority of emergency surgical patients are woken up at the end of the operation, extubated and returned to the ward for further management via the recovery room.

The volatile anaesthetic agent, for example isoflurane, sevoflurane or desflurane, is discontinued 3–5 minutes before surgery finishes. The concentration of expired volatile agent can be used to guide the emergence from anaesthesia.

The nasogastric tube, if present, should be suctioned to reduce the amount of gastric contents and the oropharnyx is cleared of secretions without inducing gagging and coughing.

Intravenous atropine 20 μg/kg and neostigmine 50 μgm/kg are administered to reverse muscle relaxation. Extubation is only undertaken when the patient is fully awake and able to respond appropriately to verbal commands, and when the protective laryngeal reflexes and muscle power (ability to cough effectively) have returned.

If there is a high risk of immediate postoperative regurgitation and vomiting, an orogastric tube should have been placed intraoperatively to suck out any fluids from the stomach. Otherwise, the patient should be extubated in the left lateral position in the Trendenlenburg position. Suction must always be readily available at extubation.

Oxygen 100% is given to the patient until a regular breathing pattern and stable vital signs are established. The monitors are then removed and the patient transferred to the recovery room for an appropriate period prior to returning to the ward.

Prophylactic mechanical ventilation in the intensive care unit is warranted for patients who have been in prolonged hypotension, severe sepsis (peritonitis, empyema), cardiorespiratory failure, overt pulmonary aspiration, and for those with severe co-morbidity like ischaemic heart disease.

Regional Anaesthesia for Emergency Surgery

The advantages of regional anaesthesia include the avoidance of problems due to difficult airway and pulmonary aspiration, the effective blunting of the endocrine metabolic stress response, reduction in the incidence of deep vein thrombosis and pulmonary embolus and provision of analgesia after the operation. The lack of systemic side-effects of general anaesthesia (drowsiness, nausea and vomiting, hypothermia, hyperthermia) and the advantage of the awake patient serving as his or her own monitor, are additional benefits.[10]

Regional techniques (spinal or epidural anaesthesia) are useful in lower abdominal and lower limb surgery. Spinal anaesthesia has the added advantages of being rapid in onset and providing reliable anaesthesia, but it is not suitable if surgery is longer than 3–4 hours because it is a one-shot technique. For longer operations, a combined spinal-epidural technique (CSE) is attractive as the epidural catheter inserted can be used to administer "top-up" boluses of local anaesthetic when the spinal anaesthetic block has worn off.

Common operations in the emergency operating theatre frequently done under regional anaesthesia include dynamic hip screw insertion, fixation of lower limb fractures, lower limb amputation, wound debridement and caesarean section.

However, when considering regional anaesthesia for an emergency surgery, the anaesthesiologist needs to exclude any contra-indications like coagulopathy, severe hypovolaemia, sepsis (particularly of the skin over the lumbar or thoracic spine), elevated intracranial pressure, and patient refusal. Severe coronary artery disease and severe stenotic aortic and mitral valve disease, back deformities, neurological disease and aspirin ingestion are relative contra-indications. Preparations for emergency surgery done under regional anaesthesia are the same as for general anaesthesia.

Postoperative Management

All patients require oxygen immediately after the operation. Pain and shivering increase oxygen consumption. Anaesthesia worsens ventilation/perfusion mismatch and depresses respiration. Furthermore, the use of nitrous oxide leads to diffusion hypoxia. *Oxygen therapy* via an oxygen mask should be continued until the patient can maintain good SpO_2 (> 95%) on room air. Certain types of patients like the obese, frail and elderly, those with significant cardiorespiratory disease, and those patients who have undergone major thoracic and major intra-abdominal surgery, may need supplementary oxygen and SpO_2 monitoring for the next 24 hours. These patients are susceptible to hypoxia because of their lower respiratory reserve. They are also often unable to compensate for the postoperative atelactasis, increased ventilation-perfusion mismatch and alveolar hypoventilation that result from surgery, anaesthesia and administration of opioids for postoperative analgesia. These hypoxic episodes have been associated with various postoperative problems, including myocardial ischaemia.

It is important to ensure that the patient receives adequate analgesia to be comfortable, cooperative, able to ventilate and cough effectively and yet be haemodynamically stable.

Analgesia can be given by regional anaesthetic, parenteral, oral or rectal routes. The dosage needs to be considered carefully if the volaemic and metabolic status of the patient is not optimal.

If an epidural has been placed, local anaesthesia (bupivacaine or ropivacine) alone or in combination with an opioid (fentanyl) can provide excellent pain relief without oversedating the patient. This method is more labour intensive as a certain degree of monitoring is needed in the High Dependency Unit (HDU) or intensive care unit (ICU).

Intravenous morphine, given as a bolus, infusion or via a patient-controlled analgesia (PCA) pump, may be just as effective. Intramuscular morphine 0.1–0.2 mg/kg four-hourly is still used in many centres, but the intermitent injections and inconsistent analgesia are common disadvantages. The route of administration of morphine analgesia depends on the cooperation of the patient, availability of equipment and medical expertise in the postoperative ward or intensive care unit.

Per rectal preparations of a non-steroidal anti-inflammatory drug (NSAID) like diclofenac 100 mgm and intravenous ketorolac 10–20 mg are effective and can lower the dose of morphine required by up to 30%, reducing the incidence of respiratory depression. It is important to avoid using NSAID in the presence of coagulopathy, unstable haemodynamic status, renal disease and upper gastrointestinal ulcers.

Oral analgesic agents are generally not given immediately postoperatively as the absorption is unreliable. The onset of analgesic effect is delayed because of reduced gastric emptying and vomiting may occur.

Postoperative nausea and vomiting, besides being unpleasant, can produce a rise in intra-cranial pressure that is undesirable in patients with head injuries. It should be treated using common anti-emetics like prochlorperazine, cyclizine, metoclopramide, droperidol or ondansetron.

Fluid management must take into account maintenance needs and fluid losses (for example, gastric aspirate, surgical drains, and third-space and intestinal losses) as well as inadequate intraoperative transfusion. Postoperatively, normal saline or Hartmann's solution at 1.5–2.0 ml/kg/hr can be used with the addition of 1 mmol/kg/day of potassium as daily replacement. The use of more than 1000 ml/day 5% Dextrose as fluid maintenance should be discouraged because with release of anti-diuretic hormone (ADH) and aldosterone. Water retention will lead to hyponatraemia. It is therefore prudent to measure serum electrolyte concentrations daily after major surgery involving large fluid shifts.

Blood transfusion is required if blood loss is significant, especially when there is hypotension, tachycardia or anaemia.

Oliguria is common in the immediate postoperative phase owing to the hormonal effects of the stress response. Oliguria is usually due to hypovolaemia. If the urine output is less than 0.5 ml/kg/hr for more than 2–3 hours, it may indicate poor renal perfusion that must be treated aggressively to prevent further deterioration. Fluid therapy guided by central venous pressure monitoring, maintenance of an adequate mean arterial blood pressure and judicious frusemide therapy, in that order, should be ordered to restore urine output.

Patients lose heat during major surgery and may remain cold for many hours unless active re-warming measures (overhead heat radiator, forced warm air blanket, warmed fluid infusion) are taken. Hypothermia causes vasoconstriction and shivering which is unpleasant, increases cardiac afterload and myocardial oxygen demand. The viability of free flaps will be threatened by vasoconstriction induced by hypothermia, hypovolaemia and pain.

Monitoring of vital signs, urine output, fluid losses and laboratory parameters (full blood count, serum creatinine and electrolyte concentrations, clotting screen) at appropriate intervals must be continued.

Conclusion

Anaesthesia for emergency surgery should be carried out only after the best possible efforts to optimise the patient's medical and surgical conditions. A suitably experienced anaesthesiologist should conduct the intraoperative anaesthetic management by employing appropriate monitoring. One of the main roles of the anaesthesiologist is to secure and maintain the airway without causing regurgitation and aspiration of gastric contents during anaesthesia. The anaesthesiologist also maintains the oxygenation and ventilation, as well as the tissue perfusion of the patient. Postoperatively, the anaesthesiologist needs to ensure that the patient is looked after in a ward that can provide suitable monitoring and support in managing fluids, analgesia and providing oxygen therapy.

References

1. Leong CK, Thaung MK (1998). The patient for emergency surgery. In *Anaesthesia: A Practical Handbook, 1st Ed.* Hwang NC (ed.) Singapore: Oxford University Press.
2. Turner DAB (1996). Emergency anaesthesia. In *Textbook of Anaesthesia, 3rd Ed.* Aitkenhead AR, Smith G (eds.) Great Britain: Churchill Livingstone.
3. MacFadyan UM (1996). Maternal and neonatal physiology. In *Textbook of Anaesthesia, 3rd Ed.* Aitkenhead AR, Smith G (eds.) Great Britain: Churchill Livingstone.
4. Steve JK, Grande CM (1994). Anesthesia for trauma. In *Anaesthesia, 4th Ed.* Miller R (ed.) USA: Churchill Livingstone.
5. Gibbs CP, Modeu JH (1994). Pulmonary aspiration of gastric contents: pathophysiology, prevention and management. In *Anaesthesia, 4th Ed.* Miller RD (ed.) USA: Churchill Livingstone.
6. Singapore Society of Anaesthesiologists (1992). Monitoring during anaesthesia. In *Safety Guidelines in Anaesthesia, 2nd Ed.* Singapore.
7. Morgan GE, Mikhail MS (eds.) (1996). *Airway Management in Clinical Anaesthesiology, 2nd Ed.* USA: Appleton and Lange.
8. Gaiger R (1993). Airway evaluation and management. In *Clinical Anaesthesia Procedures of the Massachusetts General Hospital, 4th Ed.* Davison JK, Eckhardt WF, Perese DA (eds.) USA: Little, Brown and Company.

9. Sellick BA (1961). Cricoid pressure to control regurgitation of stomach contents during induction of anaesthesia. *Lancet* **ii**, 404–406.
10. McConachie I, McGeachie J (1996). Regional anaesthetic techniques. In *Wylie and Churchill-Davidson's A Practice of Anaesthesia, 6th Ed.* Healy Thomas EJ, Cohen Peter J (eds.) Avon Great Britain: Edward Arnold The Bath Press.

39

Early Postoperative Care of the Acute Surgical Patient

Huei-Leng Chee
Claire Ang

Introduction

Surgery and anaesthesia constitute stress. The post-operative period is crucial; adequate and appropriate care is paramount in ensuring the proper recovery of the patient. It also serves to prevent and preempt complications. If complications should arise, the vigilant clinician should detect these early and institute appropriate measures. A systematic approach to reviewing the post-operative patient is advised.

Assessment of the Patient

This consists of a chart review and a physical examination.

(1) *The surgical notes*

Ascertain what operation was done. Note any intra-operative incidents or immediate post-operative complications that may have occurred.

(2) *The anaesthetic chart*

This would allow one to determine:

- the type of anaesthesia given
- how stable the patient was during the operation
- when and what medications were given
- what and how much fluids were given
- whether there was extensive blood loss and what replacements, if any, were given. The chart also records recovery room progress; for example if there were periods of hypoxia and what action was taken.

(3) *The patient's previous clinical history and medications*

There may be specific parameters which require more careful monitoring, for example, blood sugar monitoring in a diabetic patient.

(4) *The post-operative orders*

- Take note of the monitoring required, for example blood pressure, pulse rate, pulse oximetry (SpO_2), and the frequency at which these are to be recorded.
- Any specific orders, such as any drains to be put to suction.
- Investigations to be carried out. Remember to review these!
- Example 1: A chest X-ray may have been ordered because a central venous catheter was inserted intra-operatively. Check position of the central venous cathether and any possible complications that may have occurred.

  Example 2: A daily haemoglobin concentration (Hb) may have been ordered. Note the trend of the Hb. Is it falling: what is the reason? Is the patient still bleeding or is there a new site of bleeding?
- Nutrition. Is the patient to be on "nil-by-mouth" and if yes, for how long a period of time?

(5) *Post-operative medications*

- Type of analgesia. If the patient is on patient-controlled analgesia (PCA): ensure that no other opioids are ordered.

- Antibiotics. Does the patient have any allergies? Are the antibiotics for surgical prophylaxis: if so, they should be stopped after 24 to 48 hours.

Physical Examination

Perform a clinical examination. Pay particular attention to the following.

(1) *General status of the patient*

Is he alert? If the patient is drowsy after the effects of anaesthesia, is he

- easily arousable?
- in pain?
- pale?

(2) *Cardiovascular system*

- Check the pulse rate, blood pressure and heart sounds.
- Is there tachycardia or bradycardia? Check surgical drain output.

(3) *Respiratory system*

- Is the patient tachypnoeic or is he hypoventilating? One of the most common causes of tachypnoea is pain, while respiratory depression can be caused by excessive use of opioids.
- Is there equal air entry in both lungs?
- Are there crepitations audible?
- Are there rhonchi?

(4) *Check the sites where devices have been introduced*

- Make sure that intravenous drips are working. Check for inflammation and/or haematoma over insertion sites.
- If there is a urinary catheter present, make sure that it is patent. "Poor" urine output may be due to blockage, improper siting or displacement of the urinary catheter.

- If a central venous catheter is present, check the site. Ensure that there is good backflow.
- If an epidural catheter had been sited, check that it is properly connected to the relevant infusion of analgesia agent(s).

Monitoring the Post-operative Patient

In the immediate post-operative period (the first 24 hours), vital parameters should be checked and recorded hourly. The frequency can subsequently be decreased when the patient's condition has been demonstrated to be stable. As a minimum requirement, the post-operative patient requires monitoring of the cardiovascular and respiratory systems. Additional monitoring of other body systems are required depending on the type and extent of surgery, and the patient's premorbid medical condition. The greater the number of organ systems being monitored, and the greater the required intensity of monitoring, then the greater the required nurse-to-patient ratio. Admission to the intensive care unit is indicated when the patient requires a high level of monitoring of, and therapy for, any major organ system.[1]

While objective monitoring of vital signs provides information of a patient's status, it must not completely replace clinical examination. At best, numbers complement regular and careful physical examination.

Cardiovascular monitoring

Basic cardiovascular monitoring involves monitoring heart rate and blood pressure. Additional haemodynamic monitoring like central venous pressure may be required according to the needs of the patient. Pulmonary artery catheters require specialised skills for insertion and care, and are best managed in the intensive care unit.

Most healthy patients who have undergone surgery of a minimally- to moderately-invasive nature can have their pulse rate monitored as a reflection of their actual heart rate. This level of monitoring can be carried out in the general ward. For elderly patients, patients who have pre-existing heart disease, and those who have undergone major surgery, it would be prudent to have continuous *electrocardiograph* (*ECG*) monitoring in a high dependency ward.

For the vast majority of patients, *intermittent non-invasive blood pressure* (*NIBP*) monitoring will suffice. This can be done either manually or with automated techniques.

Manual measurement of blood pressure involves inflation of an occlusive cuff above the systolic blood pressure, and gradual deflation until Korotkoff's sounds are auscultated. The limitations of manual blood pressure measurement include:

(1) human operator error
(2) vasoconstriction resulting in soft sounds
(3) rapid cuff deflation resulting in erroneous readings

Automated techniques of blood pressure measurement reduce observer error and incorrect cuff inflation techniques. However, these are subject to errors resulting from:

- wrong cuff size
- dysrhythmias
- motion artefacts
- extremes of hypertension and hypotension.

Invasive arterial blood pressure (*IABP*) monitoring measures blood pressure directly by means of an indwelling arterial catheter coupled to a fluid-filled tubing to a pressure transducer. The transducer converts the pressure waveform into an electrical signal, which is then displayed on a screen together with the pressure readings.

Invasive blood pressure monitoring is indicated in:

- surgery involving significant blood loss or fluid shifts
- when frequent arterial blood sampling is necessary
- haemodynamic instability
- inotrope therapy.

Patients who have the latter two indications are best managed in the intensive care unit.

Central venous pressure (*CVP*) monitoring may be required as a guide for intravenous fluid therapy in patients who require aggressive volume loading, whose cardiac function is optimal within a narrow range of filling pressures. A central venous catheter is also indicated for administration of inotropes and parenteral nutrition.

CVP monitoring can be carried out with a transducer system that displays the central venous waveform simultaneously with pressure readings in mmHg. If a transducer system is not available, a water manometer system can be used to measure CVP in cmH_2O.

Hypertension in the early post-operative period is commonly due to pain, inadequately treated pre-existing hypertension, or a full bladder in a patient who is not catheterised. Hypercarbia, resulting from hypoventilation that is caused by the residual effects of anaesthesia, can also give rise to hypertension. In patients with an intracranial pathology, hypertension may be a sign of raised intracranial pressure.

Specific treatment of hypertension is not always indicated. An expectant approach is taken if residual effects of anaesthesia are the cause of hypoventilation. Inadequate analgesia should be addressed accordingly. It has to be remembered that excessive dosages of opioids can be the cause of respiratory depression leading to hypoventilation. Should there be any doubt, the duty anaesthesiologist should be consulted.

Post-operative *hypotension* is often due to intravascular hypovolaemia. The anaesthesia chart should be reviewed to determine the intra-operative fluid balance. Physical signs of hypovolaemia may be subtle, with only a mild tachycardia and cool peripheries to collaborate with the diagnosis. Crystalloids and colloids are usually adequate to correct post-operative volume deficits. Pallor and inspection of surgical drains may raise the suspicion of bleeding, in which case haemoglobin concentration and coagulation studies should be done even as blood transfusion is being ordered. A relative hypovolaemic state can result from vasodilatation due to rewarming.

Hypotension may also be secondary to residual effects of anaesthetic agents on the myocardium, spinal or epidural anaesthesia causing peripheral vasodilatation. Carefully titrated doses of vasopressors, such as ephedrine, may be indicated.

More serious causes of hypotension include tension pneumothorax caused by attempts at central venous cannulation or inadvertant intra-operative surgical breach of the pleura; or sepsis precipitated by surgical manipulation of an infected focus.

Respiratory monitoring

Respiratory rate monitoring is required for all patients after surgery. This basic clinical mode of monitoring is carried out at all levels of hospital wards. It is complementary to regular clinical examination.

Pulse oximetry is a non-invasive method of continuously monitoring oxygen saturation. Two wavelengths of light (660 nm and 940 nm) from a light-emitting diode are passed through a vascular bed to a photodetector. The amount of light reaching the photodetector varies according to the relative concentrations of oxyhaemoglobin and deoxy-haemoglobin. Pulse oximetry improves detection of desaturation, with an accuracy of ±4%.

Pulse oximetry in a high dependency setting is indicated in patients who are at risk of peri-operative respiratory failure. The major risk factors include:

- advanced age
- history of significant cardiorespiratory disease
- major surgery involving main body cavities of head, thorax and abdomen
- surgery involving major blood loss
- patients receiving intrathecal or epidural opioids.

Despite its accuracy, there are limitations to its use.

(1) Abnormal haemoglobins like carboxyhaemoglobin and methaemoglobin can result in significant inaccuracies in pulse oximetry readings. The former results in readings higher than that

of the actual state of oxygenation, while the latter results in an SpO_2 of 85%.

(2) Intravascular dyes (e.g. methylene blue) and pigments such as nail polish also affect the accuracy of pulse oximetry.
(3) Poor perfusion (due to low cardiac output or severe peripheral vasoconstriction) of the area where the probe is attached, produces an unreliable reading. This would be indicated by a dampened plethysmographic waveform.
(4) Motion of the part of the body where the probe is attached will disrupt a steady pulsatile waveform that is required for accurate readings.
(5) High intensity of ambient light over the probe interferes with accurate photodetection. This can be corrected by shielding.

Arterial blood gas (*ABG*) measurement provides data on oxygenation, ventilation and acid-base balance. It should be carried out if a patient's respiratory parameters are deteriorating, or a clinical examination suggests a possible respiratory complication. It should also be done as a routine post-operative blood investigation in patients who have a history of significant lung disease and those who have undergone major thoracic or upper abdominal surgery. This group of patients is at high risk of developing post-operative respiratory complications and a "baseline" record allows for earlier detection of deterioration. Effects of therapy can also be objectively measured.

Chest X-rays should be done in post-operative patients who have undergone thoracic surgery. It is also required if the patient had a central venous catheter inserted intra-operatively.

Hypoventilation in the immediate post-operative period is a common respiratory complication. Hypercarbia is manifested as an increase in arterial carbon dioxide tension ($PaCO_2$) and hypoxaemia is manifested as a decrease in arterial oxygen tension (PaO_2) (hypoxaemia).

The causes of hypoventilation include:

(1) Reduced ventilatory drive, as a result of

- the effect of respiratory depressant drugs

- intracranial pathology, such as tumour, haemorrhage
- peri-operative cerebrovascular accident

(2) Peripheral factors, such as

- pain
- tight dressings
- abdominal distension
- obesity.

A number of drugs administered in the peri-operative period can reduce the ventilatory drive. All volatile and most intravenous anaesthetic agents depress the respiratory centre. With newer anaesthetic drugs that have less residual effects, this is not as significant a problem as it was in the past.

Opioid analgesics exert a dose-dependent effect in respiratory depression. The elderly are particularly sensitive to its effects. This, however, is insufficient reason to limit opioid dosages since pain can cause reduced ventilation. Post-operative analgesia with morphine can be safely delivered by patient-controlled analgesia (PCA), provided the patient understands its correct use and is adequately monitored. When opioids are administered into the subarachnoid or epidural space, respiratory depression may occur many hours later.

Patients who have received spinal opioids should be monitored in a high-dependency ward for at least six hours after administration of the last dose.

Abdominal distension, obesity and tight dressings or abdominal binders can result in hypoventilation because these limit diaphragmatic movement during respiration.

Hypoxaemia is frequently caused by ventilation-perfusion abnormalities. Small airway closure is common after surgery and anaesthesia, especially in the dependent areas of the lung. This results in lung units that are perfused but not ventilated, causing hypoxaemia. Supplemental oxygen overcomes most cases of mild hypoxaemia. Care has to be exercised for patients with chronic obstructive lung disease whose ventilation is dependent on the hypoxic drive.

Renal monitoring

The volume of urine produced is an indicator of the adequacy of renal perfusion and, indirectly, of the adequacy of perfusion of other vital organs.[2,3] Urine output should be maintained at 0.5–1.0 ml/kg/hr. Accurate hourly measurement of urine volumes with a urometer is indicated in situations such as:

- major surgery involving large volumes of blood loss or fluid shifts
- polytrauma
- hypotension from any cause
- pre-existing renal impairment.

Oliguria is common in the early post-operative period. It may be due to the physiological response to stress-induced activation of the renin-angiotensin-aldosterone system. More often, it is due to hypovolaemia or hypotension.

Hypovolaemia should be suspected in the presence of cool peripheries and a relative tachycardia despite a normal blood pressure. In such a situation, urine output will be restored with fluid repletion. A healthy young patient will usually tolerate fairly rapid rates of volume loading (for example, 1 litre of crystalloids in 1 hour). Greater caution has to be exercised when the patient is elderly, or has limited cardiovascular reserve. Fluid repletion in such cases must not only be slower, guided by CVP monitoring if necessary; the patient must also be reviewed more frequently to assess adequacy of the fluid therapy.

Hypotension resulting in decreased urine output should be treated according to the cause. Relative hypotension may be present in an elderly patient or a patient with poorly controlled hypertension. Such patients require higher perfusion pressures to achieve adequate urine output. In the absence of hypovolaemia, vasopressors, such as adrenaline, may be needed to increase the blood pressure.

Stress Ulcer Prophylaxis[4,5]

The incidence of stress ulceration has improved considerably in the past few years, possibly because of better resuscitation, decreased use of ulcerogenic drugs, and more stringent criteria for its diagnosis. The main risk factors for the development of stress ulceration are:

- mechanical ventilation for > 48 hours
- deranged coagulation
- hypotension
- sepsis
- drugs, for example steroids, aspirin and other non-steroidal anti-inflammatory drugs.

Prophylactic therapy against stress ulceration is not indicated in all patients, only those with high risk factors. Commonly used drugs include H_2 antagonists (e.g. ranitidine), proton pump inhibitors (e.g. omeprazole), and cytoprotective agents (e.g. sucralfate).

Histamine (H_2) antagonists show similar effectiveness in gastric acid suppression. Ranitidine and famotidine are more commonly used because cimetidine inhibits the cytochrome P_{450} oxidase system, thus affecting the metabolism of other drugs.

Proton pump inhibitors are as efficacious as H_2 antagonists in suppressing gastric acid production. These appear to have fewer side effects.

Sucralfate acts by forming an inert complex with the stomach mucosa, thereby preventing erosion. It requires an acidic environment for activation, and therefore cannot be prescribed in conjunction with antacids, H_2 antagonists or proton pump inhibitors. The use of sucralfate in general surgical patients is limited because enteral feeding is restricted for various reasons, including gastrointestinal surgery, ileus and pancreatitis.

Early enteral feeding obviates the need for stress ulcer prophylaxis unless the patient has a history of peptic ulcer disease.

Infectious Issues

The acute surgical patient is at increased risk of infectious complications either because the surgical pathology has an infectious cause (for example acute cholecystitis, necrotising fasciitis) or the emergency situation required procedures to be performed in less than completely aseptic conditions (for example, exsanguination requiring emergency laparotomy).

Antibiotics have to be prescribed empirically to cover for the most common pathogens found in the surgical site in question. A detailed exposition of antibiotic prescription for different types of surgical conditions is beyond the scope of this section. However, some general principles apply.

(1) Appropriate cultures should be taken before administration of antibiotics. This is to increase the chances of a positive yield from culture specimens.

(2) Appropriate cultures should also be taken from the surgical site directly. Any positive result can then be correlated for rationalisation of antibiotic therapy.

(3) Intravenous cannulas, invasive monitoring devices, chest drains, that were placed under emergency situations should be removed or changed as soon as it is practical, without compromising patient safety. This should also be done for a patient who is repatriated from another medical facility. Should the devices have been in place for any length of time (> 5 days), the distal ends should be sent for cultures, in addition to blood cultures taken at the same time. The wounds should be examined and any discharge from the wound should be sent for culture.

(4) Empiric antibiotics should provide broad-spectrum cover until specimen cultures have been reported. Once bacteriology and antibiotic sensitivities are known, antibiotics should be changed to narrow-spectrum ones. This is done to reduce the incidence of antibiotic resistance.

(5) As far as possible, the number of antibiotics prescribed should be kept to the minimum that is consistent with adequate therapy.

Deep Vein Thrombosis Prophylaxis

Thrombosis of the deep veins of the lower limbs is often asymptomatic. Up to 95% of pulmonary emboli originate from such clots. The real incidence of deep vein thrombosis (DVT) is unknown, and appears to vary with different patient populations undergoing different types of surgeries. Appropriate prophylactic measures therefore also vary in efficacy between the varied groups of patients. Early ambulation should be encouraged in all post-operative patients to minimise the risk of DVT. Prophylaxis against thromboembolism should be particularly directed at patients with high risk factors such as:

- history of venous thromboembolism
- prolonged bed rest or inactivity
- multisystem trauma, particularly those with orthopaedic, spinal or head injury
- lower extremity or pelvic surgery
- obesity
- nalignancy
- hypercoagulable states, for example, anti-thrombin III deficiency, and presence of anti-phospholipid antibody.

DVT prophylaxis[8] includes *mechanical* and *pharmacological* measures.

Mechanical prophylaxis includes elastic stockings and pneumatic compression devices. These appear to be less effective than pharmacological measures and therefore, as far as possible, should not be used in isolation.

Low-dose subcutaneous heparin (5000 IU 12-hourly) has been found to be effective in reducing the incidence of DVT by 50–80%. Risks of excessive bleeding in patients who have undergone surgery with primary haemostasis are low (< 2%).

Low-molecular-weight heparins (LMWH)[9] are as efficacious as unfractionated heparin in reducing the risk of DVT in most types of surgical patients. However in multi-system trauma patients, LMWH's have been found to decrease the incidence of DVT by a further 30% over unfractionated heparin.

Caution must be exercised with patients who have had an epidural puncture[10] in the peri-operative period, as there is a risk of epidural haematoma. Catheter removal should not take place within six hours of administration of the last dose of heparin, and 12 hours of the last dose of a low-molecular-weight heparin. After epidural catheter removal, the patient must be monitored for persistent neurological deficits.

Conclusion

The principles of post-operative care of acute surgical patients are not markedly different from that of elective surgical patients. However, greater vigilance is often required because the acute surgical patient may not be well optimised pre-operatively, and thus is at greater risk of developing post-operative complications. Knowledge of common post-operative complications and their risk factors will determine the degree of monitoring and therapy that is required to ensure a smooth recovery.

References

1. Hutton P, Prys-Roberts C (eds.) (1994). *Monitoring in Anaesthesia and Intensive Care*. London: W.B. Saunders Company Ltd.
2. Better OS, Stein JH (1990). Early management of shock and prophylaxis of acute renal failure in traumatic rhabdomyolysis. *N Engl J Med* **332**, 825–829.
3. Thadhani R, Pascual M, Bonventre JV (1996). Acute renal failure. *N Engl J Med* **334**, 1448–1460.
4. Tryba M, Cook D (1997). Current guidelines on stress ulcer prophylaxis. *Drugs* **54**, 581–596.

5. Cook D, Guyatt G, Marshall J, *et al.* (1998). A comparison of sucralfate and ranitidine for the prevention of upper gastrointestinal bleeding in patients requiring mechanical ventilation. Canadian Critical Care Trails Group. *N Engl J Med* **338**, 791–797.
6. Nichols RL (1996). Surgical infections: prevention and treatment — 1965 to 1995. *Am J Surg* **172**, 68–74.
7. Nichols RL (2001). Preventing surgical site infections: a surgeon's perspective. *Emerg Infect Dis* **7**, 220–224.
8. Clagett GP, Anderson FA, Geerts W, *et al.* (1998). Prevention of venous thromboembolism. *Chest* **114**(suppl), S531–560.
9. Knudson MM, Morabito D, Paiement G, Shackleford S (1996). Use of low molecular weight heparin in preventing thromboembolism in trauma patients. *J Trauma* **41**, 446–459.
10. Horlecker TT, Wendel DJ (1998). Spinal and epidural blockade and perioperative low molecular weight heparin: smooth sailing in the Titanic. *Anesth Analg* **86**, 1153–1156.

Index